MEDICINE
in Quotations

◆ SECOND EDITION ◆

For a catalogue of publications available from ACP, contact:

Customer Service Center
American College of Physicians
190 N. Independence Mall West
Philadelphia, PA 19106-1572
215-351-2600
800-523-1546, ext. 2600

Visit our Web site at www.acponline.org

MEDICINE
in Quotations

◆ SECOND EDITION ◆

Views of Health and Disease
Through the Ages

Edited by

EDWARD J. HUTH, MD, MACP, FRCP (LONDON)

T. JOCK MURRAY, OC, MD, FRCPC, FRCP (LONDON), MACP

AMERICAN COLLEGE OF PHYSICIANS
PHILADELPHIA

Director, Editorial Production: Linda Drumheller
Associate Publisher: Diane McCabe
Production Supervisor: Allan S. Kleinberg
Senior Production Editor: Karen C. Nolan
System Analyst/Developer: Scott Thomas Hurd
Composition: Michael Ripca, Wendy Smith
Subject Indexer: Nelle Garrecht
Jacket Design: Elizabeth Swartz
Interior Design: Kate Nichols

Printed in the United States of America
Composition by American College of Physicians
Printing/binding by Sheridan Press

ISBN: 1-930513-67-4

06 07 08 09 10 / 10 9 8 7 6 5 4 3 2 1

Contents

Major Contributors

Kurt Aterman
Giulio J. Barbero
William K. Beatty
W. Watson Buchanan
Tsung O. Cheng
L.J. Clein
J. Russell Elkinton
John H. Felts

William S. Haubrich
Edward J. Huth
S.M. MacLeod
Ana Marusic
Robert Matz
John L. McClenahan
Owen McInerny
Matthew Menken

T. Jock Murray
Fred B. Rogers
Charles G. Roland
Mark E. Silverman
Bert Spilker
Marvin J. Stone
John Walton

Other Contributors

Janet Byron Anderson
Billy F. Andrews
John H.M. Austin
Jeremiah A. Barondess
T.F. Baskett
Ronen Ben Ami
Jim Bowers
Charles S. Bryan
John P. Bunker
Howard Burchell
Ian A. Cameron
Kathleen Case
Iain Chalmers
Mitchell H. Charap
Leighton Cluff
J.T.H. Connor
Ralph Crawshaw
Michael Cussen
Lois DeBakey
Jacalyn Duffin
Johathan Dwyer
Magdy N. Falestiny
Rudy Falk
J. Fonseca
Herbert L. Fred
W. Bruce Fye
Henry L. Galan
Richard Ganz

Toby Gelfand
Bill Gibson
Richard L. Golden
James Gray
Ralph Hauke
J. Willis Hurst
D. Geraint James
David M. Klachko
Sanford Koltonow
Daniel Kombert
Michael A. LaCombe
Mario R. Lamothe
Ronald V. Loge
James Magner
R.A. Matawaran
Wendy Mitchinson
Daniel E. Moerman
Robert H. Moser
Alistair Munro
Ann L. Murray
Shannon Murray
Earl F. Nation
Francis A. Neelon
Ben Nemeny
David M. Newman
John Noble
Jack Obeid
Nicholas Owens

Bernardine Z. Paulshock
Brian Payton
Steven J. Peitzman
Claus A. Pierach
Alan V. Pollock
H. Phelps Potter Jr.
Sundaram V. Ramanan
Dwaine Rieves
Edward C. Rosenow III
Mark E. Rupp
Alex Sakula
Max Samter
John W. Scott
Roy Selby
M.R. Shetty
Jean-Marc Soules
Deborah Spruill
Stuart Sutton
Theodore Sunao Takata
Hector O. Ventura
Emmet Ray Vick
Frederick B. Wagner, Jr.
Sigmund Weitzman
Wendell A. Wilson
Stewart Wolf
Charles F. Wooley
Henrik R. Wulff

Acknowledgments

Assembling the quotations in this collection would have been impossible, or at least very difficult, without the help of many colleagues in the United States, Canada, and abroad who sent us submissions for consideration. All who supplied quotations for the first or second edition are listed on the Contributors page whether or not their quotations were finally selected for inclusion. We cannot express strongly enough our thanks for their invaluable help.

Nor can we thank sufficiently the staff of the Editorial Production Division of the American College of Physicians for their assistance in greatly facilitating our work on this edition and in preparing it for publication: Linda Drumheller, Director, Editorial Production; Scott Thomas Hurd, Systems Analyst/Developer; and Allan S. Kleinberg, Production Supervisor. Our interest in preparing a second edition of *Medicine in Quotations* was shared by Diane McCabe, Associate Publisher; we are grateful for her support.

The library that proved most valuable in our verification efforts for both editions was that of the College of Physicians of Philadelphia, an incredibly rich source of medical history. Our work was expedited greatly by the expert guidance of two members of its staff, Richard Fraser and Lisa Gensel.

Introduction
to the Second Edition

Our Aims

Why a Book of Medical Quotations?

Compiling over 3500 medical quotations—enough to fill a substantial book—is no slight task. What might justify this labor? Can quotations help readers understand what medicine is and is not? What are the uses of a book of quotations? How do these uses determine which quotations should go into the book and which should not? And how should one make the individual in-or-out decisions? We asked ourselves these questions before we started our work. We asked them again as we sorted through the 5000 quotations initially submitted.

What Are the Uses of Quotations?

We all know the after-dinner drone who adorns his remarks with wisdom ostentatiously borrowed from Osler. We all know the chief of service who, as he perambulates on rounds, parades his knowledge by spouting pearls from an obscure 19th century Frenchman. Quotations can serve as cheaply acquired badges of erudition, but they have better uses for most of us.

You may have firm views on how a patient and a physician should relate to each other. Among the quotations here, you may find your convictions stated with a clarity and strength that reinforce your sense of what is right—or perhaps you will come across opposing or differing views that encourage thoughtful reconsideration.

A book of quotations with the right scope serves yet another purpose. It concisely shows how some medical concepts and practices have developed and changed through generations and how others have remained remarkably constant. One can see that many diseases and syndromes were identified a thousand or more years ago; here are stimuli for all physicians to observe disease closely and discerningly. Who among us will see "new" diseases with an open mind and sharper eyes? Can we write so clearly that the disease we describe today will be recognizable a thousand years from now?

The most important use of a collection such as this is seeing, in brief, what views—of physicians and patients, of diseases and treatments—were held in other times and places. Are we in medicine today what the physicians and surgeons of past centuries were? Did patients centuries ago expect of their doctors what our patients expect of us? Alan Gregg commented in 1941 that:

> The humanist is not interested in the past merely because it is the past. As the statistician likes a long series, not a short one, the humanist similarly likes the long accumulations from the past to illustrate the nature of man....
> "*Plus ça change; plus ça reste.*"[1]

Cultures change through time, but human nature probably changes little. What men and women were in centuries past they will continue to be in times to come. Such a view can help us physicians determine how we can serve the art of medicine.

Is a New Collection Needed?

We know of at least three earlier books of medical quotations. The most impressive of these is *Familiar Medical Quotations*, edited by Maurice Strauss.[2] One of us (EJH) contributed many quotations to that book, and we both still admire its scope and variety. But advances in clinical medicine and its basis in medical science have greatly increased practical medical knowledge in the past four decades. The economic setting and structure of medicine has changed radically and brought difficulties not foreseen in the time of Strauss. Furthermore, although the Strauss collection does carry some quotations detailing the growth of concepts of normal bodily functions and diseases through two millennia, it seemed to us to fall short of what could be done for that purpose. A third point is also relevant: Some of the quotations in the Strauss collection have citations exact enough to enable the reader to go directly to the quoted passage in the source, but many citations simply refer to an entire work. We felt that we must supply the exact location of each quoted passage so the curious reader could find the context that might illuminate its meaning. We concluded that a new collection—with recent entries, with a wider scope, and with more detailed references to original sources—was justified.

The Process

Step 1: Compiling the Quotations

Both of us had quotation collections; they are represented here. We also turned to colleagues who might be willing to contribute their own collections or to search for new quotations. Thanks to the willingness of Frank Davidoff, then Editor of *Annals of Internal Medicine*, to publish a Letter to the Editor inviting contributions while the first edition of *Medicine in Quotations* was being prepared, many submissions came from outside our own circle of professional friends. The responses from personal colleagues and other readers of *Annals* were deeplyy satisfying. We also searched anew ourselves. Sources included histories of medical and surgical specialties that quote important original passages, anthologies of notable excerpts from the medical literature, and important original papers identified in *Morton's Medical Bibliography*.[3] However, we certainly have not exhausted the number of usable quotations from such sources—far from it.

Step 2: Selecting the Quotations for This Book

We had no formula for what quotations should be included. The physical size of the planned book determined to some degree how many quotations we could use. But the central task remained that of looking at each quotation and asking ourselves these questions: Does the quotation represent knowledge specifically relevant to medical concepts and practice, either as they developed in the past or as they stand today? Is the quotation pithy, clear, and compelling as a truth even if it is taken out of context? Is its worth apparent even if one ignores the name of its author? Will its meaning be unmistakable to physicians, other health care professionals, and medical and nursing students without commentary? Is the quotation relevant to all human affairs, not just medicine, and is it of a kind readily found in collections of truly broad scope? Some contributors may feel that we did not always answer these questions correctly and erred in excluding some quotations they submitted. Some readers may feel that we admitted quotations we should have left out. We hope we have not erred too often.

One of the most difficult decisions that arose during our selection process concerned the relative importance of recent medical breakthroughs. As one looks farther back in time, it is easier to recognize the major advancements in medicine. However,

> In recent decades, discoveries are to a far greater extent "incremental"; this could be explained by research areas being much narrower, more and larger groups working on them, the increased speed and sophistication of the methodology of research, and faster and more frequent publication of results influenced by intense competition.[4]

Perhaps in the time between publication of the first edition and this second edition, the differences between incremental and major advances may have become clearer and may hence be better reflected in the present volume.

Step 3: Preparing the Second Edition

Those readers who say to themselves, "Why did they leave out ____?" or "Why isn't ____ quoted?" should think of this collection as a mosaic. The chips we included give some picture of medical thinking and practice—knowledge and ignorance, successes and blunders, humility and arrogance—through many centuries. But because there must be a limit to the physical size of this volume, the mosaic does have gaps. Surgeons will probably detect many missing bits from the history of their field. Dermatologists will ask why diseases of the skin are only skimpily represented. Ophthalmologists might like to have seen a history of cataract removal.

We can respond that we had no biases in assembling our medical mosaic. If quotations pertaining to the fields of internal medicine and neurology are more numerous than those in other areas, it is because we come from those backgrounds. It is hoped, however, that this edition has added pieces to the mosaic in other areas that make its total image more pleasing.

Finally, we have included numerous quotations representing views that we do not hold—a few may even be repugnant to some readers. However, we felt that a range of views on some topics was needed to depict how they can be viewed quite differently by different persons in different times.

The Future

We continue to collect quotations in the event that the reception of this work calls for a third edition. Hence we invite readers to submit quotations they feel would complement the current collection—that is, to fill in the mosaic we have begun. We seek, specifically, quotations that illustrate how medical concepts and practices have developed from ancient times to the present. Please be sure to include full bibliographic information:

From journals and magazines:
1. All author names, in full if possible
2. Full article title
3. Full journal title
4. Year of publication
5. Volume number (or give the full date of publication for journals or magazines without continuous pagination)
6. Inclusive page numbers of article

From books:
1. All author or editor names
2. Full book title (with any edition and volume numbers)
3. City of publication
4. Name of publisher
5. Year of publication
6. Page number(s) on which the quote appears

For quotations that come from secondary sources, we should have the same data to enable us to try to find them in the primary source.

To submit quotations or to request what bibliographic information to include for additional kinds of sources (e.g., newspapers, classic works of literature, unpublished material), please write to Medical Quotations, Editorial Production Division, American College of Physicians, 190 North Independence Mall West, Philadelphia, PA 19106-1572. Or you may send a fax to Medical Quotations, ACP Editorial Production Division, at 215/351-2644.

—*EJH, TJM*

References

1. **Gregg A.** Humanism and science. *Bull N Y Acad Med.* 1941;17:83-99.
2. **Strauss M (ed).** *Familiar Medical Quotations.* Boston: Little, Brown; 1968.
3. **Norman JM (ed).** *Morton's Medical Bibliography: An Annotated Check-List of Texts Illustrating the History of Medicine,* 5th ed. Aldershot, England: Scolar Press; 1991.
4. **Morton LT, Moore RJ.** *A Chronology of Medicine and Related Sciences.* Aldershot, England: Scolar Press; 1991:1.

Notes for Readers

Quotation Organization

Quotations have been grouped alphabetically by topic. Under each topic, the quotations are ordered chronologically, with the oldest quotations coming first, to give historical perspective on changes in knowledge, concepts, and practice over time. Each entry includes the quotation's date, author, and source. Each entry is numbered for easy referencing from the both the Subject Index and the Author–Citation Index. Quotations within the same year are arranged alphabetically by author name. Quotations for which a date (either specific or approximate) could not be determined have been placed at the end of their respective topics. Biblical quotations, however, have been placed at the *beginning* of their respective topics.

Topic Headings

In general, we preferred broad terms over more specific terms (e.g., *Epilepsy* over *Grand Mal Seizures*). In certain cases, however, we did use more specific topic names. For example, quotations about angina pectoris originally were placed under *Coronary Artery Disease*, but there were enough quotations dealing specifically with the symptom of angina pectoris to justify its own topic. These quotations came mainly from the years before coronary obstructive disease was seen as a major cause of angina pectoris; however, quotations that illustrate the growth of this concept were placed under *Coronary Artery Disease*. For this reason, the Subject Index is cross-referenced, so that if you look up *Coronary Artery Disease*, it will direct you to "see *Angina Pectoris*" and vice versa.

Quotations about structural properties (either normal or abnormal) of particular organs or organ systems are listed under a term representing that organ or system; however, some quotations about functional properties of organs or systems have been assigned to a functional term. This is the reason behind having separate sections of quotations about both the *Lung* and *Respiration* and the *Heart* and *Circulation*. Again, use the cross-referenced Subject Index as a guide.

Because some readers may be unfamiliar with medical terminology, such standard terms as *Renal Function* and *Pulmonary Disease* were discarded in favor of *Kidney Function* and *Lung Disease*. To bring all the quotations pertaining to cancer together, we changed headings such as *Breast Cancer* and *Stomach Cancer* to *Cancer of the Breast* and *Cancer of the Stomach*.

Attribution of Authorship

The authorship assigned to some quotations may not be entirely accurate. Some works attributed to Hippocrates, for instance, may not represent the writings by the person named Hippocrates and should be designated more properly as works in the Hippocratic canon from an unknown author. However, for the purposes of this collection, such questions were dodged, and in this case the simple, conventional authorship of "Hippocrates" was assigned.

Quotations of unknown authorship (e.g., proverbs or editorials) have been attributed to "[Anonymous]."

For some quotations, the author is not an "author" in the usual sense; rather, he or she had given a speech, written a letter, or kept a personal diary.

For the authors of medical journals (especially modern ones), up to four authors are named. If the actual number exceeded four, then three were named and the rest replaced by the phrase "and others."

Forms of Author Names

Many author names in this book have both Latin and native-language forms. In these instances, we have elected to use the form preferred in a standard reference work in English, such as *Morton's Medical Bibliography*. We have selected the form more likely to be represented in histories of medicine in the English language. If an alternative form exists (as it does with authors of classic Arabic literature), we have given the alternative name in parentheses after the more commonly used name. For authors best known by a pseudonym, we also have provided the person's proper name in parentheses. For example, above a quotation from the French playwright Molière, the author name appears as "Molière (Jean-Baptiste Poquelin)"; and for the statistician who identified his authorship as Student, the author name appears as "Student (William Sealy Gosset)."

Where possible, we have tried to give full names, even if they are not the names commonly used to refer to the author. We refer to Wilfred Trotter, the famous English surgeon, as "Wilfred Batten Lewis Trotter."

We have omitted almost all honorifics, such as "Sir" and "Baron." We realize that some authors prominent in medical history are widely referred to as "Sir" (e.g., William Osler, Thomas Browne), but many authors had honorific titles that were never widely used. Austin Bradford Hill, for example, was knighted but not widely known as "Sir," and there are others. For consistency, we decided to do without honorifics.

Attribution of Date

The publication date of the original source has been used wherever possible, even if the quotation came from a publication (e.g., translation) with a later date. Where a quotation date is unknown, we have placed the birth and death dates of the author in square brackets (such quotations are ordered by the author's death date). For anonymous quotations with no dates (e.g., various proverbs), we have not assigned *any* date. Stated simply, we could not justify the exhaustive research necessary to find an exact date for, say, a Croatian proverb, when such information would not yield any significant value. Thus, as mentioned previously, undated quotations are placed at the end of their topic group.

Quotation Language

Virtually all the quotations herein appear in English language sources, whether it is the original source or a translation. The references for quotations from translations are usually to an English language version of the original work or to English language publications that anthologize extensive translations of non–English language works. Very few quotations appear in their original language or in a translation that represents an original mix of two or more languages. Some are translations made by a submitter.

We also have aimed to retain the original spelling, capitalization, punctuation, and style of the quotations (for both English language sources and translations). Differences from present-day usage persisted well into the 19th century.

Sources

Sources at the End of Quotations

The source listed at the end of each quotation is, in most cases, the full title of the original book, journal, play, poem, or treatise. Exceptions include excessively long titles (which we shortened) and collections of aphorisms, diary entries, and letters. Occasionally, a quotation is from an author who is quoted in a book or journal article written by *another* author. This second author appears before the source, separated by a comma.

Sources in the Author–Citation Index

The full bibliographic information for each original source appears in the Author–Citation Index, which is listed alphabetically by the name of quotation's author. For sources that could not be verified—because they were either out of print or unavailable at several local medical libraries—the reference closes with the statement "[Limited data]."

Many quotations were submitted from a secondary source that had cited an original source that could not be verified. If the secondary source was judged to be a reliable scholarly work, we closed the reference by indicating its full bibliographic information in square brackets.

When various editions are available for an original or secondary source, we endeavored to provide the most recently published version.

For more information, see the Author–Citation Index on p. 429.

ABETALIPOPROTEINEMIA (BASSEN-KORNZWEIG SYNDROME)

Frank A. Bassen, Abraham L. Kornzweig; 1950   **1**

A girl, aged 18 [was] born of parents who were first cousins. She had an atypical retinitis pigmentosa with involvement of the macula. The neurological examination showed diffuse disease of the central nervous system, as seen in Friedreich's ataxia. An additional finding...was that of a malformation of the red blood-cells. These cells had a peculiar crenated appearance, due to the presence of pseudopods or protoplasmic projections.   *Blood*

H.B. Salt, O.H. Wolff, June K. Lloyd, and others; 1960   **2**

A 17-month-old girl with steatorrhea was found to have no serum β-lipoprotein.... The red blood-cells showed...acanthocytosis. In the parents and one grandparent the β-lipoprotein was reduced to about half its normal level. The syndrome, which we designate a-β-lipoprotienaemia, is regarded as an inborn error of metabolism with a recessive mode of inheritance.   *The Lancet*

ABORTION

Socrates; *circa* 450 BC   **3**

It is the midwives who have the power to bring on the pains [in childbirth], and also, if they think it fit, to relieve them; they do it by the use of simple drugs, and by singing incantations. In difficult cases, too, they can bring about the birth; or, if they consider it advisable, they can promote a miscarriage.   *Plato, The Theaetetus*

Hippocrates; [460-375 BC]   **4**

I will not give to a woman an abortive remedy.   *The Hippocratic Oath*

[Anonymous]; *circa* 50   **5**

Do not kill a fetus by abortion.   *The Didache (Teachings of the Apostles)*

Juvenal (Decimus Junius Juvenalis); 60-140   **6**

When did you ever discover
Labor pains in a golden bed? There are potent prescriptions,
Fine professional skill, to be hired for inducing abortions,
Killing mankind in the womb. Rejoice, unfortunate husband,

Give her the dose yourself. Never let her…go on to full term and deliver
Something whose hue would seem to prove you a blackamoor father.   *Satires X*

Tertullian (Quintus Septimius Tertullianus); *circa* 197   **7**
With us [Christians] murder is forbidden once for all. We are not permitted to destroy
even the fetus in the womb, as long as blood is still being drawn to form a human being.
                                                                          Apologetical Works

Hugh Lenox Hodge; 1839   **8**
All the authority of the practitioner [must] be employed; often he must… grasp the conscience of his weak and erring patient, and let her know, in language not to be misunderstood, that she is responsible to her Creator for the life of the being within her.   *Foeticide*

Charles Warrington Earle; 1888   **9**
In my judgment the value of a child in utero is not at all comparable to that of a mother, already surrounded it may be, with a family of children and whose domestic and social
responsibilities are beyond estimation.   *Transactions of the Illinois State Medical Society*

Pius XI; 1930   **10**
However we may pity the mother whose health and even life is imperiled by the performance of her natural duty, there yet remains no sufficient reason for condoning the direct
murder of the innocent.   *Casti Connubi*

American Medical Association, House of Delegates; 1970   **11**
Abortion…should not be performed when contrary to the best interests of the patient
since good medical practice requires due consideration for the patient's demands…. No
physician or other professional personnel shall be compelled to perform any act which
violates his good medical judgment. Neither physician, hospital, or hospital personnel
shall be required to perform any act violative of personally held moral principles.
                                                      Journal of the American Medical Association

American Medical Association, Judicial Council; 1970   **12**
The Principles of Medical Ethics of the AMA do not prohibit a physician from performing an abortion that is performed in accordance with good medical practice and under circumstances that do not violate the laws of the community in which he practices.
                                                            U.S. Supreme Court: Roe v. Wade

American Public Health Association; 1970   **13**
Rapid and simple abortion referral must be readily available through state and local public health departments, medical societies, or other non-profit organizations.
                                                            U.S. Supreme Court: Roe v. Wade

U.S. Supreme Court: *Roe v. Wade*; 1973   **14**
A state criminal abortion statute of the current Texas type, that excepts from criminality
only a *life-saving* procedure on behalf of the mother, without regard to pregnancy stage
and without recognition of the other interests involved, is violation of the Due Process
Clause of the Fourteenth Amendment.   *U.S. Supreme Court: Roe v. Wade*

Harley S. Smyth; 1982   **15**
It takes no seer to recognize the paradoxes inherent in today's practice. Consider one of
them. In the large urban hospital, at one end of the corridor, a highly skilled team, using
powerful technological tools, strives 24 hours a day to render safe the passage of a premature newborn from its gestational age of 26 weeks to infant maturity. At the other end
of the same corridor feticide is carried out for many non-medical reasons.
                                 Annals of the Royal College of Physicians and Surgeons of Canada

ABSCESS

[Anonymous]; *circa* 1500 BC   **16**

If you examine a swelling of pus in any limb of a man and you find it [with] its head raised and it is enclosed and it is rounded, you shall say concerning it: "a swelling of pus, an illness which will be treated by me with the knife treatment." There is something in it like mucus. Something comes forth like wax. It makes a pocket. If anything [remains] in its pocket, it recurs.   *Ebers Papyrus*

ACADEMIC HEALTH CENTERS

René Jules Dubos; 1965   **17**

The luxurious hospitals, lavish research facilities, and scientific programs of training, of which we are justifiably so proud, are likely to appear within a few decades as magnificent cenotaphs to concepts which once were vital forces but which are no longer generating truly new scientific departures.   *Man Adapting*

ACADEMIC MEDICINE

Robert G. Petersdorf; 1981   **18**

Academicians expect too much of academic medicine. They wish for the gentility of the academician of yesteryear, the income of the cardiovascular surgeon, and the kudos of the molecular biologist who clones a new gene (provided that it is the right one, of course), and they complain if they don't get all of it.   *New England Journal of Medicine*

Paul Starr; 1982   **19**

Physicians in training or engaged in research do not require their patients' good will for future business. Their professional rewards depend on the opinion of colleagues.   *The Social Transformation of American Medicine*

ACANTHOCYTOSIS

Karl Singer, Ben Fisher, Meyer A. Perlstein; 1952   **20**

A 13-and-a-half-year-old boy, the offspring of a consanguinous marriage...developed a progressive ataxic neuropathy...with a peculiar malformation of...erythrocytes.... The erythrocytic anomaly consisted of an unusual type of "crenation".... We have called them acanthrocytes (*akantha*, thorn in Greek).   *Blood*

G. Druez; 1959   **21**

We believe that the term *acanthocytosis* is etymologically more faithful than the term *acanthrocytosis* proposed by Singer.... We have shown that the erythrocytic anomaly is not due to the presence of an abnormal hemoglobin.... We believe that the [recessive hereditary] defect could modify the structure of the [erythrocytic] membrane (between lipid and protein molecules).   *Revue d'Hématologie*

ACETYLCHOLINE

Reid Hunt, René de M. Taveau; 1906   **22**

Acetyl-cholin... is a substance of extraordinary physiological activity..... I think it safe to state that as regards its effect upon the circulation, it is the most powerful substance known.... It is a hundred times more active in causing a fall of blood pressure than is adrenalin in causing a rise.   *British Medical Journal*

ACHONDROPLASIA

Samuel Thomas von Soemmerring; 1791   **23**

[The child] has a very unusual, peculiar appearance. It is of the female gender.... It is very fat and round; but the upper and lower extremities are very much too short.... The stripped bone of the forearm, elbow and wrist, I find knotty, misshapen, bent and the substance almost similar to that of a rachitic child, so that this deformity seems to me to be a true bone disease.   *Abbildungen und Beschreibungen Einiger Misgeburten*

ACID-BASE PHYSIOLOGY

Lawrence Joseph Henderson; 1908   **24**

The effectiveness of bicarbonates and phosphates to preserve neutrality in protoplasm is extraordinarily great. The bicarbonates constitute the first reserve, so to speak, in neutralizing acid. They are effective in a far greater degree than the salts of any acids in equal concentration could be because of the regulation of carbonic acid concentration by diffusion and excretion.   *American Journal of Physiology*

Lawrence Joseph Henderson; 1913   **25**

Such are the physico-chemical facts regarding neutrality regulation in heterogeneous systems by means of carbonic acid and bicarbonates.... There is, I believe, except in celestial mechanics, no other case of such accuracy in a natural regulation of the environment.
                                                    The Fitness of the Environment

Donald Dexter Van Slyke; 1921   **26**

In order to determine which one of the possible variations exists in the blood *in vivo* it is necessary to ascertain two of the involved variables, such as the pH [$BHCO_3$], and [H_2CO_3].   *Journal of Biological Chemistry*

ACQUIRED IMMUNE DEFICIENCY SYNDROME (AIDS)

Michael S. Gottlieb, Robert Schroff, Howard M. Schanker, and others; 1981   **27**

We recently treated several young, previously healthy, homosexual men for multiple episodes of *Pneumocystis carinii* pneumonia, extensive mucosal candidiasis, and severe viral infections. The clinical manifestations and studies of cellular immune function...indicated a...severe acquired T-cell defect....This syndrome represents a potentially transmissible immune deficiency.   *New England Journal of Medicine*

M.G. Sarngadharan, Mikulas Popovic, Lilian Bruch, and others; 1984   **28**

We have shown a high incidence of specific antibodies to HTLV-III in patients with AIDS [88%] and pre-AIDS [79%].   *Science*

Robert C. Gallo, S.Z. Salahuddin, Mikulas Popovic, and others; 1984   **29**

The HTLV-III produced by cultured T cells from patients with AIDS and pre-AIDS is highly infectious and can be readily transmitted to fresh umbilical blood and adult peripheral blood or bone marrow lymphocytes.   *Science*

Edwina Currie; 1987   **30**

My message to the businessmen of this country when they go abroad on business that there is one thing above all they can take with them to stop them catching AIDS, and that is the wife.   *The Observer*

Abraham Verghese; 1994   **31**

Even if I'd made no money, even if it was the pariah of specialties by virtue of its lack of procedures, an unexpected fringe benefit had become evident with the appearance of AIDS: In those early days, dealing with AIDS made us an elite group, an unexpectedly glamourous group. Even the cardiac surgeons could not approach our kind of heroism. Yes, they dealt with death every day. But it was somebody else's death they had to worry about. Never their own.   *My Own Country*

ACROMEGALY

Pierre Marie; 1885   **32**

There exists a disease specially characterised by an hypertrophy of the hands, feet, and face, which we propose to call Acromegaly; that is to say, hypertrophy of the hands and feet (not because...the hands and feet are alone affected during the course of the malady, but because their increase is an initial lesion, and constitutes the most characteristic feature of the affection).   *Essays on Acromegalia*

ACUPUNCTURE

Jacob de Bondt; 1658   **33**

The results in Japan which I will relate surpass even miracles. For chronic pains of the head, for obstruction of the liver and spleen, and also for pleurisy, they bore through [the flesh] with a stylus made of silver or bronze.   *Historia Naturalis et Medica Indias Orientalis*

James Morss Churchill; 1828   **34**

Acupuncture is now employed, not only in the Eastern Hemisphere, in France, and in America, but throughout the British dominions, and in our London hospitals.... For chronic rheumatism, it will be found a most valuable remedy.... Lumbago and Sciatica frequently disappear as if charmed away.

Cases Illustrative of the Immediate Effects of Acupuncturation

Joseph Pancoast; 1846   **35**

[Acupuncture] consists in the introduction of fine, well-tempered sharp-pointed needles, through the integuments and into the subjacent tissues at variable depths.... It is a practice borrowed from the Chinese and Japanese. No great value is now attached to it as a remedial measure, though its use has occasionally been attended with advantage in neuralgia, chronic rheumatism, indolent tumors, indurated lympatic glands.

A Treatise on Operative Surgery

Gwei-Djen Lu, Joesph Needham; 1980   **36**

The scientific rationale of acupuncture will in due course be established.   *Celestial Lancets*

ADAPTATION

René Jules Dubos; 1968   **37**

One of the unique characteristics of man is that he does not live only in the present; at his best, he has a deep sense of continuity with the past and is concerned with the future.... Adaptability must incorporate the needs of day-to-day existence subject to limitations and requirements created by the desire to preserve the past and modified by anticipations for the future.   *Man, Medicine, and Environment*

René Jules Dubos; 1968   **38**

Almost universally, man tries to eliminate the unpleasant effects of environmental forces instead of making the greater effort required to cope with them through his own adaptive physiological resources.   *Man, Medicine, and Environment*

ADOLESCENCE

Moses Maimonides; *circa* 1190   **39**

The adolescent years of man are those in which the finest temperaments occur which are the best balanced.   *Rosner F and Munter S, The Medical Aphorisms of Moses Maimonides*

Theodore Lidz; 1969   **40**

A serious source of family discord derives from keeping an adolescent boy from practicing an instrumental role within the family.... Within the family even a late adolescent is a member of the childhood generation, and the exercise of...decision making by the youth can afford a direct challenge to...paternal prerogatives.... When a male adolescent's instrumental assertiveness is squelched he seeks to break up the family social system.

Adolescence: Psychosocial Perspectives

Barry Nurcombe; 1970   **41**

Pressing home a seeming advantage, the sceptical youth asks pointed questions about the values his mentors hold so dearly. His parents react, perhaps, by tightening the rules and by demanding behaviour more circumspect than they ask of themselves.

Medical Journal of Australia

ADRENAL GLANDS

Thomas Addison; 1855   **42**

The functions of the supra-renal capsules...are almost or altogether unknown. The large supply of blood which they receive from three separate sources; their numerous nerves, derived immediately from the semilunar ganglia and solar plexus; their early development in the foetus; their unimpaired integrity to the latest period of life; and their peculiar gland-like structure; all point to the performance of some important office.

On the Constitutional and Local Effects of Disease of the Supra-renal Capsules

Charles Edouard Brown-Séquard; 1856   **43**

The facts which Addison has published seem to lead to the conclusion that these little organs are essential to life.   *Archives Général de Médecine*

ADRENERGIC RECEPTORS

Raymond Perry Ahlquist; 1948   **44**

There are two distinct types of adrenotropic receptors as determined by their relative responsiveness to the series of racemic sympathomimetic amines most closely related to epinephrine. The alpha adrenotropic receptor is associated with most of the excitatory functions (vasoconstriction, and stimulation of the uterus, nictitating membrane, ureter and dilator pupillae) and one important inhibitory function (intestinal relaxation). The beta adrenotropic receptor is associated with most of the inhibitory functions (vasodilation, and inhibitors of the uterine and bronchial musculature) and one excitatory function (myocardial stimulation).   *American Journal of Physiology*

ADRENOCORTICAL INSUFFICIENCY (ADDISON DISEASE)

Thomas Addison; 1855   **45**

The leading and characteristic features of the morbid state...are, anaemia, general languor and debility, remarkable feebleness of the heart's action, irritability of the stomach, and a peculiar change of colour in the skin, occurring in connection with a diseased condition of the "supra-renal" capsules.... This discolouration pervades the whole surface of the body, but is commonly most strongly manifested on the face, neck, superior extremities, penis, and scrotum, and in the flexures of the axillae and around the navel.

On the Constitutional and Local Effects of Disease of the Supra-renal Capsules

Thomas Addison; 1855   **46**

Her complexion was very dark, her whole person emaciated...she had bilious vomiting...and occasionally wandering a little in her intellects. [At necropsy] the only marked disease was the renal capsules, both of which were enlarged, lobulated, and the seat of morbid deposits apparently of a scrofulous character.

On the Constitutional and Local Effects of Disease of the Supra-renal Capsules

George W. Thorn, Lewis L. Engel, Harry Eisenberg; 1939   **47**

Bilaterally adrenalectomized dogs, fed a constant diet of low sodium and chloride content, may be maintained in excellent condition, by means of the subcutaneous implantation of pellets of crystalline desoxy-corticosterone acetate.

Bulletin of the Johns Hopkins Hospital

ADULTERY

Ambroise Paré; [1510-1590]   **48**
They say Hippocrates, by this explication of causes, freed a certain noble-woman from suspicion of adultery, who being white herself, and her husband also white, brought forth a child as black as an aethiopian, because in copulation she strongly and continually had in her mind the picture of the aethiope. *Collected Works*

Sacha Guitry; 1948   **49**
There are women whose infidelities are the only link they still have with their husbands.

Elles et Toi

ADVERSE DRUG EFFECTS

Ovid; [43 BC - 17 AD]   **50**
The same object will both wound and cure me. *Tristia*

Willis C. Maddrey, John K. Boitnott; 1975   **51**
When a patient [who] is on a drug—on any drug—becomes ill, the Napoleonic Code rather than the English common law should apply: the drug should be presumed guilty until proved innocent. *Hospital Practice*

AGING

Huang Ti Nei Ching Su Wen; [2697-2597 BC]   **52**
When a man grows old his bones become dry and brittle like straw, his flesh sags and there is much air within his thorax, and pains within his stomach; there is an uncomfortable feeling within his heart, the nape of his neck and the top of his shoulders (are contracted), his body burns with fever, his bones are stripped and laid bare of flesh, and his eyes bulge and sag. *The Yellow Emperor's Classic of Internal Medicine*

Hippocrates; [460-375 BC]   **53**
Old men suffer from difficulty of breathing, catarrh accompanied by coughing, strangury, difficult micturition, pains at the joints, kidney disease, dizziness, apoplexy, cachexia, pruritus of the whole body, sleeplessness, watery discharges from the bowels, eyes, and nostrils, dullness of sight, cataract, hardness of hearing. *Aphorisms*

Aristotle; [384-322 BC]   **54**
In the decline of life the power to generate ceases in males and the menstrual discharge ceases in females. *De Generatione Animalium*

Juvenal (Decimus Junius Juvenalis); 60-140   **55**
A long old age is full of continual evils:
Look, first of all, at the face, unshapely, foul, and disgusting,
Unlike its former self, a hide, not a skin, and chopfallen;
Look at the wrinkles too, like those which a mother baboon
Carves on her face in the dark shade of Numidian jungles....
The old are all alike, and they look it.
Doddering voices and limbs, bald heads, running noses, like children's,
Munching their bread...with gums that are utterly toothless... food everlastingly tasteless
. *Satires X*

Clement III; [reigned 1187-1191]   **56**
Young men be not proud in the presence of a decaying old man; he was once that which
you are, he is now that which you will be.   *Alexandrov AV, et al., Neurology*

Petrarch (Francesco Petrarca); 1373   **57**
Continued work and application form my soul's nourishment. So soon as I commenced
to rest and relax I should cease to live. I know my own powers. I am not fitted for other
kinds of work, but my reading and writing, which you would have me discontinue, are easy
tasks.   *Letter to Boccaccio*

Michel de Montaigne; 1580   **58**
Sometimes it is the body that first surrenders to age, sometimes, too, it is the mind; and
I have seen enough whose brains were enfeebled before their stomach and legs.
                                                                Essays. Of Age

William Shakespeare; 1598   **59**
And so, from hour to hour, we ripe and ripe,
And then, from hour to hour, we rot and rot;
And thereby hangs a tale.   *As You Like It, Act II, Scene vii*

Thomas Browne; 1643   **60**
Age doth not rectify, but incurvate our natures, turning bad dispositions into worser
habits, and (like diseases,) brings on incurable vices; for every day as we grow weaker in
age, we grow stronger in sin: and the number of our days doth but make our sins innumerable.   *Religio Medici*

John Milton; 1667   **61**
This is Old Age; but then, thou must outlive
Thy youth, thy strength, thy beauty, which will change
To withered, weak and gray; thy senses, then,
Obtuse, all taste of pleasure must forgo,
To what thou hast; and, for the air of youth,
Hopeful and cheerful, in thy blood will reign
A melancholy damp of cold and dry
To weight thy spirits down, and last consume
The balm of life.   *Paradise Lost*

François, Duc de la Rochefoucauld; 1678   **62**
Old age is a tyrant who prohibits all the pleasures of youth on pain of death.
                                        Moral Reflections, Sentences, and Maxims

François, Duc de la Rochefoucauld; 1678   **63**
The most dangerous weakness of old people who have been amiable is to forget that they
are no longer so.   *Moral Reflections, Sentences, and Maxims*

François, Duc de la Rochefoucauld; 1678   **64**
There are few people who at the first sign of age do not show in what respects their body
and mind will eventually fail.   *Moral Reflections, Sentences, and Maxims*

François, Duc de la Rochefoucauld; 1678   **65**
Age makes men both sillier and wiser.   *Moral Reflections, Sentences, and Maxims*

Benjamin Franklin; 1749   **66**
All would live long, but none would be old.   *Poor Richard's Almanac*

Tobias Smollett; 1771   **67**
There is...one disease...for which you [doctors] have found as yet no specific, and that is
old age, of which this tedious unconnected epistle is an infallible symptom. *What, therefore, cannot be cured, must be endured.*   *Humphry Clinker*

Samuel Johnson; [1709-1784]   **68**
It is a man's own fault, it is from want of use, if his mind grows torpid in old age.
Boswell J, The Life of Samuel Johnson

William Heberden; 1802   **69**
The love of life, or fear of death, makes most men unwilling to allow that their constitution is breaking; and for this reason they are ready to impute to any other cause what in
reality are the signs of approaching and unavoidable decay.
Commentaries on the History and Cure of Diseases

John Keats; 1820   **70**
Here, where men sit and hear each other groan;
Where palsy shakes a few, sad, last grey hairs....   *Ode to a Nightingale*

Josh Billings (Henry Wheeler Shaw); 1874   **71**
About the best thing that extreme old age kan do for us iz tew make death a relief.
Everybody's Friend

Oliver Wendell Holmes; 1887   **72**
Men born in the same year watch each other, especially as the sands of life begin to run
low, as we imagine so many damaged hour-glasses to keep an eye on each other. Women,
of course, never know who are their contemporaries.   *Our Hundred Days in Europe*

Oliver Wendell Holmes; 1891   **73**
Women find it easier than men to grow old in a becoming way.... With old men it is too
often different. They do not belong so much indoors as women do. They have no pretty
little manual occupations.... [He] smokes his pipe, but does not know what to do with his
fingers.   *Over the Teacups*

Oliver Wendell Holmes; 1891   **74**
Habits are the crutches of old age; by the aid of these we manage to hobble along after
the mental joints are stiff and the muscles rheumatic...when every act of self-determina-
tion costs an effort and a pang.   *Over the Teacups*

Oscar Wilde; 1891   **75**
The tragedy of old age is not that one is old, but that one is young.
The Picture of Dorian Gray

William Osler; 1905   **76**
I have two fixed ideas.... The first is the comparative uselessness of men above forty years
of age.... My second fixed idea is the uselessness of men above sixty years of age, and the
incalculable benefit it would be in commercial, political and in professional life if, as a
matter of course, men stopped work at this age.   *The Fixed Period*

Ambrose Bierce; 1906   **77**
Age, *n*.That period of life in which we compound for the vices that we still cherish by
reviling those that we have no longer the enterprise to commit.   *The Devil's Dictionary*

William Osler; 1913   **78**
One of two things happens after sixty, when old age takes a fellow by the hand. Either the
rascal takes charge as general factotum, and you are in his grip body and soul; or you take
him by the neck at the first encounter and after a good shaking make him go your way.
Fletcher R, Canadian Medical Association Journal

Thomas Clifford Allbutt; 1919   **79**
The stealthy foot of time carries us from youth to age so imperceptibly that we are hardly aware of the change; insensibly we shorten our arms, husband our strength, and are willing to think our prowess undiminished.   *British Medical Journal*

Santiago Ramón y Cajal; 1920　　　　　　　　　　　　　　　　　**80**
The saddest thing about old age is that its future is behind it.　　*Chatting over Coffee*

Charles Horace Mayo; 1934　　　　　　　　　　　　　　　　　**81**
Long ago I learned from my father to put old people to bed only for as short a time as was absolutely necessary, for they were like a foundered horse, if they got down it was difficult for them to get up, and their strength ebbed away very rapidly while in bed.
Annals of Surgery

Santiago Ramón y Cajal; [1852-1934]　　　　　　　　　　　　**82**
A characteristic of old age is thinking that our own ruin should coincide precisely with that of the universe.　　*Craigie EH and Gibson WC, The World of Ramón y Cajal*

Walter de la Mare; 1951　　　　　　　　　　　　　　　　　**83**
And saddest of all earth's clocks is
Others growing old....　　　　　　　　　　　　　　　　　*Winged Chariot*

Tennessee Williams; 1957　　　　　　　　　　　　　　　　　**84**
It takes character to refuse to grow old, Doctor—successfully to refuse to. It calls for discipline, abstention. One cocktail before dinner, not two, four, six—a single lean chop and lime juice on a salad in restaurants famed for rich dishes.　　*Suddenly Last Summer*

Leonard Larson; 1960　　　　　　　　　　　　　　　　　**85**
There are no diseases of the aged, but simply diseases among the aged.
Statement to the Senate Finance Committee

Louis Lasagna; 1962　　　　　　　　　　　　　　　　　**86**
Medicine,...consider forsaking the worship of the goddess Longevity. Must we be Methuselites, blindly adoring a giant hourglass on a sere and treeless plain?
The Doctors' Dilemmas

William Carlos Williams; [1883-1963]　　　　　　　　　　　　**87**
In old age
the mind
casts off
rebelliously
the eagle
from its crag.　　　　　　　　　　　　　　　　　　　　*Poem*

Theodor Reik; 1966　　　　　　　　　　　　　　　　　**88**
We can keep pace only with our generation or with our contemporaries, and we have great difficulty in understanding the generation before us and after us, and the situation becomes worse the older we become.　　*The Many Faces of Sex*

Marya Mannes; 1968　　　　　　　　　　　　　　　　　**89**
The woman who seems to be thirty-five but whom I know to be sixty, is, to me, disquieting. A life should leave its traces, and the total lack of them is a negation of experience.
Psychosomatics

Elaine M. Brody; 1971　　　　　　　　　　　　　　　　　**90**
The aging person's functioning, inpaired though it may be, can not be preserved or improved if he is assigned the role of full-time professional patient. His person and dress, the room in which he lives, the opportunity for privacy, the rhythm of his daily life...should convey the fact that the institution is his home, and should permit expression of his personal life style.　　*Journal of the American Geriatric Society*

Vannevar Bush; 1971　　　　　　　　　　　　　　　　　**91**
We all know the troubles of old age. The bones creak; the eyes get dim, one forgets names.... The spark does not ignite; adrenalin has lost its potency. But there is something

to be said on the other side. It is pleasant to rise in the morning, look out at the snow, and remark "I'm not going to the office today".... The beauty of nature has lost none of its charm; the beauty of women none of its benediction. There is...a possibility of growing old gracefully, and with content in one's heart.   *Bulletin of the New York Academy of Medicine*

Earle P. Scarlett; 1972   **92**
Since the remainder of his life is inevitably short, it is really the natural thing for an aging man to become adventurous. The aging can plead no excuse for causation, for, with every day that passes, the aging have less and less to risk or lose, so that in reality the time has now come when they may confidently practice the virtues of rashness, recklessness, and open-hearted generosity.   *Roland CG, In Sickness and in Health*

Anthony Powell; 1973   **93**
Growing old is like being increasingly penalized for a crime you haven't committed.
Temporary Kings

Robert N. Butler; 1979   **94**
It has been said that until a person is 40, his face belongs to his forebears, because its appearance is principally determined by his genes. After that time, the face mirrors the establishment of a human being distinct from the generations preceding him; it is a reflection tempered and altered by the sum total of the unique happenings that compose his life's experience.   *Annals of Internal Medicine*

Norman Cousins; 1981   **95**
Longevity by itself is indistinguishable from vegetation. A man can acquire a new pancreas, kidney, liver, heart, bone marrow and lung, but he will succumb to boredom if his mind is without a horizon.   *Human Options*

Eugene Shapiro; 1985   **96**
When you get older and enter the world of medicine, the good news is that you meet a lot of people. The bad news is that almost all of them are doctors.... When you're 64, a doctor is someone you see on a soap opera. When you're 66, you see more of them than members of your family.   *The New York Times*

Petr Skrabanek; 1986   **97**
There are fates worse than death. Longevity drags if you have buried your children. Poverty, loneliness, incontinence, dependence, and dementia are some of the final rewards. Not everybody hopes for a long life followed by death from boredom.... Why be afraid of sudden death from coronary artery heart disease if you cannot regret it the day after?   *The Lancet*

Bernard Isaacs; 1992   **98**
The "Geriatric Giants"—immobility, incontinence, instability and intellectual deterioration.   *The Challenge of Geriatric Medicine*

Sherwin B. Nuland; 1994   **99**
Surrounded by it though we may be, there is for each of us that something within that turns the face of consciousness away from the reality of our own concomitant aging.
How We Die

Robert N. Butler; 1996   **100**
Old age is a territory populated largely by women.   *New England Journal of Medicine*

John Kenneth Galbraith; 1998   **101**
Great age is not uniformly a benign experience; however, I am fully persuaded that it is much better than the alternative.   *Cassidy J, The New Yorker*

Francine Prose; 2000   102
Age and death: the unfairness of it, the daily humiliation of watching your power vanish just when you figure out how to use it.   *Blue Angel*

Croatian proverb   103
To get old is in the hands of God, but to stay young is a human skill.
Proverb

AGNOSIA

Adolf Kussmaul; 1877   104
We have discovered cases in the literature, which were known as aphasia, but should not be designated as such, inasmuch as the patients were able to express themselves in speaking and writing. They were neither inarticulate (incapable of speech) nor illiterate (incapable of writing); but despite an acute sense of hearing they could no longer comprehend words they heard or, despite good vision, they could no longer read the words they saw.
Die Störungen der Sprache

ALCOHOL

Homer; *circa* 700 BC   105
Inflaming Wine, Pernicious to Mankind
Unnerves the Limbs, and dulls the noble Mind.   *The Iliad*

Seneca; [8 BC - AD 65]   106
Drunkeness is simply voluntary insanity.   *Epistles*

Saint Basil the Great; [330-379]   107
Drunkeness, the ruin of reason, the destruction of strength, premature old age, momentary death.   *Homilies*

William Shakespeare; 1606   108
Lechery, sir, it provokes, and unprovokes; it provokes the desire, but it takes away the performance: therefore, much drink may be said to be an equivocator with lechery: it makes him, and it mars him; it sets him on, and it takes him off; it persuades him, and disheartens him; makes him stand to, and not stand to; in conclusion, equivocates him in a sleep, and, giving him the lie, leaves him.   *Macbeth, Act II, Scene iii*

John Fletcher, George Chapman, Ben Jonson, Philip Massinger; 1630   109
Wine works the heart up, wakes the wit,
There is no cure 'gainst age but it.
It helps the head-ach, cough and tissick,
And is for all diseases Physick.   *The Bloody Brother, Act II, Scene ii*

Thomas Willis; [1621-1675]   110
After a man has taken wine or other spiritous liquors he is at once revived and restored. The reason is that in the mouth, oesophagus and stomach there are certain vital and animal spirits constantly scattered, roaming and, as it were, keeping watch. [Because these spirits are] analogous and proportionate to [those] in wine...they readily mix. Then, taking their new guests by the hand, as it were, convey them to the heart and brain.
Cordials

William Penn; 1693   111
All excess is ill, but drunkenness is of the worst sort: it spoils health, dismounts the mind, and unmans men; it reveals secrets, is quarrelsome, lascivious, impudent, dangerous, and mad.   *The Fruits of Solitude*

John Wesley; 1747   112
Strong, and more especially, spirituous liquors, are a certain, though slow, poison.
The Iliac Passion

George Gordon Byron; 1819   **113**
Tis pity wine should be so deleterious,
For tea and coffee leave us much more serious.   *Don Juan*

Berton Roueché; 1960   **114**
For alcohol, in contrast to most of our cultural acquisitions, owes nothing to man's cre-
ative hand. It comes to us as a triumph not of human imagination but of human curiosity. Like fire, it is a natural phenomenon that man stumbled upon and gratefully bent to
his use.   *The Neutral Spirit*

Winston Churchill; 1963   **115**
Always remember...that I have taken more out of alcohol than alcohol has taken out of
me.   *Reynolds Q, By Quentin Reynolds*

ALCOHOLISM

François Rabelais; 1532   **116**
A hundred devils leap into my body, if there be not more old drunkards than old physi-
cians.   *Gargantua and Pantagruel*

Thomas Becon; 1558   **117**
When the wine is in, the wit is out.   *Catechism*

John Lyly; 1580   **118**
Long quaffing maketh a short life.   *Euphues and His England*

Thomas Fuller; 1732   **119**
Bacchus hath drowned more men than Neptune.   *Gnomologia*

William Heberden; 1802   **120**
The effects of hard drinking are, flatulence, loss of appetite, morning sickness, wasting of
the flesh and strength, tremblings, pains of the stomach, cough, jaundice, dropsy, forgetfulness and inattention, giddiness, diarrhoea, broken sleep.
                                                Commentaries on the History and Cure of Diseases

Edward Rowland Sill; [1841-1887]   **121**
First the man takes a drink,
Then the drink takes the man.   *An Adage from the Orient*

Charles Warrington Earle; 1891   **122**
When you talk about inebriety being a disease, you take away the very last hope of
reforming men who are addicted to the use of liquor.   *Chicago Medical Recorder*

William Styron; 1990   **123**
The storm which swept me into a hospital...began as a cloud...the previous June. And the
cloud...involved alcohol, a substance I had been abusing for forty years.... I used alcohol
as the magical conduit to fantasy and euphoria, and to the enhancement of the imagination [and] as a means to let my mind conceive visions that the unaltered, sober brain has
no access to.... I [used alcohol] to calm the anxiety and incipient dread that I had hidden
away for so long somewhere in the dungeons of my spirit.   *Darkness Visible*

ALDOSTERONE

Hilary M. Grundy, Sylvia A. Simpson, J.F. Tait; 1952   **124**
This further investigation has fully confirmed the earlier, more indirect work, which
showed that the mineral activity of beef adrenal extract was not due to any of the known
biologically active cortical steroids. Positive characterization of the [minerally active]
structure of the compound must await the isolation of larger amounts of material.
                                                                                                            Nature

Jerome W. Conn; 1955 **125**

These studies delineate a new clinical syndrome which is designated temporarily as primary aldosteronism. In its fully developed state it is characterized by the presence in the urine of excessive amounts of a sodium-retaining corticoid, by severe hypokalemia, hypernatremia, alkolosis, and a renal tubular defect in the reabsorption of water.... All of the chemical deviations...became normal within ten days following removal of the adrenal tumor. *Journal of Laboratory and Clinical Medicine*

ALLERGY

Clemens von Pirquet; 1906 **126**

For this general concept of the changed capacity for reaction, I propose the term *allergy*. "Allo" denotes the deviation from the original state, from the behavior of the normal, as in *allorhythmia, allotropy*. *Muenchener Medizinische Wochenschrift*

ALTERNATIVE MEDICINE

Ambrose Bierce; 1906 **127**

Homeopathy, *n.* A school of medicine midway between Allopathy and Christian Science. To the last both the others are distinctly inferior, for Christian Science will cure imaginary diseases, and they can not. *The Devil's Dictionary*

Edward Shorter; 1991 **128**

The last decade has seen a large flight to "alternative therapies" such as naturopathy, iridology, reflexology, and the like. Lacking any scientific basis, these alternative therapies represent a return to the eighteenth century, when all therapies, medical and nonmedical alike, were based upon anecdotal results rather than systematic demonstration of efficacy. *Doctors and Their Patients*

Edward W. Campion; 1993 **129**

Unconventional treatments often seem to make people feel more comfortable, even when their accompanying theories are silly. *New England Journal of Medicine*

Michael Baum; 1996 **130**

There is much that we can learn from complementary medicine to make our patients feel better while our science attempts to make them get better.... However, to encourage the terminally ill to spend the last few precious months of life chasing the false promise of a cure is as cruel as it is intellectually dishonest. *Journal of the Royal Society of Medicine*

Roy Porter; 1997 **131**

Alternative medicine...may be no less "medicalizing" (and risky) than the orthodox medicine they repudiate.... Modern health preoccupations have spawned a new health mysticism, spurred by big companies which profit from vitamin sales and public health preoccupation. *The Greatest Benefit to Mankind*

ALZHEIMER'S DISEASE

Alois Alzheimer; 1907 **132**

A woman, 51 years old, showed jealousy toward her husband as the first noticeable sign....Soon a rapidly increasing loss of memory could be noticed. She could not find her way around in her own apartment.... Her entire behavior bore the stamp of utter perplexity. She was totally disoriented to time and place.... The generalized dementia progressed.... After 4 1/2 years...death occurred.... The autopsy revealed a generally atrophic brain without macroscopic lesions.... Scattered through the...cortex...one found miliary foci that were caused by the deposition of a peculiar substance.

Allgemeine Zeitschrift für Psychiatrie

Norma Wylie; 1996   133

Alzheimer's can be called the long good-bye. You grieve about the loved one from the moment you begin to observe the gradual loss of memory and the speech and personality changes, because they are incurable. The person you love is gradually changing before your eyes. You say good-bye many times until the final good-bye at death.

Sharing the Final Journey: Walking with the Dying

AMAUROTIC FAMILIAL IDIOCY (TAY-SACHS DISEASE)

Bernard Parney Sachs; 1887   134

The little girl S., who was but two years at the time of death, was the first born of young and healthy parents.... We have here an agenetic condition pure and simple, affecting the highest nerve elements.   *Journal of Nervous and Mental Diseases*

AMERICAN COLLEGE OF PHYSICIANS

Rosemary Stevens; 1971   135

Internists were the next [after surgeons] to distinguish themselves above the basic education for general practice.... In 1913, Philip Mills Jones had questioned: "And what in the world is the matter with internists? Are they asleep at the switch? Are they going to let the surgeons...put it all over them again? Are they not going to organize an American Royal College of Physicians?... Up and have at them!".... [Heinrich] Stern cherished the concept of an American college of physicians as eagerly as Franklin Martin identified with the College of Surgeons.... Stern...only managed to set up the American College of Physicians in...1915.   *American Medicine and the Public Interest*

Rosemary Stevens; 1971   136

On the prompting of the American College of Physicians...a joint educational committee in internal medicine was reactivated in 1949 whose membership consisted of the College, the [AMA Council on Medical Education], and the American Board of Internal Medicine. In 1953 the name was changed to the Residency Review Committee in Internal Medicine.   *American Medicine and the Public Interest*

AMERICAN MEDICAL ASSOCIATION

Henry Jacob Bigelow; 1871   137

The American Medical Association is a body of medical gentlemen, practically volunteer delegates, having primarily in view the agreeable and commendable object of a journey to break the monotony of medical practice and give them an apology for leaving their homes and their patients at a pleasant season of the year.   *Medical Education in America*

AMERICAN MEDICINE

William Douglass; 1755   138

The physical practice in our colonies is so perniciously bad, that excepting in surgery and some very acute cases, it is better to let nature...take her course.... When I first arrived in New England, I asked G.P., a noted facetious practitioner, what was their general method of practice; he told me their practice was very uniform, bleeding, vomiting, blistering, purging.   *The Present State of the British Settlements of North America*

Abraham Flexner; 1910   139

We have indeed in America medical practitioners not inferior to the best elsewhere; but there is probably no other country in the world in which there is so great a distance and so fatal a difference between the best, the average, and the worst.

Medical Education in the United States and Canada

Rosemary Stevens; 1971   140

Physicians returned from the German clinics to practice, and to teach in American medical schools. Scientific experts jostled against the old-style practitioners. In the years between 1890 and 1914, American medical science was driven from mediocrity to eminence, paving the way for world leadership in medicine in the years following World War 1.

American Medicine and the Public Interest

AMINO ACIDS

Franz Hofmeister; 1904   141

...One may...consider the proteins as for the most part arising by condensation of *a*-amino acids, whereby the linkage through the group -CO-NH-CH= has to be regarded as the regularly recurring one.   *Ergebnisse der Physiologie*

AMYOTROPHIC LATERAL SCLEROSIS

Stephen W. Hawking; 1993   142

I am quite often asked: How do you feel about having ALS? The answer is, not a lot. I try to lead as normal a life as possible and not think about my condition or regret the things it prevents me from doing, which are not that many.

Black Holes and Baby Universes and Other Essays

ANATOMY

Aristotle; [384-322 BC]   143

The inner parts...are for the most part unknown; at least, those of man are, and hence we have to refer to those of other animals, the natural structure of whose parts those of man resemble, and examine them.   *De Partibus Animalium*

Galen; [130-200]   144

Make it rather your serious endeavour not only to acquire accurate book-knowledge of each bone but also to examine assiduously with your own eyes the human bones them-selves.   *On Anatomical Procedures*

Guido da Vigevano; 1345   145

Since it is prohibited by the Church to perform anatomies on the human body, and since it is impossible to know the medical art completely, unless one has knowledge of anato-my... I shall demonstrate patently and openly the anatomy of the human body, through properly executed illustrations.   *Anothomia Designata per Figuras*

William Harvey; 1628   146

I profess to learn and to teach anatomy, not from books but from dissections; not from the positions of philosophers but from the fabric of nature.

An Anatomical Treatise on the Movement of the Heart and Blood in Animals

Jacobus Sylvius (Jacques Dubois); 1635   147

I would have you look carefully and recognize by eye when you are attending dissections.... For my judgment is that it is much better that you should learn the matter of cutting by eye and touch than by reading and listening. For reading alone never taught anyone how to sail a ship, to lead an army, nor to compound a medicine, which is done rather by the use of one's own sight and the training of one's own hands.   *Opera Medica*

Thomas Browne; 1643   148

In our study of Anatomy there is a mass of mysterious Philosophy, and such as reduced the very Heathens to Divinity: yet, amongst all those rare discoveries and curious pieces I find in the Fabrick of Man, I do not so much content my self as in that I find not, there is no Organ or Instrument for the rational Soul.   *Religio Medici*

Thomas Sydenham; 1688   **149**

All that Anatomie can doe is only to shew us the gross and sensible parts of the body, or the vapid and dead juices all which, after the most diligent search, will be noe more able to direct a physician how to cure a disease than how to make a man.

Unpublished manuscript

William Hunter; *circa* 1750   **150**

Anatomy is the only solid foundation of medicine; it is to the physician and surgeon what geometry is to the astronomer. It discovers and ascertains truth, overturns superstition and vulgar error, and checks the enthusiasm of theorists and sects in medicine, to whom, perhaps, more of the human species have fallen a sacrifice than to the sword itself or to pestilence.   *Andrews HR, British Medical Journal*

Mark Twain (Samuel Langhorne Clemens); 1867   **151**

Anatomists see no beautiful women in all their lives, but only a ghastly sack of bones with Latin names to them, and a network of nerves and muscles and tissues inflamed by disease.   *Letter to the Alta Californian*

William Rimmer; 1890   **152**

As well...to set a person down to read a foreign language before he has learned the value of the letters which compose the words, as to ask a person to draw a human figure without some knowledge of the bones and muscles which compose it.

Bartlett TH, The Art and Life of William Rimmer

Abraham Flexner; 1910   **153**

Anatomy and physiology form but the vestibule of medical education. They teach the normal structure of the body, the normal function of the parts, fluids, organs, and the conditions under which they operate. The next step carries the student *in medial res*; he begins pharmacology—the experimental study of the response of the body to medication.

Medical Education in the United States and Canada

ANEMIA

Johannes Lange; 1554   **154**

Her face, which...was distinguished by rosiness of cheeks and redness of lips, is some how as if exsanguinated, sadly paled, the heart trembles with every movement of her body, and the arteries of her temples pulsate, and she is seized with dyspnoea in dancing or climbing the stairs...and the legs...become edematous at night.... This disease frequently attacks virgins, when now mature they pass from youth to virility. For at this time...the menstrual blood flows from the liver to the...womb.   *Medicinalium Epistolarum Miscellanea*

Nicolas Andry de Bois-Regard; 1741   **155**

The wan Complexion, otherwise called the *Green Sickness*, to which the Fair-Sex are so subject, proceeds commonly from the internal Piles, which are swelled, painful, and do not bleed, or from the Menses being suppressed...If the Chlorosis proceeds from the second Cause, you must have recourse to Broths made of Veal.   *Orthopaedia*

Gabriel Andral; 1843   **156**

There are cases...in which [the blood's] amount of globules falls much below the physiological mean, and diminishing more and more, reaches a proportion so low that we can scarcely comprehend how, with so few globules in the blood, life can still be maintained. This diminution, in different degrees, of the globular element of the blood is the fundamental character of anaemia, a condition which...is the opposite of plethora.

Essai d'Hématologie Pathologique

ANESTHESIA

Henry Jacob Bigelow; 1846   **157**
It has long been an important problem in medical science to devise some method of mitigating the pain of surgical operations. An efficient agent for this purpose has at length been discovered. A patient has been rendered completely insensible during an amputation of the thigh, regaining consciousness after a short interval.

Boston Medical and Surgical Journal

Henry Jacob Bigelow; 1846   **158**
On the 16th of Oct., 1846, an operation was performed at the [Massachusetts General] hospital, upon a patient who had inhaled a preparation prepared by Dr. Morton, a dentist of this city with the alleged intention of producing insensibility to pain.... No doubt, I think, existed in the minds of those who saw this operation, that the unconsciousness was real; nor could the imagination be accused of any share in the production of these remarkable phenomena.   *Boston Medical and Surgical Journal*

John Warren; 1846   **159**
Gentlemen, this is no humbug.   *Gordon R, The Alarming History of Medicine*

Robert Liston; 1846   **160**
I tried the ether inhalation to-day in a case of amputation of the thigh...one of the most painful operations in surgery, and with the most perfect and satisfactory results. It is a very great matter to be able thus to destroy sensibility to such an extent, and without, apparently, any bad result. It is a fine thing for operating surgeons, and I thank you most sincerely for the early information you were so kind as to give me of it.   *The Lancet*

James Young Simpson; 1847   **161**
I have never had the pleasure of watching over a series of better or more rapid recoveries; nor once witnessed any disagreeable result follow to either mother or child; whilst I have now seen an immense amount of maternal pain and agony saved by its employment. And I most conscientiously believe that the proud mission of the physician is distinctly twofold—namely, to alleviate human suffering, as well as preserve human life.

Account of a New Anaesthetic Agent

Crawford Williamson Long; 1849   **162**
Since '42, I have performed one or more surgical operations annually, in patients in a state of etherization.... From one [patient] I removed three tumours the same day.... I amputated two fingers of a negro boy.   *Southern Medical and Surgical Journal*

James Young Simpson; 1849   **163**
I am informed, that in another medical school, my conduct in introducing and advocating the superinduction of anaesthesia in labour has been publicly denounced *ex cathedra* as an attempt to contravene the arrangements and decrees of Providence, hence reprehensible and heretical in its character, and anxiously to be avoided and eschewed by all properly principled students and practitioners.   *Anaesthesia*

Crawford Williamson Long; 1853   **164**
The ether was given to Mr. Venable on a towel and fully under its influence, I extirpated the tumour....The patient continued to inhale ether during the time of the operation, and seemed incredulous until the tumour was shown to him. He gave no evidence of pain during the operation and assured me after it was over that he did not experience the least degree of pain.   *Transactions of the Georgia Medical and Surgical Association*

Queen Victoria; 1853   **165**
We are having the baby [Prince Leopold], and we shall have the chloroform.

Bennion E, Antique Medical Instruments

Silas Weir Mitchell; 1896   **166**
Whatever triumphs still shall hold the mind,
Whatever gifts shall yet enrich mankind,
Ah! here, no hour shall strike through all the years,
No hour so sweet as when hope doubt and fears,
'Mid deepening silence watched one eager brain
With Godlike will decree the Death of Pain.   *The Birth and Death of Pain*

Washington Ayr; 1897   **167**
The heroic bravery of the man who voluntarily placed himself upon the table, a subject for the surgeon's knife, should be recorded and his name enrolled upon parchment, which should be hung upon the walls of the surgical amphitheatre in which the operation was performed. His name was Gilbert Abbott.   *The Semi-Centennial of Anaesthesia*

ANEURYSM

Ambroise Paré; 1575   **168**
Great *Aneurismaes* under the Arm pits, in the Groins and other partt wherein there are large vessels, admit no cure, because so great an eruption of blood and spirit often follows upon such an incision, that death prevents both Art and Cure.... The *Aneurismaes* which happen in the internall parts are incurable. Such as frequently happen to those who have often had the unction and sweat for the cure of the French disease...it distendsit to that largeness as to hold a mans Fist.   *Works*

Jean-François Fernel; 1581   **169**
An aneurism is the dilatation of an artery full of spiritous blood. It sometimes occurs externally, as in the hands and feet, or about the throat and chest; differing in this respect from a varix, that it is large, swollen, and has an often annoying pulsation.... It also sometimes occurs in the internal arteries, especially in the chest, or about the spleen and mesentery, where a violent throbbing is frequently observable.   *Universa Medicina*

Richard Wiseman; 1676   **170**
All *Aneurisma's* are difficult of Cure. Those which are large, and arise from Arteries deep in the Muscles, to which you cannot make your Applications, are incurable: and if they be unadvisedly opened, the Patient is in great danger of his life. But if the *Aneurisma* be in such a Part as is capable of Bandage and application of Medicaments, the Cure is feasible; or the Disease may be palliated to the ease of the Patient.
    Severall Chirurgical Treatises

Thomas Bevill Peacock; 1863   **171**
In the *advanced stage of dissecting aneurism* there is found an opening through the internal coats of the vessel, leading into a sac situated within the arterial tunics, and extending to a greater or lesser distance along the course of the vessel. This sac is lined by a distinct membrane very similar to the natural lining membrane of the arteries.
    Transactions of the Pathological Society of London

ANEURYSM OF THE AORTA

Giovanni Battista Morgagni; 1761   **172**
A certain debauchee having gone into the house...and after a little time having come out...and [the strumpet] not having appear'd for two or three hours after, the neighbours...found her not only dead but cold; lying in bed with such a posture of body, that it could not be doubted what business she had been about.... I conjectur'd...that the cause of this sudden death would certainly be found to consist in the rupture of some large vessel.... [At necropsy] an orifice...communicated with a roundish aneurism, that hung to it in the form of a sacculus.... And it had been ruptured in the upper part.
    The Seats and Causes of Diseases

Jean-Nicolas Corvisart des Marest; 1806   **173**

Along with these signs, so to say, pathognomonic, I place a sort of peculiar whistling....
The whistling does not exist except when the tumor produces compression of the trachea,
that is to say, when the aneurysm is located on the arch of the aorta.

An Essay on the Organic Diseases and Lesions of the Heart and Great Vessels

William Silver Oliver; 1878   **174**

Place the patient in the erect position, and direct him to close his mouth, and elevate his chin
to the fullest extent, then grasp the cricoid cartilage between the finger and thumb, and use
gentle upward pressure on it, when if dilatation or aneurism exist, the pulsation of the aorta
will be distinctly felt transmitted through the trachea to the hand. This act of examination
will increase laryngeal distress should this accompany the disease.   *The Lancet*

William Osler; *circa* 1900   **175**

There is no disease more conducive to clinical humility than aneurysm of the aorta.

Aphorisms

ANGINA PECTORIS

Edward Hyde, Earl of Clarendon; 1759   **176**

His Father had long suffered under an Indisposition...which gave him rather frequent
Pains... He was...seized on by so sharp a Pain in the left Arm...that the Torment made him
as pale...as if He were dead; and He used to say, "that He had passed the Pangs of Death,
and he should die in one of those Fits"; as soon as it was over; which was quickly.

The Life of Edward, Earl of Clarendon

Giovanni Battista Morgagni; 1761   **177**

A mother...had been long subject to attacks of the following kind. From bodily excursions
there arose a sort of grievous anguish within the left upper part of the breast, and numbness of the left arm; all of which readily ceased when she ceased to move. This woman,
while travelling...was suddenly siezed with one of these paroxysms, and, crying out that
she was dying, immediately expired.   *The Seats and Causes of Diseases*

William Heberden; 1768   **178**

There is a disorder of the breast marked with strong and peculiar symptoms, considerable
for the...danger belonging to it.... The seat of it, and sense of strangling, and anxiety with
which it is attended, may make it not improperly be called angina pectoris. They...are
seized while they are walking (more especially if it be up a hill and soon after eating) with
a painful and most disagreeable sensation in the breast, which seems as if it would extinguish life, if it were to increase or continue; but the moment they stand still, all this
uneasiness vanishes.   *Medical Transactions of the Royal College of Physicians*

[Anonymous]; 1785   **179**

It is about five or six years since, that I first felt the disorder which you treat of; it always
attacked me when walking, and always after dinner, or in the evening....The first symptom
is a pretty full pain in my left arm a little above the elbow; and in perhaps half a minute
it spreads across the left side of my breast, and produces either a little faintness, or a thick-
ness in my breathing; at least I imagined so, but the pain generally obliges me to stop.

Medical Transactions of the Royal College of Physicians

Caleb Hillier Parry; 1799   **180**

The disease generally attacks persons of the male sex; and, of them, those who are
inclined to corpulency. The first symptom is an uneasy sensation...an anxiety, or a pain,
extending generally from about the middle of the sternum across the left breast, and, in
certain stages...usually stretching into the left arm.... The patient feels as if persisting in
the exertion would produce a total suspension of the powers of life.

An Inquiry into the Symptoms and Causes of the Syncope Anginosa

David Dundas; 1809   181

He was seized with a considerable pain at the heart, and a difficulty of respiration, great palpitation and great anxiety. He conceived that the smallest motion of the body would have instantly destroyed him, and this dread seemed to have totally bereft him of the power of utterance.   *Medical-Chirurgical Transactions*

Dominic John Corrigan; 1837   182

In some cases of what are called Angina Pectoris the paroxysms of dyspnoea, anxiety, mental distress, etc. constituting a fit of Angina Pectoris...are really the symptoms of aortitis, or inflammation of the mouth of the aorta.   *Dublin Journal of Medical Sciences*

Thomas Lauder Brunton; 1867   183

As I believed the relief [from angina pectoris] produced by the bleeding was due to the diminution it occasioned in the arterial tension, it occurred to me that a substance which possesses the power of lessening it in such an eminent degree as nitrite of amyl would probably produce the same effect.... On proceeding to try it on the wards...my hopes were completely fulfilled.   *The Lancet*

William Murrell; 1879   184

From a consideration of the physiological action of the drug [nitroglycerin] and more especially from the similarity existing between its general action and that of nitrite of amyl, I concluded that it would probably prove of service in the treatment of angina pectoris, and I am happy to say that this anticipation has been realised.   *The Lancet*

William Osler; 1892   185

It is not the delicate neurotic person who is prone to angina, but the robust, the vigorous in mind and body, the keen and ambitious man, the indicator of whose engines is always at "full speed ahead."   *The Lancet*

ANGIOKERATOMA

Vittorio Mibelli; 1890   186

The presence of small red spots could be seen, which resembled telangiectases and were covered already by a slightly elevated and horny epidermis.... The external appearance of the small tumours suggested the diagnosis of keratoma. We must however distinguish what I call Angiokeratoma from simple keratoma.

Comptes Rendus des Congrès Internationale de Dermatologie et Syphilis

ANGIONEUROTIC EDEMA (QUINCKE DISEASE)

Heinrich Irenaeus Quincke; 1882   187

I wish to identify a skin disease which does not seem to be rare; however, only a few cases of it have been described. This disease appears as oedematous swelling of the skin and the subcutaneous tissue in localized lesions from 2 to 10 cm. or more in diameter.... Patients usually have a sense of tension of the skin—pruritus is not common.

Monatlich Praktische Dermatologie

ANGIOTENSIN

Irvine Heinly Page, Oscar Marvin Helmer; 1940   188

Renin...when purified...produced no vasoconstriction when perfused with Ringer's solution through a dog's tail or rabbit's ear.... The pressor activity could be restored by addition of a protein-like substance contained in plasma.... Renin reacts with renin-activator to form a strong pressor substance.... It is suggested that this substance be called angiotonin.   *Journal of Experimental Medicine*

ANIMAL RESEARCH

George Bernard Shaw; 1911   189
If the medical profession were to outdo the Anti-Vivisection Societies in a general professional protest against the practice and principles of the vivisectors, every doctor in the kingdom would gain substantially by the immense relief and reconciliation which would follow such a reassurance of the humanity of the doctor.   *The Doctor's Dilemma, Preface*

ANOREXIA NERVOSA

William Withey Gull; 1868   190
At present our diagnosis is mostly one of inference, from our knowledge of the liability of the several organs to particular lesions; thus we avoid the error of supposing the presence of mesenteric disease in young women emaciated to the last degree through hysteric apepsia, by our knowledge of the latter affection, and by the absence of tubercular disease elsewhere.   *The Lancet*

William Withey Gull; 1874   191
In...1868, I referred to a peculiar form of disease occurring mostly in young women, and characterized by extreme emaciation.... At present our diagnosis of this affection is negative, so far as determining any positive cause from which it springs.... The subjects...are...chiefly between the ages of sixteen and twenty-three.... My experience supplies at least one instance of a fatal termination.... Death apparently followed from the starvation alone.... The want of appetite is, I believe, due to a morbid mental state.... We might call the state hysterical.   *Transactions of the Clinical Society of London*

Sheila MacLeod; 1981   192
[Anorexia nervosa] is a disease in which the concept of the whole person is so confused, so dialectically divided, that "I" can at the same time be choosing to live, as the self, and choosing to die, as the body, however unconscious those choices may be.   *The Art of Starvation*

Brian S. Turner; 1996   193
The onset of anorexia is situated in a conflict over dependence and autonomy in the relationship between mother and daughter.   *The Body and Society*

Roy Porter; 1997   194
Modern anorexia is the biopsychosocial disorder mirroring a society with specific tensions and contradictions: the bourgeois family, supportive yet suffocating, and all the paradoxical hypocrisies of modern attitudes towards youth, food, femininity, beauty and sexuality, are whipped up by the media and by multi-million pound food and style industries.

The Greatest Benefit to Mankind

ANTIBIOTICS

Alexander Fleming; 1946   195
It seems likely that in the next few years a combination of antibiotics with different antibacterial spectra will furnish a "cribrum therapeuticum" from which fewer and fewer infecting bacteria will escape.   *Chemotherapy: Yesterday, Today, and Tomorrow*

ANTIBODIES

Paul Ehrlich; 1897   196
Our knowledge of cell functions and especially of synthetic processes... lead us... to assume that in the formation of antibodies, we are dealing with the enhancement of a normal cell function, and not with the creation at need of new groups of atoms. Physiological analogues of the group of the specifically combining antibodies must exist beforehand in the organism or in its cells.   *Klinisches Jahrbuch*

ANTISEPSIS

Joseph Lister; 1867   **197**
Bearing in mind that it is from the vitality of the atmospheric particles that all the mischief arises, it appears that all that is requisite is to dress the wound with some material capable of killing these septic germs, provided that any substance can be found reliable for this purpose, yet not too potent as a caustic.   *The Lancet*

Joseph Lister; 1867   **198**
When it had been shown by... Pasteur that the septic property of the atmosphere depended...on minute organisms suspended in it...it occurred to me that decomposition in the injured part might be avoided...by applying as a dressing some material capable of destroying the life of the floating particles.... The material which I have employed is carbolic...acid.... Since the antiseptic treatment has been brought into full operation...my wards...have completely changed...so that during the last nine months not a single instance of pyaemia, hospital gangrene, or erysipelas has occurred.   *The Lancet*

William H. Byford; 1880   **199**
With reference to the question of drainage: My practice has undergone some change within a few years, since Listerism came into vogue. I cannot reconcile antiseptic practice with the use of a drainage tube.   *Transactions of the American Gynecological Society*

ANTITOXINS

Emil Adolf von Behring, Shibasaburo Kitasato; 1890   **200**
The immunity of rabbits and mice which have been immunized against tetanus rests on the capability of cell-free blood serum to render harmless the toxic substances which the tetanus bacilli produce.   *Deutsche Mediziniche Wochenschrift*

AORTIC DISSECTION

William E. Hunt, Charles F. Wooley; 1996   **201**
I...had the sudden onset of a severe pain just medial to and above the left scapula.... The intensity...rapidly reached a level I had rarely experienced.... The pain was pulsating slowly [at] my pulse rate.... I then noticed numbness and tingling in both legs.... I was beginning to believe that these symptoms could only be the result of a dissecting aneurysm of the aorta.   *American Heart Journal*

AORTIC SUBVALVULAR STENOSIS

Norman Chevers; 1842   **202**
The part of the [aortic] orifice immediately below the valve...is occasionally found coated with masses of fibrinous or other deposit; this layer of fibrinous structure is also apt to become hardened and rather contracted, after attacks of endocarditis, and in cases of disease affecting the left auricoventricular orifice; in this way forming a cause of narrowing of the lower part of the aortic ostium, which I believe to be frequently overlooked.
Guy's Hospital Reports

AORTIC VALVE DISEASE

Jean-Nicolas Corvisart des Marest; 1806   **203**
When it is considered how narrow the opening is, which these constrictions leave, it is difficult to conceive how such an organic derangement can continue for years. It is evident, if such an obstacle to the circulation were suddenly introduced into a healthy subject, death would immediately follow: but as these obstacles are slowly formed, the circulation is gradually impeded, and nature seems in some measure to be habituated to such a perversion of her laws.   *An Essay on the Organic Diseases and Lesions of the Heart and Great Vessels*

AORTIC VALVE MURMURS

James Hope; 1839   **204**
When a murmur of this kind is louder along the tract of the ascending aorta than opposite to the valves, and is...peculiarly superficial and hissing, it proceeds from disease of
that vessel.   *A Treatise on the Diseases of the Heart*

AORTIC VALVE REGURGITATION

William Cowper; 1706   **205**
The Valves of the Great Artery...were Petrify'd, insomuch that they could not approach
each other.... But an Orifice...remain'd always open by the Petrifactions...which had clog-
g'd these Valves, and hindered their application to each other.... These Valves...are rendered more or less useless: For as their Offise is to prevent the return of the Blood into
the Heart, in its Diastole...the consequences must be, not only a regurgitation of Blood
into the Heart, but they baulk its impulsive force.
Philosophical Transactions of the Royal Society

Raymond Vieussens; 1715   **206**
His pulse...appeared to be very full, very fast, very hard, unequal, & so strong that the
artery...struck the ends of my fingers just as a cord would have done which was very tightly drawn & violently shaken.... The ends [of the aortic valves] could never approach each
other closely enough to prevent any opening between them; that is why whenever the
aorta contracted, it sent back into the left ventricle a part of the blood which it had just
received.   *Traité Nouveau de la Structure et des Causes de Movement Natural du Coeur*

Giovanni Battista Morgagni; 1761   **207**
For as one of these [the aortic valve] was bony, and the others indurated, so being...less
yielding to the blood, they might encrease the obstacles to its exit, and, on the other
hand, not sufficiently prevent its return, when, soon after, repuls'd by the contraction of
the great artery; so that, as some portion of it return'd into the left ventricle of the heart.
The Seats and Causes of Diseases

Thomas Hodgkin; 1827   **208**
I shall designate by the term *retroversion of the valves* that diseased state which allows of
their dropping towards the ventricle. Instead of effectually closing the vessel against a
reflux of the blood.... The impulse of the heart was not particularly feeble, but was considerably diffused; the sound very general over the whole of the left side.... Each contraction appeared lengthened, accompanying with a purring, thrilling, or sawing kind of noise.
London Medical Gazette

Thomas Hodgkin; 1829   **209**
Thou wilt probably recollect having pointed out to me...a particular state of the valves of
the Aorta which, by admitting of their falling back towards the ventricle, unfits them
for...their function.... Auscultation often detects a prolonged and perverted sound, such
as has been compared to the stroke of a saw, the puff of a pair of bellows or the action of
a rasp.   *London Medical Gazette*

Dominic John Corrigan; 1832   **210**
When the semilunar valves...become incapable of closing the mouth of the aorta, then
after each contraction of the ventricle, a portion of the blood just sent into the
aorta...returns back into the ventricle. Hence the ascending aorta and arteries arising from
it...become...flaccid or lessened in their diameter.... The ventricle again contracts and
impels quickly into these vessels...blood, which suddenly and greatly dilates them. The
diastole of these vessels is thus marked by so sudden and so great an increase of size as to
present the visible pulsation which constitutes one of the signs of the disease.
Edinburgh Medical and Surgical Journal

James Hope; 1839   211

Aortic regurgitation produces a pre-eminently *jerking* pulse, a high degree of the pulse of unfilled arteries, as seen in anaemia from any cause. The diastole or beat of the artery is short and quick, as if the blood were smartly jerked or shot under the finger, the vessel during the intervals feeling unusually empty. This is the most remarkable, appreciable, and constant pulse produced by disease of the heart. In the immense majority of cases, the practitioner may conjecture the disease by this sign alone.

A Treatise on the Diseases of the Heart

Paul Louis Duroziez; 1861   212

In cases of uncomplicated aortic insufficiency, wherein the heart beats vigorously and the arteries pulsate and react forcefully, the double murmur [over the femoral arteries] is audible; when, contrarily, aortic insufficiency is complicated by a considerable degree of aortic or mitral stenosis...the arteries are moderately distended with blood and thus the second murmur is difficult to hear.   *Archives Générales de Médecine*

Heinrich Irenaeus Quincke; 1868   213

As far as the capillary pulse is concerned, so can one see it best on his own fingernail...between the whitish, blood-poor area and the red injected part of the capillary system of the nail-bed...there is, with each heartbeat, a forward and backward movement of the margin between the red and white part.... A large and rapidly falling pulse is seen especially in aortic insufficiency, and for this reason the capillary pulse is especially clear in this condition.   *Wiener Klinische Wochenschrift*

AORTIC VALVE STENOSIS

Jean-Nicolas Corvisart des Marest; 1806   214

When the indurated and ossified semi-lunar valves of the aorta stop a portion of this vessel, the obstacle which they form breaks the wave of blood propelled by the heart into the artery; strong and frequent palpitations supervene, because the heart is easily filled, but is difficultly emptied; thence results a more protracted residence of the blood in the left cavities, a longer application of the stimulus of the blood on the parietes of the heart, in fact, a greater irritation of the organ. The pulse, in this case, may preserve a certain degree of hardness, and rigidity, but never much fulness or regularity.

An Essay on Organic Diseases and Lesions of the Heart and Great Vessels

William Stokes; 1854   215

Strong action of the left ventricle; extremely loud and musical murmur at the aortic orifice, transmitted through the whole extent of the arterial tree; the heart's action generally regular.... The phenomena arise from extensive ossific disease of the aortic opening.

The Diseases of the Heart and Aorta

APHASIA

William Heberden; 1802   216

The inability to speak is owing sometimes not to the paralytic state of the organs of speech only, but to the utter loss of the knowledge of language and letters...by slow degrees, getting the use of the smaller words first, and being frequently unable to find the word they want, and using another for it of a quite different meaning, as if it were a language which they had once known, but by long disuse had almost forgotten.

Commentaries on the History and Cure of Diseases

APOPTOSIS

J.F.R. Kerr, A.H. Wyllie, A.R. Currie; 1972   217

This distinctive type of [cell] necrosis.... we suggest... be called *Apoptosis*.... The word... is used in Greek to describe the "dropping off"... of petals from flowers, or leaves from trees.

To show the derivation clearly, we propose that the accent should be on the penultimate syllable, the second half of the word being pronounced like "ptosis" (with the "p" silent) ... which comes from the same root, "to fall".
British Journal of Cancer

APOTHECARY

Ambrose Bierce; 1906   **218**
Apothecary, *n.* The physician's accomplice, undertaker's benefactor and graveworm's provider.
The Devil's Dictionary

APPENDICITIS

Laurence Heister; 1755   **219**
I found the small guts very red and inflamed in several places.... But, when I was about to demonstrate the situation of the great guts, I found the vermiform process of the caecum preternaturally black, adhering closer to the peritonaeum than usual. As I now was about to separate it...the membranes of this process broke...and discharged two or three spoonfuls of matter. This instance may stand as a proof of the possibility of inflammations arising, and abscesses forming, in the appendicula.
Medical, Chirurgical, and Anatomical Cases and Observations

John William Keys Parkinson; 1812   **220**
He was suddenly seized with vomiting and great prostration of strength. The abdomen became very tumid and painful upon being pressed.... Death...took place within 24 hours.... Upon examination the whole surface of the peritoneum was found inflamed.... The viscera...appeared in a perfectly healthy state, excepting the appendix vermiformis of the coecum.... About an inch of its extremity was considerably enlarged and thickened, its internal surface ulcerated, and an opening from ulceration...through which it appeared, that a thin dark-coloured and highly fetid fluid, had escaped into the cavity of the abdomen.
Medico-Chirurgical Transactions

Jean-Baptiste Louyer-Villermay; 1824   **221**
If the autopsy...presented some differences in shape and details, the foundation was the same, in that the same organ, the cecal appendix, was affected in the same way, and produced the death of the patients with a similar rapidity. In both cases, the gangrene compromised the totality of the appendix, had a very limited extension in the neighboring tissues, and did not include the peritoneum, the intestinal mass, the interior of the cecum and any of the other viscera.
Inflammatory Conditions of the Cecal Appendix

Thomas Hodgkin; 1836   **222**
The partial inflammation of the peritoneum, in the Iliac fossa, is sometimes set up by disease in the Appendix caeci.... The appendix having been perforated by ulcerations, occasioned by the lodgement of the faecal concretions in its cavity, extravasation takes place, and inflammation of a more severe and serious kind is originated.... Nature sometimes succeeds in limiting the inflammation to a part of the right side; but it is at other times diffused over the whole abdomen...and quickly proves fatal.
Lectures on the Morbid Anatomy of the Serous and Mucous Membranes

Thomas Addison; 1839   **223**
A hardness and tumefaction are soon very evident to the hand.... General symptoms of peritonitis often take place, and terminate fatally; but under careful treatment the inflammation remains circumscribed...assuming the form of a local, deep-seated abscess.... From numerous dissections it is proved that the faecal abscess thus formed in the right iliac region arises, in a large majority of cases, from disease set up in the appendix caeci.
Elements of the Practice of Medicine

Reginald Heber Fitz; 1886   **224**

As a circumscribed peritonitis is simply one event, although usually the most important, in the history of inflammation of the appendix, it seems preferable to use the term appendicitis to express the primary condition.... Sudden, severe abdominal pain is the most constant, first, decided symptom of perforating inflammation of the appendix.... The vital importance of the early recognition...is unmistakable. Its diagnosis, in most cases, is comparatively easy. Its eventual treatment by laparotomy is generally indispensable.

Transactions of the Association of American Physicians

Charles McBurney; 1889   **225**

General abdominal pain is often all that the patient will complain of during the first few hours of his attack.... But after the first few hours it becomes more evident that the chief seat of pain is at [the iliac fossa], and the general pain then usually subsides.... In every case the seat of greatest pain, determined by the pressure of one finger, has been very exactly between an inch and a half and two inches from the anterior spinous process of the ilium on a straight line drawn from that process to the umbilicus.   *New York Medical Journal*

Charles McBurney; 1894   **226**

The section of the external oblique muscle and aponeurosis should correspond, great care being taken to separate these tissues in the same line, *not cutting any fibres across....* When the edges of the wound in the external oblique are now strongly pulled apart with retractors, a considerable expanse of the internal oblique muscle is seen.... The fibres of the internal oblique and transversalis muscles can now be *separated.*   *Annals of Surgery*

Albert John Ochsner; 1901   **227**

1. Peristaltic motion of the small intestines is the chief means of carrying the infection from the perforated or gangrenous appendix to the other portions of the peritoneum.
2. This can be prevented by prohibiting the use of every kind of food and cathartics by mouth, and by employing gastric lavage....
4. This form of treatment, when instituted early, will change the most violent and dangerous form of acute perforative or gangrenous appendicitis into a comparatively mild and harmless form.   *Journal of the American Medical Association*

APPETITE

Ambrose Bierce; 1906   **228**

Abdomen, *n.* The temple of the god Stomach, in whose worship, with sacrificial rites, all true men engage. From women this ancient faith commands but a stammering assent. They sometimes minister at the altar in a half-hearted and ineffective way, but true reverence for the one deity that men really adore they know not. If woman had a free hand in the world's marketing, the race would become graminivorous [i.e., feed only on grasses].   *The Devil's Dictionary*

ARGYLL ROBERTSON PUPIL

Douglas Argyll Robertson; 1869   **229**

I could not observe any contraction of either pupil under the influence of light, but, on accommodating the eyes for a near object, both pupils contracted.

Edinburgh Medical Journal

ARGYRIA

Oliver Wendell Holmes; 1860   **230**

So we must keep doctors awake by telling them that they have not yet shaken off astrology and the doctrine of signatures, as is shown by the form of their prescriptions, and their use of nitrate of silver, which turns epileptics into Ethiopians.

The Professor at the Breakfast Table

ARTERIOSCLEROSIS

Leonardo da Vinci; [1452-1519]   231
Veins which by the thickening of their tunicles in the old restrict the passage of the blood, and by this lack of nourishment destroy their life without any fever, the old coming to fail little by little in slow death.   *MacCurdy E, The Notebooks of Leonardo da Vinci*

William Cheselden; 1756   232
Sometimes the ossifying matter flows out of the bones, and forms bony excrescences; and frequently in very old men it fixes on the arteries, and makes them grow bony; and when this happens to a degree, the arteries lose their power to propel the blood, until the extreme parts mortify.   *The Anatomy of the Human Body*

Kilmer S. McCully; 1969   233
The arterial lesions discovered in a child who has an abnormality of cobalamin metabolism resulting in homocystinemia, cystathioninemia, and methylmalonic acidemia, resemble... many of those lesions found in patients with cystathionine synthetase deficiency with homocystinemia. Since the two disorders... both result in elevation of homocysteine concentration, the arterial damage found in association with both diseases is attributed to the metabolic effects of increased concentration of homocysteine, homocystine, or a derivative of homocysteine. [There are implications] for the pathogenesis of arteriosclerosis in individuals free of known enzyme deficiencies.   *American Journal of Pathology*

ARTHRITIS

Aretaeus the Cappadocian; [81-138?]   234
Arthritis is a general pain of all the joints; that of the feet we call Podagra; that of the hip joint, Schiatica; that of the hand, Chiragra.... Arthritis fixes itself...sometimes in the hip-joints; and for the most part in these cases the patient remains lame in it.
     On Arthritis and Schiatica

Cotton Mather; 1722   235
A Rheumatism, called, A Bastard-Gout, Lies in Wandring Pains of the Joints, which proceed... from a Volatile Acid falling on the Membranes of them. The Lower Part of the Back Sometimes is more particularly Siezed with such Pains. And then, the, Sciatica, or, Hip-Gout, becomes the name of the Malady.   *The Angel of Bethesda*

William Heberden; 1802   236
The chronical differs from the acute rheumatism in being joined with little or no fever, in having a duller pain, and commonly no redness, but the swellings are more permanent, and the disease of much longer duration; for if the acute species have continued some months, the other has continued for many years.... Both kinds of the rheumatism attack indiscriminately males and females, rich and poor.   *Commentaries on the History and Cure of Diseases*

ARTHROSCOPY

Michael S. Burman; 1931   237
A new procedure for the examination of the larger joints has been described.... We believe arthroscopy to be a key procedure in the study of joint physiology and pathology. The method as yet is still in its infancy.   *Journal of Bone and Joint Surgery*

Michael S. Burman; 1934   238
Arthroscopy can be done without fear of infection or of trauma to the joint.... It has the advantages of a diagnostic arthrotomy without necessitating operation.... It has...difficulties...which necessitate the most thorough cadaver practice before arthroscopy should be attempted on a patient.   *Journal of Bone and Joint Surgery*

ARTIFICIAL RESPIRATION

Robert Hooke; 1666   239

I did heretofore give this *Illustrious Society* [the Royal Society] an account of an Experiment I formerly tryed of keeping a Dog alive...by the Reciprocal blowing up of his Lungs with *Bellowes*, and they suffered to subside, for the space of an hour or more, after his *Thorax* had been so display'd [cut open], and his *Aspera arteria* [bronchus had been] cut off just below the *Epiglottis*, and bound upon the nose of the Bellows.

Philosophical Transactions of the Royal Society

Edward Albert Sharpey-Schafer; 1904   240

To effect artificial respiration put yourself athwart or on side of the patient's body in a kneeling posture.... Place your hands flat over the lower part of the back (on the lowest ribs)...and gradually throw the weight of your body forward on to them so as to produce firm pressure...upon the patient's chest. By this means the air (and water, if there is any) is driven out of the patient's lungs. Immediately thereafter raise your body slowly so as to remove the pressure.

Medico-Chirurgical Transactions

ASCITES

Aretaeus the Cappadocian; [81-138?]   241

The symptoms are very great and very easy to see, to touch, and to hear; in Ascites, for example, to see the tumidity of the abdomen, and with the swelling about the feet; the face, the arms, and other parts are slender, but the scrotum and prepuce swell....To touch—by strongly applying the hand and compressing the lower belly; for the fluid will pass to other parts. But when the patient turns to this side or that, the fluid, in the change of posture, occasions swelling and fluctuation, the sound of which may be heard.

On Dropsy

ASPHYXIA NEONATORUM

William John Little; 1843   242

In many instances the spasmodic affection is produced at the moment of birth or within a few hours or days of that event.... In two cases the birth occurred at the full period of gestation, but owing to the difficulty and slowness of parturition, the individuals were born in a state of asphyxia, resuscitation having been obtained, at the expiration of two and four hours, through the persevering efforts of the acoucheurs.

The Lancet

ASPIRIN (ACETYLSALICYLIC ACID)

Edward Stone; 1763   243

I gathered near a pound weight [of the bark] and which I dried for more than three months, at which it was reduced to a powder.... In a few days [I] increased the dose... and the ague was soon removed.... I have continued to use it as a remedy for ague and intermitting disorders for five years... and successfully.... The tree from which this bark is taken is stiled... Salix, alba, vulgaris, the common white Willow.

Philosophical Transactions of the Royal Society

Felix Hoffman; 1897   244

When salicylic acid... is heated with acetic anhydride... for 3 hours under reflux, the salicylic acid is quantitatively acetylated. After distilling off the acetic acid, one obtains the above in the form of crystals.... By its physical properties, e.g. its sour taste without being corrosive, the acetylsalicylic acid differs favourably from salicylic acid, and is now being tested... for its usefulness.

Journal

J. Wilthauer, J. Wohlgemut; 1899   245

If we were asked to give a resumé of out results with aspirin, we would state that aspirin has the same properties as salicylic acid. However aspirin appears to be... more satisfactory... since it does not evoke gastric distress or the loss of appetite.

Therapeutische Halbmonatshefte

C.D.W. Morris; 1967   **246**

I have studied the effects of [acetylsalicyclic acid] on platelet stickiness and bleeding times.... In 25 studies there was, in all cases except one, depression of platelet stickiness of more than 10%.... Interference with physiological thrombus formation is a possible indication that acetylsalicylic acid may play a therapeutic role in the management of pathological thrombosis.   *The Lancet*

ASPIRIN IDIOSYNCRASY SYNDROME

Louis E. Prickman, Harold F. Buchstein; 1937   **247**

Hypersensitivity to acetylsalicylic acid is the most common form of drug allergy, and it is much more common than is generally supposed.... Particularly noteworthy is the high incidence of hypersensitivity...among the asthmatic, especially among asthmatic individuals with nasal polyps.... It should never be administered...to asthmatic patients with polyps.   *Journal of the American Medical Association*

Max Samter, Ray F. Beers Jr.; 1968   **248**

The clinical triad of nasal polyposis, bronchial asthma, and life-threatening reactions to acetylsalicylic acid is a disease entity, not a chance cluster of allergic symptoms and represents, in fact, the prototype of a syndrome that has not been previously described and deserves recognition.   *Annals of Internal Medicine*

ASTHMA

Aretaeus the Cappadocian; [81-138?]   **249**

If from running, gymnastic exercises, or any other work, the breathing becomes difficult, it is called Asthma.... Women are more subject to the disease than men.... Children recover more readily than these.... But if the evil gradually get worse, the cheeks are ruddy; eyes protuberant, as if from strangulation...a desire of much and of cold air; they eagerly go into the open air, since no house sufficeth for their respiration; they breathe standing, as if desiring to draw in all the air which they possibly can inhale.   *On Asthma*

Thomas Willis; 1674   **250**

Among the Diseases whereby the Region of the breath is wont to be infested, if you regard their tyranny and cruelty, an Asthma (which is sometimes by reason of a peculiar symptome denominated likewise an Orthopnoea) doth not deserve the last place; for there is scarce any thing more sharp and terrible than the fits thereof.... Breathing, whereby we chiefly live, is very much hindred by the assault of this disease, and is in danger, or runs the risque of being quite taken away.   *Pharmaceutice Rationalis*

William Heberden; 1802   **251**

The first fit of the asthma has been experienced at all times, from the earliest infancy to extreme old age, and in every intermediate stage of life.
     Commentaries on the History and Cure of Diseases

Ernst von Leyden; 1872   **252**

In the center of the just described cylindric masses we found a great number of very small crystals which were colorless, had a subdued shine, and all showed the form of pointed octahedrons.... It is with interest that I have found these same structures in four cases of the same illness.... Each case was diagnosed as bronchial asthma.   *Archiv für Pathologie und Anatomie*

ATHEROSCLEROSIS

Felix Jacob Marchand; 1904   **253**

May I be allowed to make a proposition as to the nomenclature? If, as we have seen, the processes of the primary fatty and atheromatous degeneration are intimately involved in the sclerosing processes, then the name *arteriosclerosis* is not sufficient to include the entire disease. I therefore would like to recommend for this the expression *atherosclerose* or, if you prefer, *sclero-atherosis*. *Über Arteriosclerose (Atherosclerose)*

ATRIAL FIBRILLATION

Heinrich Ewald Hering Jr.; 1903   **254**

The pulsus irregularis observed in *valvular heart diseases, coronary sclerosis*, and myocardial diseases is persistent and for that reason I have called it pulsus irregularis perpetuus; ...it is essentially the same whether the patient's heart beats *faster* or *slower*; ...it does not arise under the influence of respiration, and thus it is not identical with pulsus irregularis respiratorius. All of these facts suggest that the pulsus irregularis perpetuus has its origin within the heart and is of *cardiac origin*. *Prager Medizinische Wochenschrift*

Heinrich Ewald Hering Jr.; 1903   **255**

The pulsus irregularis perpetuus has not yet been analysed and it seems at first glance to be quite difficult to get any firm basis for analysis in the confusion of short and long cycles, small and large pulses.... How can the increased heart rate and the abnormally short cycle arise? Certainly only by some accelerating cause.... The pulsus irregularis analysed here, which is observed in *valvular heart diseases, coronary sclerosis*, and *myocardial diseases*, is *lasting*. *Prager Medizinische Wochenschrift*

James Mackenzie; 1904   **256**

As the result of a study of a large number of cases where a jugular pulse was present I have been able to establish the fact that the cause of the irregularity is due to the rhythm of the heart proceeding from the ventricles, and not, as normally, from the great veins as they debouch into the auricles. *British Medical Journal*

James Mackenzie; 1908   **257**

I was at a loss to understand the nature of the heart's action in these cases; and as I found them very frequently...with a history of rheumatism, I determined to watch individual cases with rheumatic hearts.... I [accepted] the fact that these cases owed their abnormal [electrocardiographic] action to auricular fibrillation; and...the reason those evidences of auricular activity...disappear, is because the auricle ceases to act as a contracting chamber. *Froude H, Diseases of the Heart*

James Mackenzie; 1908   **258**

All the positive evidences of auricular activity, capable of being revealed by clinical methods, showed the cessation of auricular action with the onset of this irregularity.

Froude H, Diseases of the Heart

Thomas Lewis; 1909   **259**

The irregular pulse of mitral stenosis,...already referred to, is due to fibrillation of the auricle.... The rhythm is entirely disorderly, and the sizes of the beats do not correspond to the pauses which precede them. Fibrillation of the auricle results in a similar action of the ventricle. *British Medical Journal*

Thomas Lewis; 1910   **260**

Complete irregularity of the heart is the result of auricular fibrillation. *Heart*

Thomas Lewis; 1912   **261**

The ventricle is robbed of the regular impulses which form its accustomed supply. These are replaced by numerous and hap-hazard impulses, escaping to the ventricle from the turmoil which prevails in the upper chamber; the change in the action of the ventricle...is consequently profound. Its rate of beating rises considerably and the contractions follow each other in a completely irregular fashion. *Clinical Disorders of the Heart Beat*

Thomas Lewis; 1912   **262**

When the auricle is caused to pass into fibrillation or delirium, the appearances are quite distinctive; the muscular walls are maintained in a position of diastole; systole, either complete or partial, is never accomplished; the structure as a whole rests immobile; but close observation of the muscle surface reveals its extreme and incessant activity, rapid and minute twitchings and undulatory movements are visible over the whole.

Clinical Disorders of the Heart Beat

Elliott Carr Cutler, Samuel Albert Levine, Claude Schaeffer Beck; 1924   263

The right auricle was enormously dilated, blue in color, and in complete rest, without even fibrillary motions running across it. The right auricular appendage from time to time showed irregular convulsive contractions.

Archives of Surgery

ATRIOVENTRICULAR BUNDLE

Wilhelm His Jr.; 1893   264

I have succeeded in finding a muscle bundle which unites the auricular and ventricular septum.... The bundle arises from the posterior wall of the right auricle, near the auricular septum, in the atrioventricular groove [and] proceeds...until near the aorta it forks itself into a right and left limb which latter ends in the base of the aortic cusp of the mitral valve. Whether this bundle really transmits the impulse from the auricle to the ventricle I am unable to say with certainty.

Arbeiten für Medizinische Kliniken

ATTENTION-DEFICIT DISORDER

George Frederic Still; 1902   265

A... feature in many of these cases of moral defect without general impairment of intellect is a quite abnormal incapacity for sustained attention.... [A] boy, aged six years,... was unable to keep his attention... to a game for more than a very short time, and... the failure of attention was very noticeable at school, with the result that in some cases the child was backward in school attainments, although in manner and... conversation he appeared as bright and intelligent as any child could be.

The Lancet

AUSCULTATION

René-Théophile-Hyacinthe Laennec; 1802   266

[Buisson] distinguishes two sorts of hearing, the passive or *audition*, the active or *auscultation*, a division based on equally exact observations and on which is based the difference between the words, *to hear* and *to listen*.

Journal de Médecine Brumaire

René-Théophile-Hyacinthe Laennec; 1819   267

If you place your ear against one end of a wooden beam the scratch of a pin at the other extremity is most distinctly audible. It occurred to me that this physical property might serve a useful purpose in the case with which I was then dealing. Taking a sheaf of paper I rolled it into a very tight roll, one end of which I placed over the praecordial region, whilst I put my ear to the other. I was both surprised and gratified at being able to hear the beating of the heart with much greater clearness and distinctness than I had ever done before by direct application of my ear.

Traité de l'Auscultation Médiate

René-Théophile-Hyacinthe Laennec; 1820   268

I especially like the disadvantages that [Merat] finds in a purely mechanical technique [auscultation], which will tend to turn physicians away from skillful conjectures over the pulse, the facies, and excrement. It is the same as refusing to dash around Paris in a cabriolet for fear of losing the ability to tiptoe over droppings in the street.

Letter to his cousin Meriadec

AUSTIN FLINT MURMUR

Austin Flint; 1862   **269**

In some cases in which free aortic regurgitation exists, the left ventricle becoming filled before the auricles contract, the mitral curtains are floated out, and the valve closed when the mitral current takes place, and, under these circumstances, this murmur may be produced by the current just named, although no mitral lesion exists.

American Journal of Medical Science

AUSTRALIA ANTIGEN

Baruch S. Blumberg, Harvey J. Alter; 1965   **270**

An isoprecipitin is present in the sera of many patients with hemophilia who have received transfusions. It reacts with a protein (the "Australia antigen") that is found in the sera of some normal individuals from foreign populations but is absent in sera of the United States populations studied. It is found in approximately 10% of patients with leukemia.   *Journal of the American Medical Association*

AUTOPSIES

George Eliot; 1871   **271**

Mrs Dollop became more and more convinced...Dr. Lydgate meant to let the people die in the Hospital, if not to poison them, for the sake of cutting them up without saying by your leave or with your leave; for it was a known "fac" that he had wanted to cut up Mrs Goby, as respectable a woman as any in Parley Street, who had money in trust before her marriage—a poor tale for a doctor, who if he was good for anything should know what was the matter with you before you died, and not want to pry into your inside after you were gone.   *Middlemarch*

Abraham Flexner; 1910   **272**

The physician is constantly in contact with disease processes that he is unable to correlate with the accompanying structural modifications. Occasionally the surgeon throws a stream of light upon such a situation; too often all is dark until the autopsy reveals the truth.   *Medical Education in the United States and Canada*

Abraham Flexner; 1910   **273**

The effective teaching of pathology is dependent on ease and frequency of access to the autopsy-room.... The post-mortem is in this country relatively rare and precarious [and] that not infrequently pathological courses are organized and given whose illustrative material is limited to models, to a small number of preserved specimens, or even to bits of material already cut into microscopic sections or just lacking that last touch.

Medical Education in the United States and Canada

Roscoe C. Giles; 1932   **274**

A check-up of one's clinical findings at the autopsy table is indispensable to the progress of the art and science of medicine. The public is being aroused to the importance of autopsies as a matter of self-protection. I believe it is only a matter of time before physicians as well as hospitals will be rated by the percentage of autopsies they do or see in their practices.   *Journal of the National Medical Association*

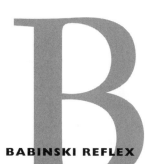

BABINSKI REFLEX

Joseph-François-Félix Babinski; 1896   **275**

In a certain number of cases of hemiplegia or crural monoplegia,...there is a disturbance of the cutaneous plantar reflex.... On the healthy side, pricking of the sole of the foot provokes, as usual in normal subjects, flexion of the thigh towards the pelvis, of the leg towards the thigh, of the foot towards the leg and of the toes upon the metatarsus. On the paralyzed side a similar excitation also results...but the toes, instead of flexing, execute a movement of extension upon the metatarsus.

Comptes Rendus des Séances de le Société de Biologie

BACTERIA

Ferdinand Julius Cohn; 1872   **276**

At last, in the most recent times, an unexpected knowledge of the secret life energies of bacteria has been revealed, through which they rule with demoniacal power over the weal and woe, and even over the life and death of man.

Bacteria: The Smallest of Living Organisms

BACTERIAL ENDOCARDITIS

Samuel Wilks; 1868   **277**

I bring this case before your notice, because it is the most marked which I have ever seen of the pyaemic process in connection with endocarditis.... The arterial blood may be...primarily infected at the very centre of the circulation. Just as, in ordinary pyaemia, the poisoned blood travels from the circumference to the centre so here the converse process is in operation, the seat of the infection being the heart itself.   *British Medical Journal*

William Osler; 1909   **278**

One of the most interesting features of [endocarditis] and one to which very little attention has been paid is the occurrence of ephemeral spots of a painful nodular erythema, chiefly in the skin of the hands and feet, the *nodosités cutanées éphémerès* of the French.... The commonest situation is near the tip of the finger, which may be slightly swollen.

Quarterly Journal of Medicine

BACTERIOPHAGE

Frederick William Twort; 1915   **279**
It seems probable... that the active transparent material is produced by the micrococcus, and since it leads to its own destruction, it might almost be considered as an acute infectious disease of micrococci.   *The Lancet*

Félix Hubert d'Herelle; 1917   **280**
In some patients recovering from dysentery, I noticed that the disappearance of the dysenteric bacillus coincided with the appearance of an invisible microbe endowed with properties antagonistic to the pathogenic bacillus. This microbe, truly a microbe of immunity, is an obligatory bacteriophage; its parasitism is strictly specific.
    Comptes Rendus Academie des Sciences

S.E. Luria, T.F. Anderson; 1942   **281**
We have undertaken an investigation of the problems of phage structure, size, reproduction and lytic activity by means of the RCA electron microcscope... Micrographs show the constant presence of particles of extremely constant and characteristic aspect. They consist of a round "head" and a much thinner "tail", which gives them a peculiar sperm-like appearance.   Proceedings of the National Academy of Sciences

BALLISTOCARDIOGRAPHY

J.W. Gordon; 1877   **282**
The body thus supported hammock-wise has a movement corresponding to that observable by means of a weighing-machine, and, with a sphygmograph adapted to the circumstances, yielding [a] curve...characteristic of the aortic flow.
    Journal of Anatomy and Physiology

Yandell Henderson; 1905   **283**
Under the influence of the mass-movements of the circulation, the body recoils at each heart beat feetward, headward, and again feetward. By means of a "swinging table" these movements can be magnified one hundred times and recorded in the form of a "recoil curve." The amplitude of these recoil movements...is held to be proportional to the volume of the systolic discharge of the heart.   *American Journal of Physiology*

Claude Gordon Douglas, John Scott Haldane, Yandell Henderson, Edward C. Schneider; 1913   **284**
The relative amplitude of the [recoil] curve of any individual at any time is taken as an index of the systolic discharge of the heart.... The curves obtained in ourselves after acclimatisation to the altitude of [Pike's] Peak were not sensibly different in size from the normals recorded in Colorado Springs.   *Philosophical Transactions of the Royal Society*

C.B. Heald, W.S. Tucker; 1922   **285**
This paper deals with a new method of measuring body recoil as the result of heart action.... A method is indicated of expressing this kinetic energy of the body in C.G.S. units.... An analysis of these curves shows that the events of a heart cycle can be recognised. The results so far obtained are consistent with accepted physiological data as to the variations in the systolic output of the heart, as affected by exercise, respiration, or the actions of vaso-constrictors and vaso-dilators.   *Proceedings of the Royal Society*

Isaac Starr, A.J. Rawson, H.A. Schroeder, Norman Ross Joseph; 1939   **286**
Apparatus is described for recording the forces set up by the heart's recoil and the blood's impacts in man.... The relation between the ballistic waves and the cardiac output has been studied empirically by comparative experiments.... When these formulae [from the theoretical study] were used...the cardiac output calculated from the ballistic waves [showed] satisfactory agreement with that estimated by the ethyl iodide method in 28 of 30 consecutive cases.   *American Journal of Physiology*

BÁRÁNY POINTING TEST

Robert Bárány; 1913   **287**

I ask the patient to close his eyes and to extend his arm and to touch my finger held directly in front of him.... Eventually, after missing the finger once or twice, a normal person can touch the finger with the eyes shut. When horizontal nystagmus to the left is produced, the patient misses my finger by past pointing to the right.... This reaction originates in the cerebellum and specifically in the ipsilateral hemisphere, and is constant and regular.   *Deutsche Medizinische Wochenschrift*

BARBITURATES

Emil Fischer; 1903   **288**

Diethylmalonylurea...surpasses all soporifics that have been studied. If this compound is readily produced and has advantages of taste and solubility, it seems to be the best among the members of the new class. Because of its complicated chemical designations, the name *Veronal* [barbitone] is suggested.   *Therapie der Gegenwart*

BARR BODY

Murray L. Barr, Ewart G. Bertram; 1949   **289**

Nerve cells of mature female cats contain a well-developed nucleolar satellite which is located... immediately adjacent to the nucleolus.... As a rule, nerve cells of mature male cats contain a poorly developed nucleolar satellite.... The morphologic distinction... is so clear that [tissue] sections [from] animals of both sexes may be readily sorted into two groups without prior knowledge of the sex.   *Nature*

BELIEF

George Bernard Shaw; 1911   **290**

There is no harder scientific fact in the world than the fact that belief can be produced in practically unlimited quantity and intensity, without observation or reasoning, and even in defiance of both, by the simple desire to believe founded on a strong interest in believing.   *The Doctor's Dilemma, Preface*

Stella Neeson; 1975   **291**

There is an ever growing hunger for mysticism to cure a sort of avitaminosis of the spirit.
                                          Journal of the American Medical Association

BELL PALSY

Charles Bell; 1821   **292**

We have proofs equal to experiments, that in the human face the actions of the muscles which produce smiling and laughing, are a consequence of the influence of this respiratory nerve [i.e., a branch of the seventh cranial nerve]. [In an afflicted patient] the side where the suppuration had affected the nerve remained placid, while the opposite side exhibited the usual distortion.   *Philosophical Transactions of the Royal Society*

Charles Bell; 1823   **293**

There is a motion of the eye-ball, which, from its rapidity, has escaped observation. At the instant in which the eye-lids are closed, the eye-ball makes a movement which raises the cornea under the upper eye-lid.... When a dog was deprived of the power of closing the eye-lids of one eye by the division of the nerves of the eye-lids, the eye did not cease to turn up when he was threatened, and when he winked with the eye-lids of the other side.
                                          Philosophical Transactions of the Royal Society

Charles Bell; 1829   **294**

The forehead of the [affected] side is without motion, the eyelids remain open, the nostril has no motion in breathing, and the mouth is drawn to the opposite side.... In this man the sensibility is perfect. *Philosophical Transactions of the Royal Society*

BENCE JONES PROTEINURIA

Henry Bence Jones; 1847   **295**

The patient was a wealthy tradesman, aged forty-five.... He died about six weeks afterward, and the only marked disease was mollities ossium.... The kidneys were healthy.... [His urine]contained an enormous quantity of [the] substance, something like albumen, but differing in very many things... especially in the solubility of the nitric acid precipitate by heat.... What is the connexion between mollities ossium and the state of urine? and to such a question I am as yet unable to give a positive answer. *The Lancet*

BENIGN MYALGIC ENCEPHALOMYELITIS

[Anonymous]; 1956   **296**

The term "benign myalgic encephalomyelitis" may be acceptable.... It does describe some of the striking features of a syndrome characterized by...symptoms and signs of damage to the brain and spinal cord,...protracted muscle pain with paresis and cramp,...emotional disturbances in convalescence,...a protracted course with relapses in severe cases,...and a benign outcome. *The Lancet*

BERIBERI

Jacobus Bontius; 1629   **297**

The inhabitants of the East Indies are much afflicted with a troublesome disorder which they call the Beriberii (a word signifying a sheep). The disease has, probably, received this denomination on account that those who are seized with it, from a tottering of the knees, and a peculiar manner of walking, exhibit to the fancy a representation of the gait of that animal. *An Account of the Diseases, Natural History, and Medicines of the East Indies*

Nicholas Tulp; 1652   **298**

The youth became sick.... The inordinate cold, repercussing excessively in the nerves, produced that species of paralysis, which is called India Beri-Beri, or *ovem* [sheep], which disease has a small amount of danger, is however cured with difficulty.

Observationes Medicae

Graham Steell; 1906   **299**

Capricious distribution of dropsy is specially apt to occur in cases of the cardiac muscle failure of beer-drinkers and of the disease known as Beri-Beri, of both of which diseases, it is curious to note, peripheral neuritis is a clinical feature.

Textbook on Diseases of the Heart

BILIARY TRACT DISEASE

Aretaeus the Cappadocian; [81-138?]   **300**

If the passages which convey the bile to the intestine, be obstructed from inflammation or scirrhus, the bladder gets over-distended, and the bile regurgitates; it therefore becomes mixed with the blood, and the blood, passing over the whole system, carries the bile to every part of the body, which acquires the appearance of bile. But the hardened faeces are white and clayey, as not being tinged with bile, because the bowels are deprived of this secretion. *On Jaundice, or Icterus*

BIOLOGY

Lewis Thomas; 1979   **301**

The only solid piece of scientific truth about which I feel totally confident is that we are profoundly ignorant about nature. Indeed, I regard this as the major discovery of the past hundred years of biology.   *The Medusa and the Snail. Hazards of Science*

BIORHYTHMS

Richard Llewellyn Jones Llewellyn; 1885   **302**

The tendency to rhythm is deep ingrained in protoplasm—write as plain in the systole and diastole of the heart, the inspiratory and expiratory phases of respiration as in the recurrence of the menstrual cycle. Do not our body cells, too, like the "laughing soil," respond to the call of the seasons, the biologic action of light, heat, and electrical stakes or disturbances?   *Aspects of Rheumatism and Gout*

BIRTH

Hildegard of Bingen; *circa* 1150   **303**

When birth is approaching, the vessel in which the child is enclosed is torn, and then comes the eternal energy that took Eve from Adam's side... and turns upside down all the corners of the shelter in the woman's body. All the structures of the woman's body rush toward this energy, receive it, and open up to it. They do so until the child emerges.... After the child has emerged, it soon gives forth a wailing sound because it senses the darkness of the world.   *Causae et Curae*

Cotton Mather; 1724   **304**

The Terrors of *Child-bearing*, which are now upon you, do very properly lead you to Bewayl your Share in the *Sin of your first Parents*; and to Bewayl as with a *Fountain of Tears*, that *Corrupt Nature* which by a Derivation from your *Next Parents* you brought into the World with you. Think, *Lord*, I was *conceived in Sin; I was born a Leper; and my poor Child will be so too.*   *The Angel of Bethesda*

George Frank Lydston; 1912   **305**

Not to be born is by no means always a misfortune. Being born may be a calamity.
                                                       New York Medical Journal

BLADDER STONE

William Heberden; 1802   **306**

The signs of a stone in the bladder are, great and frequent irritations to make water, a stoppage in the middle of making it, and a pain with heat just after it is made; a tenesmus, pain in the extremity of the urethra, incontinence or suppression of urine, together with a quiet pulse, and the health in no bad state.

Commentaries on the History and Cure of Disease

BLOOD GASES

Donald D. Van Slyke, James M. Neill; 1924   **307**

The apparatus can be used for a convenient and fairly accurate gas analysis. It is not in the present form devised to yield results as accurate as those by the Haldane apparatus, but we have found it convenient and satisfactory in analyzing gas mixtures with CO_2 or O_2 contents outside the range of the Haldane apparatus.   *Journal of Biological Chemistry*

BLOOD GROUPS

Karl Landsteiner, Alexander Wiener; 1940   308

The capacity possessed by some rabbit immune sera produced with blood of Rhesus monkeys, of reacting with human bloods that contain the agglutinogen M has been reported previously. Subsequently it has been found that another individual property of human blood (which may be designated as Rh) can be detected by certain of these sera.

Proceedings of the Society for Experimental Biology and Medicine

BLOOD PRESSURE

Stephen Hales; 1733   309

Then untying the ligature on the artery, the blood rose in the tube 8 feet 3 inches...above the level of the left ventricle of the heart.... When it was at its full height, it would rise and fall at and after each pulse two, three, or four inches, and sometimes it would fall 12 or 14 inches, and have there for a time the same vibrations up and down, at and after each pulse. *Statical Essays. Haemastaticks*

Jean-Leonard-Marie Poiseuille; 1828   310

The instrument...which may be termed a Haemodynamometer, having been introduced into the common carotid artery of a dog, the blood of the artery...impelled the mercury upwards...to the height of 4.15 inches.... Immediately afterwards...it stood at 3.35 inches above its original level...and continued to oscillate between those two points.... The Haemodynamometer [will be] of great use in determining...the modifications which the respiratory movements produce in the arterial as well as the venous circulation [and] the modifications from age [and from] the blood being rendered watery [from] particular substances. *Edinburgh Medical and Surgical Journal*

Leonard Erskine Hill, Harold Leslie Barnard; 1897   311

The armlet is strapped round the upper arm.... By means of the pump, the pressure is raised within the rubber bag until the pulsation indicated by the index of the pressure gauge becomes of maximal excursion. At this point the pressure indicated by the gauge is read, and this pressure is the mean arterial pressure.... The accuracy of this index has been proved by repeated experiment. *British Medical Journal*

James Mackenzie; 1902   312

If we possessed instruments delicate enough we might be able to determine what the normal arterial pressure of a given individual was, and to note any variation from it.... We are...driven to depend upon the most treacherous of all methods, the impressions conveyed to our minds through the sensory nerves of the fingers.... By constant practice and study, each physician makes for himself a standard of arterial pressure which he recognizes as normal. *The Study of the Pulse*

Nikolai Sergeievich Korotkov; 1905   313

The sleeve of Riva-Rocci is put on the middle third of the arm; the pressure in this sleeve rises rapidly until the circulation below...stops completely. At first there are no sounds whatsoever. As the mercury in the manometer drops...there appear the first...faint tones.... The reading on the manometer [then] corresponds to the maximum blood pressure.... Finally all sounds disappear.... The reading of the manometer at this time corresponds to the minimum blood pressure. *Izvestiya Voennomeditsinskaie Akademiia*

Committee for the Standardization of Blood Pressure Readings; 1939   314

The systolic pressure is the highest level at which successive sounds are heard.... The point where the loud clear sounds change abruptly to the dull and muffled sounds should be taken as the diastolic pressure. The American Committee recommend that if there is a difference between this point and the level at which the sounds disappear completely the latter reading should be regarded also as a measure of the diastolic pressure.

British Heart Journal

BLOOD TRANSFUSION

Samuel Pepys; 1666   **315**

This noon I met with Mr. [Robert] Hooke, and he tells me the dog which was filled with another dog's blood at the [Gresham] College the other day, is very well, and like to be so as ever. And doubts not its [i.e., blood transfusion] found being of great use to men.   *Diary*

Richard Lower; 1667   **316**

Then we...inserted Quils between the two Pipes already advanced in the two subjects, to convey the *Arteriall* bloud from the Sheep into the Veine of the Man.... And as to the quantity of Blood receiv'd into the Man's Veine, we Judge, there was about 9, or 10, ounces. The man *after* this operation, as well as *in* it, found himself very well.... He urged us to have the Experiment repeated upon him within three or four dayes after this; but it was thought advisable, to put it off somewhat longer.

Philosophical Transactions of the Royal Society

Richard Lower; 1669   **317**

I selected one dog of medium size, opened its jugular vein, and drew off blood, until...its strength was nearly gone.... I ligatured the artery from which the blood was passing, and withdrew blood again.... This was repeated...until there was no more blood or life.... In the meantime blood had been repeatedly withdrawn from this smaller animal and injected into it.... Once [the dog's] jugular vein was sewn up and its binding shackles cast off, it promptly jumped down from the table [and rolled itself] on the grass to clean itself of blood.   *A Treatise on the Heart*

James Blundell; 1829   **318**

Although the description of the instrument must appear complex, its use is simple; in truth, when the transfusion is once begun, the operator has little to do; his principal cares are—first, to see that the cup never empties itself entirely otherwise air might be carried down along with the blood. Secondly, to make sure that blood which issues by dribbling, from the arm of the person who supplies it, may not be admitted into the receiver, as its fitness for use is doubtful.   *The Lancet*

Francis Peyton Rous, J.R. Turner; 1915   **319**

It is only necessary to obtain citrated bloods from a finger-prick, make two mixtures of them in capillary pipets, and, by reading with the microscope [for agglutination], the test is finished in a few minutes. The test...enables one to determine within a few minutes...whether or not the blood of a donor is suitable for transfusion.   *Journal of Experimental Medicine*

Francis Peyton Rous, J.R. Turner; 1915   **320**

In the exsanguinated rabbit at least, transfusions of cells kept for a long time *in vitro* may be used to replace the blood loss, and...when the cells have been kept too long but are still intact, they are disposed of without harm. The indications are that kept human cells could be profitably employed in the same way.   *Journal of Experimental Medicine*

Hugh Leslie Marriott, Alan Kekwick; 1935   **321**

We have now performed 17 large drip transfusions.... We believe that the method which has been described, or one similar in principle, will be found to have important applications in the treatment of both medical and surgical conditions. It is our conviction that blood transfusion is to-day exploited only to a very small extent of its potentiality, because it is still being employed in homeopathic doses.   *The Lancet*

Bernard Fantus; 1937   **322**

This preliminary report on the establishment of a "blood bank" at the Cook County Hospital is perhaps justified by the interest displayed in this development, the inquiries received from various parts of the country, and the importance of the promptest and most generous exchange of experience in a new field of life-saving endeavor.

Journal of the American Medical Association

BLOODLETTING

Cintio D'Amato; 1669   **323**

Palpation being satisfactory, and the vein to be bled having been located with the left hand, and taken in a linen napkin for a firmer hold, so that the patient's hand cannot free itself, his hand is held by the finger and stretched somewhat while the vein is pierced longitudinally.... After making the incision the hand is again dipped in hot water so that blood will flow more freely instead of slowly, heat having the property of opening the vein and liquefying the blood. When sufficient blood has been drawn off, the wound is bound up.   *On the Correct Method of Making Incisions in Veins of the Hand*

BODY FLUIDS

Robert Boyle; 1663   **324**

If the juices of the body were more chymically examined,...it is not improbable, that many things relating to the nature of the humours, and to the ways of sweetening, actuating, and otherwise altering them, may be detected, and the importance of such discoveries may be discerned.   *Divulging of Useful Truths in Physick*

Archibald Byron Macallum; 1910   **325**

It [is] extremely probable that the inorganic composition of the blood plasma of vertebrates is an heirloom of life in the primeval ocean.   *Proceedings of the Royal Society of London*

Wallace O. Fenn; 1940   **326**

Potassium is of the soil and not the sea; it is of the cell but not the sap.   *Physiological Reviews*

BOHR EFFECT

Christian Bohr, K. Hasselbalch, Schack August Steenberg Krogh; 1904   **327**

In experiments with high carbonic acid pressures, no appreciable influence on the oxygen uptake of blood is recorded when the oxygen pressure is high as in the pulmonary blood. However, when blood reaches the tissues where the oxygen tension is low and the carbonic acid pressure is high, enhanced oxygen dissociation leads to increased utilization of oxygen.   *Scandanavian Archives of Physiology*

BONE SETTING

Hippocrates; [460-375 BC]   **328**

In treating fractures and dislocations, the physician must make the extension as straight as possible, for this is the most natural direction. But if it inclines to either side, it should rather turn to that of pronation, for there is thus less harm than if it be towards supination.   *On Fractures*

BOOKS

William Osler; 1901   **329**

To study the phenomena of disease without books is to sail an uncharted sea, while to study books without patients is not to go to sea at all.   *Books and Men*

Joseph-François Malgaigne; 1905   **330**

The physician without medical books, the lawyer without law books, manage their affairs poorly.   *Advice on the Choice of a Library*

BOWEL MOVEMENTS

Hippocrates; [460-375 BC]   **331**

The excrement is best which is soft and consistent, is passed at the hour which was customary to the patient when in health, in quantity proportionate to the ingesta; for when the passages are such, the lower belly is in a healthy state.   *The Book of Prognostics*

John Harington; 1596   **332**

A good stoole might move as great devotion in some man as a bad sermon... He that makes his belly his God, I wold have him make a Jakes his chappell.

The Metamorphosis of Aiax: A New Discourse of a Stale Subject

William Heberden; 1802   **333**

A very great difference is observable in different constitutions in regard to the evacuation by stool. One man never went but once in a month: another had twelve stools every day for thirty years, and afterwards seven in a day for seven years, and in the mean time did not fall away, but rather grew fat.   *Commentaries on the History and Cure of Diseases*

Alistair Cooke; 1986   **334**

Before I started a trip around the world, a doctor said to me that I ought... "to equip yourself with appropriate cathartics and also with some handy provision against dysentery." He was really not saying any more than a friend of mine, a layman,... "You've got," he said, "to load up with stoppers and starters."   *The Patient Has the Floor*

BRADYCARDIA

Robert Adams; 1827   **335**

An officer in the revenue, aged 68 years...was just then recovering from the effects of an apoplectic attack, which had suddenly seized him three days before.... What most attracted my attention was...the...remarkable slowness of the pulse, which generally ranged at the rate of 30 in a minute. Mr. Duggan...had seen him...in not less than twenty apoplectic attacks.... When they attacked him, his pulse would become even slower than usual; his breathing loudly stertorous.   *Dublin Hospital Reports*

William Stokes; 1846   **336**

[Fainting fits over a three-year period]always left [the patient] without any unpleasant effects.... The duration of the attack is seldom more than four or five minutes.... The pulse was varied from twenty-eight to thirty in the minute.

Dublin Quarterly Journal of Medical Science

BRAIN

[Anonymous]; *circa* 1550 BC   **337**

If you examine a man [having] a gaping wound in his head, reaching the bone, smashing his skull and breaking open [the viscera] of his skull, you should feel [palpate] his wound. You find that smash which is in his skull [like] the corrugations which appear on [molten] copper in the crucible, and something therein throbs and flutters under your fingers like the weak place in the crown of the head of a child when it has not become whole.

Ebers Papyrus

Niels Stensen; 1669   **338**

We need only view a Dissection of that large Mass, the Brain, to have ground to bewail our ignorance.... We admire... the Fibres of every Muscle, and ought still more to admire their disposition in the Brain, where an infinite number of them contained in a very small Space, do each execute their particular Offices without confusion or disorder.

Dissertation on the Anatomy of the Brain

Richard Lower; 1669   **339**

Although the brain is master of the organs of the body...it is not so placed that it can survive or have any power in the absence of their help.... On the contrary, the animal spirits, and life itself, are so dependent on the continuous supply of blood to the brain, that every...suppression...soon leads to syncope and unconsciousness, and, further, if such processes persist unduly long, the life ceases completely.   *A Treatise on the Heart*

John Hughlings Jackson; 1898   **340**

I divide the central nervous system into two Sub-systems—Cerebral and Cerebellar. The two have what I call the Lowest Level in common, or in other words this level is the lowest of the cerebral sub-system and also of the cerebellar sub-system. The Lowest Level extends, it is suggested, from the tuber cinereum to the conus medullaris.... The Rolandic region of the cortex cerebri and the prefrontal lobe (region in front of the pre-central sulcus) are the motor provinces of, respectively, the middle and highest levels of the cerebral sub-system.

The Lancet

Ambrose Bierce; 1906   **341**

Brain, *n*. An apparatus with which we think that we think. That which distinguishes the man who is content to *be* something from the man who wishes to *do* something. A man of great wealth, or one who has been pitchforked into high station, has commonly such a headful of brain that his neighbors cannot keep their hats on. In our civilization, and under our republican form of government, the brain is so highly honored that it is rewarded by exemption from the cares of office.   *The Devil's Dictionary*

Fred Plum; 1971   **342**

Man's brain is his uniquely human organ. Damage it and life loses its meaning in direct proportion, no matter what other physiologic benefits may occur in the process. The brain cannot be regenerated, repaired or homo-transplanted. It accumulates no metabolic debts and, unless supplied continuously by an effective circulation carrying large amounts of oxygen and glucose, it digests itself irreparably. This means that one cannot "let the brain go" while solving other medical problems....The integrity of the nervous system must be the first goal of therapeutics.   *Disorders of the Nervous System and Behavior*

Lewis Thomas; 1974   **343**

The human brain is the most public organ on the face of the earth, open to everything, sending out messages to everything. To be sure, it is hidden away in bone and conducts internal affairs in secrecy, but virtually all the business is the direct result of thinking that has already occurred in other minds.   *New England Journal of Medicine*

Carl Sagan; 1979   **344**

We are an intelligent species, and the use of our intelligence quite properly gives us pleasure. In this respect, the brain is like a muscle. When we think well, we feel good. Understanding is a kind of ecstasy.   *Broca's Brain*

Roger W. Sperry; 1982   **345**

The nonvocal hemisphere appears to be cognizant of the person's daily and weekly schedules: the calendar, seasons, and important dates of the year. The right hemisphere also makes appropriate discriminations that show concern with regard to the thought of possible future accidents and personal or family losses. The need for life, fire, and theft insurance, for example, seems to be properly appreciated by the extensively tested mute hemspheres of these patients.   *Science*

Richard Restak; 1995   **346**

One of the reasons that [the brain] remains so mysterious is that it is governed by both mechanical and quantum principles. As a result, the brain is inherently indeterminate, unpredictable, and uncertain.   *Brainscapes*

BRAIN DEATH

Conference of the Medical Royal Colleges and their Faculties in the United Kingdom; 1976   347

All of the following [conditions] should coexist [for considering a diagnosis of brain death]. The patient is deeply comatose.... The patient is being maintained on a ventilator because spontaneous respiration had previously become inadequate or had ceased altogether.... There should be no doubt that the patient's condition is due to irremediable structure brain damage. The diagnosis of a disorder which can lead to brain death should have been fully established.... All brainstem reflexes should be absent.

British Medical Journal

BRAIN TUMOR

Felix Platter; 1614   348

There was discovered on [the corpus callosum] of the brain a remarkable round fleshy tumor like an acorn. It was hard and full of holes and was as large as a medium-sized apple. It was covered with its own membrane and was entwined with veins.... We perceived that this ball by compressing the brain and its ducts with its mass and by flooding them, had been the occasion of the lethargy and listlessness and finally of death.

Observationes in Hominis Affectibus

BREAST FEEDING

Galen; [130-200]   349

In the uterus, we are wont to be nourished by blood, and the source of milk is from blood undergoing a slight change in the breasts. So that those children who are nourished by their mother's milk enjoy the most appropriate and natural food.   *Hygiene*

John Evelyn; 1688   350

After long trials of the Doctors, to bring up the little P. of Wales by hand (so many of her Majesties Children having died Infants) not succeeding: A country Nurse (the wife of a Tilemaker) is taken to give it suck.   *Diary*

Croatian proverb   351

The mother is not the one that gives birth, but the one that nurses her child.   *Proverb*

BRUCELLOSIS

M. Louis Hughes; 1896   352

It has occurred to me that the term "Undulant Fever" by referring to the peculiar pyrexial curve so characteristic of the disease, might prove a serviceable name.   *The Lancet*

BRUXISM

[Anonymous]; *circa* 2000 BC   353

If a man grinds...his teeth in his sleep, you will take a human skull, wash and anoint it with oil, and for seven days it shall be kept in the place at the head of his bed. Before he lies down he shall kiss it seven times and lick it seven times—so he will recover.

Kinnier WJV, Journal of the Royal Society of Medicine

BUBONIC PLAGUE

Giovanni Boccaccio; 1353   354

At the onset of the disease both men and women were afflicted by a sort of swelling in the groin or under the armpits which sometimes attained the size of a common apple or egg. Some of these swellings were larger and some smaller, and all were commonly called boils.... Afterwards, the manifestation of the disease changed into black or livid spots on the arms, thighs and the whole person.... Like the boils, which had been and continued to be a certain indication of coming death, these blotches had the same meaning for everyone on whom they appeared. *The Decameron*

Guy de Chauliac; 1363   **355**
The great mortality...was of two kinds: the first lasted two months, with continued fever & expectoration of blood. And they died of it in three days. The second was all the rest of the time, also with continued fever & apostems & carbuncles on the external parts...& they died of it in five days. And was of such great contagiousness (especially that which had expectoration of blood) that not only in visiting but also in looking at it, one person took it from another. *La Grande Chirurgie de M. Guy de Chauliac*

Ambroise Paré; 1575   **356**
The Plague is a cruel and contagious diseas, which everie-where, like a common diseas, invadeing Man and Beast, kill's verie manie, being attended, and as it were associated with a continual fever, botches, carbuncles, spots, nauseousness, vomitings, and other such malign accidents. *Works*

Athanasius Kircher; 1680   **357**
Fearful symptoms and effects result, as for example harmful abscesses, tumors, boils and bumps, carbuncles and buboes of various forms, spots and eruptions, which project from the skin and seem sown throughout the body, like hempseed. Then there comes to the patient loss of the senses and unconsciousness, weakness and vomiting.... The poisonous corpuscula are thrown off, become more poisonous and the contagion is spread still further. *Naturliche und Medicinalische Durchgrundung*

Daniel Defoe; 1722   **358**
Wherefore, were we ordered to kill all the Dogs and Cats.... All possible Endeavours were us'd also to destroy the Mice and Rats, especially the latter; by laying Rats-Bane, and other Poisons for them, and a prodigious multitude of them were also destroy'd. *A Journal of the Plague Year*

BULIMIA

Gerald F.M. Russell; 1979   **359**
[In] 30 patients whose illness bears a close resemblance to anorexia nervosa,...episodes of overeating constituted the most constant feature of the disorder.... Overeating was often overshadowed by more dramatic clinical phenomena—intractable self-induced vomiting or purgation.... The constancy and significance of overeating invite a new terminology for description of this symptom—bulimia nervosa. *Psychological Medicine*

BURKITT TUMOR (AFRICAN LYMPHOMA)

Denis Parsons Burkitt; 1958   **360**
Thirty-eight cases of a sarcoma involving the jaws of African children are described. This is a syndrome which has not previously been fully recognized. It is by far the commonest malignant tumour of childhood seen at Mulago Hospital. *British Journal of Surgery*

BURN THERAPY

Gustav Riehl; 1925   **361**
The infusion of large quantities of fluid, mainly a salt solution, as many as 3-4 liters daily, has proved satisfactory. Sometimes a life is saved if not more than one-quarter of the body surface has received a third-degree burn.... I have given blood transfusions to two patients with severe burns, with recovery in one case and postponement of death in the other. *Wiener Klinische Wochenschrift*

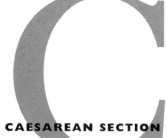

CAESAREAN SECTION

William Shakespeare; 1606 **362**
Tell thee, Macduff was from his Mother's womb
Untimely ripp'd. *Macbeth, Act V, Scene viii*

CAFFEINE

Thomas Willis; [1621-1675] **363**
Coffee disposes to wakefulness...from its stypticity which impedes the ebullition of the
blood, and thereby confines in the brain the material filling the passages. *Lecture*

John Wesley; 1747 **364**
Coffee and tea are extremely hurtful to persons who have weak nerves. *The Iliac Passion*

CALCITONIN

D. Harold Copp, E.C. Cameron; 1961 **365**
A dose of 300 to 1000 international units [of commercial parathyroid extract] was given
to the dogs by intravenous injection over a period of less than a minute.... In seven dogs.
the plasma calcium fell promptly after injection of the extract.... The data suggest that
commercial parathyroid extract may contain both parathyroid hormone and calcitonin
activity. *Science*

D. Harold Copp, E.C. Cameron, Barbara A. Cheney, and Others; 1962 **366**
Using a very precise method for measuring calcium, it has been shown that perfusing high
calcium blood through the thyroid and the parathyroids causes a prompt fall in systemic
plasma calcium that cannot be explained on the basis of suppressed parathormone production, since the effect is significantly different from the effect of total parathyroidec-
tomy. Since no effect is obtained when the thyroid alone is perfused, the fall in serum calcium apparently is due to the action of a hypocalcemic factor released only from the
parathyroid as a result of hypercalcemia. *Endocrinology*

G.C. Foster, A. Baghdiantz, M.S. Kumar, and Others; 1964 **367**
The thyroid is essential for the calcitonin effect. Since the parathyroid perfusion had no

effect, it appears that the thyroid is the source of calcitonin. It also seems likely that "thyro-calcitonin," the hypocalcaemic substance extracted from the thyroid by Hirsch et al., and calcitonin are identical. *Nature*

CANCER

Hippocrates; [460-375 BC] **368**
It is better not to apply any treatment in cases of occult cancer; for, if treated, the patients die quickly; but if not treated, they hold out for a long time. *Aphorisms*

Aulus Cornelius Celsus; 25 BC - AD 50 **369**
A carcinoma does not give rise to the same danger [as a carbuncle] unless it is irritated by imprudent treatment. This disease occurs mostly in the upper parts of the body, in the region of the face, nose, ears, lips, and in the breasts of women, but it may also arise in an ulceration, or in the spleen.... At times the part becomes harder or softer than natural.... After excision, even when a scar has formed, none the less the disease has returned, and caused death. *On Medicine*

Galen; [130-200] **370**
Of blacke cholor, without boylying (that is to say melancholic) cometh cancers, and if the humor be sharpe, it maketh ulceration, and for this cause, these tumors are more black-er in colour, then those that cometh of inflamation.... For lesse matter goeth out of the veines, into the fleshy partes, whiche compasseth them about, through the grossnes of the humor, whiche breadeth the Cancers. *De Tumoribus*

Galen; [130-200] **371**
When the tumor extends its feet from all sides of its body into the veins, the sickness pro-duces the picture of a crab. *Complete Works*

Paul of Aegina (Paulus Aegineta); [625-690] **372**
Cancer is an uneven swelling, rough, unseemly, darkish, painful, and sometimes without ulceration...and if operated upon, it becomes worse...and spreads by erosion; forming in most parts of the body, but more especially in the female uterus and breasts. It has the veins stretched on all sides as the animal the crab (cancer) has its feet, whence it derives its name. *The Seven Books of Paulus Aegineta*

Avicenna (Abu- Ali al-Husayn ibn Abdallah ibn Sina); [980-1037] **373**
The difference between cancerous swelling and induration. The latter is a slumbering silent mass which...is painless, and stationary.... A cancerous swelling progressively increases in size, is destructive, and spreads roots which insinuate themselves amongst the tissue-elements. *Liber Canonis*

Albucasis (Abul Qasim); *circa* 1050 **374**
The Ancients said that when a cancer is in a site where total eradication is possible, such as a cancer of the breasts or of the thigh, and in similar parts where complete removal is possible, and especially when in the early stage and small, then surgery was to be tried. But when it is of long standing and large you should leave it alone. For I myself have never been able to cure any such, nor have I seen anyone else succeed before me. *Cyrurgia Albucasis cum cauteriis*

Theodoric, Bishop of Cervia; 1267 **375**
The older a cancer is, the worse it is. And the more it is involved with muscles, veins and nutrifying arteries, the worse it is, and the more difficult to treat. For in such places inci-sions, cauteries and sharp medications are to be feared. *The Surgery of Theodoric*

John Hunter; [1728-1793] **376**
[Cancer] most commonly attacks the conglomerate glands, the first the female breast; also the uterus, the lips, the external nose, the pancreas, and the pylorus; besides which

the testicle is very subject to it.... The predisposing Causes of Cancer are three,...viz., age, parts, and hereditary disposition; perhaps climate.... I would, in most cases, where the lymphatic glands are...enlarged, advise that the case should be let alone.   *Of Poisons*

Johannes Müller; 1838   **377**
Carcinoma differs from simple induration both in structure and intrinsic nature.... Carcinoma also differs essentially from ulceration of indurated parts.... The peculiar productive and destructive activity of carcinoma...does give rise to general anatomical features, which are recognizable even with the naked eye.... Every form of cancer appears to occur at all times of life and in all organs, but at certain times of life some organs are more prone to cancer than others.
Über den Feinern Bau und die Formen der Krankhaften Geschwulste

Carl Wedl; 1855   **378**
We hear sometimes of cancer-cells and should, therefore, be justified in demanding such information respecting them as will place us in a condition to distinguish a cancer-cell from any other.   *Rudiments of Pathological Histology*

Armand Trousseau; 1865   **379**
Should you, when in doubt as to the nature of an affection of the stomach; should you when hesitating between chronic gastritis, simple ulcer, or cancer, observe a vein become inflamed in the arm or leg, you may dispel your doubt, and pronounce in a positive manner that there is cancer.   *Clinique Médicale de l'Hôtel Dieu de Paris*

Francis Peyton Rous; 1910   **380**
In this paper is reported the first avian tumor that has proved transplantable to other individuals. It is a spindle-celled sarcoma of the hen.... The tumors which result from the injection of a cell-free filtrate take much longer to appear.
Journal of Experimental Medicine

William Ewart Gye; 1925   **381**
These researches have led me to look upon cancer...as a specific disease caused by a virus (or group of viruses). Under experimental conditions the virus alone is ineffective; a second specific factor, obtained from tumour extracts, ruptures the cell defences and enables the virus to infect. Under natural conditions continued "irritants" are known, such as coal-tar, paraffin oils, etc. The virus probably lives and multiplies in the cell and provokes the cell to continued multiplication.   *The Lancet*

Charles Horace Mayo, William A. Hendricks; 1926   **382**
While there are several chronic diseases more destructive to life than cancer, none is more feared.   *Annals of Surgery*

Maud Slye; 1928   **383**
In thousands of mice bred in the laboratory, the tendency to be exempt from spontaneous cancer was transmitted as a simple dominant character along Mendelian lines.... The tendency to be susceptible to cancer is also inheritable, but it is inheritable as a recessive character.... There are apparently two factors necessary to induce cancer. If either of these could be wholly avoided, it might be possible to prevent cancer. These factors are (1) an inherited local susceptibility to the disease, and (2) irritation of the appropriate kind and the appropriate degree applied to the cancer-susceptible tissues.
Annals of Internal Medicine

D. Steheli, Harold E. Varmus, J. Michael Bishop, P. Vogt; 1976   **384**
We suggest that part or all of the transforming gene(s) of [avian sarcoma virus] was derived from the chicken genome or a species closely related to chicken.... We are testing the possibilities that [the nucleotide sequences that anneal with cDNAsarc] are involved in the normal regulation of cell growth and development or in the transformation of cell behaviour by physical, chemical, or viral agents.   *Nature*

Michael Baden; 1979   **385**

A cancer is not only a physical disease, it is a state of mind.

Johnston L, The New York Times

Sherwin B. Nuland; 1994   **386**

In the community of living tissues, the uncontrolled mob of misfits that is cancer behaves
like a gang of perpetually wilding adolescents. They are the juvenile delinquents of cellular society.   *How We Die*

George Zimmer; 1997   **387**

We who are struggling to escape cancer do not, obviously, want to die of it. We do prefer
death in the struggle to life under cancer's untender rule. The enemy is not pain or even
death, which will come for us in any eventuality. The enemy is cancer, and we want it
defeated and destroyed.   *Annals of Internal Medicine*

CANCER CHEMOTHERAPY

**Louis Sanford Goodman, Maxwell M. Wintrobe, William Dameshek,
and others;** 1946   **388**

This...communication presents the clinical results obtained for 67 patients treated with the
nitrogen mustards (halogenated alkyl amine hydrochlorides) for Hodgkin's disease, lymphosarcoma, leukemia and certain related and miscellaneous disorders.... Salutary results
have been obtained, particularly in Hodgkin's disease, lymphosarcoma and chronic
leukemia... In the first two... dramatic improvement has been observed.... Clinical remissions
[have lasted] from weeks to months.   *Journal of the American Medical Association*

CANCER METASTASIS

Joseph-Claude-Anthelme Récamier; 1829   **389**

The case of M. Parent leads to the admission of cancer metastases: here a spontaneous
eruption of carcinoma is succeeded by an identical eruption at another site.

Récherches sur le Traitement du Cancer

CANCER OF THE BREAST

Galen; [130-200]   **390**

Cancerous tumors develop with greatest frequency in the breast of women.... Such unnatural tumors have their source in the black bile, a superfluous residue of the body.

Opera Omnia

Aetius of Amida; [502-575]   **391**

I personally am in the habit of operating for cancer arising in the breast thusly: I make the
patient lie down; then I incise the healthy part of the breast beyond the cancerous area
and I cauterize the incised parts.... Following amputation of the entire breast, I cauterize
again all areas until all bleeding has ceased.   *Liborum Medicinalium Tomus Primus*

Theodoric, Bishop of Cervia; 1267   **392**

The signs of [cancer of the breast] are that a hot abscess begins at the size of a hazel nut
or smaller, and then increases in size little by little, with notable hardness, darkness of col-
oring, round shape, and some warmth to the touch. When it begins to grow larger, green
veins appear in it, and it has roots penetrating into the body.   *The Surgery of Theodoric*

Ambroise Paré; 1585   **393**

Mme. de Montigny...had a cancer the size of a nut in the left breast.... [Houllier] considered the tumor to be cancerous and we decided upon a palliative course, fearing to irri-
tate this Hydra, and cause it to burst in fury from its lair. He ordered...certain purga-
tions...and on the tumor was placed a sheet of lead covered with quick-silver.... A more
aggressive treatment...terminated with ulceration.... The heart failed and death followed.

Hamby WB, The Case Reports and Autopsy Records of Ambroise Paré

John Hunter; [1728-1793]   **394**
When cancer occurs in the breast of women under forty, it is more rapid in its progress
then when the patient is older, and also more extensive; remote sympathy likewise takes
place more readily in them than in the old, so that the operation succeeds better in the
latter on this account.   *Of Poisons*

Charles Hewitt Moore; 1867   **395**
Recurrent Cancer begins near the scar.... It tends toward the axilla earlier than to the
residue of the breast.... Centrifugal dispersion, not organic origin determines the recurrence of Cancer.... Cancer of the breast requires the careful extirpation of the entire
organ.... Unsound adjoining textures, especially skin, should be removed in the same mass
with the principal disease.   *Medico-Chirurgical Transactions*

Alice James; 1891   **396**
As the ugliest things go to the making of the fairest, is it not wonderful that this unholy
granite substance in my breast should be soil for the perfect flowering of Katherine's
unexampled genius for friendship and devotion...but the pain and discomfort seem a feeble price to pay for all the happiness and peace with which she fills my days.... I am being
ground slowly on the grim grindstone of physical pain and on two nights I had almost
asked for K's lethal dose.   *Her Brothers; Her Journal*

William Stewart Halsted; 1894   **397**
In fifty cases operated upon by what we call the complete method we have been able to
trace only three local recurrences [6 per cent].... In 34 (73 per cent)...there has never been
a local or regionary recurrence. 24 are living and 10 are dead. In 43 of the 46 cases (93 per
cent) there has been no true local recurrence.... These statistics are so remarkably good
that we are encouraged to hope for a much brighter...future for operations for cancer of
the breast.   *Annals of Surgery*

Robert McWhirter; 1948   **398**
When radical mastectomy is the only method of treatment available...the five year survival rate is unlikely to exceed 25 per cent.... The five year survival rate of all cases [treat-
ed by simple mastectomy and radiotherapy] coming to the Royal Infirmary in the period
1941-45 is 43.7 per cent.   *British Journal of Radiology*

E.V. Jensen, H.I. Jacobson, S. Smith, and Others; 1972   **399**
By making judicious use of estrogen antagonists in tissue uptake and sedimentation studies, it was possible to demonstrate that, if a human breast cancer specimen shows no distinct evidence of estrogen receptor, the patient has little chance of response from
endocrine ablation, whereas most but not all patients with receptor-containing cancers
can expect benefit from endocrine therapy.   *Gynecologic Investigation*

H.W. Ward; 1973   **400**
Tamoxifen (ICI 46474) was given by mouth to patients with advanced, recurrent or
metastatic breast carcinoma. At a dosage of 10 mg twice daily, 60% of patients showed
arrest or reversal of tumour growth. At a dosage of 20 mg twice daily, 77% showed arrest
or reversal of tumour growth. Side effects were usually trivial, and their incidence was the
same at both dose levels. No patients showed virilization or fluid retention.
                                                             British Medical Journal

Barbara Ehrenreich; 2001   **401**
To the extent that current methods of detection and treatment fail or fall short, America's
breast-cancer cult can be judged as an outbreak of mass delusion, celebrating survivor-
hood by downplaying mortality and promoting obedience to medical protocols known to
have limited efficacy.   *Harper's Magazine*

Barbara Ehrenreich; 2001   **402**

It is the very blandness of breast cancer, at least in mainstream perceptions, that makes it an attractive object of corporate charity and a way for companies to brand themselves friends of the middle-aged female market.   *Harper's Magazine*

CANCER OF THE LIP

Ambroise Paré; 1585   **403**

One may...cure cancers of the lip without applying caustics or any similar thing.... Pass a threaded needle through the cancer so the thread held in the left hand can lift and control the cancer without any of its escaping. One can then cut to good flesh with scissors in the right hand; and so cut that a layer of good flesh of the lip remains to serve as a base and foundation for regeneration of flesh in place of the portion amputated, supposing the cancer has not taken root and spread from top to bottom.

Hamby WB, The Case Reports and Autopsy Records of Ambroise Paré

CANCER OF THE LUNG

William George Barnard; 1926   **404**

Setting aside the squamous-celled carcinomata, there is no essential difference in macroscopic appearance or distribution between obvious carcinomata and "oat-celled" tumors, both the part of the lung affected and the metastases being exactly similar in many cases. *The so-called "oat-celled sarcoma" of the posterior mediastinum is a medullary carcinoma of bronchi.*   Journal of Pathology and Bacteriology

Evarts Ambrose Graham, Jacob Jesse Singer; 1933   **405**

The left lung and many of the tracheobronchial mediastinal glands were removed in a one stage operation because of a carcinoma that originated in the bronchus of the upper lobe but which was so close to the bronchus of the lower lobe that, in order to remove it completely, it was necessary to remove the entire lung. This is apparently the first case in which an entire lung has been removed successfully at one stage.

Journal of the American Medical Association

**Oscar Auerbach, Arthur Purdy Stout, Edward Cuyler Hammond,
Lawrence Garfinkel;** 1964   **406**

In men who die of lung cancer (squamous and undifferentiated), all of whom were smokers, the remainder of the epithelial lining shows changes that may be considered as preliminary stages to the development of lung cancer, including early invasion.... There are few such changes in nonsmokers, but they increase rapidly with the amount of cigarette smoking.   *Proceedings of the National Cancer Conference*

CANCER OF THE PROSTATE GLAND

George Langstaff; 1817   **407**

During the last six months[I.B.] had suffered...excruciating pain in the region of the kidnies and bladder, attended with almost constant desire to void urine, which was effected with the greatest difficulty.... An examination per rectum proved that there existed an enlarged...prostate gland, and slight pressure occasioned great pain.... The bladder was found [at autopsy] to contain a tumor as big as a large orange...discovered to derive its origin from the prostate gland.... The fungus...plugged up both ureters.... In the liver there were several tumours [and] several...in the lungs.   *Medico-Chirurgical Transactions*

John Adams; 1851   **408**

A schirrhous prostate conveys to the finger, passed per anum, a sense of gristly hardness, and is usually irregularly nodulated, one lobe being especially affected.... The...bladder becomes more intolerant of its contents, or retention of urine arises, blood frequently escapes with the urine, pain and restlessness become more constant.... The disease makes its appearance either in the inguinal glands or in other parts of the body.... Of the treatment, unfortunately, little of a satisfactory nature can be said.

The Anatomy and Diseases of the Prostate Gland

Hugh Hampton Young; 1905   409
Carcinoma of the prostate is more frequent than is usually supposed—occurring in about 10% of the cases of prostatic enlargement.... Cure can be expected only by radical measures and the routine removal of the seminal vesicles, vasa deferentia and most of the vesical trigone with the entire prostate as carried out in four cases.

Bulletin of the Johns Hopkins Hospital

Charles Brenton Huggins, Clarence Vernard Hodges; 1941   410
In prostatic cancer with marked elevation of acid phosphatase, castration or injection of large amounts of estrogen caused a sharp reduction of this enzyme to or towards the normal range.... In 3 patients with prostatic cancer, androgen injections caused a sharp rise of serum acid phosphatase.

Cancer Research

CANCER OF THE RECTUM

John of Arderne; 1414   411
Bubo is an apostem breeding within the anus in the rectum with great hardness but little aching. This I say, before it ulcerates, is nothing else than a hidden cancer.... Out of bubo [cancer] goes hard excretions and sometime they may not pass, because of the constriction caused by the bubo, and they are retained firmly within the rectum....I never saw nor heard of any man that was cured...but I have known many that died of the foresaid sickness.

De Arte Phisicale et de Cirurgia

CANCER OF THE STOMACH

Antonio Benivieni; 1507   412
My kinsman, Antonio Bruno, retained the food he had eaten for too short a time, and then threw it up undigested.... His body wasted away through lack of nourishment till little more than skin and bone remained. At last he was brought to his death. The body was cut open for reasons of public welfare. It was found that the opening of his stomach had closed up and it had hardened...with the result that nothing could pass through to the organs beyond, and death inevitably followed.

De Abditis Nonnulus ac Mirandis Morborum et Sanationum Causis

Giovanni Battista Morgagni; 1761   413
A man [had become] somewhat emaciated...when...a troublesome vomiting came on, of a fluid which resembl'd water, tinctur'd with soot.... Death took place.... In the stomach...was an ulcerated cancerous tumour.... Betwixt the stomach and the spleen were two glandular bodies, of the bigness of a bean, and in their colour, and substance, not much unlike that tumour which I have describ'd in the stomach.

The Seats and Causes of Diseases

Matthew Baillie; 1793   414
When the...stomach, or a portion of it, is scirrhous, it is much thicker than usual, as well as much harder.... It frequently happens that this thickened mass is ulcerated upon its surface, and then a stomach is said to be cancerous. Sometimes the inner membrane... throws out a process which terminates in a great many smaller processes.... The absorbent glands in the neighborhood are at the same time commonly enlarged, and have a very hard white structure.

Morbid Anatomy

CANCER OF THE UTERUS

Aretaeus the Cappodocian; [81-138?]   415

Ulcers, too, are formed in the womb; [some] are mild. But there are others deeper and worse than these.... Febrile heat, general restlessness, and hardness is present, as in malignant diseases; the ulcers, being of a fatal nature, obtain also the appellation of cancers.... These carcinomatous sores are chronic and deadly.

Adams F, The Extant Works of Aretaeus the Cappadocian

Aetius of Amida; [502-575]   416

Of the cancerous tumors of the uterus, some are ulcerated; some are not ulcerated, much in the same way as we have mentioned...about breast tumors.... Sometimes there is frank bleeding.... This is, as Hippocrates thought, an incurable disease.

Liborum Medicinalium Tomus Primus

George Nicholas Papanicolaou, Herbert Frederick Traut; 1941   417

In presenting this method of diagnosis at this time, we hope that it may prove to be a dependable means whereby the principal malignant diseases of the uterus can be recognized; and further that because of its simplicity, it may eventually be applied widely so that the incipient phases of the disease may come more promptly within the range of our modern modes of treatment which have been proved highly effective in early carcinoma.

American Journal of Obstetrics and Gynecology

CANNON WAVES

William Stokes; 1846   418

A new symptom has appeared, namely, a very remarkable pulsation in the right jugular vein. This is most evident when the patient is lying down. The number of the reflex pulsations is difficult to be established, but they are more than double the number of the manifest ventricular contractions. About every third pulsation is very strong and sudden, and may be seen at a distance; the remaining waves are much less distinct, and some very minor ones can also be perceived.   *Dublin Quarterly Journal of Medical Science*

CAPILLARIES

Aristotle; [384-322 BC]   419

As the blood-vessels advance, they become gradually smaller and smaller, until at last their tubes are too fine to admit blood. This fluid can therefore no longer find its way through them, though they still give passage to the humour which we call sweat.

De Partibus Animalium

Antony von Leeuwenhoek; 1688   420

I observed the young frogs...and I...discovered in them small blood-vessels.... These blood vessels, called "arteries and veins" (being nevertheless identical), were exceedingly numerous at the ends of [the] fingers.... All these vessels were so small or thin that no more than one corpuscle could pass through it at a time.   *Letter*

Ernest Henry Starling; 1895   421

Although the osmotic pressure of the proteids of the plasma is so insignificant, it is of an order of magnitude comparable to that of the capillary pressures; and whereas capillary pressure determines transudation, the osmotic pressure of the proteids of the serum determines absorption.... At any given time, there must be a balance between the hydrostatic pressure of the blood in the capillaries and the osmotic attraction of the blood for the surrounding fluids.   *Journal of Physiology*

Schack August Steenberg Krogh; 1924   422

When the muscle...is stimulated to contractions, a large number of capillaries become visible and dilated, and the rate of circulation through them is greatly increased. When the stimulus has lasted only a few seconds, the circulation returns in some minutes to the resting state.... Since capillaries, even in a group fed by the same arteriole, do not all behave in the same way, the changes obviously cannot be due to arterial pressure changes.

The Anatomy and Physiology of the Capillaries

CAPILLARY PULSE

Heinrich Irenaeus Quincke; 1868   **423**

There are...places in the human body where...one frequently observes the transmission of the pulse wave from the heart reaching to the capillaries and then into the veins: these sites are the fingernails, hand, forearm, and foot.... It can be observed in one's own fingernails, but clearer still in those of another, in the region between the white, anemic area and the redder, more injected part of the capillary system of the nail bed...there occurs...a to-and-fro movement of the margin between the red and the white portion.

Wiener Klinische Wochenschrift

CARBONIC ANHYDRASE INHIBITORS

Thaddeus Mann, David Keilin; 1940   **424**

[We tested] the effect of sulphanilamide on the catalytic activity of carbonic anhydrase in blood, in gastric mucosa and in pure enzyme preparations. The results... clearly show that sulphanilamide acts as a very powerful inhibitor of carbonic anhydrase, exhibiting marked effect even in a concentration so low as 2×10^{-6} mol.   *Nature*

William B. Schwartz; 1949   **425**

Sulfanilamide is capable of producing an increased sodium, potassium and water excretion in patients with congestive heart failure.... It appears that the inhibition of carbonic anhydrase in the cells of the renal tubules is responsible for this phenomenon.

New England Journal of Medicine

CARDIAC ARREST

Samuel Shem; 1978   **426**

At a cardiac arrest, the first procedure is to take your own pulse.   *The House of God*

CARDIAC THRILL

Jean-Nicolas Corvisart des Marest; 1806   **427**

[Constriction of the valves of the heart is marked by] a peculiar rushing like water, difficult to be described, sensible to the hand applied over the precordial region, a rushing which proceeds, apparently, from the embarrassment which the blood undergoes in passing through an opening which is no longer proportioned to the quantity of fluid which it ought to discharge.   *Organic Diseases and Lesions of the Heart and Great Vessels*

CARDIOLOGY

Lofty L. Basta; 1996   **428**

As a cardiologist, I may panic when I see somebody bleed from his nose, but not when I see a heart fibrillate. This is my territory.   *A Graceful Exit*

CARETAKERS

George M. Andes; 1998   **429**

Her responsibilities increase as my abilities decline. We who carry the cane get attention. They who walk beside us with tired steps, weary faces, and sad eyes, they who care for us, get none. Yet they bear a heavy burden, and they need support and recognition.

Annals of Internal Medicine

CAROTID SINUS

Heinrich Irenaeus Quincke; 1875   **430**
I have gained the conviction through repeated and careful observations, that the slowing of the pulse when pressure is applied on the carotid is a frequent finding, in healthy as well as in sick persons.   *Wiener Klinische Wochenschrift*

CASE HISTORIES

Rufus of Ephesus; *circa* 50   **431**
One must put questions to the patient, for thereby certain aspects of the disease can be better understood, and the treatment rendered more effective. And I place interrogation of the patient himself first, since in this way you can learn how far his mind is healthy or otherwise; also his physical strength and weakness; and you can get some idea of the disease and the part affected.   *Greek Medicine*

Paul R. McHugh; 1995   **432**
The medical report is an account of nature's power over human life through infections, neoplasms, genes, and the like.   *The American Scholar*

CASE RECORDS

John Howard; 1792   **433**
This examination may be made by a medical gentleman of the hospital, with the patient before him, his notes to be corrected by himself, and kept as a record of the history and circumstances of each case, to be referred to...by any intelligent or scientific person.... If anything extraordinary or worthy of more particular notice arises from these sources, let them be published to the world at large.   *The History of the Middlesex Hospital*

William Osler; 1903   **434**
Record what you have seen; make a note at the time; do not wait.   *Aphorisms*

CASE REPORTS

Asha Senapati; 1996   **435**
Many diseases, now well recognized, with an established pattern of symptoms and signs started out with the reporting of a single case.... Should we have said to these [authors], "I am sorry your case report is not acceptable and your description of this unusual condition or operation has no place in the established medical literature"?
                                    Journal of the Royal Society of Medicine

CASES

Denslow Lewis; 1894   **436**
No two cases are ever identical; no two cases ever agree in symptomatology or pathology; no two cases ever require exactly the same treatment; nor can you expect to ever see in any case that may come under your observation a perfect facsimile of cases previously observed.   *Chicago Clinical Review*

A. Mitscherlich, F. Mielke; 1949   **437**
There is not much difference whether a human being is looked on as a "case" or as a number to be tattooed on the arm [in a concentration camp]. These are but two aspects of the faceless approach of an age without mercy.   *Doctors of Infamy*

[Anonymous]; 1995   **438**
The use of typical as a synonym for atypical echoes a moment from my student days when a surgical registrar, called to see a patient in casualty, told us: "We must get this chap in for the firm to see. He shows the typical picture and we don't see that very often."
                                    Journal of the Royal College of Physicians

CATARACT SURGERY

Charles D. Kelman; 1967   **439**

A technique for emulsifying and aspirating a hard, senile-type cataract through a 2 to 3 mm incision is described. This procedure would shorten recuperation, minimize hospitalization and give almosy immediate rehabilitation.... A subsequent report will give the details of the instrument and the results of phaco-emulsification in humans.... ADDENDUM: Since the preparation of this manuscript, this technique of cataract removal was performed on two patients with blind eyes, demonstrating the eventual feasibility of phaco-emulsification.   *American Journal of Ophthalmology*

CATARRH

Richard Lower; 1672   **440**

Call your Catarrh a Rheum, whene'er it flows
Towards the chest; if to the throat it goes,
A Cough; and a Coryza, if to th' nose.   *De Catarrhis*

CATHETERIZATION

Werner Theodor Otto Forssmann; 1929   **441**

After the experiments in the cadavers had been successful, I undertook the first experiments in living man by *experimenting on myself*.... I carried out under local anesthesia a venesection in my left elbow and introduced the catheter without resistance in its whole length of 65 cm.... I checked *the position of the catheter in the roentgen picture* and I observed the forward advance of the catheter in a mirror held in front of the fluoroscope screen by a nurse.... The method...has opened numerous prospects for metabolic studies and for studies of cardiac activity.   *Wiener Klinische Wochenschrift*

CAUSATION (ETIOLOGY)

Jean-François Fernel; [1497-1588]   **442**

Misbalance of the Constitution is the illness, yet the cause is the practical point. There are causes we do not know.   *Sherrington CS, The Endeavor of Jean Fernel*

René-Théophile-Hyacinthe Laennec; 1819   **443**

[Pathology] is the only basis of positive knowledge in medicine and one should never lose sight of it in etiological research for fear of chasing chimeras or creating phantoms to combat.... But I also believe that it is dangerous to study local conditions exclusively and to the extent that their difference from the causes on which they depend is lost from view.... The necessary shortcomings of a limited outlook is often to take the effect for the cause, or to fall into the even greater error of considering them as identical.

Traité de l'Auscultation Médiate

Robert Koch; 1882   **444**

The facts obtained in this study may possibly be sufficient proof of the causal relationship, that only the most sceptical can raise the objection that the discovered microorganism is not the cause but only an accompaniment of the disease.... It is necessary to obtain a perfect proof to satisfy oneself that the parasite and the disease are...actually causally related, and that the parasite is the...direct cause of the disease. This can only be done by completely separating the parasite from the diseased organism [and] introducing the isolated parasite into healthy organisms and induce the disease anew with all its characteristic symptoms and properties.   *Berliner Klinische Wochenschrift*

Aubrey J. Lewis; 1934   **445**
One does not call the last straw the cause of the camel's broken back, at any rate if one is talking scientific language.   *Journal of Mental Science*

CELIAC DISEASE

W.K. Dicke, H.A. Weijers, J.H. van de Kamer; 1953   **446**
If [in cases of celiac disease] wheat is banished from the diet and rice flour, maize starch, peeled, boiled potatoes are given instead, the anorexia, vomiting, and abdominal pain disappear, the acute attacks of diarrhoea cease, the faeces become darker in colour, the patient gains in weight, and finally the growth in height becomes normal, or even more than normal.   *Acta Paediatrica*

CELLS

Robert Hooke; 1665   **447**
Our Microscope informs us that the substance of Cork is altogether fill'd with Air, and that the Air is perfectly enclosed in little Boxes or Cells distinct from one another.   *Micrographia*

CELLULAR BASIS OF LIFE

Rudolf Ludwig Karl Virchow; 1860   **448**
Where a cell arises, there a cell must have previously existed (*omnis cellula e cellula*), just as an animal can spring only from an animal, a plant from a plant.   *Cellular Pathology as Based upon Physiological and Pathological Histology*

CEREBELLUM

Pierre Fourens (Marie Jean-Pierre Flourens); 1824   **449**
A slight injury to the cerebellum invariably produces a corresponding derangement of the power of motion in animals of all ages which increases in proportion to the injury; while complete removal of the cerebellum always causes total loss of the power of regulating movement.... The intellectual faculties and the senses are not affected.   *Recherches Expérimentales sur les Propriétés du Système Nerveux, dans les Animaux Vertébrés*

Jean-Baptiste Bouillaud; 1827   **450**
In examining the clinical facts and comparing them with experiments on animals, I was able to prove that the cerebellum is a nervous center which controls diverse acts of standing, of maintaining the equilibrium, and of locomotion—in brief, the cerebellum coordinates the functions which help the animal stand and walk upright and move from one place to another.   *Archives de Médecine Général*

CEREBRAL EMBOLISM

William Senhouse Kirkes; 1852   **451**
A loud systolic murmur was heard all over the cardiac region.... While sitting up in bed eating her dinner, she suddenly fell back as if fainting...and when attended to was found speechless, though not unconscious, and partially hemiplegic on the left side.... On examining the body...the right middle cerebral artery just at its commencement was plugged up by a small nodule of firm, whitish, fibrinous-looking substance.... The mitral valve was much diseased, the auricular surface of its large cusp being beset with large warty excrescences of adherent blood-stained fibrine.   *Medico-Chirurgical Transactions*

CHANGE

Wilfred Batten Lewis Trotter; 1939   **452**
The mind likes a strange idea as little as the body likes a strange protein, and resists it with

a similar energy. It would not perhaps be too fanciful to say that a new idea is the most quickly acting antigen known to science. If we watch ourselves honestly we shall often find that we have begun to argue against a new idea even before it has been completely stated. I have no doubt that that last sentence has already met with repudiation—and shown how quickly the defence mechanism gets to work.

The Lancet

CHARACTER

Ambrose Bierce; 1906   **453**

Physiognomy, *n*. The art of determining the character of another by the resemblances and differences between his face and our own, which is the standard of excellence.

The Devil's Dictionary

John Chalmers Da Costa; 1915   **454**

Oh, for some x-ray which would show us in the human the glass from the diamond, the plate from the gold!

New York Medical Journal

CHAUVINISM

William Osler; 1897   **455**

At any rate, whether he goes abroad or not, let him early escape from the besetting sin of the young physician, *Chauvinism*, that intolerant attitude of mind, which brooks no regard for anything outside his own circle and his own school.

Internal Medicine as a Vocation

CHEYNE-STOKES RESPIRATION

Hippocrates; [460-375 BC]   **456**

Philiscus...took to bed on the first day of acute fever.... About the middle of the sixth day he died. The respiration throughout, like that of a person recollecting himself.

Fourteen Cases of Disease

John Cheyne; 1818   **457**

The only peculiarity in the last period of his illness, which lasted eight or nine days, was in the state of the respiration: For several days his breathing was irregular; it would entirely cease for a quarter of a minute, then it would become perceptible, though very low, then by degrees it became heaving and quick, and then it would gradually cease again: this revolution in the state of his breathing occupied about a minute, during which there were about thirty acts of respiration.

Dublin Hospital Reports

William Stokes; 1854   **458**

There is a symptom which appears to belong to a weakened state of the heart, and...may be looked for in many cases of the fatty degeneration.... The symptom in question was observed by Dr. Cheyne, although he did not connect it with the special lesion of the heart. It consists in the occurrence of a series of inspirations, increasing to a maximum, and then declining in force and length, until a state of apparent apnoea is established.

The Diseases of the Heart and Aorta

CHICKEN POX

William Heberden; 1802   **459**

These pocks break out in many without any illness or previous sign: in others they are preceded by a little degree of chillness, lassitude, cough, broken sleep, wandering pains, loss of appetite, and feverishness for three days.... On the first day of the eruption they are reddish. On the second day there is at the top of most of them a very small bladder, about the size of a millet-seed.

Commentaries on the History and Cure of Diseases

CHILDREN

Henry Leber Coit; 1910   **460**

The gift of children is the most precious gift of God to mankind. It is the natural right of every child born into the world to remain and grow to years of efficiency.   *Help Bringers*

Benjamin Spock; 1946   **461**

The children who are appreciated for what they are, even if they are homely, or clumsy, or slow, will grow up with confidence in themselves, happy.... But the children who have never been quite accepted by their parents, who have always felt that they were not quite right, grow up lacking confidence. They'll never be able to make full use of what brains, what skills, what physical attractiveness they have.   *Baby and Child Care*

Cesare Pavese; [1908-1950]   **462**

One stops being a child when one realizes that telling one's trouble does not make it better.   *This Business of Living: Diaries 1933-50*

Kingsley Amis; 1963   **463**

It was no wonder that people were so horrible when they started life as children.   *One Fat Englishman*

Billy F. Andrews; 1968   **464**

The level of civilization attained by any society will be determined by the attention it has paid to the welfare of its children.   *The Children's Bill of Rights*

Billy F. Andrews; 1968   **465**

That proper shelter, nutrition, clothes, education, and health measures be provided each child to assure that each, with maturity, can assume the full responsibilities of adulthood and citizenship.   *The Children's Bill of Rights*

Billy F. Andrews; 1968   **466**

That each newborn has the inalienable right to be born wanted, loved, and protected; and while growing to maturity within and without the womb that every measure possible, as is known, be undertaken to afford the very best environment, nutrition and opportunity for growth and development.   *The Children's Bill of Rights*

CHOLECYSTOGRAPHY

Evarts Ambrose Graham, Warren Henry Cole; 1924   **467**

Definite and distinct shadows of the gallbladder [containing a radiopaque substance excreted in bile] are obtained on exposure to the roentgen ray. Up to date, shadows have been obtained on all patients who presumably had a normal gallbladder. It is more difficult to obtain a shadow of a pathologic gallbladder. We believe, however, that this fact will be almost as much aid to diagnosis as a good shadow, since we feel that virtually all normal gallbladders can be made to cast a shadow if proper methods are used.   *Journal of the American Medical Association*

CHOLELITHIASIS

Matthew Baillie; 1808   **468**

It frequently happens that gall-stones are found in the gall-bladder after death, where there was not the least suspicion of their existence during life.   *Morbid Anatomy*

CHOLERA

Aretaeus the Cappadocian; [81-138?]   **469**

Cholera is a retrograde movement of the *materiel* in the whole body on the stomach, the belly, and the intestines.... Those matters, then, which collect in the stomach, rush upwards by vomiting; but those humours in the belly, and intestines, by the passages downward...those by the anus, liquid and fetid excrement.... If the disease tend to death, the patient falls into a sweat.... Sometimes neither is there any urine collected in the bladder, owing to the metastasis of the fluids to the intestine...pulse very small.... A painful and most piteous death from spasm, suffocation, and empty vomiting. *On Cholera*

Alexandre-Jacques-François Brierre de Boismont; 1831   470

The blood in patients with cholera undergoes remarkable changes, it becomes black, thickened, viscous, and frequently forms a compact mass, separating with great difficulty into serum and coagulum. When the disease has lasted any length of time no serocity is found in the blood. *The Lancet*

William Brooke O'Shaughnessy; 1831   471

When absorption is entirely suspended as in those desperate cases which are unhappily now of daily occurrence in this metropolis, the author recommends the injection into the veins of tepid water holding a solution of normal salts of the blood. *The Lancet*

John Snow; 1849   472

I found that nearly all the deaths had taken place within a short distance of the [water] pump. There were only ten deaths in houses situated decidedly nearer to another street pump. In five of these cases the families of the deceased persons informed me that they always sent to the pump in Broad Street, as they preferred the water to that of the pump which was nearer. *On the Mode of Communication of Cholera*

Theodore Koch; 1884   473

In accordance with the cholera-material that I have so far examined, I think I can now assert that comma-bacilli are never found absent in cases of cholera; they are something that is specific to cholera. *British Medical Journal*

CHOLESTEROL

K. Bloch, D. Rittenberg; 1942   474

The feeding of deuterio acetate to mice and rats leads to the formation of deuterio cholesterol. By degradation of the sterol isolated from the animals, isotope was shown to be present in both the side chain and the nucleus of the cholesterol molecule. A minumum of 13 percent of the hydrogen atoms of cholesterol was derived from the acetate ion. The actual value must be higher. *Journal of Biological Chemistry*

CHROMOSOMES

Wilhelm Waldeyer-Hartz; 1888   475

I must beg leave to propose a separate technical name, *chromosome*, for those things which have been called by Boveri *chromatic elements*, in which there occurs one of the most important acts in karyokinese, viz. the londitudinal splitting. *Paper*

CHRONIC FATIGUE SYNDROME

Björn Sigurdsson, Kjartan R. Gudmundsson; 1956   476

Six years after an attack of Akureyri disease...many of the patients still complain of nervousness, tender muscles, pains, and tiredness. *The Lancet*

Gary P. Holmes, J.E. Kaplan, N.M. Gantz, and others; 1988   477

We propose a new name for the chronic Epstein-Barr virus syndrome—the chronic fatigue syndrome—that more accurately describes this symptom complex as a syndrome of unknown cause characterized primarily by chronic fatigue. *Annals of Internal Medicine*

Peter Manu, T.J. Lane, D.A. Matthews; 1988   478

The chronic fatigue syndrome, as [currently] defined, is uncommon, even with patients with chronic fatigue, and rare if the patients are carefully evaluated and followed up.

Annals of Internal Medicine

Gary P. Holmes; 1991   **479**

Because [the chronic fatigue syndrome] appears not to be a single disease, it is expected
that cases that represent subsets of [the syndrome] will be identified and studied as possibly separate entities.   *Reviews on Infectious Disease*

Keiji Fukuda, Stephen E. Straus, Ian Hickie, and others; 1994   **480**

The chronic fatigue syndrome is a clinically defined condition...characterized by severe
disabling fatigue and a combination of symptoms that prominently features self-reported
impairments in concentration and short-term memory, sleep disturbances, and muscu-
loskeletal pain. Diagnosis...can be made only after alternative medical and psychiatric
causes of chronic fatiguing illness have been excluded. No pathognomonic signs
or...tests...have been validated.... No definitive treatments for it exist.... Some persons
affected...improve with time but...most remain functionally impaired for several years.
                                                                  Annals of Internal Medicine

Edward Shorter; 1995   **481**

Feeling perpetually weary and unable to concentrate? You've got [myalgic
encephalomyelitis] or Chronic Fatigue Syndrome, the result of a mystery virus that seems
to affect mainly middle-class females. Thus the patients troop to the doctor, ailing with
the kinds of non-specific symptoms—pain and fatigue, vertigo and dysphoria—that have
afflicted humankind since the dawn of time.   *Journal of Psychosomatic Research*

Kenneth C. Hyams; 1998   **482**

Research studies have repeatedly demonstrated that patients with chronic somatic complaints are ill, often with debilitating fatigue and other severe symptoms that cannot be
explained by well-recognized disorders.... What remains to be established is whether
afflicted patients are suffering from unique, scientifically definable illnesses.
                                                                        Epidemiologic Reviews

CIRCLE OF WILLIS

Thomas Willis; [1621-1675]   **483**

We have elsewhere shewed, that the *Cephalick* arteries, viz. the *Carotides*, and the
Vertebrals, do so communicate one with another, and all of them in several places, are so
ingraffed one in another mutually, that if it happen, that many of them should be stopped
or pressed together at once, yet the blood being admitted to Head, by the passage of one
Artery only, either the *Carotid* or the *Vertebral*, it would presently pass through all those
parts both exterior and interior.   *The Practice of Physick*

CIRCULATION

[Anonymous]; *circa* 2500 BC   **484**

There are canals (or vessels) in it (the heart) to [every] member. Now if the priests of
Sekhmet or any physician put his hands (or) his fingers [upon the head, upon the back of
the] head, upon the two hands, upon the pulse, upon the two feet[he] measures the
heart, because its vessels are in the back of the head and in the pulse; and because its [pul-
sation is in] every vessel of every member.   *The Edwin Smith Surgical Papyrus*

Imhotep; *circa* 1550 BC   **485**

In the Heart are the vessels to the whole of the body. As to these, every physician...will
feel them when he lays his finger on the head, on the back of the head, on the hands, on
the stomach (? heart) region, on the arms, on the legs. Everywhere he feels his Heart
because its vessels run to all his limbs.... When the heart is sad, behold, it is the morose-
ness of the Heart or the vessels of the Heart are closed up insofar as they are not recognizable under thy hand.... When his Heart trembles and there is much Fat under the Left
breast, behold it is his Heart which causes a little of the sinking because his disease is
spreading.   *Ebers Papyrus*

Galen; [130-200]   **486**

Just as the pulsatile vessel which originates from the left of the two cavities of the heart is like a tree trunk for all the pulsatile vessels in the entire body...so then all of the non-pulsatile vessels in the body arise and branch off from the vena cava, like boughs from a tree trunk.   *On Nerves, Veins, and Arteries*

Galen; [130-200]   **487**

One large pulsatile vessel...arises...like a tree trunk from the left cavity of the two cavities of the heart. Then branches come off it and disperse into the entire body, like the branches, boughs and shoots which branch out from a tree trunk. This...vessel, at the time it originates from the heart branches out into two portions. One...goes toward the spine, and there branch off from it pulsatile vessels which are dispersed into all the parts below the heart. The other portion ascends to the head, and there branch off from it pulsatile vessels which are dispersed into all the parts above the heart.

On Nerves, Veins, and Arteries

Galen; [130-200]   **488**

The heart and the arteries pulsate with the same rhythm, so that from one you can judge of all.... There is swiftness and slowness...regularity and irregularity...violence, feebleness...and so on.   *On the Pulse*

William Harvey; 1628   **489**

Blood passes through the lungs and heart by the action of the [auricles and] ventricles, and is sent for distribution to all parts of the body, where it makes its way into the veins and pores of the flesh, and then flows by the veins from the circumference on every side to the centre, from the lesser to the greater veins, and is by them finally discharged into the vena cava and right auricle of the heart...in such a quantity...as cannot...be supplied by the ingesta.... It is necessary to conclude that the blood...is impelled in a circle...in a state of ceaseless motion...and that is the sole...end of the motion and contraction of the heart.   *An Anatomical Treatise on the Movement of the Heart and Blood in Animals*

William Harvey; 1628   **490**

For a long time I turned over in my mind such questions as, how much blood is transmitted, and how short a time does its passage take. Not deeming it possible for the digested food mass to furnish such an abundance of blood, without totally draining the veins or rupturing the arteries, unless it somehow got back to the veins from the arteries and returned to the right ventricle of the heart, I began to think there was a sort of motion as in a circle. This I afterwards found true.

An Anatomical Treatise on the Movement of the Heart and Blood in Animals

John McMichael, Edward Peter Sharpey-Schafer; 1944   **491**

Serial estimations of cardiac output and right auricular pressure can be made by means of a ureteric catheter passed along the veins in the right auricle. Normal resting values for arterio-venous oxygen differences were rather lower than those obtained previously by the acetylene method. Cardiac output in the supine posture showed a 33 per cent increase over that in the erect.   *British Heart Journal*

CIRCUMCISION

The Bible   **492**

And God said to Abraham, "As for you, you shall keep my covenant, you and your descendants after you throughout their generations. This is my covenant.... Every male among you shall be circumcised. You shall be circumcised in the flesh of your foreskins, and it shall be a sign of the covenant between me and you. He that is eight days old among you shall be circumcised."   *Genesis 17:9-12*

CIRRHOSIS OF THE LIVER

John Browne; 1685   **493**

[The liver] consisted, in its concave, convex, and inward Parts of *Glands*, which (with the Vessels) made up the whole Substance thereof. These *Glands* contained a yellowish *Ichor*, like so many *Pustles*, and was, I suppose, Part of the bilious Humour lodged in the same.

Philosophical Transactions of the Royal Society

Matthew Baillie; 1793   **494**

This disease is hardly ever met with in a very young person, but frequently takes place in persons of middle or advanced age: it is likewise more common in men than women. This would seem to depend upon the habit of drinking being more common in the one sex than in the other; for this disease is most frequently found in hard drinkers.

The Morbid Anatomy

Matthew Baillie; 1797   **495**

The process by which [the tubercles] are formed is very slow...and it is commonly produced by a long habit of drinking spiritous liquors. When the liver has undergone this change, it is commonly said to be scirrhous, but the morbid appearance is very different from what is observed in the genuine scirrhous of other glands. It should rather be considered as a disease *sui generis*.

The Morbid Anatomy

William Heberden; 1802   **496**

Men are more commonly affected with scirrhous livers than women, because they are more given to intemperate drinking, which is the principal cause of this disorder.

Commentaries on the History and Cure of Diseases

René-Théophile-Hyacinthe Laennec; 1819   **497**

When cut, it [a specimen of liver] seemed to be composed of a multitude of small round or oval lobules; the size varied from a grain of mustard to a grain of hemp. Between these lobules, no normal liver tissue could be seen; their color was brownish or reddish-yellow. In areas they seemed almost green. The remaining tissue presented a sensation of small pieces of soft leather.... This structure was similar to a number of conditions which we call *scirrhous*. I would like to name it *cirrhosis* because of its color.

Traité de l'Auscultation Médiate

CLASSIFICATION

René-Théophile-Hyacinthe Laennec; 1802   **498**

In the natural sciences, when observation and experiment have gathered facts, destroyed or rectified old ideas, it becomes necessary to create new classifications which link the elements of the newly acquired knowledge and distribute them in a methodical order.

Journal de Médecine Brumaire

Wilfred Batten Lewis Trotter; 1941   **499**

The air of caricature never fails to show itself in the products of reason applied relentlessly and without correction. The observation of clinical facts would seem to be a pursuit of the physician as harmless as it is indispensable. [But] it seemed irresistibly rational to certain minds that diseases should be as fully classifiable as are bettles and butterflies. This doctrine...bore perhaps its richest fruit in the hands of Boissier de Sauvages.... This Linnaeus of the bedside grouped diseases into ten classes, 295 genera, and 2400 species.

British Medical Journal

Thomas Addis; 1948   **500**

Practice is entirely concerned with the individual, whereas classification abstracts from the individual and considers the group. Classification is, therefore, at first disowned even while implicitly it is continuously in operation. But as time passes and decisions are reached on the treatment of each of these unique individuals, we begin to think of them less as people and more as instances of a series of general rules. Ultimately the detachment from individual considerations is complete, for disease in individuals has an end—they recover or they die. *Glomerular Nephritis*

CLERGYMEN

William McMichael; 1827   **501**
The Doctor should go out at one door when the Clergyman enters at the other. *The Gold-Headed Cane*

CLINICAL CHEMISTRY

J. Willis Hurst; 1995   **502**
Each organ "speaks" its own foreign language.... The language of the kidney is usually detected in the urine and blood. The language of the liver is found in the blood chemistry. *Organ Language*

CLINICAL EPIDEMIOLOGY

Pierre-Charles-Alexandre Louis; 1836   **503**
Let us bestow upon observation the care and time which it demands; let the facts be rigorously analyzed in order to a just appreciation of them; and it is impossible to attain this without classifying and counting them; and then therapeutics will advance not less than other branches of science. *Researches on the Effects of Bloodletting*

John Rodman Paul; 1938   **504**
Clinical epidemiology...is the name I would like to propose for a new science.... It is a science concerned with circumstances, whether they are "functional" or "organic," under which human disease is prone to develop. It is a science concerned with the ecology of disease. *Journal of Clinical Investigation*

CLINICAL EXPERIENCE

Michael Crichton; 1971   **505**
"In my experience" is a phrase that usually introduces a statement of rank prejudice or bias. The information that follows it cannot be checked, nor has it been subjected to any analysis other than some vague tally in the speaker's memory. *New England Journal of Medicine*

CLINICAL OBSERVATION

Thomas Sydenham; [1624-1689]   **506**
Experience is the sole guide. This we attain by observing...the method that right reason dictates—the suggestions of common sense rather than of speculation. *Works*

Thomas Jefferson; 1807   **507**
I believe we may safely affirm, that the inexperienced and presumptuous band of medical tyros let loose upon the world, destroys more of human life in one year, than all the Robinhoods, Cartouches, & Mcheaths do in a century.... I wish to see a reform, an abandonment of hypothesis for sober facts, the first degree of value set on clinical observation, and the lowest on visionary theories. *Letter to Dr. Caspar Wistar*

Richard Bright; 1832   **508**
It is quite impossible for any man to gain information respecting acute disease, unless he watch its progress. Day after day it must be seen; the lapse of eight-and-forty hours will so change the face of disease. Acute disease must be seen at least once a-day by those who wish to learn; in many cases twice a-day will not be too often. *Address*

Peter Mere Latham; 1845   **509**

Clinical observation, with a view of keeping a man up to what is known, and perfecting him in its accustomed uses, may be an affair of sober industry only, of patient and almost passive looking on. But clinical observation, with a view of knowing more than is known, and turning new knowledge to its uses, belongs to an industry of another kind, to an energy ever active and stirring, and drawing upon, and working with, the highest faculties of the mind.   *Aphorisms*

Armand Trousseau; 1868   **510**

To know the natural progress of diseases is to know more than half of medicine.... There is a sufficiently easy method of acquiring this knowledge so important to the practitioner. Observe the practice of many physicians; do not implicitly believe the mere assertion of your master; be something better than servile learners; go forth yourselves to see and compare!... Knowing, henceforth, the physiognomy of the disease when allowed to run its own course, you can, without risk of error, estimate the value of the different medications which have been employed.   *Lectures on Clinical Medicine*

Samuel Wilks; 1877   **511**

It is an easier task for a man to sit in his study and write about medicine than to walk through the wards and observe facts for himself.   *Guy's Hospital Reports*

Jean-Martin Charcot; 1889   **512**

Let someone say of a doctor that he really knows his physiology or anatomy, that he is dynamic—these are real compliments; but if you say he is an observer, a man who knows how to see, this is perhaps the greatest compliment one can make.   *Leçons du Mardi*

Silas Weir Mitchell; 1889   **513**

The world of the sick-bed explains in a measure some of the things that are strange in daily life.   *Doctor and Patient*

William Osler; 1894   **514**

The important thing is to make the lesson of each case tell on your education. The value of experience is not in seeing much, but in seeing wisely.   *The Army Surgeon*

William Osler; *circa* 1900   **515**

Don't touch the patient—state first what you see; cultivate your powers of observation.
                                                                                Aphorisms

William Osler; 1903   **516**

Half of us are blind, few of us feel, and we are all deaf.   *Aphorisms*

William Osler; 1903   **517**

Each case has its lesson—a lesson that may be, but is not always, learnt, for clinical wisdom is not the equivalent of experience. A man who has seen 500 cases of pneumonia may not have the understanding of the disease which comes with an intelligent study of a score of cases, so different are knowledge and wisdom, which, as the poet truly says, "far from being one have oft-times no connecion."   *Boston Medical and Surgical Journal*

William Osler; 1903   **518**

There is no more difficult art to acquire than the art of observation, and for some men it is quite as difficult to record an observation in brief and plain language.
                                                         Boston Medical and Surgical Journal

Abraham Flexner; 1910   **519**

It becomes a serious question of professional etiquette, who should speak first or loudest—the pathologist, armed with his microscope, or the clinician, branding his stethoscope.... The way to be unscientific is to be partial—whether to the laboratory or to the hospital, it matters not. The test of a good education in medicine is the thorough interpenetration of both standpoints in their product, the young graduate.
                                          Medical Education in the United States and Canada

Charles Horace Mayo; 1916   **520**

As a profession we are probably less acute in our general observation than was the practitioner of the old school.   *The Lancet*

William Osler; 1919   **521**

Always note and record the unusual. Keep and compare your observations. Communicate or publish short notes on anything that is striking or new.

Thayer LS, Bulletin of the Johns Hopkins Hospital

William Osler; 1919   **522**

Learn to see, learn to hear, learn to feel, learn to smell, and know that by practice alone can you become expert. Medicine is learned by the bedside and not in the classroom. Let not your conceptions of the manifestations of disease come from words heard in the lecture room or read from the book. See, and then reason and compare and control. But see first.   *Thayer LS, Bulletin of the Johns Hopkins Hospital*

John Alfred Ryle; 1939   **523**

One of the Guy's surgeons had a case of ununited fracture...and decided one day...to waylay [Sir William] Gull and ask his advice on the case.... Gull took a look at the man and said "Feed him on tomatoes"—nothing more. The instruction was obeyed and the fracture united. When asked later by the surgeon his reasons for this advice, he replied that the surgeon and his house-surgeon might know all about fractures but had failed to observe that the man had signs of scurvy.   *The Lancet*

Dickinson Woodruff Richards; 1962   **524**

One might appropriately consider the stethoscope as a symbol of another skill or set of skills, that appears to be fast disappearing from our medical scene. This is the use of our five senses, the use of simple perception, or observation.

Transactions of the Association of American Physicians

Maxwell M. Wintrobe; 1980   **525**

Many look, but few see.   *Blood, Pure and Eloquent*

CLINICAL RESEARCH

John Bacot; 1829   **526**

Mr. Rose, an army surgeon...adopted the only rational plan—that of putting the question to the test of experiment, discarding all preconceived notions, and looking solely at the natural progress of the disease itself.   *A Treatise of Syphilis*

Pierre-Charles-Alexandre Louis; 1836   **527**

Let those, who engage hereafter in the study of therapeutics,...labor to demonstrate, rigorously, the influence and the degree of influence of any therapeutic agent on the *duration, progress, and termination of a particular disease*. Let them not forget that nothing is more difficult than to verify a fact of this nature; that it can be effected only by means of an extensive series of observations, collected with exactness.

Researches on the Effects of Bloodletting

[Anonymous]; 1921   **528**

Arithmetic...is a bad master, but it is a good servant. When this truth has been realized, the question of [the value of] medical records will appear in better perspective and the possibility of clinical research, not for the gifted few alone, but for all, will be admitted.

The Lancet

Jean-Martin Charcot; 1929   **529**

I firmly believe that in medicine there are areas that belong solely to the doctor, that only he can properly cultivate and bring these areas to fruition. These domains are necessarily closed to the physiologist, who day in and day out is confined to his laboratory and would disdain the teaching methods of the hospital. *Revue Deux Monde*

CLINICAL TRIALS

Ambroise Paré; 1537   **530**

I raised myself early to visit them, when beyond my hope I found those [with wounds] to whom I had applied the digestive medicament, feeling but little pain, their wounds neither swollen nor inflamed, and having slept through the night. The others to whom I had applied the boiling oil were feverish with much pain and swelling about their wounds. Then I determined never again to burn thus so cruelly the poor wounded by arquebuses.

The Apology and Treatise Containing the Voyages Made into Divers Places

Jean-Baptiste van Helmont; 1648   **531**

Let us take out of the hospitals, out of the camps, or from elsewhere, 200, or 500 poor people, that have fevers, pleurisies, etc. Let us divide them in halfes, let us cast lots, that one halfe of them may fall to my share, and the other to yours. *Ortus Medicinae*

John Haygarth; 1800   **532**

A trial may be accomplished in the most satisfactory manner, and ought to be performed without any prejudice. Prepare a pair of false, exactly to resemble the true [Perkin's] Tractors. Let the secret be kept inviolable, not only from the patient, but every other person. Let the efficacy of both be impartially tried [in patients with chronic rheumatism]; beginning always with the false Tractors.... The reports of the effects produced by the true and false Tractors [should] be fully given, in the words of the patients.

Of the Imagination

Pierre-Simon Laplace; 1820   **533**

By means of the calculus of probabilities one can appreciate the advantages and disadvantages of the methods employed in the speculative sciences. Thus, to recognize the best of the treatments in use for curing a disease, it is sufficient to test each of them on the same number of patients, making all the circumstances completely similar. The superiority of the most advantageous treatment will manifest itself more and more as this number is increased, and a calculation will lead to the probability corresponding to its advantage, and to the ratio according to which it is superior to the others.

Philosophical Essay on Probabilities

Anselme-Balthasar Richerand; 1825   **534**

In order to get out of...a labyrinth of contradictory opinions, and to fix at last such an important point of doctrine in surgery, there is only one way:... A certain number of patients should be brought together in a suitable place, and there be operated on comparatively, placing as far as possible the individual patients... chosen to undergo the operation in the same circumstances. Only an academic body whose sole interest is truth can undertake and pursue successfully such an experiment.

Historie des Progrès Récens de la Chirurgie

Carl Emil Fenger; 1839   **535**

The best method to find out which treatment may be used to the greatest advantage would be, first to determine the ratio between those who were cured and those who died among cases where no treatment was given, then to compare this result with that obtained using each single treatment and next to make similar comparisons between the effect of different treatments in different classes of cases. *Ugeskrift for Laeger*

Louis-Dominique-Jules Gavarret; 1840   **536**

For a statistic...to be considered reliable as a measure of the value of a medication, the observer must adhere to the following conditions: *a)* The patients have to be drawn exclusively from the same locality and...classes of the population... *b)* The disease under investigation must have a clearly and perfectly detectable diagnosis distinguishable from diseases that most resemble it... c) Statistics bearing on the totality of a disease ought to contain a precise indication of the number of cases comprising each of its varieties... d) The medication must be clearly formulated as well as...modifications for each variety of the disease.

Principes Généraux de Statistique Médicale, ou, Développement des Règles qui Doivent à Son Emploi

Elisha Bartlett; 1844   537

The first condition, in the establishment of a therapeutical principle...is this—that the facts, or phenomena, the relationships of which are to be investigated, shall be sufficiently fixed and definite to be comparable.... The subjects of the disease...ought to be taken from the same classes of populations.... The disease should be susceptible of a clear and positive diagnosis.... *Every case of the disease that presents itself* should be taken into account.... The method of treatment...should be defined as distinctly and as clearly as possible .   *An Essay on the Philosophy of Medical Science*

Thomas Graham Balfour; *circa* 1860   538

There were 151 boys [with evidence] they had not had scarlatina; I divided them in two sections, taking them alternately from the list, to prevent imputation of selection. To the first [76] I gave belladonna; to the second [75] I gave none;... two in each section were attacked by the disease. The numbers are too small to justify deductions... but the observation is good because it shows how apt we are to be misled by imperfect observation. Had I given the remedy to all the boys, I should probably have attributed to it the cessation of the epidemic.   *Letter to Charles West*

Claude Bernard; 1865   539

To be valid, comparative experiments have...to be made at the same time and on as comparable patients as possible.... Comparative experiment is the *sine qua non* of scientific experimental medicine; without it a physician walks at random and becomes the plaything of endless illusions. A physician, who tries a remedy and cures his patients, is inclined to believe that the cure is due to his treatment. But the first thing to ask them is whether they have tried doing nothing, i.e., not treating other patients; for how can they otherwise know whether the remedy or nature cured them?   *An Introduction to the Study of Experimental Medicine*

Johannes Andreas Grig Fibiger; 1898   540

In many cases a trustworthy verdict can only be reached when a large number of randomly selected patients are treated with the new remedy and, at the same time, an equally large number of randomly selected patients are treated as usual...   *Hospitaltidende*

Adolf Bingel; 1918   541

To make the trial [of diphtheria antitoxin serum] as objective as possible... I have sought the views of the assistant physicians of the diphtheria ward, without informing them about the nature of the serum under test.... Their judgement was thus completely without prejudice.   *Deutsches Archiv für Klinische Medizin*

William Hallock Park, J.G.M. Bullowa, M.B. Rosenbluth; 1928   542

Patients were...taken alternatively for antibody treatment or control, depending only on the order of their admission to the service. It was believed that with a sufficiently large series the distribution of cases by type would be equalized between the treated and the untreated group.   *Journal of the American Medical Association*

J. Burns Amberson Jr., B.T. McMahon, Max Pinner; 1931   543

On the basis of clinical, X-ray and laboratory findings the 24 patients were divided...into two approximately comparable groups of 12 each. The cases were individually matched, one with another, in making this division.... The matching could not be precise, but it was as close as possible.... Then by a flip of the coin, the group became identified as group I (sanocrysin-treated) and the other as group II (control).... The patients were not aware of any distinction in the treament administered. *American Reviews on Tuberculosis*

Thomas Lewis; 1934   544

To ascertain if a remedy succeeds or fails, two groups of cases should be selected being composed as similarly as possible; the patients of the groups are then treated in exactly the same way and simultaneously, except in one group they receive the remedy and the other they do not. The latter or control group serves to determine the natural course of the malady tested at the same time and under simple basal conditions. These are the conditions required by the experimental method. *Clinical Science*

Ronald Aylmer Fisher; 1935   545

The simple precaution of randomization will suffice to guarantee the validity of the test of significance, by which the result of the experiment is to be judged.

The Design of Experiments

Joseph A. Bell; 1941   546

The...problem was...locating...a group of children to be vaccinated, identical, in all attributes which might influence the occurrence and recognition of pertussis, with another group to receive no vaccine. It is impossible to select such identical groups because many of the attributes involved are not known, and many of those that are known cannot be quantitatively assessed.... The only practical approach appeared to rest in the selection of two groups, each of which is a random sample of the combined groups in the exact sense of the word. *Public Health Reports*

Medical Research Council; 1948   547

Determination of whether a patient would be treated by streptomycin and bed-rest (S case) or by bed-rest alone (C case) was made by reference to a statistical series based on random sampling numbers drawn up for each sex at each centre by Professor Bradford Hill; the details of the series were unknown to any of the investigators or to the co-ordinator and were contained in a set of sealed envelopes.... The appropriate numbered envelope was opened at the central office.... It was important for the success of the trial that the details of the control scheme remain confidential. *British Medical Journal*

Austin Bradford Hill; 1952   548

It appears sometimes to be thought that there is some necessary antagonism between the clinical assessment of a few cases and the "cold mathematics" of the statistically analyzed trial dealing with a larger number. It is difficult to see how in fact there can be any such antagonism. The clinical assessment, or the clinical impression, must itself be numerical in the long run—that patients are reacting in a way different from the way the clinician believes was customary in the past. In the control trial an attempt is made to systematize those impressions (and other measurements) and to add them up.

New England Journal of Medicine

Austin Bradford Hill; 1971   549

The variability of human beings in their illnesses and their reactions to them is a fundamental reason *for* the planned clinical trial and not *against* it.

Principles of Medical Statistics

Archibald Leman Cochrane; 1972   550

It appears in general it is Catholicism, Communism, and underdevelopment that appear to be against RCTs [randomized clinical trials]. In underdeveloped countries this can be understood, but what have Communism and Catholicism against RCTs? Is authoritarianism the common link, or is Communism a Catholic heresy?

Effectiveness and Efficiency

Archibald Leman Cochrane; 1972   551

There is something extraordinarily satisfying in designing an RCT [randomized clinical trial] of "place of therapy," writing the protocol in such a way as to avoid all the ethical pitfalls, persuading all the necessary people to participate, and checking to see that no one cheats.   *Effectiveness and Efficiency*

Archibald Leman Cochrane; 1972   552
I was trying to persuade a headmaster to randomize caning and detention for boys who were caught smoking. He answered my arguments by claiming that the trial was unnecessary as he always knew which boy should be caned and which should not. I checked as far as I could later and it looked as though his method was simple. He caned them all.
Effectiveness and Efficiency

Archibald Leman Cochrane; 1979   553
It is surely a great criticism of our profession that we have not organized a critical summary, by specialty or subspecialty, adapted periodically, of all relevant randomized controlled trials.   *Medicines for the Year 2000*

Thomas Clark Chalmers; 1984   554
I firmly believe that it's more ethical to do a randomized control trial when you don't know than to act as if you did; and I base that conclusion on the fact that I've made so many mistakes by acting as if I did know and then finding out that I didn't.
Spencer S, Healthy News

Thomas Clark Chalmers; 1984   555
I think the major ethical principle is that you shouldn't be involved in a trial unless you would be willing to be randomized yourself if you had the disease.
Spencer S, Healthy News

Archibald Leman Cochrane; 1989   556
It was [in the 1950s] that I began to wonder and discuss with my colleagues how [various] forms of medical treatment would stand up to the test of a randomised controlled trial. Looking back, this is undoubtedly the point at which [its] immense potential...began to dawn on me. It offered clinical medicine, and health services generally, an experimental approach to questions of effectiveness and efficiency, and a massive step forward from "validation" by clinical opinion and essentially subjective observations.
One Man's Medicine

Bert Spilker; 1991   557
Good data in a few patients are far better than mediocre or poor data in many patients.
Guide to Clinical Trials

Thomas Clark Chalmers; 1992   558
Why did I get into this field? I killed too many people when I was in practice.
Maguire J, Harvard Public Health Review

International Committee of Medical Journal Editors; 2004   559
Altruism and trust lie at the heart of research on human subjects. Altruistic individuals volunteer for research because they trust that their participation will contribute to improved health for others and that researchers will minimize risks to participants. In return for the altruism and trust that makes research possible, the research enterprise has an obligation to conduct research ethically and to report it honestly. Honest reporting begins with revealing the existence of all clinical studies, even those that reflect unfavorable on a research sponsor's product.   *Annals of Internal Medicine*

The Bible   560
Prove thy servants, I beseech thee, ten days; and let them give us pulse to eat, and water to drink; Then let our countenances be looked upon before thee, and the countenance of the children that eat of the portion of the king's meat: and as thou seest deal with thy servants; So he consented to them in this matter, and proved them ten days; And at the end

of ten days their countenances appeared fairer and fatter in flesh than all the children which did eat the portion of the king's meat. *Daniel 1:12-15*

CLITORIS

Nicholas Culpeper; 1660   561
The Clytorus is a sinewy and hard body, full of spongy and black matter within, as the side ligaments of the Yard are, in form it represents the Yard of a Man, and suffers erection and falling as doth that; this is that which causes lust in Women, and gives delight in copulation, for without this, a Woman neither desires copulation, or hath pleasure in it, or conceives by it. *A Directory for Midwives*

COCAINE

Sigmund Freud; 1884   562
The psychic effect...consists of exhilaration and lasting euphoria, which does not differ in any way from the normal euphoria of a healthy person.... One senses an increase of self-control and feels more vigorous and more capable of work; on the other hand, if one works, one misses that heightening of the mental powers which alcohol, tea, or coffee induce.... One...finds it difficult to believe that one is under the influence of any drug at all.... I have tested this effect of coca...some dozen times on myself. *On Cocaine*

COLITIS

Axel Munthe; 1929   563
It soon became evident that appendicitis was on its last legs, and that a new complaint had to be discovered to meet the demand. The Faculty was up to the mark, a new disease was dumped on the market, a new word was coined, a gold coin indeed, COLITIS! *The Story of San Michele*

COLLAGEN VASCULAR DISEASE

Paul Klemperer, Abou D. Pollack, George Baehr; 1942   564
The apparent heterogeneous involvement of various organs in [disseminated lupus] had no logic until it became apparent that the widespread lesions were identical in that they were mere local expressions of a morbid process affecting the entire collagenous tissue system.... A similar widespread alteration of collagen has also been noted in certain cases of diffuse scleroderma. *Journal of the American Medical Association*

COLLES FRACTURE

Abraham Colles; 1814   565
The posterior surface of the limb presents a considerable deformity; for a depression is seen in the forearm, about an inch and a half above the end of this bone, while a considerable swelling occupies the wrist and the metacarpus.
Edinburgh Medical and Surgical Journal

COLOR VISION

James Clerk Maxwell; 1861   566
The only satisfactory method of explaining our perception of colours is to suppose that we have in our eyes several different sets of nerves, one set being most affected by one kind of light and another set by a different kind of light. *Scientific Letters and Papers*

COMMUNITY LIFE

William Osler; 1891   **567**

In this country doctors are, as a rule, bad citizens, taking little or no interest in civic, state or national politics. Let me...tell of one of us...who...has found time to serve his city and his country. For more than twenty years Virchow has sat in the Berlin City Council as an alderman, and to no feature in his extraordinary life does the Berliner point with more justifiable pride. It is a combination of qualities only too rare, when the learned professor can leave his laboratory and take his share in practical, municipal work.

Boston Medical and Surgical Journal

COMPASSION

Norman Maclean; 1992   **568**

In a journey of compassion what we have ultimately as our guide is whatever understanding we may have gained along the way of ourselves and others, chiefly those close to us, so close to us that we have lived daily in their sufferings. From here on, then, in the blinding smoke it is no longer a "seeing world" but a "feeling world"—the pain of others and our compassion for them.   *Young Men and Fire*

COMPASSION FATIGUE

David Lodge; 1995   **569**

Perhaps it's what they call "compassion fatigue," the idea that we get so much human suffering thrust in our faces every day from the media that we've become sort of numbed, we've used up all our reserves of pity, anger, outrage, and can only think of the pain in our own knee.   *Therapy*

COMPLAINTS

Nun's prayer; *circa* 1650   **570**

Keep my mind free from the recital of endless details; give me wings to get to the point. Seal my lips on my aches and pains. They are increasing, and love of rehearsing them is becoming sweeter as the years go by. I dare not ask for grace enough to enjoy the tales of others' pains, but help me endure them with patience.

Museum of the Guild of Glostershire Craftsman

CONCEPTION

Soranus of Ephesus; *circa* 200   **571**

The best time for fruitful intercourse is when menstruation is ending and abating, when urge and appetite for coitus are present, when the body is neither in want nor too congested from drunkenness and indigestion,...and when a pleasant state exists in every respect.   *Gynecology*

CONCUSSION

D. Parkinson; 1977   **572**

Most of our knowledge of concussion comes from observations on the human model, and down through the ages he has been a most obliging model up to a point. He has waged almost continual warfare, and even in current peacetime North America he goes aggressively to and from work in a high powered vehicle, usually just a little faster than he should. He goes forth to compete at the various rings, and rinks, and fields, and arenas, and for other forms of amusement he attends bars and political rallies. From these sources alone we harvest 1500 well-documented cases of concussion at our center each year.   *Mayo Clinic Proceedings*

CONFIDENTIALITY

William Shakespeare; 1606   **573**
I think, but dare not speak.   *Macbeth, Act V, Scene i*

CONGENITAL HEART DISEASE (ROGER DISEASE)

Henri-Louis Roger; 1879   **574**
A *developmental defect of the heart occurs* from which *cyanosis* does not ensue in spite of
the fact that a communication exists between the cavities of the two ventricles and in
spite of the fact that admixture of venous blood and arterial blood occurs. This congenital defect...is even compatible with a long life.
Bulletin de l'Académie Nationale de Médecine

CONGENITAL HEART DISEASE (TETRALOGY OF FALLOT)

Thomas Bevill Peacock; 1846   **575**
In this case there existed extreme contraction of the orifice of the pulmonary artery, with
a deficiency in the interventricular septum, and the aorta arose in part from the right ventricle.... The heart was taken from a child two years and five months old, who had exhibited well-marked symptoms of cyanosis, which commenced three months after birth.
Transactions of the Pathological Society of London

Ètienne-Louis-Arthur Fallot; 1888   **576**
Cyanosis, especially in the adult, is the result of a small number of cardiac malformations
well determined.... One...is much more frequent than the others.... This malformation
consists of a true anatomopathologic type represented by the following tetralogy: (1)
Stenosis of the pulmonary artery; (2) Interventricular communication; (3) Deviation of
the origin of the aorta to the right; and (4) Hypertrophy, almost always concentric in type,
of the right ventricle. Failure of obliteration of the foramen ovale may occasionally be
added in a wholly accessory manner.   *Marseilles Médecine*

CONGESTIVE HEART FAILURE

Abraham Colles; 1842   **577**
It may be of some benefit, not only to my own family, to society at large, to ascertain by
examination the exact seat and anature of my last disease.... I would direct particular
attention to the heart and lungs...and the swelling in the hypochodrium.... I suspect that
there is some connection between this swelling of the hypochodrium and the diseased
state of the heart.   *Stokes W, The Diseases of the Heart and the Aorta*

CONNECTIVE TISSUE

Rudolf Ludwig Karl Virchow; 1859   **578**
Rarely has a scientific question provoked in such a short time such a great volume of
simultaneously varied and contradictory work as has the question of the nature, structure
and formation of the connective tissue.   *Virchow Archiv*

CONSCIOUSNESS

John of Mirfield; *circa* 1380   **579**
If there is any doubt as to whether a person is or is not dead, apply lightly roasted onion
to his nostrils, and if he is alive, he will immediately scratch his nose.
Aldridge HR, Johannes de Mirfield: His Life and Works

Homer William Smith; 1954   **580**
I would say that any animal is conscious if it shows self-serving neuromuscular activity

which involves a choice between two or more courses of action and which can relate past experience to anticipated future.   *Proceedings of the Charaka Club*

CONSTIPATION

Cotton Mather; 1724   **581**
For Costiveness. Take stewed *Prunes*.   *The Angel of Bethesda*

Henry Louis Mencken; 1920   **582**
There has [never] lived a poet...ancient or modern, near or far, who ever managed to write good poetry...at a time when he was suffering from stenosis at any point along the thirty-foot *via dolorosa* running from the pylorus to the sigmoid flexure.... The more he tries, the more vividly he will be conscious of his impotence.
Prejudices, 2nd series. The Divine Afflatus

CONSULTANTS

William Shakespeare; 1606   **583**
This disease is beyond my practice.   *Macbeth, Act V, Scene i*

Kurt Kroenke; 1985   **584**
Polyphysicians. Where physicians gather, opinions gather likewise. Doctors make poor fellow travelers. Confronted with a single disease,...although arriving at the same destination, they choose alternate routes. The patient consulting several pilots thus accumulates road maps. Like cooks in a kitchen or generals in a war, doctors may interfere with each other in close quarters. The ideal physician-patient ratio is often 1.
American Journal of Medicine

CONSULTATION

Henri de Mondeville; *circa* 1315   **585**
When they [consulting physicians] have asked the patient all the questions necessary, they should all leave the patient's room and go into another where they can be private, since in every consultation masters disagree [and may] burst into such language that a bystander would think they were quarreling...as indeed they sometimes are.
McVaugh MR, Bulletin of the History of Medicine

John Halle; *circa* 1565   **586**
When thou arte call'd at anye time,
A patient to see,
And dost perceave the cure too gerate,
And ponderous for thee:
See that thou laye disdeyne aside,
And pride of thyne own skyll,
And thinke no shame counsell to take,
But rather wynth good wyll.
Get one or two of experte men,
To help thee in that nede;
And make them partakers wyth thee,
In that worke to procede.   *Goodly Doctrine and Instruction*

Arthur Conan Doyle; 1894   **587**
Your husband appears to be dead, madame, and no doubt he is dead, but I have no objection to meeting anyone in consultation.   *Round the Red Lamp. The Romance of Medicine*

William Osler; *circa* 1900   **588**
The chief function of the consultant is to make a rectal examination that you have omitted.
Aphorisms

William Osler; 1903   **589**
Advice is sought to confirm a position already taken.   *Aphorisms*

George W. Thorn; 1987   **590**
Patients appreciate the physician who seeks another opinion even when he thinks he knows the answer.   *Manning PR and DeBakey L, Medicine: Preserving the Passion*

CONTINUING EDUCATION

John Hamilcar Hollister, E.P. Cook, J.L. Hamilton; 1873   **591**
It seems to us a criminal neglect, if physicians fail to keep themselves posted with reference to the advances made in pharmaceutical research.
    Transactions of the Illinois State Medical Society

John Shaw Billings; 1894   **592**
The education of the doctor which goes on after he has his degree is, after all, the most important part of his education.   *Boston Medical and Surgical Journal*

William Osler; 1900   **593**
If the license to practice meant the completion of his education how sad it would be for the practitioner, how distressing to his patients! More clearly than any other the physician should illustrate the truth of Plato's saying that education is a life-long process. The training of the medical school gives a man his direction, points him the way and furnishes a chart, fairly incomplete, for the voyage, but nothing more. Post-graduation study has always been a characteristic feature of our profession.   *The Lancet*

William Osler; 1903   **594**
We doctors do not "take stock" often enough, and are very apt to carry on our shelves stale, out-of-date goods. The society helps to keep a man "up to the times," and enables him to refurbish his mental shop with the latest wares…. It keeps his mind open and receptive, and counteracts that tendency to premature senility, which is apt to overtake a man who lives in a routine.   *Boston Medical and Surgical Journal*

Abraham Flexner; 1910   **595**
The one person for whom there is no place in the medical school, the university, or the college, is precisely he who has hitherto generally usurped the medical field—the scientifically dead practitioner, whose knowledge has long since come to a standstill and whose lectures, composed when he first took his chair, like pebbles rolling in a brook get smoother and smoother as the stream of time washes over them.
    Medical Education in the United States and Canada

John Benjamin Murphy; 1911   **596**
When a license to practice has been granted a graduate of a medical school it should be only for a period of, say five to ten years, at the end of which time he should be required to pass an examination or take a prescribed course of study. This provision is necessary to keep the general profession abreast of the times.
    Journal of the American Medical Association

George T. Harrell; 1958   **597**
The physician's continuing education…is largely a process within himself, one he pursues on his own. Most of his true learning—the part that sticks with him—is what he does for himself, by himself.   *Journal of Medical Education*

CONTRACEPTION

Tertullian (Quintus Septimius Tertullianus); *circa* 197   **598**
To prevent the birth of a child is a quicker way [than abortion] to murder. It makes no difference whether one destroys a soul already born or interferes with its coming to birth.

It is a human being and one who is to be a man, for the whole fruit is already present in the seed. *Apologetical Works*

Saint Augustine; *circa* 450   **599**
Intercourse even with one's legitimate wife is unlawful and wicked when the conception of the offspring is prevented. *Pope Pius XI, Casti Connubi*

Francis Place; 1823   **600**
A soft sponge about the size of a small ball attached to a narrow ribbon and slightly moistened... is introduced previous to sexual intercourse, and is afterwards withdrawn, and thus by an easy, simple, clearly and not indelicate method, in no ways injurious to health, not only much unhappiness and many miseries be prevented, but benefits to an incalcuable amount be conferred on society. *Handbill*

Ludwig Haberlandt; 1921   **601**
Of all the methods available, hormonal sterilization, based on a biological principle, if it can be applied unobjectionably in the human, is the ideal method for practical medicine and its future task of birth control. *Münchener Medizinische Wochenschrift*

Margaret Sanger; 1928   **602**
The... prejudice of centuries transmit from one generation to the next a vague idea that contraception is a sin. The harsh realities of life relentlessly challenge this inherited idea.... While theologians, moralists, legislators and jurists have been splitting theoretical hairs, and medical science has remained content to stand aloof from the problem of contraception, necessity has compelled men and women—and in the vast majority of cases women without the aid of men—to seek such fragmentary knowledge of Birth Control as may be available to them. *Motherhood in Bondage*

Pius XI; 1930   **603**
Since the conjugal act is designed primarily by nature for the begetting of children, those who in exercising it deliberately frustrate its natural power and purpose, sin against nature and commit a deed which is shameful and intrinsically vicious. *Casti Connubi*

CONTROVERSY

Thomas M. Durant; 1961   **604**
In clinical battles, the physician can have several theories shot from under him. *Temple University Medical Center Bulletin*

CONVALESCENCE

W.U. McClenahan; 1974   **605**
A loneliness persists and a peculiar sadness that is increased, if anything, during recovery. There are no hurrahs when one's feet touch the floor! Such depression is nothing new to me—I've seen it in many patients—but in hospitals no one ever talks about it. I wonder why. *G.P.*

COOLEY ERYTHROBLASTIC ANEMIA

Thomas Benton Cooley, E.R. Witwer, O. Pearl Lee; 1927   **606**
These children...resembled the Mongolian race distinctly. This characteristic...proved to be due partly to a muddy, yellowish discoloration of the skin and partly to a thickening of the cranial bones.... These cases seem to belong to a fairly definite clinical group.... We should define them as a form of hemolytic anemia...dependent probably on some congenital defect in the hemolytopoietic system.... That the bone change is not primary seems to be shown. *American Journal of Diseases of Children*

CORONARY ARTERY DISEASE

[Anonymous]; *circa* 1500 BC   **607**
If you examine a man because of suffering in his stomach, and he suffers in his arm, his breast and the side of his stomach, one says concerning him: It is the *wadj*-disease. Then you shall say concerning it: Something has entered his mouth. Death is approaching.

Ebers Papyrus

Fabrizio Bartoletti; 1633   **608**
I proceeded therefore to the description of the characteristic features of this dyspnoea from which sudden death can be predicted.... [The patients] are forced to stop because they experience a sort of suffocation, accompanied by a certain annoying sensation around the sternum which is indescribable and gradually ascends towards the jugulum. Rest only is the remedy for this distress, and if at rest the patients appear well.

Methodus in Dyspnoeam

William Harvey; [1578-1657]   **609**
Sir Robert Duray, when he reached about the middle period of life, made more frequent complaints of a certain distressing pain in the chest...so that dreading at one time syncope, at another suffocation in his attacks, he led an unquiet and anxious life. He...became cachetic and dropsical...and died in one of his paroxysms.

Dock G, The Medical and Surgical Reporter

John Fothergill; 1768   **610**
H.R. Esq. aged sixty-three...complained to me...that he often found a difficulty...to walk up a moderate ascent, especially if he attempted to do it hastily.... On the 13th of March 1775, in the evening, in a sudden and violent transport of anger, he fell down and expired immediately. His family were prevailed upon to allow the body to be opened.... "The two coronary arteries, from their origin to many of their ramifications upon the heart, were become one piece of bone."

Medical Observations and Inquiries

Everard Home; 1796   **611**
The attack...came on one morning...and lasted above two hours.... The pain became excruciating at the apex of the heart.... The affections above described were, in the beginning, readily brought on by exercise...but they at last seized him when laying in bed.... Upon inspecting the body after death, the following were the appearances.... The coronary arteries had their branches...in the state of bony tubes, which were with difficulty divided by the knife.

Hunter J, Treatise on the Blood

Caleb Hillier Parry; 1799   **612**
It appears, that [angina pectoris] is a case of syncope, preceded by a notable anxiety or pain in the region of the heart.... The tendency to this disorder arises from mal-organization in the heart itself; which mal-organization seems to be chiefly induration of the coronary arteries.

An Inquiry into the Symptoms and Causes of the Syncope Anginosa

Edward Jenner; 1799   **613**
I was making a transverse section of the heart pretty near its base, when my knife struck against something so hard and gritty, as to notch it. I well remember looking up to the ceiling, which was old and crumbling, conceiving that some plaister had fallen down. But on a further scrutiny the real cause appeared: the coronaries were become bony canals.

Parry CH, An Inquiry into the Symptoms and Causes of the Syncope Anginosa

Matthew Baillie; 1808   **614**
Ossification of the Coronary Arteries would seem to produce, or to be intimately connected with, the Symptoms which constitute Angina Pectoris. These consist of a pain which shoots from the middle of the sternum across the left breast, and passes down the left arm to near the elbow.

Morbid Anatomy

Allan Burns; 1809   **615**

If, however, we call into vigorous action, a limb, round which, we have with a moderate degree of tightness applied a ligature, we find that then the member can only support its action for a very short time; for now its supply of energy and its expenditure, do not balance each other. A heart, the coronary vessels of which are cartilaginous or ossified, is in nearly a similar condition.

Observations on Some of the Most Frequent and Important Diseases of the Heart

Robert Adams; 1827   **616**

A gentleman...suddenly felt severe pain in his chest, extending down his right arm, accompanied by a sensation of numbness: his sight became dim, he had vertigo, but did not fall.... [at autopsy] the semilunar valves of the aorta were completely ossified; but this bony or earthy deposition was not confined to the aorta; it extended to the coronary arteries, which were so completely converted into bone as to be quite solid.

Dublin Hospital Reports

Julius Friedrich Cohnheim; 1877   **617**

In fact Bezold by closing the coronary arteries with a clamp and Panum by producing an embolus in the same with a thin wax emulsion were able to stop the heart; but whether a similar event in human pathology will ever be observed, is to me improbable enough.

Vorlesungen über Allgemeine Pathologie

Adam Hammer; 1878   **618**

The patient suddenly collapsed in his chair. Dr. Wichmann...found that he had a weak pulse of only 40 beats/min with pale lips and was somewhat cyanotic.... I wondered if a disturbance of the nourishment of the heart could explain such a condition.... We were only permitted to take the heart out.... The uppermost layers consisted of a soft white and yellow bloody fibrin that reached all the way into the takeoff of the (right) coronary artery.

Deutsche Medizinische Wochenschrift

George Dock; 1896   **619**

In the fall of 1893 [he] noticed sharp pain under the sternum radiating to the back and down the left arm and into the left hand. This recurred at intervals.... The pain is worse after exertion.... The patient complained of nausea and pain in the heart, and soon died.... The autopsy showed...the right coronary artery was completely occluded at the orifice, being involved in the atheromatous process. The orifice of the left coronary artery was narrow.

Medical and Surgical Reporter

William Osler; 1903   **620**

Angina pectoris may be precipitated by: muscular exertion, violent mental states, stomach upsets or cold weather.

Aphorisms

James Mackenzie; 1909   **621**

A definite class of hearts...give rise to pain when the blood supply to the muscle is defective on account of narrowing or obliteration of the coronary artery, or when the heart muscle is so damaged that it is unequal to the task of maintaining an efficient circulation, so that...it becomes exhausted and pain results.

Angina Pectoris

William Osler; 1910   **622**

Angina results from an alteration in the working of the muscle fibres in any part of the cardio-vascular system, whereby painful afferent stimuli are excited.... Spasm or narrowing of a coronary artery...may so modify the action...of the heart that it works with disturbed tension.

The Lancet

William Osler; 1910   **623**

What is angina pectoris?.... A disease, characterised by paroxysmal attacks of pain, pectoral or extrapectoral, associated with changes in the arterial walls, organic or functional.

The Lancet

William Osler; 1910   **624**

There is, indeed, a frame and facies at once suggestive of angina—the well "set" man of from 45 to 55 years of age, with military bearing, iron grey hair, and florid complexion.... There are two primary features of the disease, pain and sudden death—pain, paroxysmal, intense, peculiar, usually pectoral, and with the well-known lines of radiation—death in a higher percentage than any known disorder, and usually sudden.... A very large proportion of all of the cases show changes in these [coronary] vessels.   *The Lancet*

James Bryan Herrick; 1912   **625**

The clinical manifestations of coronary obstruction will evidently vary greatly, depending on the size, location and number of vessels occluded. The symptoms and end-results must also be influenced by blood pressure, by the condition of the myocardium not immediately affected by the obstruction, and by the ability of the remaining vessels properly to carry on their work, as determined by their health or disease. No simple picture of the condition can, therefore, be drawn.   *Journal of the American Medical Association*

Fred M. Smith; 1918   **626**

The early exaggeration of the T-wave, its marked negative drop below the line within twenty-four hours and its more gradual return to its positive position and its final iso-electric or negative location were so characteristic in dogs...that similar changes in the wave in man might reasonably be supposed to be due to similar lesions.   *Archives of Internal Medicine*

James Bryan Herrick; 1919   **627**

The thought has been that...with a certain artery obstructed there is a definite lesion in the heart muscle...and if with that lesion there is a definite electrocardiogram, may we not...be able to state with a reasonable degree of certainty that the patient has had obstruction in a particular portion of the coronary system? May it perhaps be possible to localize a lesion in the coronary system with an accuracy comparable to that with which we locate obstructive lesions in the cerebral arteries?   *Journal of the American Medical Association*

Harold Ensign Bennett Pardee; 1920   **628**

A patient who had just had an attack typical of occlusion of a coronary artery showed a very remarkable electrocardiogram. The patient recovered and the electrocardiogram had changed on the fourth day to a form which it retained for four months during which he remained under observation.... It is concluded that this electrocardiographic sign indicates the presence of a rather large area of muscle degeneration.   *Archives of Internal Medicine*

Oscar Auerbach, Edward Cuyler Hammond, Lawrence Garfinkel; 1965   **629**

A study was made of the degree of atherosclerosis in the coronary arteries of 1372 men who died of diseases other than coronary heart disease.... The percentage of men with an advanced degree of coronary atherosclerosis was higher among cigarette smokers than among nonsmokers and increased with amount of cigarette smoking.   *New England Journal of Medicine*

William Dock; 1984   **630**

Tinsley Harrison's father was one of [William Osler's] patients and had severe angina at the age of thirty-eight. He went up to visit the great professor at Hopkins who took a very careful history.... After getting all this down and doing a physical examination, Osler said, "Well, I think you'll get over your angina all right when you lose the fifty-five pounds you put on between the time of your marriage and the time this began." Doctor Harrison did this and lived to the age of ninety-one.   *Weisse AB, Conversations in Medicine*

David E. Rogers; 1986   **631**

What I felt from the outset and continued to feel through about two hours of what seemed absolutely inolerable pain was that if I remained absolutely immobile, not moving even an eyelash, perhaps it would let go of me.... It was a dreadful, deep, nauseating ache.... It was an absolutely, monstrously, awful sensation, and it was totally untouched by 20, or 30 or 40 miligrams of morphine.   *The Pharos*

David E. Rogers; 1986   **632**
Most people... who were having genuine cardiac pain seemed instinctively to wish to remain very quiet, even when their pain was not particularly severe. Thus, I have gener- ally felt that when patients told me they had to keep "wiggling about" to find a comfort- able position or were "writhing with pain"... their chest pain was probably noncardiac.
                                                                          The Pharos

Nanette K. Wenger; 1999   **633**
The widespread misconception is that breast cancer is the major health problem for women in the United States.... Their lifetime mortality risk from CAD is 31% compared with 2.8% for both hip fracture...and breast cancer. Stated otherwise, a postmenopausal woman is ten times as likely to die from CAD as from breast cancer.
                                                        Coronary Artery Disease in Women

CORONARY CARE UNITS

Hughes W. Day; 1963   **634**
Using ward-type facilities, we are studying the impact of electronic equipment upon the care of patients...and upon patterns of nursing service.... Early experience proved that development of such an area is practical and that it is an ideal method for caring for the acute cardiac patient during the early stages of his critical illness.   *The Lancet*

CORRIGAN PULSE

Dominic John Corrigan; 1832   **635**
When a patient affected...is stripped, the arterial trunks of the head, neck, and superior extremities immediately catch the eye by their singular pulsation. At each diastole the subclavian, carotid, temporal, brachial and in some cases even the palmar arteries, are suddenly thrown from their bed, bounding up under the skin...when the semilunar valves,...become incapable of closing the mouth of the aorta, then after each contraction of the ventricle, a portion of the blood just sent into the aorta, greater or less, according to the degree of the inadequacy of the valves, turns back into the ventricle.
                                                        Edinburgh Medicine and Surgery

CORTISONE

Edward Calvin Kendall; 1971   **636**
The name compound E was laboratory jargon.... A distinctive name needed to be select- ed for the compound.... The chemical name of compound E is 17-hydroxy-11-dehydro- corticosterone. Since the name should contain not more than two or three syllables, it was reduced to "corticosterone." Removal of "ticoster" left "corsone." Dr. Hench made the point that in "corsone" the stress fell on the syllable "cor" which implied action on the heart. He added the letters "ti" and the word "cortisone" was coined. The name...was launched...on June 1, 1949.   *Cortisone*

COSMETIC SURGERY

Sara Murray Jordan; 1958   **637**
A much more effective and lasting method of face-lifting than surgical technique is happy thinking, new interests, and outdoor exercise.   *Reader's Digest*

CRANIAL TRAUMA

[Anonymous]; *circa* 2500 BC   **638**
Now as soon as thou findest that smash which is in his skull like those corrugations which
form on molten copper, (and) something therein throbbing and fluttering under thy fingers like the weak place of an infant's crown before it knits together—when it has happened there is no throbbing and fluttering under thy fingers, until the brain of his (the
patient's) skull is rent open—(and) he discharges blood from both his nostrils and both
his ears, (and) he suffers stiffness in his neck.   *The Edwin Smith Surgical Papyrus*

CREUTZFELDT-JAKOB DISEASE

Hans Gerhard Creutzfeldt; 1920   **639**
We are dealing with a disease process...characterized by the following features:
...unknown cause...relapsing course with remissions...cortical symptoms referable to the
motor and sensory centers...mental symptoms of the type of intellectual defect with predominance of psychomotor manifestations...progressive course...a noninflammatory focal
disintegration at the neural tissue of the cerebral cortex...a noninflammatory diffuse cell
disease with cell outfall throughout almost the entire gray substance.
                                                Zeitschrift die Gesamte Neurologie und Psychiatrie

Maura N. Ricketts; 1997   **640**
CJD [Creutzfeldt-Jakob disease] may be but the first of a number of theoretical or very
slight risks that will challenge, and even threaten, regulators, policy-makers, blood banks,
and physicians in the post-HIV era. We need methods that will free us from decision-
making paralysis when demands for answers lead only to more questions.
                                                         Canadian Medical Association Journal

Maura N. Ricketts; 1997   **641**
Evidence indicates that the risk of transmission of CJD [Creutzfeldt-Jakob disease]
through blood and blood products is not simply rare or even exceedingly rare. It is theoretical. Nonetheless, an impartial review of the available information still leaves us with
uncertainty, doubt, and suspicion. It is difficult to imagine a more problematic issue: the
agent is theorized but not identified; there is no test for exposure; there is no test for the
agent; and there is no phenotypic, neuropathologic or pathophysiologic feature that clearly differentiates between blood-borne and sporadic CJD. Epidemiologic studies are
almost crippled by difficulties in determining whether a true exposure occurred and by
the complex relationship between route of exposure, dose, and genetic susceptibility in
determining incubation period. A prolonged incubation period makes the identification
of point-source outbreaks extremely difficult.   *Canadian Medical Association Journal*

CROHN DISEASE

Burrill Bernard Crohn, Leon Ginzburg, Gordon D. Oppenheimer; 1932   **642**
We propose to describe, in its pathologic and clinical details, a disease of the terminal
ileum, affecting mainly young adults, characterized by a subcutate or chronic necrotizing
and cicatrizing inflammation. The ulceration of the mucosa is accomplished by a disproportionate connective tissue reaction...a process which frequently leads to stenosis of the
lumen of the intestine, associated with the formation of multiple fistulas.
                                                Journal of the American Medical Association

CULTURE

Stanley A. Rudin; 1963   **643**
Frustrate a Frenchman, he will drink himself to death; an Irishman, he will die of angry
hypertension; a Dane, he will shoot himself; an American, he will get drunk, shoot you,

then establish a $1,000,000 dollar aid program for your relatives. Then he will die of an ulcer.   *Harrison E, The New York Times*

CURLING ULCER

Thomas Blizard Curling; 1842   **644**
In no part of the alimentary canal are the diseases to which it is liable, so obscure, both in their origin and diagnosis, as in the duodenum; and as the following cases of ulceration of this portion of the small intestines in connection with burns, may be interesting, as tending to throw some light on its pathology, and to awaken attention to a source of danger in these accidents not generally suspected.   *Medico-Chirurgical Transactions*

CUSHING SYNDROME

Harvey Cushing; 1932   **645**
While...a disorder of...similar aspect may occur in association with pineal, with gonadal, or with adrenal tumors, the fact, that the peculiar polyglandular syndrome...may accompany a [pituitary] basophil adenoma in the absence of any apparent alteration in the adrenal cortex other than a possible secondary hyperplasia, will give pathologists reason in the future more carefully to scrutinize the anterior-pituitary for lesions of similar composition.   *Bulletin of the Johns Hopkins Hospital*

CYSTINURIA

William Hyde Wollaston; 1810   **646**
[A new species of urinary calculus] had been taken [by Dr. Reeve] from his brother when he was five years old.... These calculi have a yellowish semi-transparency; and they have also a peculiar glistening lustre.... I am...inclined to consider it as an oxide; and...it may be convenient to give it the name of *cystic oxide*.
                                            Philosophical Transactions of the Royal Society

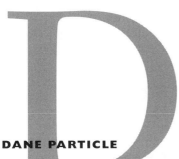

DANE PARTICLE

David S. Dane, C.H. Cameron, Moya Bruggs; 1970   647

Virus-like particles about 42 nm in diameter have been found in multiple serum specimens from Australia-antigen-positive hepatitis patients. It is suggested that these particles may be complete virus and that the much more numerous 22 nm particles and long
forms of Australia antigen are surplus virus-coat material.... [This] is a hypothesis which
cannot be proved until the virus is cultured in the laboratory.   *The Lancet*

DE TONI-FANCONI-VON ALBERTINI-ZELLWEGER SYNDROME

Giovanni de Toni; 1933   648

The patient... represents... a case of dwarfism... associated with serious rachitic manifestations.... We have found hypophosphataemia... There [was] a permanent glycosuria,
accompanied by a normal glycaemia.... The acidosis in the blood... was found by us to be
marked.... We noted that the parents of the child were first cousins, and although in renal
diabetes a hereditary dominance is generally admitted, we cannot exclude... the possibility that in some cases heredity is recessive.... It is not rash to admit the possibility of a
functional miopragia of the epithelial tubules.   *Acta Paediatrica*

Guido Fanconi, Ambrosius von Albertini, H. Zellweger; 1948   649

The authors report the case of a 2-year-old infant, normally intelligent but somewhat difficult in character... who was suffering from marked acidosis due to a metabolic acidosis
and associated with a high-grade osteoporosis with spontaneous fractures (Milkman's
fractures) and curvature of the long bones, with anaemia, changes in the cerebrospinal
fluid and poor growth. The acidosis, disturbances of calcification, blood and cerebrospinal
fluid changes could be markedly improved by vitamin D in high doses.
                    Helvetica Paediatrica Acta

DEAFNESS

Ludwig von Beethoven; 1801   650

I have often cursed my Creator and my existence. Plutarch has shown me the path of resignation.   *Letter to Dr. F.G. Wegeler*

DEATH

Martial (Marcus Valerius Martialis); 40-104   **651**
Neither fear your death's day nor long for it.   *Epigrams X, 47*

Pierre de Ronsard; *circa* 1560   **652**
Time goes, you say? Ah no!
Alas, Time stays, We go.   *Vogel K, Proceedings of the Charaka Club*

Michel de Montaigne; 1580   **653**
Death is the condition of your creation, it is part of you; you are fleeing from your own selves.... The constant work of your life is to build death.
    Essays. That to Philsophize is to Learn How to Die

Michel de Montaigne; 1580   **654**
Death of old age is a rare, singular, and extraordinary death, and hence less natural than the others; it is the last and ultimate sort of death; the farther it is from us, the less it is to be hoped for.   *Essays. Of Age*

Miguel de Cervantes; 1605-1615   **655**
There is no remembrance which time will not deface, nor no pain to which death will not put a period.   *Don Quixote*

Thomas Browne; 1643   **656**
I can cure Vices by Physicke, when they remaine incurable by Divinity; and shall obey my Pils, when they contemne their precepts. I boast nothing, but plainely say, we all labour against our owne cure; for death is the cure of all diseases.   *Religio Medici*

Thomas Browne; 1643   **657**
Men that look no farther than their outsides, think health an appurtenance unto life, and quarrel with their constitutions for being sick; but I, that have examined the parts of man, and know upon what tender filaments that Fabrick hangs, do wonder that we are not always so; and, considering the thousand doors that lead to death, do thank my God that we can die but once.   *Religio Medici*

Thomas Browne; 1658   **658**
But the iniquity of oblivion blindely scattereth her poppy, and deals with the memory of men without distinction to merit of perpetuity.... Oblivion is not to be hired. The greater part must be content to be as though they had not been, to be found in the Register of God, not in the record of man.   *Hydriotaphia or Urne Buriall*

Edward Young; 1742   **659**
All men think all men mortal but themselves.   *Night Thoughts. Night I*

Benjamin Rush; 1789   **660**
[Death] relieves the world of old men who keep the minds of men in chains to old prejudices. These men do not die half fast enough. Few Clergymen, Physicians, or Lawyers beyond 60 do any good to the world. On the contrary, they check innovation and improvement.   *Autobiography*

René-Théophile-Hyacinthe Laennec; 1810   **661**
I live among the dead and the dying. That is the best in the world for a physician, but when it lasts too long, it becomes overwhelming.   *Letter to his cousin Christophe*

Alexandre Dumas; 1845   **662**
Oh, man, the most selfish of all animals, the most personal of all creatures, who believes the earth turns, the sun shines, and death strikes for him alone—an ant cursing God from the top of a blade of grass!   *The Count of Monte Cristo*

Jan Evangelista Purkyně; *circa* 1850   **663**
Pauper ubique iacet: Everyone views the poor with contempt. But there is one thing he
has in common with the rich—the grave.   *Opera Omnia*

Alfred, Lord Tennyson; [1809-1892]   **664**
Old men must die; or the world would grow moldy, would only breed the past again.
                                                                            Nuland SB, How We Die

Edith Wharton; 1902   **665**
We are but stray atoms on the wind,
A dancing transiency of summer eves,
Till we become one with our purpose, merged
In that vast effort of the race which makes
Mortality immortal.   *Vesalius in Zante (1564)*

William James; 1902   **666**
Our civilization is founded on the shambles, and every individual existence goes out in a
lonely spasm of helpless agony.   *The Varieties of Religious Experience*

Mark Rutherford; 1910   **667**
To die is easy when we are in perfect health. On a fine spring morning, out of doors, on
the downs, mind and body sound and exhilarated, it would be nothing to lie down on the
turf and pass away.   *More Pages from a Journal*

Henry Louis Mencken; 1920   **668**
[Dr. George W.] Crile said that death was acidosis—that it was caused by the failure of
the organism to maintain the alkalinity necessary to its normal functioning—and in the
absence of any proofs or even argument to the contrary I accepted his notion forthwith
and have cherished it ever since. Thus think of death as a sort of deleterious fermentation, like that which goes on in a bottle of Château Margaux when it becomes corked.
Life is a struggle, not against sin, not against the Money Power, not against malicious animal magnetism, but against hydrogen ions.   *Prejudices, 2nd series. Exeunt Omnes*

Thomas Stearns Eliot; 1920   **669**
Webster was much possessed by death
And saw the skull beneath the skin.   *Whispers of Immortality*

Harvey Cushing; 1925   **670**
The truth is, an immense majority of all die as they are born—oblivious. A few, very few,
suffer severely in the body, fewer still in the mind.   *The Life of William Osler*

Santiago Ramón y Cajal; [1852-1934]   **671**
How supremely tragic seems this abandonment of the spirit and the unresisting surrender of our organs to all the disintegrating effects of cosmic forces! And what distressing
indifference is that of nature as it casts away, like vile dross, the masterpiece of creation,
the sublime cerebral mirror, in which it acquires consciousness of itself.
                                                                        The World of Ramón y Cajal

Miroslav Krleza; 1936   **672**
God is a wondrous and horrifying word, made up from fear from death.   *Essays*

Allan Duncan; 1947   **673**
The Indians I met were used to death and dying. They saw it daily as they slaughtered
and trapped animals for their livelihood. For them everything had its time, ending in
death, and they could not understand our fear of dying. "Why do white men fear death?"
they often asked me. "Nobody fears the onset of the unconsciousness called sleep yet you
are afraid of the sleep, death."   *Medicine, Madams and Mounties*

Giuseppe di Lampedusa; 1958   **674**

Death, oh yes, it existed of course, but it was something that happened to others. The thought occurred...that it was ignorance of this supreme consolation that made the young feel sorrows much more sharply than the old; the latter are nearer the safety exit.

The Leopard

James Baldwin; 1963   **675**

Life is tragic simply because the earth turns and the sun inexorably rises and sets, and one day, for each of us, the sun will go down for the last, last time. Perhaps the whole root of our trouble, the human trouble, is that we will sacrifice all the beauty of our lives, will imprison ourselves in totems, taboos, crosses, blood sacrifices, steeples, mosques, races, armies, flags, nations, in order to deny the fact of death, which is the only fact we have.

The Fire Next Time

Committee on Human Studies; 1968   **676**

An organ, brain or other, that no longer functions and has no possibility of functioning again is for all practical purposes dead. Our first problem is to determine the characteristics of a permanently nonfunctioning brain.... No spontaneous muscular movements or spontaneous respiration or response to stimuli such as pain, touch, sound, or light.... Irreversible coma with abolition of central nervous system activity.... The flat or isoelectric EEG.... No electroencephalographic response to noise or to pinch.

Journal of the American Medical Association

Stewart Alsop; 1973   **677**

One learns to live with death by not thinking about it too much.   *Stay of Execution*

Richard Selzer; 1976   **678**

You do not die all at once. Some tissues live on for minutes, even hours, giving still their little cellular shrieks, molecular echoes of the agony of the whole corpus.

Mortal Lessons. The Corpse

Philip Larkin; 1977   **679**

The mind blanks at the glare...
...at the total emptiness for ever,
The sure extinction that we travel to
And shall be lost in always. Not to be here,
Not to be anywhere....
Death is not different whined at than withstood.   *Aubade*

Kenneth Rexroth; 1980   **680**

All men have to die, and one would think a sane man would want to take that into account, at least a little. But our whole civilization is a conspiracy to pretend that it isn't going to happen.   *Introduction to Selected Poems of D.H. Lawrence*

Philippe Ariès; 1981   **681**

Death has ceased to be accepted as a natural, necessary phenomenon. Death is a failure, a "business lost."   *The Hour of Our Death*

Robertson Davies; 1994   **682**

The relationship of the patient to Death is not by any means the same thing as the medical probability of recovery.   *The Cunning Man*

Sherwin B. Nuland; 1994   **683**

None of us seems psychologically able to cope with the thought of our own state of death, with the idea of a permanent unconsciousness in which there is neither void nor vacuum—in which there is simply nothing.   *How We Die*

Sherwin B. Nuland; 1994   **684**

If one were to name the universal factor in all death, whether cellular or planetary, it would certainly be loss of oxygen.   *How We Die*

Lofty L. Basta; 1996   **685**

I do not want to relinquish control over how I will die; I do not want to be "treated to death."   *A Graceful Exit*

Daniel J. Baxter; 1997   **686**

I have come to believe that a content life is one that gracefully carries death on its shoulder as a friend and not a feared adversary.   *The Least of These My Brethren*

George Soros; 1999   **687**

Death is clearly a problem that has no solution. But the way we treat death can make it better or worse. If we deny the fact and refuse to deal with the circumstances of death, which many Americans do, that makes it worse.   *New York Review of Books*

John Updike; 2000   **688**

All mortals are mounting the gallows steps, but how near we have come only God knows.
                                                                             Gertrude and Claudius

Wendell Berry; 2000   **689**

The crudest manifestation of modern medicine is its routine, stubborn and finally cruel resistance to death.   *Life is a Miracle*

DECISION MAKING

George Bernard Shaw; 1906   **690**

You are asking me to kill another man for his sake; for as surely as I undertake another case, I shall have to hand back one of the old ones to the ordinary treatment. Well, I don't shrink from that. I have had to do it before; and I will do it again if you can convince me that his life is more important than the worst life I am now saving. But you must convince me first.   *The Doctor's Dilemma, Act I*

Harold M. Schoolman; 1977   **691**

A physician who is 90 per cent "certain" about any decision will always seek additional information in the hope that it will increase the "confidence" with which he makes such a decision. The decision...will be either correct or incorrect, and the outcome is independent of the confidence with which the decision is reached. When additional information cannot possibly alter the decision, but only gives rise to a greater sense of comfort on the part of the physician, such additional information is of no benefit to the patient. Its only benefit is in reducing the discomfort of the physician.   *New England Journal of Medicine*

Eric J. Cassell; 1984   **692**

Physicians should define their diagnostic and therapeutic goals in terms of the everyday life and function of individual patients.... Unfortunately, that ideal is seldom met.... In part the problem arises because physicians are trained from the first days of medical school to disregard the knowledge they bring with them of everyday life and human function as irrelevant to medicine.... Doctors are not trained to include in their decision making the kind of "soft" and often subjective information that is relevant to the everyday life and function of sick persons.   *The Place of the Humanities in Medicine*

Raymond Tallis; 1998   **693**

Physicians will always have to rely on often quite primitive intuitions of the right thing to do, based on a sense of clinical probability, and informed by their humanity and their sense of responsibility, and instructed by what they have learned from conversations with patients and their supporters, and with their medical and nursing colleagues, from their training and from their personal and professional experiences. By this means, despite their insolubility in theory, ethical dilemmas are resolved in practice; or, at least, in praxis. Decisions are made; or they, somehow, happen.   *Times Literary Supplement*

DEFORMITY

William Shakespeare; 1592   **694**
I, that am curtail'd of this fair proportion,
Cheated of feature by dissembling nature,
Deform'd, unfinish'd, sent before my time
Into this breathing world, scarce half made up
And that so lamely and unfashionable
That dogs bark at me as I halt by them....   *Richard III, Act I, Scene i*

Francis Bacon; 1625   **695**
Deformed persons are commonly even with nature; for as nature hath done ill by them, so do they by nature—; being for the most part (as the Scripture saith) void of naturall affection; and so they have their revenge of nature.   *Essays. Of Deformity*

DELIRIUM

Hippocrates; [460-375 BC]   **696**
When in acute fevers, pneumonia, phrenitis, or headache, the hands are waved before the face, hunting through empty space, as if gathering bits of straw, picking the nap from the coverlet, or tearing chaff from the wall—all such symptoms are bad and deadly.
           The Book of Prognostics

DEMENTIA

Philippe Pinel; 1801   **697**
Rapid succession or uninterrupted alternation of isolated ideas, and evanescent and unconnected emotions [unconnected either to each other or to external real events]. Continually repeated acts of extravagance; complete forgetfulness of every previous state; diminished sensibility to external impressions; abolition of the faculty of judgement; perpetual activity.   *Treatise on Insanity*

Jean-Ètienne-Dominique Esquirol; 1838   **698**
They entertain...perfect indifference towards objects that were once most dear. They see their relatives and friends without pleasure and leave them without regret. They are uneasy in...the privations that are imposed on them, and rejoice little at the pleasures which are procured for them. What is passing around them, no longer awakens interest.... The events of life are of little account, because they can connect themselves with no remembrances, nor any hope. Indifferent to everything, nothing affects them.... He who is in a state of dementia imagines not, nor indulges in thought. He has few or no ideas.
           Des Maladies Mentales

DENTAL HEALTH

American Dental Association; 1985   **699**
Brush [your teeth] and floss them and take them to the dentist. Care for them and they will stay with you. Ignore them, and they'll go away.   *Advertisement*

Croatian proverb   **700**
The best tooth brush is the one often used.   *Proverb*

Croatian proverb   **701**
White sugar, black teeth.   *Proverb*

DENTISTS

Ambrose Bierce; 1906   702
Dentist, *n.* A prestidigitator who, putting metal into your mouth, pulls coins out of your pocket.   *The Devil's Dictionary*

DEOXYRIBONUCLEIC ACID (DNA)

Johann Friedrich Miescher; 1871   703
I have recovered by treating [pus] cells... with diluted hydrochloric acid.... a fine powder.... consisting of completely clean nuclei.... I believe that from the analyses [of them] presented... the conclusion can be drawn that we are... dealing... with a chemical entity.... In favor of this is the approximate agreement in the N-content of the soluble nuclein and of the whole nuclei.   *Ueber die Chemische Zusammensetzung der Eiterzellen*

Frederick Griffith; 1928   704
The most attentuated pneumococcus may develop the full equipment of virulence. The first essential is a situation in which it can multiply, unchecked by the inhibitory action of a healthy mucous membrane. In the nidus thus formed the pneumococcus gradually builds up from material furnished by its distintegrating companions an antigenic structure with invasive properties sufficient to cope with the resistance of its host. [The "material" was shown in 1944 by Avery, MacLeod, and McCarty to be DNA.]   *Journal of Hygiene*

O. T. Avery, C.M. MacLeod, M. McCarty; 1944   705
From type III pneumococcus a biologically active fraction has been isolated... which in exceedingly minute amounts is capable... of inducing the transformation of unencapsulted R-variants of pneumococcus Type II into fully encapsulated cells of the same specific type as that of the heat-killed microorganisms from which the inducing material was recovered.... The active fraction... consists principally... of a highly polymerized, viscous form of deoxyribonucleic acid.   *Journal of Experimental Medicine*

Erwin Chargaff; 1950   706
The desoxypentose nucleic acids from animal and microbial cells contain varying proportions of the same four nitrogenous constituents, namely, adenine, guanine, cytosine, thymine. Their composition appears to be characteristic of the species.... They could very well serve as one of the agents, or possibly the agent, concerned with the transmission of inherited properties.   *Experientia*

A.D. Hershey, M.C. Chase; 1952   707
Our experiments show clearly that a physical separation of the phage T_2 into genetic and non-genetic parts is possible. A corresponding functional separation is seen in the partial independence of phenotype and genotype in the same phage. The chemical identification of the genetic part must wait, however, until some of the questions asked above have been answered.   *Journal of General Physiology*

James Dewey Watson, Francis Harry Compton Crick; 1953   708
It has not escaped our notice that the specific pairing [of bases in the double helical structure] we have postulated immediately suggests a possible copying mechanism for the genetic material.   *Nature*

J.H. Matthaei, M.W. Nirenberg; 1961   709
Cell-free extracts have been obtained which actively incorporate amino acids into proteins.... The initial rate of amino acid incorporation was not inhibited by DNAase; subsequent incorporation was greatly inhibited.... Inhibition by DNAase observed in this cell-free system may be due to the destruction of DNA and its resultant inability to serve as templates for the synthesis of template RNA.   *Proceedings of the National Academy of Sciences*

M.J. Zoller, Michael Smith; 1982   **710**

The paper presents a versatile and efficient procedure for the construction of oligodeoxyribonucleotide directed site-specific mutations in DNA fragments cloned into M13 derived vectors.... The recombinants are screened for mutant molecules.... Double-stranded DNA is isolated from the mutant and the production of the desired mutation is verified by DNA sequencing.   *Nucleic Acids Research*

DEPENDENCY

Dorothy Dinnerstein; 1976   **711**

Few of us ever outgrow the yearning to be guided as we were when we were children, to be told what to do, for our own good, by someone powerful who knows better and will protect us. Few of us even wholeheartedly try to outgrow it.   *The Mermaid and the Minotaur*

DEPRESSION

Robert Burton; 1621   **712**

[Never despair.] It may be hard to cure, but not impossible for him that is most grievously affected, if he be but willing to be helped.   *The Anatomy of Melancholy*

Thomas Willis; [1621-1675]   **713**

Tho the delirious affect of universal Melancholy contains manifold symptoms, yet they consist chiefly in these three things; first, that the affected are almost continuously occupied in thinking, so that their Fancy is scarce ever idle, and at rest. Secondly, in thinking they comprehend fewer things in their minds than they were wont before, so that they often roul in their minds the same Object day and night... thirdly, the Idea of Objects or Conceptions appear often deform'd... so that every small thing seems to them great and most difficult.   *The Practice of Physick*

Samuel Johnson; 1781   **714**

He languished some years under that depression of mind which enchains the faculties without destroying them, and leaves reason the knowledge of right without the power of pursuing it.   *Lives of the Poets. Collins*

William Heberden; 1802   **715**

It is a sort of waking dream, which, though a person be otherwise in sound health, makes him feel symptoms of every disease; and, though innocent, yet fills his mind with the blackest horrors of guilt.   *Commentaries on the History and Cure of Diseases*

Wilhelm Nero Pilatus Barbellion (Bruce Frederick Cummings); 1919   **716**

Suffering from depression,...the melancholy fit fell very suddenly. All the colors went out of my life, the world was dirty grey.... All looked dreary and cheerless.   *The Journal of a Disappointed Man*

William Styron; 1990   **717**

In depression...faith in deliverance, in ultimate restoration, is absent. The pain is unrelenting, and what makes the condition intolerable is the foreknowledge that no remedy will come—not in a day, an hour, a month, or a minute.... It is hopelessness even more than pain that crushes the soul.   *Darkness Visible*

William Styron; 1990   **718**

The madness of depression is...the antithesis of violence. It is a storm indeed, but a storm of murk. Soon evident are the slowed-down responses, near paralysis, psychic energy throttled back close to zero. Ultimately, the body is affected and feels sapped, drained.   *Darkness Visible*

Joel P. Smith; 1997   **719**
Our energy is radically reduced. We feel flaccid.... We lack self-starting qualities.... We lack interest in others, whether family, friends, or colleagues, and in those activities...which were the day-to-day agendas of our lives. Our hope is gone.... We are profoundly pessimistic and preoccupied with death...darkness or emptiness—life without meaning and therefore spiritually bereft.... We are contemptuous of ourselves.
The American Scholar

Andrew Solomon; 1998   **720**
When you are depressed, the past and the future are absorbed entirely by the present, as in the world of a three-year-old. You can neither remember feeling better nor imagine that you will feel better.... Depression means that you have no point of view.   *The New Yorker*

DERMATOLOGY

Vincent Joseph Derbes; 1981   **721**
I have long had the idea that God created psoriasis and warts to teach dermatologists the merits of humility.   *Rational Drug Therapy*

John V. Alcott; 1986   **722**
If it's dry, make it wet,
If it's wet, make it dry,
Your patients don't get well,
But, then, they don't die!   *World Medical News*

DIABETES INSIPIDUS

Johann Peter Frank; 1794   **723**
The subdivisions of diabetes depend on the quality and external modifications of the excreted urine which at times may be insipid, clear as water, at other times as sweet as honey.... The main illness becomes worse if diarrhea sets in—I have seen this in one case of diabetes insipidus—but, on some occasions, as other observers have maintained, the poluria may subside with benefit to the patient.   *De Curandis Hominum Morbis Epitomie*

DIABETES MELLITUS

Aretaeus the Cappadocian; [81-138?]   **724**
Diabetes is a wonderful affection, not very frequent among men, being a melting down of the flesh and limbs into urine.... The patients never stop making water, but the flow is incessant, as if from the opening of acqueducts. The nature of the disease, then, is chronic, and it takes a long period to form; but the patient is short-lived, if the constitution of the disease be completely established; for the melting is rapid, the death speedy.
On Diabetes

Thomas Willis; 1674   **725**
Diabetes is called so from... *Transeo*, or passing through too swift a passage of the matter that is drunk.... Those labouring with this Disease, piss a great deal more than they drink, or take of any liquid ailment; and moreover they have always joyned with it continual thirst.... The Urine in all...was wonderfully sweet as it were imbued with Honey or Sugar.... I remember two Women...to whom accrued...a great flood of Urine and languor, and wasting away of the Flesh.   *Pharmaceutice Rationalis*

Matthew Dobson; 1776   **726**
Two quarts of this [patient's] urine were, by a gentle heat, evaporated to dryness.... There remained...a white cake.... This cake was granulated, and broke easily between the fingers; it smelled sweet like brown sugar, neither could it from the taste be distinguished from sugar.   *Medical Observations and Inquiries*

Adolf Kussmaul; 1874   **727**

Since I have seen three diabetics in the course of a year die, with remarkably similar symptoms in which there was a *peculiar comatose condition preceded and accompanied by dyspnoea*, I believe that it...has to do with a form of death which...bears the closest relationship to the disturbances in the metabolism in diabetes... [Kussmaul breathing]

Deutsche Archiv für Klinische Medizin

Joseph von Mering, Oscar Minkowski; 1890   **728**

After complete removal of the [pancreas], the dogs became diabetic. It has not to do simply with a transient glycosuria, but a genuine lasting diabetes mellitus, which in every respect corresponds to the most severe form of this disease in man.... The dogs...showed an abnormal hunger and an abnormally increased thirst [and] a marked polyuria.... The sugar content of the blood was very markedly increased.

Archiv für Experimentell Pathologie und Pharmakologie

Eugene Lindsay Opie; 1900   **729**

It has been suggested by several observers that the islands of Langerhans may furnish an internal secretion to the blood.... Where diabetes is the result of pancreatic disease, do the islands exhibit lesions? I have examined microscopically the pancreas from eleven cases of diabetes, and in four instances such marked change was found [in the islands] that one could not doubt the relationship of the general disease to the lesion of the organ.

Journal of Experimental Medicine

Frederick Grant Banting, Charles Herbert Best; 1922   **730**

Intravenous injections of extract from dog's pancreas, removed from seven to ten weeks after ligation of the ducts, invariably exercises a reducing influence upon the percentage sugar of the blood and the amount of sugar excreted in the urine.... The extent and duration of the reduction varies directly with the amount of extract injected.

Journal of Laboratory and Clinical Medicine

DIAGNOSIS

Chang Chung-Ching; *circa* 150   **731**

The skilful doctor knows what is wrong by observing alone, the middling doctor by listening, and the inferior doctor by feeling the pulse.

Wong KC and Lien-Teh W, History of Chinese Medicine

Galen; [130-200]   **732**

It is always necessary to speak first of the organ exhibiting a damaged function, then to search for the type of damage and whether the condition is persistent or still developing but will never remain stable; further, if it has already developed, whether the active cause of the disease remains attached to this organ or is transient.   *On the Affected Parts*

Galen; [130-200]   **733**

Diseases can be diagnosed from the specific character of the symptoms of each. The nails become bent in wasting diseases. A chill of no [evident] reason and followed by fever is a sign that an inflammation changes into an abscess; a blackened tongue is a sign of a burning fever; a particular type of discoloration of the whole body indicates in some cases a disease of the liver...and cannot escape the knowledgeable physician.

On the Affected Parts

Arnald of Villanova; [1240-1311]   **734**

Physician! When you shall be called to a sick man, in the name of God seek the assistance of the Angel who has attended the action of the mind and from inside shall attend the departures of the body. You must know from the beginning how long the sick has been laboring, and in what way the illness has befallen him, and by inquiring about the symptoms, if it can be done, ascertain what the disease is.   *Bedside Manners in the Middle Ages*

William Ockham; 1318   **735**

Plurality must not be posited without necessity (*Pluralitas non est ponenda sine necessitate*). ["Ockham's razor"—sometimes phrased as "Among competing hypotheses, favor the simplest one."] *In Libros Sententiarum*

Henry Fielding; 1749   **736**

To say the truth, every physician almost hath his favourite disease, to which he ascribes all the victories obtained over human nature. *Tom Jones*

William Heberden; 1802   **737**

Whatever probability there may be, that the bladder is empty, and that the disease is in the kidneys, it will still be advisable in every suppression to make the matter certain by the introduction of a catheter. *Commentaries on the History and Cure of Diseases*

René-Théophile-Hyacinthe Laennec; 1826   **738**

I have tried to place the internal organic lesions on the same plane as the surgical diseases with respect to diagnosis. *Traité de l'Auscultation Médiate*

Peter Mere Latham; 1845   **739**

Oftentimes, in particular cases, we catch ourselves at work fabricating a sort of fictitious faith, and setting it up against all the experience of our lives, sooner than give the disease up for incurable. *Aphorisms*

Peter Mere Latham; 1878   **740**

The diagnosis of disease is often easy, often difficult, and often impossible. *Collected Works*

James Paget; 1885   **741**

To treat a sick man rightly requires the diagnosis not only of the disease but of all the manner and degrees in which its supposed essential characters are modified by his personal qualities, by the mingled inheritances that converge in him, by the changes wrought in him by the conditions of his past life, and by many things besides. *Address to the Abernethian Society*

William Osler; 1894   **742**

There are, in truth, no specialties in medicine, since to know fully many of the most important diseases a man must be familiar with their manifestations in many organs. *The Army Surgeon*

William Osler; 1895   **743**

To confess ignorance is often wiser than to beat about the bush with a hypothetical diagnosis. *Ephemerides*

William Osler; *circa* 1900   **744**

Absolute diagnoses are unsafe, and are made at the expense of the conscience. *Aphorisms*

William Osler; *circa* 1900   **745**

Probability is the rule of life, especially under the skin. Never make a positive diagnosis. *Aphorisms*

William Osler; 1902   **746**

In the fight which we have to wage incessantly against ignorance and quackery among the masses and follies of all sorts among the classes, *diagnosis*, not *drugging*, is our chief weapon of offence. Lack of systematic personal training in the methods of the recognition of disease leads to the misapplication of remedies, to long courses of treatment when treatment is useless, and so directly to that lack of confidence in our methods which is apt to place us in the eyes of the public on a level with empirics and quacks. *The Army Surgeon*

William Osler; 1919   **747**

Observe, record, tabulate, communicate. Use your five senses.

Thayer LS, Johns Hopkins Hospital Bulletin

Thomas Addis; 1948   **748**

[The physician] will use scientific methods, he will for a time dismember his patient—isolate, for instance, his kidneys or his heart and observe their action under very specialized conditions—but in the end he has to put these parts together again in his "diagnosis"...his total conception of the relationships between the patient as a person, the disease as a part of the patient, and the patient as a part of the world in which he lives.

Glomerular Nephritis

John L. McClenahan; 1962   **749**

A sick man may wear a wrong diagnosis around his neck like a millstone, and the doctor's job may be first to undiagnose him so recovery can begin.   *Medical Affairs*

Karl Menninger; 1963   **750**

We disparage labeling of all kinds in psychiatry insofar as these labels apply to supposed diseases or conditions of specific etiological determination. We deplore the tendency of psychiatry to retain its old perjorative name-calling function. Patients who consult us because of their suffering and their distress and their disability have every right to resent being plastered with a damning index tab. Our function is to help these people, not to further afflict them.   *The Vital Balance*

Henry George Miller; 1968   **751**

The most valuable diagnostic instrument is the passage of time.   *World Neurology*

Lawrence L. Weed; 1969   **752**

The student or physician should list *all* the patient's problems, past as well as present, social and psychiatric as well as medical. The list should not contain diagnostic guesses; it should simply state the problems at a level of refinement consistent with the physician's understanding, running the gamut from the precise diagnosis to the isolated, unexplained finding.   *Medical Records, Medical Education, and Patient Care*

Archibald Leman Cochrane; 1972   **753**

[Diagnosis] grew up in advance of therapy. For a considerable period able clinicians had little else to do but refine the art of diagnosis. It became in this way almost dissociated from treatment and became regarded, consciously or unconsciously, as an end in itself.

Effectiveness and Efficiency

Harry Klinefelter; 1973   **754**

[Physicians] should try to rule in rather than rule out diseases.... [Physicians] are interested in determining what is wrong with their patients rather than what is *not* wrong with them.... One can never rule out a disease; one simply puts it farther back in his mind.

Resident and Staff Physician

Sydney Walker III; 1996   **755**

Diagnosis means finding the cause of a disorder, not just giving it a name.

A Dose of Sanity

Jerome Lowenstein; 1997   **756**

Odors, bedside photographs, the patient's gestures and body language, and the emotional tone of the initial greeting reveal much about the patient and help to bridge the uncomfortable gap between the student or physician and the patient.

The Midnight Meal and Other Essays

DIAPHRAGM

Ambrose Bierce; 1906   **757**
Diaphragm, *n.* A muscular partition separating disorders of the chest from disorders of the bowels.   *The Devil's Dictionary*

DIET

Hildegard of Bingen; *circa* 1150   **758**
If human beings consume meat or other food that is rich in fats, or if they eat foods containing too much blood, they will incur infirmity rather than health.   *Causae et Curae*

[Anonymous]; 1490   **759**
Great suppers do the stomacke much offend,
Sup light if quiet you to sleep intend.   *The School of Salernum*

Cotton Mather; 1724   **760**
There is nothing under the Sun, that can render the Blood and Juices, *Thin* and *Sweet* and *Right*, and constantly in a Flowing State, but keeping to a *Spare, Lean, Fluid* sort of a *Diet*.   *The Angel of Bethesda*

Benjamin Franklin; 1733   **761**
Cheese and salt meat, should be sparingly eat.   *Poor Richard's Almanac*

William Stark; 1788   **762**
Doctor B— Franklin, of Philadelphia, informed me, that he himself, when a journeyman Printer, lived a fortnight on bread and water, at the rate of 10 pounds of bread per week, and that he found himself stout and hearty with this diet.   *Works*

William Heberden; 1802   **763**
Many physicians appear to be too strict and particular in the rules of diet and regimen, which they deliver as proper to be observed by all who are solicitous either to preserve or recover their health....The common experience of mankind will sufficiently acquaint any one with the sorts of food which are wholesome to the generality of men; and his experience will teach him which of these agrees best with his particular constitution.
Commentaries on the History and Cure of Diseases

The Bible, The Apocrypha   **764**
Many have died of gluttony, but he who is careful to avoid it prolongs his life.
Ecclesiasticus 37:31

DIGESTION

Thomas Willis; [1621-1675]   **765**
From the memory of some particularly appetising food there often arises an agreeable sensation for gentle motion of the spirits in...the brain...(which) even expand outwards and provoke saliva in the mouth, as though keen to meet a pleasant guest, in the shape of some highly desired food.   *Lecture*

Theodor Schwann; 1836   **766**
Free acid is...essential in digestive action [but is] however not the only active element.... Since [another substance] active in very small amounts carries on the digestion of the most important animal nutrients, one might with justice apply to it the name pepsin.
Archiv für Anatomie und Physiologie Wissenschaft Medizinische

Ivan Petrovich Pavlov; 1897   **767**
A dog...possesses an ordinary gastric fistula with [a] metallic cannula, and has had its oesophagus divided as well, so that the mouth is cut off from all communication with the cavity of the stomach.... I give the dog food. The animal eats greedily, but the whole of

the food swallowed, comes out again at the oesophageal opening in the neck.... Perfectly pure gastric juice makes its appearance at the fistula.... It is obvious that the effect of the feeding is transmitted by nervous channels to the gastric glands.

The Work of the Digestive Glands

DIGITALIS

William Withering; 1785   768

My opinion was asked concerning a family receipt for the cure of the dropsy.... It had long been kept a secret by an old woman in Shropshire, who had sometimes made cures after the more regular practitioners had failed. I was informed also, that the effects produced were violent vomiting and purging; for the diuretic effects seemed to have been overlooked.... It was not very difficult for one conversant in these subjects, to perceive that the active herb could be no other than the Foxglove.   *An Account of the Foxglove*

William Withering; 1785   769

The Foxglove...given in very large and quickly-repeated doses, occasions sickness, vomiting, purging, giddiness, confused vision, objects appearing green or yellow; increased secretion of urine, with frequent motions to part with it, and sometimes inability to retain it; slow pulse, even as slow as 35 in a minute, cold sweats, convulsions, syncope, death.... *Let the medicine...be given in the doses, and at the intervals mentioned above—until it either acts on the kidneys, the stomach, the pulse, or the bowels; let it be stopped upon the first appearance of any one of these effects.*   *An Account of the Foxglove*

William Stokes; 1854   770

The Method of Bouillaud consists in the application of a blister to the praecordial region, and then sprinkling the vesicated surface every day with from six to fifteen grains of the powder of digitalis. Thus,...we may diminish the number and force of the pulsations of the heart.... Should experience confirm the efficacy of this treatment, it has advantages over the internal exibition of the remedy, which is so apt to cause a weakened state of the stomach.   *The Diseases of the Heart and Aorta*

DIPHTHERIA

Aretaeus the Cappadocian; [81-138?]   771

Ulcers occur on the tonsils; some...mild and innocuous; but others...pestilential, and fatal.... Such as are broad, hollow, foul, and covered with a...black concretion, are pestilential.... If it [the disease] extend to the tongue, the gums, and the alveoli, the teeth also become loosened and black; and the inflammation seizes the neck; and these die within a few days from the inflammation, fever, foetid smell, and want of food.

On Ulcerations About the Tonsils

Nicholas Tulp; 1641   772

The types of angina are various, but none is more pernicious than...an inflammation of the muscles on the inside of the larynx. A deep swelling of which, if indeed it should compress the narrow top of the trachea; & pressing upon its cord...not only the voice itself is suppressed; but moreover the passage of air is shut off; or rather of life itself. Which without air [the patient] does not last a single day.   *Observationes Medicae*

Guillaume de Baillou (Ballonius); 1740   773

The greatest difficulty was in breathing.... The surgeon said he sectioned the body of the boy with this difficult breathing and with the disease...of unknown cause; sluggish resisting phlegm was found which covered the trachea like a membrane and the entry & exit of air to the exterior was not free: thus sudden suffocation.

Epidemiorum et Ephemeridium Libri Duo

Armand Trousseau; 1833   **774**

"The child, almost breathing his last, let himself be placed on a dining-room table. With a burned match I traced on his neck a line so that my bistoury should not go astray." The operation is then described. The child had a stormy time; there was evidently wound infection. Twelve days after operation the cannula was removed, he breathed through the larynx, and three days later the wound in the neck was healed.

Journal des Connaissances Médico-chirurgicales

William Henry Welch; 1892   **775**

It may be considered as established now that the toxic products and not the bacilli themselves invade the tissues in diphtheria. This fact would at once suggest that the general lesions (those produced at a distance from the seat of inoculation in animals, and the situation of the local process in human beings) were the effects of the soluble poison diffused through the body.   *Bulletin of the Johns Hopkins Hospital*

Emil Adolf von Behring; 1893   **776**

The response to the disease [diphtheria] can be segregated into three groups, each defined by the proper and sufficient use of the antitoxin serum. 1) Prevention of disease, if the serum is administered before the appearance of symptoms. 2) Prevention of progression of the disease when it is apparent clinically. 3) Reversal of severe and advanced affliction leaving only a mild and benign illness.   *Deutsche Medizinische Wochenschrift*

DISCOVERY

William Dock; 1980   **777**

The most remarkable fact about the Korotkoff sound is that it was discovered. Its observation confirmed Pasteur's thesis that "chance favors the prepared mind"—meaning that chances are innumerable or infrequent but prepared minds are very rare.

New England Journal of Medicine

DISEASE

Hippocrates; [460-375 BC]   **778**

The human body contains blood, phlegm, yellow bile and black bile. These...make up its constitution and cause its pains and health. Health is...that state in which these...substances are in the correct proportion to each other.... When one of these is separated from the rest and stands by itself, not only the part from which it has come, but also that where it collects and is present in excess, should become diseased, and because it contains too much of the particular substance, cause pain and disease.   *Hippocratic Writings*

Plato; [427-347 BC]   **779**

Since the body is compacted of four ingredients, earth, fire, water and air, disorders and diseases arise from abnormal usurpation or deficiency of these ingredients, or from their moving from their own place to a foreign one.   *Dialogues. Timaeus*

Moses Maimonides; *circa* 1190   **780**

The most important consideration in the causation of disease is the body constitution which becomes afflicted. Therefore, not all people will die during an epidemic.

Rosner F and Munter S, The Medical Aphorisms of Moses Maimonides

John Donne; [1573-1631]   **781**

Put all the miseries that man is subject to together, *sicknesse* is more than all. It is the *immediate* sword of God.... In *poverty* I lack but other things; in *banishment* I lack other men; but in *sicknesse*, I lack my self.... How shall I put a just value upon God's great *blessings* of *Wine*, and *Oyle*, and *Milke*, and *Honey*, When my taste is gone, or of *Liberty*, when the *gout* fetters my feet?   *Sermon XX*

Thomas Sydenham; [1624-1689]   **782**
Acute disease is an act of God; of chronic disease the patient himself is the author.
Works

Hermann Boerhaave; 1715   **783**
Whatever State of the human Body doth disorder the vital, the natural, or even the animal functions of the same, is called a Disease.   *Aphorisms*

Henry David Thoreau; 1851   **784**
Is not disease the rule of existence? There is not a lily pad floating on the river but has been riddled by insects. Almost every shrub and tree has its gall, oftentimes esteemed its chief ornament and scarcely to be distinguished from the fruit. If misery loves company, misery has company enough. Now, at midsummer, find me a perfect leaf or fruit.
Journal

William Osler; 1903   **785**
Variability is the law of life, and as no two faces are the same, so no two bodies are alike, and no two individuals react alike and behave alike under the abnormal conditions which we know as disease.   *Boston Medical and Surgical Journal*

David Riesman; 1936   **786**
Diseases, at least many of them, are like human beings. They are born, they flourish and they die. Some may be ternal or at least coeval with the race, but seeing how many have disappeared or are in the process of disappearing, it would hardly be a wise prophecy to predict eternity for any of them.... [Some] have disappeared because they were really not diseases at all but symptoms wrongly interpreted as clinical entities.
Annals of Medical History

Alan Gregg; 1941   **787**
The perpetual enemies of the human race, apart from man's own nature, are ignorance and disease.   *Bordley J and Harvey AM, Two Centuries of American Medicine*

Ivo Andri; 1945   **788**
Disease is a fate of the poor, but also a punishment of the rich.   *The Chronicle of Travnik*

Thomas Addis; 1948   **789**
We are accustomed to speak of"disease entities" as though they had an independent, individual existence and could be recognized as friends—or better, perhaps, as enemies. This is...one of those abstractions that do violence to the reality of the...situation, for there is no disease aside from the patient. The disease is the change produced in the patient by a pathological process. Diagnosis involves the observation of the patient as he is, and...a reconstruction in imagination of the patient as he was, before afflicted. The disease is the difference between those two pictures.   *Glomerular Nephritis*

René Jules Dubos; 1961   **790**
It can be said that each civilisation has a pattern of disease peculiar to it. The pattern of disease is an expression of the response of man to his total environment (physical, biological, and social); this response is, therefore, determined by anything that affects man himself or his environment.   *Indiana Medicine and Surgery*

Charles E. Rosenberg; 1962   **791**
[A] disease is no absolute physical entity but a complete intellectual construction, an amalgam of biological state and social definition.   *The Cholera Years*

René Jules Dubos; 1968   **792**
Complete and lasting freedom from disease is but a dream remembered from imaginings of a Garden of Eden.   *Man, Medicine, and Environment*

René Jules Dubos; 1968 **793**
The difficulty of defining disease is implied in the very structure of the word: "dis-ease." So many different kinds of disturbances can make a person feel not at ease and lead him to seek the aid of a physician that the word ought to encompass most of the difficulties inherent in the human condition. *Man, Medicine, and Environment*

Bernard Straus; 1970 **794**
Almost as fast as one disease is conquered new ones are discovered and sometimes created. We exchange new ones for old. The balance is clearly on the credit side and it is a fact that many of the old scourges, real or imaginary, are gone or are vanishing.
Medical Counterpoint

Lewis Thomas; 1976 **795**
We do go about curing a substantial number of ailments.... But there is another part of the mystique. It's the great secret of doctors, known only to their wives, but still hidden from the public. Most things get better by themselves; most things, in fact, are better in the morning. *New York Times Magazine*

Susan Sontag; 1978 **796**
Nothing is more punitive than to give a disease a meaning—that meaning being invariably a moralistic one...the subjects of deepest dread (corruption, decay, pollution, anomie, weakness) are identified with the disease, that horror is imposed on other things. The disease becomes adjectival. *Illness as Metaphor*

Susan Sontag; 1978 **797**
Theories that diseases are caused by mental states and can be cured by will power are always an index of how much is not understood about the physical terrain of a disease.
Illness as Metaphor

Robert P. Hudson; 1983 **798**
Diseases are not immutable entities but dynamic social constructions that have biographies of their own. *Disease and Its Control*

Robert P. Hudson; 1983 **799**
If a medical and social consensus defined freckles as a disease, this benign and often winsome skin condition would become a disease. Patients would consult physicians complaining of freckles, physicians would diagnose and treat freckles, and presumably, in time, we would have a National Institute of Freckle Research. *Disease and Its Control*

Charles E. Rosenberg, Janet Golden; 1992 **800**
"Disease" is an elusive entity. It is not simply a less than optimum physiological state. The reality is obviously a good deal more complex; disease is at once a biological event, a generation-specific repertoire of verbal constructs reflecting medicine's intellectual and institutional history, an occasion of and potential legitimation for public policy, an aspect of social role and individual—intrapsychic—identity, a sanction for cultural values, and a structuring element in doctor and patient interactions. In some ways disease does not exist until we have agreed that it does, by perceiving, naming, and responding to it.
Framing Disease

Sherwin B. Nuland; 1994 **801**
The quest to achieve true dignity fails when our bodies fail. *How We Die*

Barton Childs; 1995 **802**
Disease cannot be described simply as a consequence of a chance encounter with an inimical environment. Rather, it is individual variation in homeostatic range and flexibility that differentiates the disease-prone individual. *A Logic of Medicine*

Gerald I. Byrne; 2001   **803**

Disease is a genotypic or phenotypic state, often influenced by enviromental factors, that places individuals at risk for internally derived adverse consequences.   *Science*

L.K.F.Temple, R.S. McLeod, S. Gallinger, J.G.Wright; 2001   **804**

Disease is a state that places individuals at increased risk of adverse consequences.

Science

DISLOCATIONS

[Anonymous]; *circa* 2500 BC   **805**

If thou examinest a man having a dislocation in his mandible, shouldst thou find his mouth open (and) his mouth cannot close for him, thou shouldst put thy thumb(s) upon the ends of the two rami of the mandible in the inside of his mouth, (and) thy two claws (meaning two groups of fingers) under his chin, (and) thou shouldst cause them to fall back so that they rest in their places.   *The Edwin Smith Surgical Papyrus*

DIURETICS

William Dock; 1984   **806**

The mercurial treatment for diuresis...was discovered by the nurses. They used to give mercurials intravenously for the treatment of syphilis, and frequently the syphilitic patients had congestive heart failure resulting from syphilitic aortic insufficiency. They kept jugs at the end of the beds to measure the urine output, and the nurses kept pointing out to the doctors that whenever they gave mercurials to one of these patients in heart failure he'd have one hell of a diuresis.   *Weisse AB, Conversations in Medicine*

DIZZINESS

Henry George Miller; 1968   **807**

Dizziness covers anything from severe aural vertigo to a housewife feeling nervous in the supermarket.   *World Neurology*

DOCTORS

Martial (Marcus Valerius Martialis); *circa* 50   **808**

Doctor Diaulus has changed his trade:
He is now a mortician—
With the same results he got before
As a practicing physician.   *Epigrams I, 47*

Su Shih (Su Tung-po); *circa* 1050   **809**

To be a writer requires the wasting of paper: to be a doctor requires the sacrificing of lives.   *Garrison FH, Bulletin of the New York Academy of Medicine*

Petrarch (Francesco Petrarca); *circa* 1365   **810**

I once heard a physician of high standing in his profession say:.... If a hundred men, or a thousand, of the same age and general constitution and accustomed to the same diet should all fall victim to a disease at the same time, and if half of them should follow the prescriptions of our contemporary doctors, and if the other half should be guided by their natural instinct and common sense, with no doctors at all, I have no doubt that the latter group would do better.   *Letter to Boccaccio*

Paracelsus (Theophrastus Bombastus von Hohenheim); [1493-1541]   **811**

A clear conscience.
Desire to learn and gain experience.
A gentle heart and a cheerful spirit.

Moral manner of life and sobriety in all things.
Greater regard for his honor than for money.
More interest in being useful to his patient than to himself.
You must not be married to a bigot. *Doctors and Patients*

Michel de Montaigne; 1580 **812**
Who ever saw a doctor use the prescription of his colleague without cutting out or adding something? Thereby they clearly enough betray their art and reveal to us that they consider their reputation, and consequently their profit, more than the interest of their patients. *Essays. Of the Resemblance of Children to Fathers*

Michel de Montaigne; 1588 **813**
If your doctor does not think it good for you to sleep, to drink wine, or to eat such-and-such a food, don't worry: I'll find you another who will not agree with him.
Essays. Of Experience

Molière (Jean-Baptiste Poquelin); 1673 **814**
They [physicians] know rhetoric and grammar, and can talk the finest Latin and give Greek names to all diseases and define them and class them. But as for curing them, that's what they know nothing about. *Le Malade Imaginaire, Act III, Scene 3*

Molière (Jean-Baptiste Poquelin); 1673 **815**
Ego, cum isto boneto
Venerabili et docto,
Dono tibi et potestaten
Medicandi,
Purgandi,
Bleedandi,
Pierceandi,
Cutandi,
Chopandi,
Et assassinandi—
Impune per totam terram! *Le Malade Imaginaire*

Philander Misaurus [pseudonym]; 1720 **816**
If the Devil ever created any Thing, it was the Doctor. *The Honour of the Gout*

Jonathan Swift; 1731 **817**
The doctors, tender of their fame,
Wisely on me lay all the blame:
"We must confess his case was nice;
But he would never take advice.
Had he been rul'd, for aught appears,
He might have liv'd these twenty years;
For, when we open'd him, we found
That all his vital parts were sound." *Verses on the Death of Dr. Swift*

Alexander Pope; 1732] **818**
Who shall decide when doctors disagree? *Moral Essays. Epistle III, To Lord Bathurst*

Benjamin Franklin; 1733 **819**
Beware of the young Doctor & the old Barber. *Poor Richard's Almanac*

Benjamin Franklin; 1736 **820**
God heals, and the Doctor takes the Fees. *Poor Richard's Almanac*

Jonathan Swift; 1738 **821**
The best doctors in the world are Doctor Diet, Doctor Quiet, and Doctor Merryman.
Polite Conversation

Thomas Percival; 1803   **822**

The strictest temperance should be incumbent on the [medical] faculty; as the practice of both physic and surgery at all times requires the exercise of a clear and vigorous understanding: And on emergencies, for which no professional should be unprepared, a steady hand, and acute eye, and an unclouded head, may be essential to the well being, and even to the life, of a fellow creature.   *Medical Ethics*

René-Théophile-Hyacinthe Laennec; 1816   **823**

Here [my cousin Ambroise] is "docteur," but so little "docte" [learned].

Letter to his uncle Guillaume Laennec

George Eliot; 1871   **824**

For my own part, I like a medical man more on a footing with the servants; they are often all the cleverer.   *Middlemarch*

Robert Arthur Talbot Gascoyne-Cecil, Marquess of Salisbury; 1877   **825**

You should never trust experts. If you believe the doctors, nothing is wholesome; if you believe the theologians, nothing is innocent; if you believe the soldiers, nothing is safe. They all require to have their strong wine diluted by a very large admixture of insipid common sense.   *Letter to Lord Lytton, Viceroy of India*

Josh Billings (Henry Wheeler Shaw); 1881   **826**

When a doctor looks me square in the face and can't see no money in me, then I am happy.   *Works*

Mark Twain (Samuel Langhorne Clemens); 1883   **827**

I have pitied doctors from my heart. What does a lovely flush in a beauty's cheek mean to a doctor but a break that ripples above some deadly disease? Are not all her visible charms sown thick with what are to him the signs and symbols of hidden decay? Does he ever see her beauty at all, or doesn't he simply view her professionally, and comment upon her unwholesome condition all to himself? And doesn't he sometimes wonder whether he has gained most or lost most by learning his trade?   *Life on the Mississippi*

Jean-Martin Charcot; 1888   **828**

Let someone say of a doctor that he really knows his physiology or anatomy, that he is dynamic—these are not real compliments; but if you say he is an observer, a man who knows how to see, this is perhaps the greatest compliment one can make.   *Lecture*

Oliver Wendell Holmes; 1891   **829**

There is also a young Doctor, waiting for his bald spot to come, so that he may get into practice.   *Over the Teacups*

Oliver Wendell Holmes; 1893   **830**

Talk of your science! after all is said
There is nothing like a bare and shiny head;
Age lends the graces that are sure to please;
Folks want their doctors mouldy, like their cheese.   *Rip Van Winkle, MD*

Arthur Conan Doyle; 1894   **831**

No doctor has a right to be a pessimist. If you are conscious of that temperament, you should fly the profession. A reasoned optimism is essential for a doctor.

Round the Red Lamp. The Romance of Medicine

Arthur Conan Doyle; 1894   **832**

He has the healing touch—that magnetic thing which defies explanation or analysis.... His mere presence leaves the patient with more hopefulness and vitality. The sight of disease affects him as dust does a careful housewife. It makes him angry and impatient. "Tut, tut, this will never do!" he cries, as he takes over a new case.... Dying folk cling to his hand as if the presence of his bulk and vigour gives them more courage to face the change; and that kindly, wind-bitten face has been the last earthly impression which many a sufferer has carried into the unknown. *Round the Red Lamp. Behind the Times*

William Withey Gull; 1896   **833**
There are many good general practitioners, there is only one good universal practitioner—
"a warm bed." *A Collection of the Published Writings*

William Osler; 1902   **834**
To wrest from nature the secrets which have perplexed philosophers in all ages, to track to their sources the causes of diseases, to correlate the vast stores of knowledge, that they may be quickly available for the prevention and cure of disease—these are our ambitions.
Chauvinism in Medicine

William Osler; 1906   **835**
There are only two sorts of doctors: those who practice with their brains, and those who practice with their tongues. *Counsels and Ideals*

William Osler; 1909   **836**
We doctors have always been a simple, trusting folk! Did we not believe Galen implicitly for fifteen hundred years and Hippocrates for more than two thousand years?
Address to the Ontario Medical Association

Albert V. Harmon; 1911   **837**
It's a mighty conscientious doctor who will tell a rich man that his trouble is imaginary.
Large Fees and How To Get Them

Albert V. Harmon; 1911   **838**
A full beard is an efficient badge of the doctor's calling, and is essential in establishing his professional identity among the people.... A physician should never dress flashily, but he should be garbed well. It creates a good impression. *Large Fees and How To Get Them*

George Bernard Shaw; 1911   **839**
Doctors are just like other Englishmen: most of them have no honor and no conscience: what they commonly mistake for these is sentimentality and an intense dread of doing anything that everybody else does not do, or omitting to do anything that everybody else does. *The Doctor's Dilemma, Preface*

George Bernard Shaw; 1911   **840**
Doctors, if no better than other men, are certainly no worse.
The Doctor's Dilemma, Preface

George Bernard Shaw; 1911   **841**
Even the fact that doctors themselves die of the very diseases they profess to cure passes unnoticed. *The Doctor's Dilemma, Preface*

George Bernard Shaw; 1911   **842**
Make it compulsory for a doctor using a brass plate to have inscribed on it, in addition to the letters indicating his qualifications, the words "Remember that I too am mortal."
The Doctor's Dilemma, Preface

George Bernard Shaw; 1911   **843**
Nothing is more dangerous than a poor doctor: not even a poor employer or a poor land-lord. *The Doctor's Dilemma, Preface*

George Bernard Shaw; 1911   **844**
Thus everything is on the side of the doctor. When men die of disease they are said to die from natural causes. When they recover (and they mostly do) the doctor gets the credit of curing them. *The Doctor's Dilemma, Preface*

George Bernard Shaw; 1911   **845**

Treat persons who profess to be able to cure disease as you treat fortune tellers.

The Doctor's Dilemma, Preface

Ernest Hemingway; 1929   **846**

I have noticed that doctors who fail in the practice of medicine have a tendency to seek one another's company and aid in consultation. A doctor who cannot take out your appendix properly will recommend to you a doctor who will be unable to remove your tonsils with success.   *A Farewell to Arms*

Sidney Kingsley; 1933   **847**

A doctor should not have to worry about money! That's one disease he's not trained to fight. It either corrupts him, or it destroys him.   *Men in White, Act 1, Scene iv*

Merrill Moore; 1938   **848**

Doctors must die, too; all their knowledge of
Digitalis, adrenalin, henbane,
Matters little if death raps again—
Once he may be forestalled, but their great love
Or little love of life is merely human:
Doctors must die like other men and women.   *Sonnet*

Alfred North Whitehead; 1941   **849**

One of the most advanced types of human being on earth today is the good American doctor.... He is skeptical toward the data of his own profession, welcomes discoveries which upset his previous hypotheses, and is still animated by humane sympathy and understanding.   *Dialogues of Alfred North Whitehead*

Fuller Albright; 1951   **850**

As with eggs, there is no such thing as a poor doctor; doctors are either good or bad.

Diseases of the Ductless Glands

Thomas Merton; 1953   **851**

I am surprised to find how much of the artist there is in doctors, for medicine is an art as well as a science and therefore its techniques demand a certain skill that is not abstract but born of connatural intuition.   *The Sign of Jonas: The Journal of Thomas Merton*

Albert Denti di Pirajno; 1955   **852**

"Whence come disease and healing?" asked the prophet Moses of God.
"From me," was the reply.
"What purpose do doctors serve?"
"They earn their living and cultivate hope in the heart of the patient until I either take away his life or give him back his health."   *A Cure for Serpents*

Sylvia Plath; 1963   **853**

Sunday—the doctor's paradise! Doctors at country clubs, doctors at the sea side, doctors with mistresses, doctors with wives, doctors in church, doctors in yachts, doctors everywhere resolutely being people, not doctors.   *The Bell Jar*

Theodore Fox; 1965   **854**

With all its faults the profession to which he belongs is not a body of technologists interested solely in the means by which physical or mental processes can be restored to normal: it is a body of doctors seeking to use these means to an end—to help patients to cope with their lives.... The doctor has learnt more about disease,...but he is, and must always be, a human being devoted first to human beings.   *The Lancet*

Alvan R. Feinstein; 1967   **855**

Unlike other types of scientific equipment, a clinician is not easily tested, compared, or calibrated in the act of getting clinical evidence. He can markedly improve the scientific quality of his performance, however, if he is willing to recognize the importance of what he does, to acknowledge himself as the apparatus to be improved, and to revise many minor and some major aspects of the way he works. *Clinical Judgment*

Eugene A. Stead Jr.; 1968 **856**
What the patient needs is a doctor. *Just Say for Me*

Earle P. Scarlett; 1972 **857**
The average doctor is something of a scientist, something of an artist, something of a priest, but nothing at all of a civil servant or dull bureaucrat. He is living in a tumultuous world.... He is trying to keep his balance as a human being in a civilization that conducts its worship in automobile showrooms, does its singing in commercials, lives on catch-words, gathers various impedimenta about him and calls it "gracious living."
Roland CG, In Sickness and in Health

Eugene A. Stead Jr.; 1983 **858**
We know that any doctor who knows what he or she knows and can comfortably say, "I don't know" is a safe doctor. *Address to the Duke Medical Association*

Peter Richards; 1985 **859**
A doctor must accept and live with uncertainty and fallibility, inescapable parts of any walk of life but harder to bear in matters of life or death. *Learning Medicine*

Phil R. Manning; 1987 **860**
An inquiring, analytical mind; an unquenchable thirst for new knowledge; and a heartfelt compassion for the ailing—these are prominent traits among the committed clinicians who have preserved the passion for medicine.
Manning PR and DeBakey L, Medicine: Preserving the Passion

Anatole Broyard; 1992 **861**
A doctor, like a writer, must have a voice of his own, something that conveys the timbre, the rhythm, the diction, and the music of his humanity that compensates us for all the speechless machines. *Intoxicated by My Illness. The Patient Examines the Doctor*

Barton Childs; 1995 **862**
The best of all worlds is attained in the doctor who cleaves to the Oslerian ideal in prac-tice and the Garrodian in thinking. *A Logic of Medicine*

Eric J. Cassell; 1995 **863**
We want doctors to function as well when they are tired as when they are rested, to admit error freely to themselves and others, to care more about the patients' being okay than about whether they are right, to put their patients' interests ahead of their own (the unknowing think this is about money; how about time, family, privacy, or freedom?). Surprisingly, over the years this is generally what we have gotten from our doctors, prob-ably because the rewards have, in the past, been so great that they overwhelmed the price.
New England Journal of Medicine

Sherwin B. Nuland; 1998 **864**
Self-awareness has never been the strong suit of those who choose to become doctors. When so much fuel is readily available for stoking the fires of ego, there is little inclina-tion to apply it in raising the candlepower of the searching light that might illumine the inner man or woman. *American Scholar*

Sherwin B. Nuland; 2001 **865**
A distinguished medical historian, now long dead, once told me that doctors are the only real philosophers, because only doctors know how people actually behave.

American Scholar

[Anonymous]; Unknown   **866**
[In a bathroom in the House of the Seven Sages, Ostia Antica, Italy:] Bene caca et declina medicos. [Shit well and avoid doctors.]   *The American Scholar*

The Bible, The Apocyrpha   **867**
Honor the physician with the honor due him...for the Lord created him; for healing comes from the Most High, and he will receive a gift from the king. The skill of the physician lifts up his head, and in the presence of great men he is admired.

Ecclesiasticus 38:1-3

DOCTORS AS PATIENTS

Richard Gordon; 1953   **868**
A layman is told to stay in bed for an extra week, and take a fortnight at the seaside; but a doctor, after taking his temperature every half-hour for a day or so, suddenly discovers he is completely cured. He at once gets up and puts on his clothes, and either goes downstairs and takes the evening surgery or makes for the garden to catch up with his digging. [Doctors] can't afford to be ill: they're not registered as patients under the National Health Service.   *Journal of the American Medical Association*

Richard Gordon; 1953   **869**
The public always appear surprised that doctors should fall ill, as though hearing a policeman's house had been burgled or the fire station had gone up in flames. Doctors go sick fairly often, though they suffer differently from anyone else: they have only one disease, which presents both a mitis and a gravis form.   *Journal of the American Medical Association*

DOCTORS' WIVES

Earle P. Scarlett; 1972   **870**
The doctor's wife...must realize proudly that her husband is in the privileged class—privileged to have duodenal ulcer, coronary thrombosis, and a lonely life. She must never be jealous, a virtue that harks back to the pre-stethoscope days when the doctor laid his bearded face on the lily-white bosom and listened with one ear for rales and with the other for the patient's husband. She must be sympathetic with her husband, for no one else ever will be.   *Roland CG, In Sickness and in Health*

DOGMATISM

William Harvey; *circa* 1650   **871**
I tremble lest I have mankind at large for my enemies, so much doth wont and custom become a second nature. Doctrine, once sown, strikes deep its root, and respect for antiquity influences all men. Still, the die is cast, and my trust is in my love of truth, and the candour of cultivated minds.   *Asher R, Richard Asher Talking Sense*

William Osler; 1902   **872**
The greater the ignorance, the greater the dogmatism.   *Chauvinism in Medicine*

Abraham Flexner; 1910   **873**
Men possessed of vague preconceived ideas are strongly disposed to force facts to fit, defend, or explain them. And this tendency both interferes with the free search for truth and limits the good which can be extracted from such truth as is in its despite attained.

Medical Education in the United States and Canada

DREAMS

Lucretius (Titus Lucretius Carus); [99-55 BC]   **874**
Each of us in sleep most often seems to follow the activity to which he is most closely

bound, to carry out the occupation to which he has been devoting the most time, to pursue the line of thinking on which his mind has been most intent.

On the Nature of Things

Jules Renard; 1887 **875**

How odd is the world of dreams! Thoughts, inner speech crowd and swarm—a little world hastening to live before the awakening that is its end, its particular death. *Journal*

Peter B. Medawar; 1967 **876**

There should be no need to emphasize, in this century of radio sets and electronic devices, that many dreams may be assemblages of thought-elements that convey no information whatsoever: that they may be just noise. *The Art of the Soluble*

DRUG INTERACTIONS

Kenneth Lloyd Melmon, Howard Fred Morreli; 1978 **877**

Drug interactions per se are no threat to a patient; a physician's ignorance either through lack of knowledge of interaction or through lack of adequate observation of the patient and proper interpretation of new events is dangerous. *Clinical Pharmacology*

DRUGS

Galen; [130-200] **878**

All who drink of this remedy recover in a short time, except those whom it does not help, who all die. Therefore, it is obvious that it fails only in incurable cases.

Strauss MB, Familiar Medical Quotations

Paracelsus (Theophrastus Bombastus von Hohenheim); *circa* 1538 **879**

All substances are poisonous, there is none which is not a poison; the right dose differentiates a poison from a remedy. *Seven Defensiones*

Michel de Montaigne; 1580 **880**

I think of physic as much good or ill as any one would have me: for...we have no traffic together. I am of a quite contrary humour to other men, for I always despise it; but when I am sick, instead of recanting, or entering into composition with it, I begin...to hate and fear it, telling them who importune me to take physic, that at all events they must give me time to recover my strength and health, that I may be the better able to support and encounter the violence and danger of their potions.

Essays. Various Events from the Same Counsel

James I; 1604 **881**

Medicine hath that virtue, that it never leaveth a man in that state wherein it findeth him; it makes a sick man whole but a whole man sick. *A Counter Blaste to Tobacco*

Molière; 1673 **882**

Nearly all men die of their remedies, and not of their diseases.

Le Malade Imaginaire, Act III, Scene iii

Benjamin Franklin; 1733 **883**

He's the best physician that knows the worthlessness of the most medicines.

Poor Richard's Almanac

Peter Mere Latham; 1836 **884**

Poisons and medicines are oftentimes the same substances given with different intents.

General Remarks on the Practice of Medicine

Henry David Thoreau; 1860 **885**

If you look over a list of medicinal recipes in vogue in the last century, how foolish and useless they are seen to be! And yet we use equally absurd ones with faith today.

Journal

Oliver Wendell Holmes; 1860   **886**

No families take so little medicine as those of doctors, except those of apothecaries.

Currents and Counter-Currents in Medical Science

Oliver Wendell Holmes; 1860   **887**

I firmly believe that if the whole materia medica, as now used, could be sunk to the bottom of the sea, it would be all the better for mankind—and all the worse for the fishes.

Currents and Counter-Currents in Medical Science

Oliver Wendell Holmes; 1861   **888**

The disgrace of medicine has been that colossal system of self-deception, in obedience to which mines have been emptied of their cankering minerals, the vegetable kingdom robbed of all its noxious growths, the entrails of animals taxed for their impurities, the poison-bags of reptiles drained of their venom, and all the inconceivable abominations thus obtained thrust down the throats of human beings suffering from some fault of organization, nourishment, or vital stimulation.   *Border Lines of Knowledge*

William Osler; 1895   **889**

But know also, man has an inborn craving for medicine. Generations of heroic dosing have given his tissues such a thirst...for drugs. As I once before remarked, the desire to take medicine is one feature which distinguishes man, the animal, from his fellow creatures. It is really one of the most serious difficulties with which we have to contend. Even in minor ailments, which would yield to dieting or to simple home remedies, the doctor's visit is not thought to be complete without the prescription.   *Teaching and Thinking*

William Osler; 1903   **890**

Remember how much you do not know. Do not pour strange medicines into your patients.   *Aphorisms*

William Osler; 1903   **891**

The young physician starts life with twenty drugs for each disease, and the old physician ends life with one drug for twenty diseases.   *Aphorisms*

Ambrose Bierce; 1906   **892**

Medicine, *n.* A stone flung down the Bowery to kill a dog in Broadway.

The Devil's Dictionary

Henry Louis Mencken; 1956   **893**

A fool who, after plain warning, persists in dosing himself with dangerous drugs should be free to do so, for his death is a benefit to the race in general.

Minority Report: H. L. Mencken's Notebooks

Henry Louis Mencken; 1956   **894**

[It] is undoubtedly a proper function of government to protect people against impostures that they cannot penetrate themselves. [On the Pure Food and Drugs Act]

Minority Report: H.L. Mencken's Notebooks

Eugene A. Stead Jr.; 1968   **895**

The weller you are the more drugs you can take without getting sick. That's why doctors don't get into more trouble than they do with therapy.   *Annals of Internal Medicine*

John Lister; 1975   **896**

I remembered an Irish woman who once said to me, "You know, if only you doctors could find a cure for these wretched antibiotics, you would be doing us all a good turn, and anyway all of my family in Ireland died wither of T. B. or D.T.'s and they were a damned sight happier than us lot being kept alive with your lousy drugs."

New England Journal of Medicine

Kurt Kroenke; 1985   **897**
The human's "desire to take medicine" carries, however, a price tag. Nature's maladies are succeeded by iatrogenic hazards. Arising out of a restorative instinct, polypharmacy becomes itself an affliction.   *American Journal of Medicine*

Zeljko Poljak   **898**
Polypharmacy is a prosthesis for the physician's incompetence. The less he knows, the more prescriptions he writes.   *Loknar V, Croatian Medical Quotations*

Russian proverb   **899**
Expensive medicines are always good: if not for the patient, at least for the druggist.
    Proverb

DUPUYTREN CONTRACTION

Guillaume Dupuytren; 1833   **900**
Individuals pre-disposed to the affection we are describing, observe that it is more difficult to extend the fingers of the affected hand.... The first [interphalangeal joint] is flexed at nearly a right angle...the most powerful efforts are insufficient to extend it.... Hence, it was natural to conclude, that the commencement of the disease was in the unusual tension of the palmar aponeurosis.   *Permanent Retraction of the Fingers*

DYING

Aesop; *circa* 500 BC   **901**
An Old Man was employed in cutting wood in the forest, and, in carrying the faggots to the city for sale one day, became very wearied with his long journey. He sat down by the wayside, and throwing down his load, besought Death to come. "Death" immediately appeared in answer to his summons and asked for what reason he had called him. The Old Man hurriedly replied, "That, lifting up the load, you may place it again on my shoulders."   *The Old Man and Death*

Plato; [427-347 BC]   **902**
That which takes place according to nature is pleasant, but that which is contrary to nature is painful. And thus death, if caused by disease or produced by wounds, is painful and violent; but that sort of death which comes with old age and fulfils the debt of nature is the easiest of deaths, and is accompanied with pleasure rather than with pain.
    Dialogues. Timaeus

Desiderius Erasmus; 1518   **903**
The road leading up to death is harder than death itself. If a man dismisses from his thought the horror and imagination of death, he will have rid himself of a great part of the evil.... Awareness of death... is either nonexistent or else an extremely low-grade awareness, because before Nature reaches this point it dulls and stuns all areas of sensation.   *Colloquies. The Funeral*

Michel de Montaigne; 1580   **904**
In the judgement I make of another man's life, I always observe how he carried himself at his death; and the principal concern I have for my own is that I may die well—that is, patiently and tranquilly.   *Essays. That We Should Not Judge of Our Happiness Until After Death*

John Webster; 1612   **905**
Death hath ten thousand several doors
For men to take their exits.   *The Duchess of Malfi*

William Hunter; 1783   **906**
If I had strength enough left to hold a pen,...I would write how easy and pleasant a thing it is to die.   *British Medical Journal*

Johann Wolfgang von Goethe; [1749-1832]   **907**
My bundle [is] packed, and I am waiting for the order to march off.

Nager F, Der Heilkundige Dichter

Søren Kierkegaard; [1813-1855]   **908**
To die well is the height of wisdom of life.   *Basta LL, A Graceful Exit*

Joseph W. Freer; 1862   **909**
Even in the stage of dying the physician should not forsake the sick, for even then he may
become a benefactor, and if he cannot save, may at least relieve departing life.

Valedictory address

Matthew Arnold; 1867   **910**
Nor bring, to see me cease to live,
Some doctor full of phrase and fame,
To shake his sapient head and give
The ill he cannot cure a name.   *A Wish*

Oliver Wendell Holmes; 1891   **911**
Old age leaps upon [the nose] as his saddle, and rides triumphant, unchallenged, until
the darkness comes which no glasses can penetrate. Nature is pitiless in carrying out the
universal sentence, but very pitiful in her mode of dealing with the condemned on his way
to the final scene.   *Over the Teacups*

William Osler; 1897   **912**
Cease then, and let me alone. For generations has not this been [the sick man's]
immemorial privilege, a privilege with vested rights as a deep-seated animal instinct—to
turn his face to the wall, to sicken in peace and, if he so wishes, to die undisturbed.

Aequanimitas. Nurse and Patient

William Osler; 1904   **913**
I have careful records of about five hundred death-beds.... Ninety suffered bodily pain or
distress of one kind or another, eleven showed mental apprehension, two positive terror,
one expressed spiritual exaltation, one bitter remorse. The great majority gave no sign one
way or the other; like their birth their death was a sleep and a forgetting.

A Study of Death

Maria Rainer Rilke; 1905   **914**
God, give us each our own death,
the dying that proceeds
from each of our lives:
the way we loved,
the meanings we made,
our need.   *On Poverty and Death*

Thomas Mann; 1922   **915**
A man's dying is more the survivors' affair than his own.   *The Magic Mountain*

Santiago Ramón y Cajal; [1852-1934]   **916**
It is the great privilege of children to die without knowing that they are dying.

Craigie EH and Gibson WC, The World of Ramón y Cajal

Dylan Thomas; 1951   **917**
Do not go gentle into that good night,
Old age should burn and rave at close of day;
Rage, rage against the dying of the light.   *Do Not Go Gentle into That Good Night*

Richard A. Kern; 1951 **918**

Death comes oftenest at night, especially in the small hours after midnight, when vital forces seem to be at their lowest ebb. In the very old, death often takes over from his brother, sleep. *The Care of the Aged*

Wilder Penfield; 1963 **919**

There are times when compassion should prompt us to forgo prolonged and costly treatment. If a man must die, he has the right to die in peace, as he would prefer to do if asked. Positive action to take a life is not permitted. But the negative decisions that ease and shorten suffering have always been ours to make. *The Second Career*

Elisabeth Kübler-Ross; 1969 **920**

Watching a peaceful death of a human being reminds us of a falling star; one of a million lights in the vast sky that flares up for a brief moment only to disappear into the endless night forever. *On Death and Dying*

Elisabeth Kübler-Ross; 1970 **921**

Those who have the strength and the love to sit with a dying patient in the *silence that goes beyond words* will know that this moment is neither frightening nor painful, but a peaceful cessation of the functioning of the body. *On Death and Dying*

Earle P. Scarlett; 1972 **922**

Moliere...the great dramatist and actor, who detested doctors and pilloried them for the amusement of posterity, when asked if he wanted the doctor to come, replied (as they say) with his last breath: "No, I'm too ill to see him." *Roland CG, In Sickness and in Health*

Stewart Alsop; 1973 **923**

A dying man needs to die, as a sleepy man needs to sleep, and there comes a time when it is wrong, as well as useless, to resist. *Stay of Execution*

Norman Cousins; 1981 **924**

The unbearable tragedy is not death but dying in an alien arena—separated from dignity, separated from the warmth of familiar things, separated from the ever-present ministrations of a loving relationship and an outstretched hand. *Human Options*

Philip Roth; 1983 **925**

Most doctors are frightened of death and the dying. People need an incredible amount of support when they die. And the doctor who is frightened can't give it to them.

The Anatomy Lesson

Norman Cousins; 1989 **926**

It is not uncommon for seriously ill patients, when talking among themselves, to recognize a hierarchy of longevity. Those who have been informed by their physicians that they probably have only three months to live are envious of those who have a year. Patients set goals for themselves.... Attaining these goals can be a great victory—even though a grim outcome is only being postponed. *Head First*

Anthony Burgess; 1990 **927**

If there is only darkness after death, then that darkness is the ultimate reality and that love of life that I intermittently possess is no preparation for it. In face of the approaching blackness, which Winston Churchill facetiously termed black velvet, concerning oneself with a world that is soon to fade out like a television image in a power cut seems mere frivolity. *You've Had Your Time*

Sherwin B. Nuland; 1994 **928**

Modern dying takes place in the modern hospital, where it can be hidden, cleansed of its organic blight, and finally packaged for modern burial. We can now deny the power not only of death but of nature itself. *How We Die*

Sherwin B. Nuland; 1994   **929**

This hope, the assurance that there be no unreasonable efforts, is an affirmation that the dignity to be sought in death is the appreciation by others of what one has been in life. It is a dignity that proceeds from a life well lived and from the acceptance of one's own death as a necessary process of nature that permits our species to continue in the form of our own children and the children of others.... The "real" event taking place at the end of our life is our death, not the attempts to prevent it.   *How We Die*

Lofty L. Basta; 1996   **930**

I know how I do not want to die. I do not want to die in a hospital bed, hooked up to a multitude of tubes that are connected to machines that breathe for me, produce urine on my behalf, or beat in place of my heart. I have had a great life, and I am enjoying the best years of my life. I want to preserve the remainder of it as long as I can, but not at any cost.
                                                                               A Graceful Exit

Philip Roth; 2000   **931**

I began... to envisage the fatal malady that, without anyone's recognizing it, was working away inside us, within each and every one of us: to visualize the blood vessels occluding under the baseball caps, the malignancies growing beneath the permed hair, the organs misfiring, atrophying, shutting down, the hundreds of billions of murderous cells surreptiously marching this entire audience toward the improbable disaster ahead.
                                                                               The Human Stain

Croatian proverb   **932**

When gulps start rattling in the throat, death is close.   *Proverb*

DYSENTERY

William Heberden; 1802   **933**

The Dysentery is common in camps.   *Commentaries on the History and Cure of Diseases*

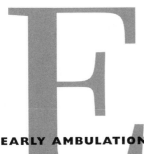

EARLY AMBULATION

Richard Asher; 1947 **934**
Teach us to live that we may dread
Unnecessary time in bed.
Get people up and we may save
Our patients from an early grave. *British Medical Journal*

EATING

Benjamin Franklin; 1733 **935**
Eat to live, and not live to eat. *Poor Richard's Almanac*

[Anonymous]; *circa* 1750 **936**
Who eats slowly, works longer. *Kekez J, Svaki je Kamen da se Kuca Gradi*

ECLAMPSIA

John Charles Weaver Lever; 1843 **937**
In NO cases have I detected albumen, except in those in which there have been convulsions, in or which symptoms have presented themselves, and which are readily recognised
as the precursors of puerpural fits. *Guy's Hospital Report*

EDEMA

William Heberden; 1802 **938**
Where persons after having laboured for some time under complaints of the lungs, or of
the bowels, begin to find a swelling in the legs, it is a sign of some deep mischief in the
breast or abdomen, the swelling will most probably increase to a just dropsy, and the case
end fatally. *Commentaries on the History and Cure of Diseases*

EDUCATION

René-Théophile-Hyacinthe Laennec; 1821   939
People need to have things trumpeted into their ears several times and from all directions. The first sound pricks up the ear, the second shakes it, and with the third, it goes in.

Letter to his cousin Meriadec

Oscar Wilde; 1895   940
I do not approve of anything that tampers with natural ignorance. Ignorance is like a delicate exotic fruit; touch it and the bloom is gone.   *The Importance of Being Earnest, Act I*

William Osler; 1905   941
When a simple, earnest spirit animates a college, there is no appreciable interval between the teacher and the taught—both are in the same class, the one a little more advanced than the other.   *The Student Life*

Henry E. Sigerist; 1943   942
[U]niversity education becomes sterile the moment it is divorced from research.... The professor becomes older every year but his students remain eternally young, and this contact...is a great stimulus to him. It makes him look beyond the boundary of his generation, and he who in his research is working for the future, with and through his students, can help in shaping tomorrow's world.... When he follows them up in their professional life and sees the seed germinating, he feels a satisfaction equal to that of having procreated children.   *The University's Dilemma*

Henry E. Sigerist; 1944   943
Graduate schools, to be sure, must train students for professions, must prepare them to play their part in society as teachers, physicians, scientists, lawyers, ministers, or engineers. But graduate education must be infinitely more than the imparting of technical knowledge. It must be education.   *The University at the Crossroads*

Frances D. Fergusson; 1990   944
What does an undergraduate, liberal arts education offer? I will identify four elements. A liberal arts education emphasizes (1) historical awareness, (2) the ability to think creatively and take risks, (3) an international perspective and global awareness, and (4) ethical responsibility. These guiding goals and values of a liberal arts education are also basic prerequisites to successful engagement in your professions as physicians and researchers.

Mayo Clinic Proceedings

ELECTROCARDIOGRAPHY

Augustus Désiré Waller; 1887   945
If a pair of electrodes (zinc covered by chamois leather and moistened with brine) are strapped to the front and back of the chest, and connected with a Lippmann's capillary electrometer, the mercury in the latter will be seen to move slightly but sharply at each beat of the heart.... The electrical variation precedes the heart's beat.

Journal of Physiology

Willem Einthoven; 1903   946
This instrument—the string galvanometer—is essentially composed of a thin silver-coated quartz filament, which is stretched like a string, in a strong magnetic field. When an electric current is conducted through this quartz filament, the filament reveals a movement which can be observed and photographed by means of considerable magnification.

Archiv für Gesundheit Physiologie

EMBOLISM

William Senhouse Kirkes; 1852   947

The effects produced and the organs affected will be...determined by the side of the heart from which the fibrinous masses have been detached; for if the right valves have furnished the source of the fibrine, the lungs will bear the brunt of the secondary mischief, displaying it in coagula in the pulmonary arteries...but if...the left valves are affected, the mischief...may fall on any systemic part, but especially...the brain, spleen, and kidneys.

Medico-Chirurgical Transactions

Rudolf Ludwig Karl Virchow; 1860   948

Secondary disturbances certainly are very frequently occasioned, but not so much by the immediate introduction of the softened masses as fast as they become liquid into the blood, as by the detachment of larger or smaller fragments from the end of the softening thrombus which are carried along by the current of blood and driven into remote vessels. This gives rise to the very frequent process upon which I have bestowed the name of Embolia.

Cellular Pathology

Thomas Lewis; 1922   949

Many years ago I witnessed for the first time a curious and fatal accident. It occurred in a woman suffering from mitral stenosis and heart failure. This woman acquired an attack of fibrillation of the auricles which lasted for several days and then suddenly ended; when it ended, clots were detached from the heart, which produced multiple embolism of the lungs and brain, and these led quickly to a fatal termination. Fibrillation of the auricles predisposes to clotting in the auricular appendices.

American Journal of the Medical Sciences

EMBRYO

Hildegard of Bingen; *circa* 1150   950

After the man's semen has fallen into its place so that it must be molded into a human form, from the woman's menstrual blood a fine skin, like a small vessel, will grow around that form and hold and surround it so that it may not be moved or fall, because the coagulated blood collects there so that this form lies in its middle, like a person in the shelter of his house.

Causae et Curae

EMBRYOLOGY

Kaspar Friedrich Wolff; 1759   951

From the theory of epigenesis we deduce that the parts of the body have not pre-existed but that they were formed gradually. This does not happen through an accumulation of small particles, or through any type of fermentation, or due to mechanical causes, or through the action of the soul. The basis for development of the parts...are only rudiments which later will be transformed into the differentiated structures of the body.

Theoria Generationis

EMOTIONAL DISORDERS

George Cheyne; 1733   952

The Title I have chosen... is a Reproach... thrown on this Island by Foreigners... by whom nervous Distempers, Spleen, Vapours, and Lowness of Spirits, are in Derision, called the ENGLISH MALADY.... The Richness and Heaviness of our Food, the Wealth and Abundance of the Inhabitants... the Inactivity and Sedentary Occupations of the better Sort... and the Humor of living in great, populous and consequently unhealthy Towns, have brought forth a Class and Set of Distempers... scarce known in our Ancestors.... These nervous disorders being computed to make almost one third of the Complaints of the People of Condition in England.

The English Malady

EMOTIONAL GROWTH

Sigmund Freud; 1924   **953**

The little girl likes to regard herself as what her father loves above all else; but the time comes when she has to endure a harsh punishment from him and she is cast out of her fool's paradise. The boy regards his mother as his own property; but he finds one day that she has transferred her love and solicitude to a new arrival.

The Dissolution of the Oedipus Complex

EMPATHY

Charles D. Aring; 1958   **954**

The act or capacity of entering into or sharing the feelings of another is known as sympathy. Empathy, on the other hand, not only is an identification of sorts but also connotes an awareness of one's separateness from the observed. One of the most difficult tasks put upon man is reflective commitment to another's problem while maintaining his own identity.... A subtle and significant feature of a happy medical practice is to remain unencumbered by the patient's problems. *Journal of the American Medical Association*

Howard Spiro; 1992   **955**

Empathy is the "almost magical" emotion that persons or objects arouse in us as projections of our feelings.... Medical students lose some of their empathy as they learn science and detachment, and hospital residents lose the remainder in the weariness of overwork and in the isolation of the intensive care units that modern hospitals have become.

Annals of Internal Medicine

Howard Spiro; 1992   **956**

Empathy is the feeling that persons or objects arose in us as projections of our feelings and thoughts. It is evident when "I and you" becomes "I *am* you," or at least "I might be you." *Annals of Internal Medicine*

EMPYEMA

Hippocrates; [460-375 BC]   **957**

If sufferers from pleurisy do not cough up material within fourteen days, the inflammation produces empyema... If those patients in whom pleurisy has resulted in empyema evacuate the abscess by expectoration within forty days following its bursting, they recover. If this is not so, they become consumptive. *Aphorisms*

Hippocrates; [460-375 BC]   **958**

Empyema may be recognized in all cases by the following symptoms: In the first place, the fever does not go off, but is slight during the day, and increases at night, and copious sweats intervene, there is a desire to cough, and the patients expectorate nothing worth mentioning, the eyes become hollow...the nails of the hand are bent, the fingers are hot.

The Book of Prognostics

ENDOCARDITIS

Jean-Baptiste Bouillaud; 1841   **959**

[The name] *endocarditis*, which I have given to inflammation of the inner membrane of the heart in general, appears to me, according to all reports, to conform to the principles of nomenclature universally adopted today. I will propose that of cardiovalvulitis to designate especially inflammation of the valves of the heart, which are, as everyone knows, essentially formed of a fibrous tissue upon which is folded back the endocardium or internal membrane of the heart. One can thus give to this local disease the name valvular endocarditis. *Traité Clinique de Maladies du Coeur*

ENVIRONMENT

Aldous Huxley; 1961   960
We ought to love the whole planet and treat it as though it were a vulnerable living organ-ism, refraining scrupulously from all those outrages against nature which have turned so much of the once fertile earth into treeless and eroded deserts, have befouled so much of what was once beautiful with excrement, industrial wastes and slums. Love is as neces-sary for human survival and growth as are bread on the physical and knowledge on the symbolic level.   *The Humanist Frame*

René Jules Dubos; 1968   961
Man is more the product of his environment than of his genetic endowment. The health of human beings is determined not by their race but by the conditions under which they live.   *Man, Medicine, and Environment*

René Jules Dubos; 1968   962
Physiologists, psychologists, psychiatrists, and writers have described, each in his own way, a seemingly endless variety of acquired responses, ranging from the salivation of dogs at the sound of a bell to the pathological effects of the Freudian complexes, or the remem-brance of things past evoked by a madeleine dipped into a cup of tea.
Man, Medicine, and Environment

René Jules Dubos; 1968   963
It is a dangerous error to believe that disease and suffering can be wiped out altogether by raising still further the standards of living, increasing our mastery of the environment, and developing new therapeutic procedures. The less pleasant reality is that, since the world is ever changing, each period and each type of civilization will continue to have its burden of diseases created by the unavoidable failure of biological and social adaptation to counter new environmental threats.   *Man, Medicine, and Environment*

Robertson Davies; 1994   964
I make house calls.... I want to see where my patients live...which tell[s] much about the quality of life they experience.... All these details are to me elements in a diagnosis.... The doctor who refuses to make house calls cannot hope for my sort of medical awareness.
The Cunning Man

ENVIRONMENTAL ILLNESS

René Jules Dubos; 1968   965
During recent decades we have gone far toward controlling microbial spoilage of food, but some of the new synthetic products ubiquitous in modern life are responsible for an end-less variety of allergic and toxic effects.   *Man, Medicine, and Environment*

ENZYMES

Frederick Gowland Hopkins; 1913   966
We have arrived... at a stage when, with a huge array of examples before us, it is logical to conclude that all metabolic tissue reactions are catalyzed by enzymes.   *Lecture*

EPIDEMICS

John Brownlee; 1908   967
Epidemics are caused by various kinds of organisms both plant and animal. It is to be noticed that the same law applies indifferently whatever the source of the infection. It applies to the bacilli of plague and enteric fever, to the spirillum of cholera, to the para-sites of small pox, probably protozoal, and to those of yellow fever almost certainly pro-tozoal.   *Germinal Vitality*

EPIDEMIOLOGY

Paul Dudley White; 1959   968
Nature has for centuries been conducting gigantic experiments as to the effect of climate, of type of work, of diet, and of local or worldwide diseases on men, women, and children of different races, that are spread out before our very eyes for us to record and to analyze, quite readily yielding information that might never be obtainable by our own experiments on man.   *Patterns of Incidence of Certain Diseases*

EPILEPSY

Hippocrates; [460-375 BC]   969
The patient loses his speech, and chokes, and foam issues from the mouth, the teeth are fixed, the hands are contracted, the eyes distorted, he becomes insensible, and in some cases the bowels are evacuated.   *On the Sacred Disease*

Hippocrates; [460-375 BC]   970
The disease called Sacred...appears to me to be nowise more divine nor more sacred than other diseases, but has the natural cause from which it originates like other affections. Men regard its nature and cause as divine from ignorance and wonder, because it is not at all like to other diseases.   *On the Sacred Disease*

Aretaeus the Cappadocian; [81-138?]   971
The person lies insensible.... The tongue protrudes, so as to incur the risk of a great wound, or of a piece of it being cut off, should the teeth come forcibly together with the spasm.... The utterance a moaning and lamentation.... When they come to the termination of the illness, there are unconscious discharges of the urine, and watery discharges from the bowels.... At the termination, they are torpid in their members at first, experience heaviness in the head...and are languid, pale, spiritless and dejected.   *On Epilepsy*

Galen; [130-200]   972
Certainly epilepsy is a convulsion of all parts of the body, not continuous as...tetanus, but occurring at intervals. Epilepsy is not only different in this manner from spasm but also because the intellect and sensory perception are damaged. From this it becomes evident that the origin of this ailment resides somewhere high up in the brain.   *On the Affected Parts*

Hildegard of Bingen; *circa* 1150   973
The body falls to the ground and remains there as if dead until the soul has regained its powers.... When they fall to the ground, thrown down by this illness, they sometimes let out a sound that sounds rather mournful and natural and they froth a lot at the mouth.   *Causae et Curae*

William Shakespeare; 1599   974
Cassius. But soft, I pray you: what, did Caesar swound?
Casca. He fell down in the market-place, and foamed at mouth, and was speechless.
Brutus. 'Tis very like: he hath the falling sickness.   *Julius Caesar, Act I, Scene ii*

Cotton Mather; 1724   975
The *Spectator*, beholding one arrested with an *Epilepsy*, thrown down on the Ground with a Sudden Abolition of Sense, the Eyes distorted, the Mouth perhaps foaming, the Face with an Aspect full of Agony, and *Convulsive Motions* of the Limbs, from a depraved *Lympha* mixing with the Animal Spirits in the *Brain*, and thence issuing forth with an Irritation of the Nerves.... How can he but say, *Mine Eye affecteth mine Heart.... Lord, How Thankful should I be, in that I am Spared*!   *The Angel of Bethesda*

William Heberden; 1802   976
The fit makes the patient fall down senseless; and without his will or consciousness presently every muscle is put in action, as if all the powers of the body were exerted to free

itself from some great violence.... The urine, excrements, and seed, are sometimes forced away, and the mouth is covered with foam, which will be bloody, when the tongue has been bitten, as it often is in the agony.   *Commentaries on the History and Cure of Diseases*

John Hughlings Jackson; 1864   977
I have recorded the case of a man who had fits beginning in his left foot. The first shock was from the base of the great toe; he became insensible and was not, he told me, locally paralysed after the paroxysms. At length he found that he could stop his fits, prevent the convulsions spreading, or rather that his son could, by rubbing the calf (the spasm being by the procedures adopted kept to the leg); then the leg was always temporarily paralysed after each seizure.   *The Medical Times and Gazette*

John Hughlings Jackson; 1864   978
I suppose that in cases of epilepsy and of epileptiform seizures there is a very local discharge-lesion (physiological fulminate) of a few highly unstable cells of one half of the brain.   *The Medical Times and Gazette*

John Shaw Billings; [1838-1913]   979
If [the operation] does not prove immediately fatal, and he reports the case early, say within the first month, it will in very many cases come into the list of cases of epilepsy cured by surgical treatment.   *Garrison FH, John Shaw Billings: A Memoir*

Henry George Miller; 1968   980
A fit during sleep is epilepsy unless proved otherwise.   *World Neurology*

EPINEPHRINE (ADRENALINE)

George Oliver; 1895   981
The suprarenal capsules yield to water (cold or hot), to alcohol or to glycerine a substance which exerts a most powerful action upon the blood vessels, upon the heart, and upon the skeletal muscles.... *The effect upon the blood vessels* is to cause extreme contraction of the arteries, so that the blood-pressure is enormously raised.   *Journal of Physiology*

John Jacob Abel, Albert Cornelius Crawford; 1897   982
We have now obtained the active [blood-raising] principle [of the suprarenal capsule] in the form of a sulfate.... Our sulfate is very active physiologically. A small quantity suffices to raise the blood pressure... and it is therefore evident that we have isolated the active principle.   *Bulletin of the Johns Hopkins Hospital*

John Jacob Abel; 1899   983
The principle produced by the adrenal body that raises and supports blood-pressure is a special basic substance whose percentage composition is expressed by $C_{17}H_{15}NO_4$ and which I name *epinephrin*.   *Hoppe-Seyl Z. Physiol. Chem.*

Thomas Bell Aldrich; 1901   984
The most recent and in many respects the most important principle of the suprerenal gland, although not exhaustive, is from Dr. Jokichi Takamine [Takamine: Therapeutic Gazette, 1901:221] who has isolated the blood-pressure raising principle of the gland in a stable and pure crystalline form, by a method which he claims to be entirely different from any employed. To this body which is very active in raising the blood pressure, he has given the name *Adrenalin*.   *American Journal of Physiology*

EPONYMS

William R. Gowers; 1884   985
I have avoided the use of these [eponymic] terms. This system of nomenclature is full of inconvenience, increasing the difficulties of the student, and leading to frequent mistakes in scientific writings. There are very few observations in medicine regarding which it is not

obvious that they would speedily have been made by some one other than the actual observer; that it was very much of an accident that they were made by certain individuals.

The Diagnosis of Diseases of the Spinal Cord

Fuller Albright; 1947   **986**

The use of a person's name for the designation of a syndrome has objections, the chief one being that no one can decide whose name to use. One can always go to the literature and find some preceding reference to a case which in all likelihood had the syndrome in question. Often each language produces its own "first" describer.

Journal of Clinical Endocrinology

EQUANIMITY

William Osler; 1889   **987**

From its very nature this precious quality [imperturbability] is liable to be misinterpreted, and the general accusation of hardness, so often brought against the profession, has here its foundation.   *Aequanimitas. Aequanimitas*

William Osler; 1889   **988**

One of the first essentials in securing a good-natured equanimity is not to expect too much of the people amongst whom you dwell.   *Aequanimitas. Aequanimitas*

William Osler; 1903   **989**

Things cannot always go your way. Learn to accept in silence the minor aggravations, cultivate the gift of taciturnity and consume your own smoke with an extra draught of hard work, so that those about you may not be annoyed with the dust and soot of your complaints.   *The Master-word in Medicine*

Howard Spiro; 1992   **990**

Should equanimity be so widely praised for all physicians? Detachment has been much lauded since Osler, but is it as helpful to the internist as to the surgeon? Whom does it help? Too much emotion in medical practice can be destructive; passion needs control. However, these matters need discussion as much as do somatostatin receptors.

Annals of Internal Medicine

Alfred Cox; Unknown   **991**

Like most preachers[William Osler] did not always practice what he preached. His wife, in a memoir she wrote of him, says.... "It was all very well of William to preach Aequanimitas but I notice that when there was trouble at home,...he invariably had important engagements elsewhere and left me to cultivate the quiet mind—if I could."

Manning PR, Medicine: Preserving the Passion

ERGOT

John Stearns; 1808   **992**

It expedites lingering parturition, and saves to the accoucheur a considerable portion of time, without producing any bad effects on the patient.... In most cases you will be surprised with the suddenness of its operation.... Since I have adopted the use of this powder I have seldom found a case that detained me more than three hours.... It is a vegetable, and appears to be a spurious growth of rye.   *New York Medical Repository*

ERRORS

Hippocrates; [460-375 BC]   **993**

I know that the common herd of physicians, like the vulgar, if there happen to have been any innovation made about that day, such as the bath being used, a walk taken, or any unusual food eaten, all which were better done than otherwise, attribute notwithstanding the cause of these disorders, to some of these things, being ignorant of the true cause, but proscribing what may have been very proper.   *On Ancient Medicine*

Galen; [130-200]   **994**
Many physicians who clearly see a fact they cannot explain simply deny that it exists.
On the Affected Parts

William Osler; 1892   **995**
Start out with the conviction that absolute truth is hard to reach in matters relating to our fellow creatures, healthy or diseased, that slips in observation are inevitable even with the best trained faculties, that errors in judgement must occur in the practice of an art which consists largely in balancing probabilities—start, I say, with this attitude of mind.... You will draw from your errors the very lessons which may enable you to avoid their repetition.   *Teacher and Student*

ERYTHROBLASTOSIS FETALIS

Philip Levine, Lyman Burnham, E.M. Katzin, Peter Vogel; 1941   **996**
In 93 per cent of the cases investigated, erythroblastosis fetalis results from the iso-immunization of the Rh-mother by the Rh factor in the red blood cells of the fetus.
American Journal of Obstetrics and Gynecology

Louis Klein Diamond; 1948   **997**
The removal of as much as possible of the baby's own blood should theoretically help diminish the damage resulting from the presence of this free and bound [maternal anti-Rh agglutinins] in the circulation and in the tissues. Such reasoning led to the trial of replacement transfusion.... For an evaluation of our present mode of therapy, we have statistics collected over the past 15 years or more.... Of the 85 infants treated by umbilical vein replacement transfusion, 65 are now living and well and show no evidence of residual damage.... Our statistics...show close to a 90% recovery rate.   *Pediatrics*

ERYTHROMELALGIA (MITCHELL'S DISEASE)

Silas Weir Mitchell; 1878   **998**
The patient...begins to suffer with pain in the foot or feet.... In the mass of instances...the pain is of a burning character.... The next striking peculiarity...is the flushing of the part upon exertion.... In the worst cases, when the patient is at rest, the limbs are cold, and even pale.
Philadelphia Medical Times

ESMARCH BANDAGE

Johann Friedrich August von Esmarch; 1873   **999**
We wrap the legs tightly from the toes to above the knees, with elastic bandages made from woven rubber, forcing the blood out of the vessels of the limb by an even compression. Then we apply rubber tubing tightly, four or five times around the upper thigh...where the bandage stops,...in such a manner that not one drop of blood can enter the parts below it.... The patient [in the course of operation on the limb] has lost no more than a teaspoonful of blood!   *Sammlung von Klinische Vorträge*

ESOPHAGEAL ACHALASIA

Henry Stanley Plummer; 1908   **1000**
The symptom-complex in cardiospasm [the term by which esophageal achalasia was formerly known] is as a rule almost pathognomonic. It may be divided into the three stages...first, cardiospasm without food regurgitation; second, cardiospasm with immediate food regurgitation; third, cardiospasm with dilated esophagus, the retention of food in the dilated portion and its regurgitation at irregular intervals after taking.
Journal of the American Medical Association

ESOPHAGEAL TUBE FEEDING

Thomas Willis; 1674   1001

At length the Disease having overcome all remedies, he was brought into that condition, that growing hungry he would eat until the *Oesophagus* was filled up to the Throat, in the mean time nothing sliding down into the Ventricle.... Presently putting this [device] down in the *Oesophagus*, he did thrust down into the Ventricle, its Orifice being opened, the Food which otherwise would have come back again.... Without doubt in this case the Mouth of the Stomach being always closed, either by a Tumour or Palsie, nothing could be admitted into the Ventricle unless it were violently opened.   *Pharmaceutice Rationalis*

ETHNIC STEREOTYPING

Richard C. Cabot; 1909   1002

[T]he chances are ten to one that I shall look out of my eyes and see, not Abraham Cohen, but a Jew.... I do not see this man at all. I merge him in the hazy background of the average Jew.... He [is] no more real than the thousands of others whom I had seen and forgotten—because I never saw *them*, but only their ghostly outline, their generic type, the racial background out of which they emerged.   *Social Service and the Art of Healing*

EUGENICS

William E. Seidelman; 1991   1003

Eugenics arose from a scientific curiosity about human differences: poverty, health, height, intelligence, behavior. Scientific inquiry extended itself into what were considered to be racial differences, which included not only physical differences, but also cultural and religious differences. Scientific racism predated, paralleled, and eventually merged with eugenics. While not all eugenicists were necessarily racist, the eugenic rationale provided an acceptable intellectual and scientific basis for scientific racism. Physicians played important roles in the development of scientific racism.

International Journal of Health Services

EUTHANASIA

William Shakespeare; 1595   1004

Now put it, God, in the physician's mind
To help him to his grave immediately!   *Richard II, Act I, Scene iv*

Richard A. Kern; 1951   1005

Should the physician ever speed the end and so reduce the patient's suffering? No. Custom, tradition, experience, social sanction, law, and religion are unanimous in this, and rightly so. Euthanasia would be a long step backward in civilization.

The Care of the Aged

Sherwin B. Nuland; 1994   1006

The guild of Hippocrates should not develop a new specialty of accoucheurs to the grave so that conscience-stricken oncologists, surgeons, and other physicians may refer to others those who wish to exit the planet.   *How We Die*

EVIDENCE

Kathryn Montgomery Hunter; 1991   1007

The danger as always is anecdotalism, the inherent deception of drawing a broad generalization from very few cases. A perjorative cloud hangs over the anecdote in medicine. Exceptions are allowed: there seems to be little danger in the illustrative use of a similar case during the discussion of a differential diagnosis or in the citation of a notable exception as a cautionary example that marks the limits of a topic under discussion.   *Doctor's Stories*

Sherwin B. Nuland; 1998   **1008**

What of the allegedly indisputable nature of the evidence on which so much of the so-called scientific medicine is based? On close inspection, much of that turns out to be disputable and even undependable. In a word, uncertain.   *The Uncertain Art: Prooemium*

EVOLUTION

Peter Mark Roget; 1834   **1009**

Thus we find that each new form which arises, in following the ascending scale of creation, retains a strong affinity to that which had preceded it, and also tends to impress its own features on those which immediately succeed.   *Animal and Vegetable Physiology*

William Osler; 1894   **1010**

In no way has biological science so widened the thoughts of men as in its application to social problems. That throughout the ages, in the gradual evolution of life, one unceasing purpose runs; that progress comes through unceasing competition, through unceasing selection and rejection; in a word, that evolution is the one great law controlling all living things, "the one divine event to which the whole creation moves," this conception has been the great gift of biology to the nineteenth century.   *The Leaven of Science*

René Jules Dubos; 1968   **1011**

Modern man can so manipulate his environment and the conditions of his life to minimize the effects of genetic abnormalities and postpone death from the diseases they cause. Needless to say, such manipulations interfere with or prevent altogether the operation of natural selective processes.   *Man, Medicine, and Environment*

Lewis Thomas; 1977   **1012**

We need now to be examining more closely the evolution of the whole system of living things, the entire spectacularly coherent structure of the biosphere. There is a grand harmony in this massive arrangement, and we are all aware of it.

New England Journal of Medicine

Matko Marusic; 1987   **1013**

There is no life without death because there is no adaptation without selection.

Lijecnicki Vjesnik

EWING SARCOMA

James Ewing; 1921   **1014**

There is a rather common tumor occurring in young subjects, commonly identified with osteogenic sarcoma, and usually called round cell sarcoma, which is really of endothelial origin, and which is marked by such peculiar gross anatomical, clinical, and therapeutic features as to constitute a specific neoplastic disease of bone.

Proceedings of the New York Pathological Society

EXAMINATION

Archimathaeus; *circa* 1100   **1015**

The fingers should be kept on the pulse at least until the hundredth beat in order to judge of its kind and character; the friends standing round will be all the more impressed because of the delay, and the physician's words will be received with just that much more attention.   *The Coming of a Physician to His Patient*

John A. Kolmer; 1961   **1016**

No clinical or laboratory examination can be better than the thoroughness and skill with which it is conducted.   *Clinical Diagnosis by Laboratory Examinations*

EXERCISE

Moses Maimonides; 1198   **1017**

Nothing is to be found that can substitute for exercise in any way.... Exercise will expel the harm done by most of the bad regimens that most men follow. Not all motion is exercise. Exercise is powerful or rapid motion or a combination of both, vigorous motion which alters breathing and increases its rate.   *Regimen of Health*

John Dryden; 1700   **1018**

Better to hunt in fields, for health unbought,
Than fee the doctor for a nauseous draught.
The wise, for cure, on exercise depend;
God never made his work for man to mend.   *Epistle to John Driden of Chesterton*

Tobias Smollett; 1771   **1019**

I am persuaded that all valetudinarians are too sedentary, too regular, and too cautious— We should sometimes increase the motion of the machine, to unclog the wheels of life.   *Humphry Clinker*

George Frank Lydston; 1893   **1020**

Athletics for health should be the motto of the man who trains. Athletics for big muscles and competitive feats of strength and endurance are pernicious, illogical, and dangerous.   *Journal of the American Medical Association*

George Frank Lydston; 1893   **1021**

A man may use dumb bells and think of the price of wheat; if, however, he is engaged in boxing, wrestling, fencing, base ball, hand ball or tennis, he is apt to pay strict attention to the subject in hand.   *Journal of the American Medical Association*

Bruce B. Dan; 1984   **1022**

Sedentary people have shriveled hearts and most of us who do not exercise have an atrophied body.   *Lyons RD, The New York Times*

Barbara Ehrenreich; 1990   **1023**

Exercise is the yuppie version of bulimia.   *Worst Years of Our Lives*

EXOPHTHALMOS

Carl Adolph von Basedow; 1840   **1024**

Exophthalmos is to be differentiated from prolapsus bulbi caused by injury to the muscular retention apparatus (always associated with swelling and disease of the neighboring soft and hard coats of the eye ball), from osteomalacia, periostitis, exostosis, polypous disease of the frontal, antrum, and ethmoidal sinuses, tumors of the brain, cystic tumors of the orbit, scirrhous tumor of the lacrymal glands, trauma, ecchymosis and inflammatory swellings of the cellular tissue in the orbit.   *Wochenschrift für die Gesamte Heilkunde*

EXPERIENCE

Paracelsus (Theophrastus Bombastus von Hohenheim); *circa* 1538   **1025**

The book of Nature is that which the physician must read; and to do so he must walk over the leaves.   *Seven Defensiones*

Michel de Montaigne; 1588   **1026**

And physic itself professes always to have experience for the test of its operations; so Plato had reason to say that, to be a right physician, it would be necessary that he who would become such, should first himself have passed through all the diseases he pretends to cure.... I should put myself into such hands; the others but guide us, like him who paints seas and rocks and ports sitting at table, and there makes the model of a ship sailing in all security; but put him to the work itself, he knows not at which end to begin.   *Essays. Of Experience*

Peter Mere Latham; 1836   1027

We physicians had need be a self-confronting and a self-reproving race; for we must be ready, without fear or favour, to call in question our own Experience and to judge it justly; to confirm it, to repeat it, to reverse it.   *General Remarks on the Practice of Medicine*

George Bernard Shaw; 1906   1028

Mind you, that you have a sound scientific theory to correlate your observations at the bedside. Mere experience by itself is nothing. If I take my dog to the bedside with me, he sees what I see. But he learns nothing from it. Why? Because he's not a scientific dog.   *The Doctor's Dilemma, Act I*

John Chalmers Da Costa; 1915   1029

Each one of us, however old, is still an undergraduate in the school of experience. When a man thinks he has graduated, he becomes a public menace.   *New York Medical Journal*

William J. Mayo; 1921   1030

Experience is the great teacher; unfortunately, experience leaves mental scars, and scar tissue contracts.   *Journal of the American Medical Association*

Wilfred Batten Lewis Trotter; 1932   1031

An event experienced is an event perceived, digested, and assimilated into the substance of our being, and the ratio between the number of cases seen and the number of cases assimilated is the measure of experience.   *Art and Science in Medicine*

EXPERIMENTS

Claude Bernard; 1878   1032

We must not deceive ourselves, morals do not forbid making experiments on one's neighbor or on one's self; in everyday life men do nothing but experiment on one another. Christian morals forbid only one thing, doing ill to one's neighbor. So, among the experiments that may be tried on man, those that can only harm are forbidden, those that are innocent are permissible, and those that may do good are obligatory.   *An Introduction to the Study of Experimental Medicine*

Wilhelm Conrad Röntgen; 1894   1033

The experiment is the most powerful and most reliable lever enabling us to extract secrets from nature.... The experiment must constitute the final judgment as to whether a hypothesis should be retained or be discarded.   *Glasser O, The Early History of the Roentgen Rays*

William Maddock Bayliss, Ernest Henry Starling; 1899   1034

Although in many cases we have been able to explain the results obtained by previous observers by reference to one or other of the disturbing conditions mentioned above [i.e., to the physiology of the intestine], we must confess that in some instances we have been absolutely unable to reproduce effects described by physiologists of repute, however we might vary our method of experiment; and we have had to come to the unsatisfactory conclusion that these results [i.e., of earlier authors] were due to fallacy of observation or experimental methods.   *Journal of Physiology*

EXTRASYSTOLES

James Mackenzie; 1902   1035

In many cases the finger fails to recognize the small pulse beat due to an early occurring systole. In such cases it is usual to assume that either the heart has missed a beat, or that it has sent on a wave too small to be recognized. What usually happens is that the ventricle has made a premature systole, but the force has been so small that it has not been able to overcome the pressure in the aorta...or that having done so, the wave of blood sent forth has not been of sufficient strength to be felt by the finger.   *The Study of the Pulse*

James Mackenzie; 1902 **1036**

The ventricle has made a premature systole, but the force has been so small that it has not been able to overcome the pressure in the aorta and open the aortic valves.... If the heart be auscultated there will be heard the two short, sharp sounds...occurring at the beginning of the long pause, and caused by the rapid premature systole of the ventricle.

The Study of the Pulse

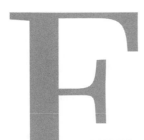

FALLOPIAN TUBES

Gabriele Falloppio; 1561   **1037**

That slender and narrow seminal passage arises from the horn of the uterus very white
and sinewy but after it has passed outward a little way it becomes gradually broader and
curls like the tendrils of a vine until it comes near the end when the tendril-like curls
spread out and it terminates in a very broad ending which appears membranous and
fleshy on account of its reddish colour.

Fulton JF, Selected Readings in the History of Physiology

FAMILIES

Benjamin Rush; 1801   **1038**

Our business leads us daily into the abodes of pain and misery. It obliges us likewise, frequently to witness the fears with which our friends leave the world, and the anguish which
follows, in their surviving relatives. A pious word, dropped from the lips of a physician in
such circumstances of his patients, often does more good than a long, and perhaps an
ingenious discourse from another person, inasmuch as it falls upon the heart, in the
moment of its deepest depression from grief.   *The Vices and Virtues of Physicians*

Santiago Ramón y Cajal; 1920   **1039**

Try to honor your children lest they dishonor you.   *Chatting over Coffee*

Edward Shorter; 1975   **1040**

The nuclear family is crumbling—to be replaced...by the free-floating couple, a marital
dyad subject to dramatic fissions and fusions, and without the orbiting satellites of puber-
tal children, close friends, or neighbors...just the relatives, hovering in the background,
friendly smiles on their faces.   *The Making of the Modern Family*

Joseph Bellina, Josleen Wilson; 1986   **1041**

Call it cosmic spark or spiritual fulfillment, biological need or human destiny—the desire
for a family rises unbidden from our genetic souls. In centuries past, to multiply was to
prevail—the family was stronger, and better able to survive than the individual.

The Fertility Handbook

Robert Pope; 1991   **1042**

When I was told that my cancer had left me with a twenty per cent chance of living, I began to evaluate my life seriously for the first time.... I came to see that I had placed too much importance on work and discovered that the real value in my life came from relationships with family and friends. Our lives can easily become rote: we can often act like somnambulists rather than being fully alive. A disease can wake us up and make us want to enrich our lives.   *Illness and Healing*

John Updike; 1998   **1043**

Love takes many forms outside the narrow groove of copulative heterosexual relations. Any close family seethes with it, and with jealousy, possessiveness, and the resentments bred of interdependence.   *The New Yorker*

FAMILY DOCTORS

John Hamilcar Hollister; 1908   **1044**

Specialists are a necessity and are not to be ruled out, but for the all-round needs of the family the old family doctor will have the last smile. He may disappear for the time, but he will come back again, and when he does he will come to stay.
Memories of Eighty Years

Jerome J. Rubin; 1963   **1045**

The good old "family doc" or "country doc" has no reason to exist in this modern age. Let's face it. He was a wonderfully affable, understanding man, who replaced his lack of knowledge with human kindness and human warmth. When medicine encompassed a broad, but not a collosal [sic], quantity of knowledge the old fashioned general practitioner could practice with some degree of success and achievement.
Philadelphia Medicine

FAT

Rachmiel Levine; *circa* 1970   **1046**

Every carbon in fat is derived from sugar that man ate or that the cow ate. Oil or fat is nothing more than congealed candy.   *Lecture*

FEES

Euripides; [485-406 BC]   **1047**

In times like these, when wishes soar but power fails,
I contemplate the steady comfort found in gold:
Gold you can spend on guests;
Gold you can pay the doctor when you get sick.   *Electra*

Hippocrates; *circa* 400 BC   **1048**

I urge you not to be too unkind, but to consider carefully your patient's superabundance or means. Sometimes give your services for nothing, calling to mind a precious benefaction or present satisfaction.   *Precepts*

FETAL ALCOHOL SYNDROME

Christy N. Ulleland; 1972   **1049**

We have presented a group of infants wuth intrauterine growth failure whose mothers had one thing in common: that is, relatively severe chronic alcoholism. Viewed another way, intrauterine growth failure occurred in 83% of the offspring of women whose alcoholism was readily recognized.   *Annals of the New York Academy of Sciences*

Kenneth L. Jones, David W. Smith; 1973   1050

The first necropsy performed on a patient with fetal alcohol syndrome disclosed serious dysmorphogenesis of the brain, which may be responsible for some of the functional abnormalities and the joint malposition seen in this syndrome.   *The Lancet*

Kenneth L. Jones, David W. Smith, Christy N. Ulleland,
Ann Pytkowicz Streissguth; 1973   1051

Eight unrelated children and three different ethnic groups, all born to mothers who were chronic alcoholics, have a similar pattern of craniofacial, limb, and cardiovascular defects associated with prenatal-onset growth deficiency and developmental delay.   *The Lancet*

FETAL HEART

Jacques Alexandre Lejumeau (de Kergaradec); 1822   1052

Will it not be possible to judge the state of health or disease of the fetus from the variations that occur in the beat of the fetal heart?   *Memoire sur l'Auscultation*

FETAL TRANSFUSION

Albert William Liley; 1963   1053

The aim of the exercise is simply to arrest deterioration if possible and gain a few extra weeks of gestation so that the skilled paediatric care of severe haemolytic disease is not nullified by gross prematurity.   *British Medical Journal*

FEVER

Samuel Shem; 1978   1054

If you don't take a temperature, you can't find a fever.   *The House of God*

FIBEROSCOPY

H.H. Hopkins, N.S. Kapany; 1954   1055

An optical unit has been devised which will convey optical images along a flexible axis. The unit comprises a bundle of fibres of glass, or other transparent material, and it therefore appears appropriate to introduce the term "fibrescope" to denote it.   *Nature*

FLUID-ELECTROLYTE DISORDERS

Alexandre-Jacques-François Brierre de Boismont; 1831   1056

The blood in patients with cholera undergoes remarkable changes. It becomes black, thickened, viscous, and frequently forms a compact mass, separating with great difficulty into serum and coagulum. When the disease has lasted any length of time, no serocity is found in the blood.   *The Lancet*

William Brooke O'Shaughnessy; 1831   1057

The blood drawn in the worst of cases of the cholera, is unchanged in its anatomical or globular structure.... It has lost a large proportion of its water, 1000 parts of...serum having but the average of 860 parts of water.... It has lost also a great proportion of its neutral saline ingredients.... Of the free alkali contained in healthy serum, not a particle is present in some...cases, and barely a trace in others.... All the salts deficient in the blood...are present in large quantities in the peculiar white dejected matters.   *The Lancet*

FLUID THERAPY

Thomas Latta; 1832   1058

The great disideratum of restoring the natural current in the veins and arteries, of improving the colour of the blood, and recovering the functions of the lungs, in Cholera Asphyxia, may be accomplished by injecting a weak saline solution into the veins of the patient. To Dr.

Thomas Latta...is due the merit of first having recourse to this practice.... To produce the effect referred to, a large quantity must be injected, from *five to ten pounds in an adult*.

Lewins R, The Lancet

Francis Rynd; 1861   1059

The subcutaneous introduction of fluids, for the relief of neuralgia, was first practised in this country by me, in the Meath Hospital, in the month of May, 1844. The cases were published in the "Dublin Medical Press" of March 12, 1845. Since then, I have treated very many cases, and used many kinds of fluids and solutions, with variable success. The fluid I have found most beneficial is a solution of morphia in creosote, ten grains of the former to one drachm of the latter.   *Dublin Quarterly Journal*

FLUORIDATION

Peter B. Medawar; 1979   1060

Every time the mayor of an American municipality finds against fluoridation or someone in England pronounces it inefficacious or even downright harmful, there is a clamor of rejoicing in the corner of Mount Olympus presided over by Gaptooth, the God of Dental Decay.

Advice to a Young Scientist

FOCAL GLOMERULONEPHRITIS (BERGER-HINGLAIS DISEASE)

J. Berger, N. Hinglais; 1968   1061

It appears... that in most cases of "focal" chronic glomerulonephritis, there are in most of the focal lesions, diffuse intercapillary deposits. This observation, aside from its theoretical interest, has a practical value: the immunofluorescence allows an easy diagnosis of this variety of glomerulonephritis in the cases where optical microscopy leads wrongly to the conclusion that the kidney is normal or has other kinds of lesions.   *Journal of Urology (Paris)*

FOCAL INFECTION

Benjamin Rush; 1809   1062

I have been made happy...in pointing out a connection between the extraction of decayed and diseased teeth and the cure of general diseases.... Our success in the treatment of all chronic diseases would be very much promoted, by directing our inquiries into the state of the teeth in sick people, and by advising their extraction in every case in which they are decayed.   *Medical Inquiries and Observations*

FOLIC ACID

Lucy Wills; 1931   1063

In marmite, and probably in other yeast extracts, there appears to be a curative agent for this dread [tropical macrocytic anaemia] which equals liver extract in potency, and has the advantage in India of being comparatively cheap and of vegetable origin.

British Medical Journal

Tom Douglas Spies, C.F. Vitter, M.B. Koch, M.H. Caldwell; 1945   1064

Persons with macrocytic anemia in relapse have a significant response following the administration of synthetic folic acid.... In every instance the number of reticulocytes increased in the peripheral blood, and the red blood cell counts and hemoglobin content rose toward normal levels.   *Southern Medical Journal*

Robert Crane Angier; 1946   1065

After acid hydrolysis of the aromatic amine fraction [derived from the fermentation *L. casei* factor], a compound was isolated and identified as *p*-aminobenzoic acid.... For the compounds formed from *p*-aminobenzoic acid and *p*-aminobenzoyl-l(+)-glutamic acid, the names pteroic acid and pteroylglutamic acid are suggested.   *Science*

FRÖHLICH SYNDROME (DYSTROPHIA ADIPOSOGENITALIS)

Alfred Fröhlich; 1901   1066

A boy of 14 years, has been under our observation since November 1899.... I wish to stress the obesity in the body of our patient.... The most marked collections of fat are in the skin of the trunk especially the abdomen and in the region of the genitalia.... We can conclude that with symptoms, which point to a tumor in the neighborhood of the brain stem, with the absence of acromegalic symptoms, the presence of other trophic symptoms, such as rapidly developing obesity or skin changes suggesting myxedema, points to the hypophysis as the point of origin of the tumor.   *Wiener Klinische Rundschau*

FRENCH MEDICINE

Kenneth M. Ludmerer; 1985   1067

Ironically, astute observation—the great strength of the French clinical school—became the cause of its ultimate eclipse, insofar as it led French clinicians to distrust experimental laboratory investigation. French medical science did not investigate the causes of disease, and by the time of the European revolutions of 1848 it had lost its former ascendancy.   *Learning to Heal*

FRONTIER MEDICINE

Frances Trollope; 1832   1068

The city is full of physicians... When a medical man intended settling in a new situation, he...walked the streets at night... If he saw the dismal twinkle of the watch-light from many windows...disease was busy, and the "location" might suit him well.... Cincinnati was far from healthy.   *Domestic Manners of the Americans*

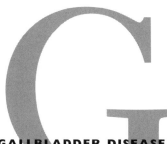

GALLBLADDER DISEASE

Jean-François Fernel; 1554   1069
Obstruction, calculus, fullness and emptiness attack the gall bladder. The obstruction is either of the duct by which the bile is led away from the liver, or of that by which it is discharged from the gall bladder into the intestine.... In both [the] feces [are] whitish [and] the bile diffused with the blood throughout the whole body disfigures the skin with jaundice.   *Medicina*

Ludwig Courvoisier; 1890   1070
With stone obstruction of the common duct, dilatation of the gallbladder is rarely observed; the organ has already undergone contraction; with obstruction from other causes, dilatation is to be expected.   *The Pathology and Surgery of the Biliary Tract*

GALLOP SOUNDS

Pierre-Carl-Èdouard Potain; 1876   1071
We find in the heart in patients suffering from interstitial nephritis, a special sound which is the bruit designated by Professor Bouillaud with the name "Gallop rhythm" [*bruit de galop*]. This sound results from the abruptness with which the dilation of the ventricle takes place during the pre-systolic period.... It appears to be an indirect consequence of the excessive arterial tension which interstitial nephritis produces.
       Bulletin of the Society of Medical Hospitals (Paris)

GALLSTONES

Antonio Benivieni; 1507   1072
There died...a noble woman...with the prostrating pain of a stone.... It seemed advisable to open the body of the dead, and a great many stones were found, not only in the bladder, as was thought, besides one, which was contained in the wall of the gall bladder of a black color and the size of a dried chestnut, all the others in the lining, by which the liver is covered, from which besides they had formed a little bag, as it were, in a dependent skin.
       De Abditis Nonnulus ac Mirandis Morborum et Sanationum Causis

Matteo Realdo Colombo; 1559   1073

Moreover I have taken out innumerable stones with my own hands, with various colors found in the kidneys, in the lungs, in the liver, in the portal vein.... Also in the gall bladder...I found stones of various shapes and of various colors and very many in some others.

De re Anatomica Libri

Gentile da Foligno; 1586   1074

In the gall bladder many stones were seen, Gentile himself testifies, in a certain woman, whose viscera were removed, so that the body could be embalmed they found in the duct of the gall bladder at its mouth, a stone tending to green, from which the moderns with right remark that there was jaundice present.   *De Medica Historia Mirabili Libri Sex*

Giovanni Battista Morgagni; 1761   1075

Carolus Stephanus has asserted that [gallstones] have been seen by him "chiefly in women who were pretty far advanc'd in life"; and, in this age, Frederick Hoffman has said that "they are found very rarely in men, who are in the flourishing time of life, but more frequently in old men, and still more frequently in women than in men." The first thing pronounced by Hoffman, therefore, is much more true than the last.   *The Seats and Causes of Diseases*

GANGRENE

[Anonymous]; *circa* 2000 BC   1076

If the tips of [the patient's] fingers are falling off and are black, he will die.

Wilson JVK, Journal of the Royal Society of Medicine

GASTRIC ACID SECRETION

William Prout; 1823   1077

That a free, or at least an unsaturated acid usually exists in the stomach of animals, and is in some manner connected with the important process of digestion, seems to have been the general opinion of physiologists.... The object of the present communication is to show, that the acid in question is the muriatic acid, and that the salts usually met with in the stomach, are the alkaline muriates.   *Philosophical Transactions of the Royal Society*

Charles F. Code; 1977   1078

It is unlikely that histamine is the only route of stimulation to the parietal cells of all species. It would be hard to imagine, after all the millions of years it has taken to develop this mechanism from fish and reptiles on up through mammals to man, that nature would not have developed alternatives to histamine.   *New England Journal of Medicine*

GASTRIC FUNCTION

Jacob Anton Helm; 1801   1079

I repeated the experiment [in a 56-year-old woman who had long suffered with a spontaneous gastric fistula] with milk and noticed that it always turned sour and coagulated. The sole exception was immediately after the patient had flushed her stomach [by drinking water]; the milk which she drank immediately after did not coagulate for some time, presumably for the lack of gastric juice. That [i.e., secretion of gastric juice] could be hastened always by stimulating the inner surface of her stomach with the finger.

Gesundheits Taschenbuch

William Prout; 1824   1080

These results thus seem to demonstrate that free, or at least unsaturated, muriatic acid in no small quantity exists in the stomach of three animals during the digestive process; and... in the stomach of the horse, the calf. and the dog. I have also quite uniformly found free muriatic acid in great abundance in the acid fluid ejected from the human stomach in severe cases of dyspepsia.   *Philosophical Transactions of the Royal Society*

Walter Bradford Cannon; 1898   1081

The mixing of a small quantity of subnitrate of bismuth with the food allows not only the contractions of the gastric wall, but also the movements of the gastric contents to be seen with the Rontgen rays in the uninjured animal during normal digestion. An unsuspected nicety of mechanical action and a surprising sensitiveness to nervous conditions have thereby been disclosed.   *American Journal of Physiology*

GASTRIC INTUBATION

Adolf Kussmaul; 1869   1082

Often when I observed the patient in the wretched prodromal stage of vomiting, the thought occurred to me that I might relieve her suffering by the employment of the stomach-pump, as the removal of large masses of decomposed acid gastric contents should cause relief from agonizing burning and retching at once.   *Deutsche Archiv für Klinische Medizin*

GASTRIC SURGERY

Christian Albert Theodor Billroth; 1881   1083

The problem of the anastomosis between the considerably larger stomach lumen with the smaller opening of the duodenum arose [upon resection of a tumor in the distal stomach]. Inasmuch as it was desirable to avoid wedges and folds, the stomach walls themselves were sutured together first, beginning at the greater curvature namely from below until the remaining lumen of the stomach could be easily united with the opening of the duodenum.

Wien Medizinische Wochenschrift

GASTRIC ULCER

Matthew Baillie; 1793   1084

Opportunities occasionally offer themselves of observing ulcers of the stomach.... They appear very much as if some little time before a part had been cut out from the stomach with a knife, and the edges had healed, so as to present an uniform smooth boundary round the excavation which had been made.   *Morbid Anatomy*

Jean Cruveilier; 1829   1085

Anatomically considered, the simple chronic ulcer of the stomach consists of a spontaneous loss of substance, ordinarily circular, with the margins cut perpendicularly, the bottom gashed and thick and of variable dimensions. Almost always single, the ulcer is situated most commonly either on the small curvature or upon the posterior wall of the stomach.... Its advance is slow and progressive, it spreads out on the surface, but especially it excavates deeply; and if helpful adhesions do not oppose, sooner or later the stomach is perforated and the contents are scattered throughout the peritoneal cavity.

Anatomie Pathologique du Corps Humain

GASTROENTEROLOGY

Gerald S. Foster; 1977   1086

When dealing with an intra-abdominal problem the clinician's greatest ally is the radiologist. As a matter of fact, gastroenterology without expert radiology is like lox without a bagel.

New England Journal of Medicine

Howard Spiro; 1985   1087

I do not know how dosages of H_2-blockers were calculated in this country, but I imagine that the objective was to eradicate every trace of acid—an approach entirely in keeping with the long Calvinist tradition of U.S. gastroenterology.   *Hospital Practice*

GASTROSCOPY

Rudolf Schindler; 1922   1088

Gastroscopic examination...permits repeated differential diagnosis, which is not possible by other methods, for interpreting pictures of disease conditions, which formerly could not be diagnosed at all. The different forms of chronic gastritis and ventricular polyposis especially belong in this class.   *Munchen Medizinische Wochenschrift*

Basil Isaac Hirschcowitz, L.E. Curtiss, C.W. Peters,
H. Marvin Pollard; 1958   1089

The principle of fiber optics has been applied in the development and construction of a completely flexible optical instrument which allows direct visualization of the cavity of the duodenum.... The esophagus, stomach, and duodenum all can be visualized in one instrumentation.   *Gastroenterology*

GENERALISTS

Rosemary Stevens; 1971   1090

[A generalist] would not be a general practitioner, in the sense of being willing to treat patients over the whole range of medicine, including areas preempted by specialists. Rather, he would be a generalist by virtue of his function as the selector, initiator, orchestrator, and interpreter of the services of specialists.   *American Medicine and the Public Interest*

Rosemary Stevens; 1971   1091

The role of the generalist in medicine has been, and remains, the most important single issue in modern medicine, for the structure of the medical profession hinges on whether—and how—general practice is recognized.   *American Medicine and the Public Interest*

GENES

Wilhelm Ludwig Johanssen; 1911   1092

I have proposed the terms *gene* and *genotype*... to be used in the science of genetics. *Gene* is nothing but a very applicable little word, easily combined with others, and hence it may be useful as an expression for the "unit-factors," "elements" or "allelomorphs" in the gametes, demonstrated by modern Mendelian researches.   *American Naturalist*

Alfred Henry Sturtevant; 1913   1093

It has been found possible to arrange six sex-lined factors in *Drosophila* in a linear series, using the number of cross-overs per 100 cases as an index of the distance between any two factors.... These results form a new argument in favor of the chromosome view of inheritance, since they strongly indicate that the factors are arranged in a linear series, at least mathematically.   *Journal of Experimental Zoology*

GENETIC CODE

Francis Harry Compton Crick, L. Burnett, S. Brenner,
R.J. Watts-Tobin; 1961   1094

We report genetic experiments which... suggest that the genetic code is of the following general type: (*a*) A group of three bases... codes one amino-acid. (*b*) The code is not of the overlapping type... (*c*) The sequence of the bases is read from a fixed starting point.... If the starting point is displaced by one base, then the reading into triplets is displaced and thus becomes incorrect.   *Nature*

GENETICS

Gregor Johann Mendel; 1866   1095

The theory is confirmed that the pea hybrids form egg and pollen cells which, in their constitution, represent in equal numbers all constant forms which result from the combination of the characters united in fertilisation.   *Versuche öber Pflanzen-hybriden*

Gregor Johann Mendel; 1866   **1096**

The constant characters which appear in the several varieties of a group of plants may be obtained in all the associations which are possible according to the [mathematical] laws of combinations, by means of repeated artificial fertilization.

Proceedings of the Natural History Society of Brunn

Francis Galton; 1876   **1097**

Nature prevails enormously over nurture when the differences of nurture do not exceed what is commonly to be found among persons of the same rank of society and in the same country.   *Journal of the Anthropological Institute of Great Britain and Ireland*

Wilhelm Ebstein; 1885   **1098**

We cannot be too particular in the choice of our ancestors.

The Regimen to be Adopted in Cases of Gout

William Withey Gull; 1896   **1099**

We could wish that...*life-histories* were found in every family, showing the health and diseases of its different members. We might thus in time find evidences of pathological connections and morbid liabilities not now suspected.   *Memoir*

Archibald Edward Garrod; 1908   **1100**

The chemical error pursues an even course and shows no tendency to become aggravated as time goes on, and, they are little likely to be influenced by any therapeutic measures at our disposal. Yet they are characterized by wide departures from the normal of the species far more conspicuous than any ordinary individual variations, and one is tempted to regard them as metabolic sports, the chemical analogues of structural malformations.

Inborn Errors of Metabolism

Archibald Edward Garrod; 1908   **1101**

Nor can it be supposed that the diversity of chemical structure and process stops at the boundary of the species, and that within that boundary, which has no real finality, rigid uniformity reigns. Such a conception is at variance with any evolutionary conception of the nature and origin of species. The existence of chemical individuality follows of necessity from that of chemical specificity, but we should expect the differences between individuals to be still more subtle and difficult of detection.   *Inborn Errors of Metabolism*

John Scott Haldane; 1914   **1102**

All the evidence points to the nuclear germ-plasm as the essential carrier of hereditary characters. We are thus compelled, on the mechanistic hypothesis, to attribute to the germ-plasm, or germinal nuclear substance, a structure so arranged that in presence of suitable pabulum and stimuli it produces the whole of the vast and definitely ordered assemblage of mechanisms existing in the adult organism.

Mechanism, Life, and Personality

Sigmund Freud; 1924   **1103**

Even at birth the whole individual is destined to die, and perhaps his organic disposition may already contain the indication of what he is to die from.

The Dissolution of the Oedipus Complex

Thomas Hunt Morgan; 1926   **1104**

The characters of the individual are referable to paired elements (genes) in the germinal matter that are held together in a definite number of linkage groups.... The members of each pair of genes separate when germ cells mature.... Each germ-cell comes to contain only one set.... These principles...enable us to handle problems of genetics in a strictly numerical basis, and allow us to predict...what will occur.... In these respects the theory [of the gene] fulfills the requirements of a scientific theory in the fullest sense.

The Theory of the Gene

Thomas Hunt Morgan; 1926   1105

It is difficult to resist the fascinating assumption that the gene is constant because it represents an organic chemical entity. This is the simplest assumption that one can make at present, and since this view is consistent with all that is known about the stability of the gene it seems, at least, a good working hypothesis.   *The Theory of the Gene*

René Jules Dubos; 1968   1106

So obvious are cultural forces in human activities that social scientists tend to believe that man has escaped from the clutches of biology. In reality...biological forces still profoundly affect most of his individual and social life.... Some of the differences between exceptionally gifted persons and ordinary human beings certainly rest on a genetic basis.... History is, in part at least, the outcome of forces set in motion by the peculiar genetic endowment of a few innovators.   *Man, Medicine, and Environment*

Frank Macfarlane Burnet; 1969   1107

Twelve days ago, I reached the age conventionally regarded as the allotted span of human life.... I am an old man and...in a certain sense I am immortal. Nearly seventy-*one* years ago a genetic programme came into being in the zygote—the newly fertilized egg—from which there developed that fantastic four-dimensional clone of cells in spacetime, which is, has been, and always [will] be ME.   *Australasian Annals of Medicine*

Lewis Thomas; 1974   1108

The cloning of human beings is on most of the lists of things to worry about from science, along with behavior-control, genetic engineering, transplanted heads, computer poetry, and the unrestrained growth of plastic flowers.   *New England Journal of Medicine*

Edward O. Wilson; 1978   1109

The question of interest is no longer whether human social behavior is genetically determined; it is to what extent.   *On Human Nature*

Edward O. Wilson; 1978   1110

Human nature is...a hodge podge of specific genetic adaptations to an environment largely vanished.   *On Human Nature*

Ian Lloyd; 1990   1111

When the full map of the human genome is known...we shall have passed through a phase of human civilization as significant as, if not more significant than, that which distinguished the age of Galileo from that of Copernicus, or that of Einstein from that of Newton.... We have crossed a boundary of unprecedented importance.... There is no going back.... We are walking hopefully into the scientific foothills of a gigantic mountain range.   *Official Record, House of Commons*

GENOMICS

Victor A. McKusick, Frank H. Ruddle; 1987   1112

For the newly developing discipline of mapping/sequencing (including analysis of the information) we have adopted the term *genomics*. We are indebted to T. H. Roderick of the Jackson Laboratory. Bar Harbor, Maine, for suggesting the term. The new discipline is born from a marriage of molecular and cell biology with classical genetics and is fostered by computational science.   *Genomics*

GERIATRICS

François Ranchin; 1627   1113

Not only physicians, but everybody else attending old people, being accustomed to their constant complaints, and knowing their ill-tempered and difficult manners, realize how noble and important, how serious and difficult, how useful and even indispensable is that part of practical Medicine, called Gerocomica, which deals with the conservation of old people and the healing of their diseases.   *Opscula Medica*

Richard A. Kern; 1962   **1114**
The most effective therapeutic weapon at the disposal of a physician in the care of the aged is sympathy. The oldsters don't get too much of it at best.... Absence of sympathy may render weak the most powerful measures that science affords.
Temple University Medical Center Bulletin

Robertson Davies; 1994   **1115**
The disease is the signal, that comes late in the day, that a life has become hard to bear.
The Cunning Man

GERM THEORY

John Hamilcar Hollister; 1885   **1116**
Far be it from me to speak disparagingly of these [Koch's] investigations. As never before the advocates and opponents of the germ theory of disease are marshalled in conflict. The smoke of the battle is yet too intense for us to determine where final victory shall rest, but one thing is certain. From such prolonged and skillful investigations by such able observers we shall date a new era in the advancement of medical science.
Journal of the American Medical Association

GINSENG

Samuel Stearns; 1801   **1117**
This is a small plant growing in Canada, Vermont, Virginia, and some other parts of America.... The Chinese call the root a restorative.... They drink an infusion of the leaves instead of tea.... The Author has found it beneficial for coughs, consumptions, and spasmodic disorders. This plant ought to be cultivated in gardens.   *The American Herbal*

GLAUCOMA

Friedrich Wilhelm Ernst Albrecht von Graefe; 1857   **1118**
It seemed to me that all the characteristic symptoms [of glaucoma] tended to one point—*increase of the intra-ocular pressure*.... Supported by these facts and considerations, I considered myself perfectly justified iridectomy in glaucoma; for I knew the favorable action of the operation on the condition of the choroid in regard to its circulation.
Archives of Ophthalmology

GLOBUS HYSTERICUS

William Heberden; 1802   **1119**
The hysteric globe in the throat is scarcely ever heard of among men, but is one of the most familiar symptoms with hysteric women.   *Commentaries on the History and Cure of Diseases*

GOITER

Juvenal (Decimus Junius Juvenalis); 60-140   **1120**
Would a goiter surprise anybody
If it appeared in the Alps?   *Satires X*

Thomas Prosser; 1769   **1121**
The Bronchocele, Derby-neck, is a tumor arising on the fore part of the neck; it generally first appears some time betwixt the age of eight and twelve years, and continues gradually to increase for three, four, or five years.... It generally occupies the whole front of the

neck, as the whole thyroid gland is here enlarged…This disease...affects the inhabitants about the Alps, and other parts of Italy.

An Account and Method of Cure of the Bronchocele, or, Derby-Neck

GONOCOCCAL OPHTHALMIA

Philippe Ricord; 1838   1122
Its development must be attributed to the direct application of the gonorrheal matter to the conjunctiva.... The first thing to be urged is speed and energy.... Hesitation and uncertainty are often followed by loss of the eyes.... One must always insist on applications of silver nitrate.   *A Practical Treatise on Venereal Diseases*

Carl Sigmund Franz Crede; 1884   1123
All the sebaceous matter clinging to the eyelids was removed. Then on the table where the child is swathed *before* clothes are put on the child, each eye is opened by means of two fingers, *a single drop of a two percent solution of silver nitrate hanging on a little glass rod* is brought close to the cornea until it touches it, and is dropped on the middle of it. *There is no further care given to the eyes.*   *Prophylaxis of the Inflammation of the Eye of the Newborn*

GONORRHEA

Aretaeus the Cappadocian; [81-138?]   1124
From satyriasis a transition takes place to an attack of gonorrhoea.   *On Gonorrhea*

Raymundus Mindererus; 1620   1125
If you be troubled with the *Gonorrhaea*, take *House-leek* growing on old walls (call'd by the Latins, *Semper vivum minus*), put it into your shoes, and go bare-foot upon it; anoint your loyns and privy parts with *Henbane-owl*; and take mornings the quantity of two big hasel-nuts of well washed Turpentine, for some days together, avoiding all aromatic, hard, and salt meat.   *Medicina Militaris*

Albert Ludwig Siegmund Neisser; 1879   1126
If gonorrheal pus is spread out in... a layer, allowed to dry, stained by ... methyl violet... a number of... masses of micrococci are seen.... They have a... characteristic, typical form.... These characteristic micrococci... appear to be a constant mark of all gonorrheal affections.
Centralblatt für die Medicinischen Wissenschaften

GOUT

Hippocrates; [460-375 BC]   1127
A young man does not take the gout until he indulges in coition.   *Aphorisms*

Hippocrates; [460-375 BC]   1128
Eunuchs do not take the gout, nor become bald.   *Aphorisms*

Hippocrates; [460-375 BC]   1129
A woman does not take the gout, unless her menses be stopped.   *Aphorisms*

Hildegard of Bingen; *circa* 1150   1130
Those who have soft and rich flesh on their bodies and who frequently eat incompatible and exquisite foods will easily contract gout... Bad humors... descend to the lower parts of the bodies and begin to rage in the legs and feet.... Women do not incur gout so easily. These humors become part of the menstrual purgation and so women remain free of gout.
Causae et Curae

Anton von Leeuwenhoek; 1679   1131
There was...a hole in his arm on his elbow from which the chalk had come during quite six months on end.... I asked him to let me have some of the chalk.... [Under the lens] I

observed the solid matter which to our eyes resembles chalk and saw to my...astonishment that...it consisted of nothing but long, transparent little particles, many pointed at both ends and about 4 "axes" of the globules in length. *Letter to Lambert Velthuysen*

Thomas Sydenham; 1683   1132

The victim goes to bed and sleeps in good health. About two o'clock in the morning he is awakened by a severe pain in the great toe; more rarely in the heel, ankle, or instep. This pain is like that of a dislocation, and yet the parts feel as if cold water were poured over them.... The night is passed in torture, sleeplessness, turning of the part affected, and perpetual change of posture. *Tractatus de Podagra et Hydrope*

Cotton Mather; 1722   1133

Examine, Sir, Whether your Gout be not the Natural and probable Effect, of some Intemperance, wherein you have indulged yourself.... It may be that you have not been so careful about your Diet as you should have been.... As Hippocrates observed so long ago, Men have not the Gout before the use of Venus. You may charge yourself with some Venereal Irregularities. *The Angel of Bethesda*

William Stukeley; 1734   1134

I doubt not but the poisonous drop of the gout is similar to that of a venomous bite, as Dr. Mead observ'd it upon a microscopic glass; a parcel of small salts nimbly floating in a liquor and striking out into crystals of incrediable tenuity and sharpness, he calls them spicula and darts. *Of the Gout*

Giovanni Battista Morgagni; 1761   1135

As the gout is generally a disorder of the rich, and very seldom of the poor; and the carcasses of the latter, not the former, are delivered to anatomists; or as, if at any time the bodies of the rich are to be opened, the viscera only are subjected to examination, for the most part, and scarcely ever the limbs; it happens from hence, that observations which properly relate to the gout, are far more rare in the books of anatomists, than those of a great number of other diseases. *The Seats and Causes of Diseases*

William Rowley; 1770   1136

Causes of the gout are: hereditary disease,...high living and exercises,...overabundance of wine and venery, Bacchus pater, Venus mater, ira obstetrix arthriditis.
A Treatise on the Regular, Irregular, Atonic, and Flying Gout

Samuel Johnson; 1783   1137

The Gout has within these four days come upon me with a violence, which I never experienced before. It has made me helpless as an infant. *Letter to Bennet Langton*

William Hyde Wollaston; 1797   1138

Instead of a mere concrete acid, the gouty material is a neutral compound, consisting of lithic acid and mineral alkali.... Such...are the essential ingredients of the gouty concretions.
Philosophical Transactions of the Royal Society

William Heberden; 1802   1139

The gout is derived from gouty ancestors, or is created by intemperance, or arises from some unknown causes, which are sometimes found in the sober and abstemious, none of whose family had previously been afflicted with this distemper. Women are less subject to it than men; yet examples of gouty women are by no means rare: it has even spared all the children of gouty parents except one of the daughters; and I have known a female who suffered by the gout to the degree of having numerous sores from chalkstones, though it had never been heard of among any of her relatives.
Commentaries on the History and Cure of Diseases

William Heberden; 1802   1140

Most gouts continue to return to the end of life. I never knew a certain instance of their beginning before the years of puberty. *Commentaries on the History and Cure of Diseases*

William Heberden; 1802   **1141**

The gout most usually begins with a pain in the first joint of the great toe, which soon looks very red, and after a little while begins to swell.

Commentaries on the History and Cure of Diseases

William Heberden; 1802   **1142**

[Gouty pains] are for the most part transmitted to the descendants of those who have suffered in any considerable degree.   *Commentaries on the History and Cure of Diseases*

Sydney Smith; 1840   **1143**

I am pretty well except gout, asthma, and pains in all the bones, and all the flesh, of my body.   *Virgin P, Sydney Smith*

Alfred Baring Garrod; 1848   **1144**

Thus it appears that the kidneys [in gout] had almost entirely lost their power of excreting uric acid, but not the other solids of the urine.... Uric acid is not a product of the action of the kidneys.... It is merely excreted from the system by these organs.... Urea and uric acid are separately eliminated.... Gout would...appear partly to depend on a loss...of the "uric-acid-excreting function" of the kidneys; the [symptoms that] constitute the paroxysm, arising from an excess of this acid in the blood.

Medico-Chirurgical Transactions

Alfred Baring Garrod; 1859   **1145**

That colchicum in its various forms has a most powerful influence upon the progress of gouty inflammation is undeniable, and this action is not simply limited to the removal of gout when it attacks the joints, but it proves efficacious even in its masked and irregular forms.... I would even go to the length of asserting that we may sometimes diagnose gouty inflammation from any form by noting the influence of colchicum upon its progress.

A Treatise on Gout and Rheumatic Gout

Alfred Baring Garrod; 1863   **1146**

Gout would thus appear at least partly to depend on a loss of power...of the "uric-acid-excreting function" of the kidneys.... Any undue *formation* of this compound would favour the occurrence of the disease; and hence the connection between gout and uric acid, gravel and calculi...and the influence of high living, wine, porter, want of exercise, etc., in inducing it.   *The Nature and Treatment of Gout and Rheumatic Gout*

Richard Llewellyn Jones Llewellyn; 1885   **1147**

Gout is an hereditary disorder, the *intrinsic* element of which is an inborn instability of nuclein metabolism which may remain latent, but under the influence of *extrinsic* factors, *infections*, becomes manifest, as betokened by local inflammatory tissue reactions in joints or elsewhere the specific character of which is attested by the associated uratic deposition.   *Gout*

Ambrose Bierce; 1906   **1148**

Gout, *n.* A physician's name for the rheumatism of a rich patient.   *The Devil's Dictionary*

Wilhelm His Jr.; 1909   **1149**

Experience shows that gout can in most cases be favorably influenced by diet.... Food poor in purin is rational and may be tried if it proves agreeable to the digestive organs.... There is no reason why this diet should be persisted in, if there is no distinct effect after a few weeks or months.   *Post-Graduate*

GRAHAM STEELL MURMUR

Graham Steell; 1888   **1150**

In cases of mitral obstruction there is occasionally heard over the pulmonary area...and below this region, for the distance of an inch or two along the left border of the sternum,...a soft blowing diastolic murmur immediately following, or, more exactly, running off from the accentuated second sound, while the usual indications of aortic regurgitation afforded by the pulse, etc., are absent.... The murmur of high-pressure in the pulmonary artery is not peculiar to mitral stenosis, although it is most commonly met with, as a consequence of this lesion. *The Murmur of High-Pressure in the Pulmonary Artery*

GRANT APPLICATIONS

Gideon Koren; 1997   1151

After spending weeks writing a grant application for a peer-reviewed competition, and several months worrying about it, you may receive a letter informing you that you have failed, with a couple of your anonymous colleagues telling you how stupid you actually are. This happens to all of us. *Annals of the Royal College of Physicians and Surgeons of Canada*

GRAVE ROBBING

Ambrose Bierce; 1906   1152

Body-snatcher, *n.* A robber of grave-worms. One who supplies the young physicians with that with which the old physicians have supplied the undertaker. *The Devil's Dictionary*

GROUP THERAPY

Joseph H. Pratt; 1907   1153

[The weekly meeting] is held every Friday in a large, cheerful room at the Massachusetts General Hospital.... Made up as our membership is of widely different races and different sects, the members have a common bond in a common disease. A fine spirit of camaraderie develops. The favorable cases that are making rapid progress toward recovery infuse a spirit of hope in all. *Journal of the American Medical Association*

Carl Gustav Jung; 1939   1154

The identification of an individual with a number of people who, as a group. have a collective experience of transformation [can lead to] a positive enthusiasm which spurs the individual to noble deeds, and an equally positive feeling of human solidarity.... The group can give the individual a courage, a bearing, and a dignity which may easily get lost in isolation. *Concerning Rebirth*

GUILLOTINE

Earle P. Scarlett; 1972   1155

It was Joseph Ignace Guillotin who achieved a certain type of immortality by having his name attached to the machine.... [He] later brought forward to the Assembly the proposition that all capital punishment should be by decapitation and by this machine, arguing that death in these circumstances should be swift and painless.... This proposal was in keeping with the character of the man, for Guillotin was a placid individual, a philanthropist and humanitarian. *Roland CG, In Sickness and in Health*

GULF WAR SYNDROME

R.W. Haley, T.L. Kurt, J. Hom; 1997   1156

These [survey] findings support the hypothesis that clusters of symptoms of many Gulf War veterans represent discrete factor analysis-derived syndromes that appear to reflect a spectrum of neurologic injury involving the central, peripheral, and autonomic nervous systems. *Journal of the American Medical Association*

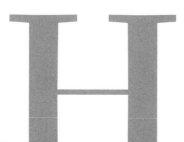

HANTAVIRUS PULMONARY SYNDROME

Stuart T. Nichol, C.F. Spiropoulou, S. Morzunov, and others; 1993   **1157**

A mysterious respiratory illness with high mortality rate was recently reported in the southwestern United States. Serologic studies implicated the hantaviruses.... A genetic detection assay amplified hantavirus-specific DNA fragments from RNA extracted from the tissues of patients and deer mice... caught at patient residences. Nucleotide sequence analysis revealed the associated virus to be a new hantavirus and provided a direct genetic link between infection in patients and rodents.   *Science*

HAY FEVER

Leonardo Botallo; 1564   **1158**

I know men in health, who directly after the odor of roses have a severe reaction from this, so that they have a headache, or it causes sneezing, or induces such a troublesome itching in the nostrils that they can not, for a space of two days, restrain themselves from rubbing them.   *De Catarrho Commentarius*

Johann Nikolaus Binninger; 1673   **1159**

The worthy Matron...of an ample and fleshy body, suffered from a Coryza many weeks at the season of roses.   *Observationum et Curationum Medicinalium*

John Bostock; 1819   **1160**

About the beginning or middle of June in every year the following symptoms make their appearance.... A sensation of heat and fullness is experienced in the eyes.... There is a slight degree of redness and a discharge of tears.... This state gradually increases, until the sensation becomes converted into...the most acute itching and smarting.... A general fullness is experienced in the head.... To this succeeds irritation of the nose, producing sneezing.... To the sneezings are added a farther sensation of tightness of the chest.... All the acute symptoms disappear about the end of July.   *Medico-Chirurgical Transactions*

HEADACHE

Henry George Miller; 1968   1161
The patient who complains of headaches for 20 years—"something must be done about them"—deserves what she is asking for.   *World Neurology*

HEALERS

Charles M. Anderson; 1989   1162
In its earliest forms, medicine was an adjunct to myth and religion. Its "cures" were based largely upon rituals, medications, and surgical procedures designed to appease various deities and to drive evil spirits, demons, devices, and so forth from the bodies of sick persons.... To change a ritual or to alter a procedure in any way was to endanger the patient and to risk further offending the forces involved in the disease, an offense that had immediate implications for the community as a whole.   *Richard Selzer and the Rhetoric of Surgery*

HEALING

Hippocrates; [460-375 BC]   1163
Healing is a matter of time, but it is sometimes also a matter of opportunity.   *Precepts*

Plato; [427-347 BC]   1164
So neither ought you to attempt to cure the body without the soul; and this is the reason why the cure of many diseases is unknown to the physicians of Hellas, because they are ignorant of the whole which ought to be studied also; for the part can never be well unless the whole is well... For this is the great error of our day in the treatment of the human body, that physicians separate the soul from the body.   *Dialogues. Charmides*

Ambroise Paré; [1510-1590]   1165
I dressed him, and God healed him.   *Keynes G, The Apologie and Treatise of Ambroise Paré*

Johann Wolfgang von Goethe; [1749-1832]   1166
Great thanks are due to Nature for putting into the life of each being so much healing power.   *Nager F, Der Heilkundige Dichter*

John Updike; 1984   1167
A scab is a beautiful thing—a coin
the body has minted, with an invisible motto:
In God We Trust.
Our body loves us,
and, even while the spirit drifts dreaming,
works at mending the damage that we do.   *Ode to Healing*

HEALTH

Huang Ti Nei Ching Su Wen; [2697-2597 BC]   1168
Nowadays people are not like this [i.e., temperate in eating and drinking]; they use wine as beverage and they adopt reckless behavior.... Their passions exhaust their vital forces; their cravings dissipate their true (essence); they do not know how to find contentment within themselves; they are not skilled in the control of their spirits. They devote all their attention to the amusement of their minds, thus cutting themselves off from the joys of long (life). Their rising and retiring is without regularity. For these reasons they reach only one half of the hundred years and then they degenerate.
The Yellow Emporer's Classic of Internal Medicine

Juvenal (Decimus Junius Juvenalis); [60-140]   1169
You should pray for a sound mind in a sound body.   *Satires X*

[Anonymous]; 1490   **1170**
Use three Physicians still; first Doctor Quiet,
Next Doctor Merry-man, and Doctor Dyet.   *The School of Salernum*

Thomas More; 1516   **1171**
Health is the greatest of bodily pleasures. Since pain is inherent in disease...and pain is
the bitter enemy of pleasure, while disease is the enemy of health, then pleasure must be
inherent in quiet good health.   *Utopia*

Martin Luther; *circa* 1566   **1172**
Alack for him that depends upon the aid of physic. I do not deny that medicine is a gift
of God, nor do I refuse to acknowledge science in the skill of many physicians; but, take
the best of them, how far are they from perfection?.... I have no objection to the doctors
acting upon certain theories, but, at the same time, they must not expect us to be the
slaves of their fancies.   *Of Sickness*

Francis Bacon; 1625   **1173**
There is a wisdome in this; beyond the rules of physic: a man's own observation, what he
finds good of, and what he finds hurt of, is the best physic to preserve health.
                                                                 Essays. Of Regimen of Health

Baltasar Gracián y Morales; 1637   **1174**
Three things make [a man] happy: Health, Wisdom, and Holiness.
                                                                 The Art of Worldly Wisdom

Mr. Tut-Tut; *circa* 1650   **1175**
The blessing of health is realized on the sickbed.   *One Hundred Proverbs*

Izaak Walton; 1676   **1176**
Look to your health; and if you have it praise God, and value it next to a good Conscience;
for, health is the second blessing that we Mortals are capable of: a blessing that money
cannot buy, and therefore value it, and be thankful for it.   *The Compleat Angler*

François, Duc de la Rochefoucauld; 1678   **1177**
Preserving the health by too strict a regimen is a wearisome malady.
                                                          Moral Reflections, Sentences, and Maxims

Benjamin Franklin; 1746   **1178**
A good Wife & Health, is a Man's best Wealth.   *Poor Richard's Almanac*

Henry David Thoreau; 1850   **1179**
As for health, consider yourself well, and mind your business. Who knows but you are
dead already? ... Men die of fright and live of confidence.   *A Writer's Journal*

Max von Pettenkofer; 1873   **1180**
Health and sickness, like strength and weakness, are not simple, sharply divided conditions, but very complex, highly involved and relative conditions, with no sharp border-
lines. No one is absolutely or completely healthy, and no one is absolutely sick; every one
is in such a condition only more or less.   *The Value of Health to a City*

Benjamin Disraeli; 1877   **1181**
The health of the people is really the foundation upon which all their happiness and all
their power as a State depend.   *Speech*

Josh Billings (Henry Wheeler Shaw); [1818-1885]   **1182**
There ain't much fun in medicine, but there's a heck of a lot of medicine in fun.
                                                                         Cousins N, Head First

Josh Billings (Henry Wheeler Shaw); [1818-1885]   **1183**
When a man loses his health, then he first begins to take care of it.
                                                            Day D, Uncle Sam's Uncle Josh

Oscar Wilde; 1895   **1184**

I think it is high time that Mr. Bunbury made up his mind whether he was going to live or to die. This shilly-shallying with the question is absurd. Nor do I in any way approve of the modern sympathy with invalids. I consider it morbid. Illness of any kind is hardly a thing to be encouraged in others. Health is the primary duty of life.

The Importance of Being Earnest, Act I

Mark Twain (Samuel Langhorne Clemens); 1897   **1185**

The only way to keep your health is to eat what you don't want, drink what you don't like, and do what you'd rather not.   *Following the Equator. Pudd'nhead Wilson's New Calendar*

Gilbert Keith Chesterton; 1905   **1186**

The mistake of all that medical talk lies in the very fact that it connects the idea of health with the idea of care. What has health to do with care? Health has to do with carelessness.

Heretics. Mr H.G. Wells and the Giants

Gilbert Keith Chesterton; 1905   **1187**

When everything about a people is for the time growing weak and ineffective it begins to talk about efficiency. So it is that when a man's body is a wreck he begins, for the first talk about efficiency. So it is that when a man's body is a wreck he begins, for the first time, to talk about health.   *Transactions and Studies of the College of Physicians of Philadelphia*

Joseph-François Malgaigne; 1905   **1188**

Man is a trinity composed of three elements: the body, the heart, and the mind. To each of these elements corresponds some need. The satisfaction of these needs, in full measure, constitutes the science of life and assures the greatest sum of happiness which we can enjoy.   *Advice on the Choice of a Library*

George Bernard Shaw; 1911   **1189**

Use your health, even to the point of wearing it out. That is what it is for. Spend all you have before you die; and do not outlive yourself.   *The Doctor's Dilemma, Preface*

Katherine Mansfield; [1888-1923]   **1190**

By health I mean the power to live a full, adult, living, breathing life in close contact with what I love—the earth and the wonders thereof.... I want to be all that I am capable of becoming.   *Journal*

Henry Louis Mencken; 1930   **1191**

What is the thing called health? Simply a state in which the individual happens transiently to be perfectly adapted to his environment. Obviously, such states cannot be common, for the environment is in constant flux.... Uninterrupted health is probably possible only to creatures of very simple structure, beginning, say, with Rhozopoda and running up to the common lot of college boys.   *The American Mercury*

World Health Organization; 1947   **1192**

Health is a complete state of physical, mental, and social well-being and not merely absence of disease.... The health of all peoples is fundamental to the attainment of peace and security and is dependent upon the fullest cooperation of individuals and States.

Chronicle of the World Health Organization

Hans Selye; 1958   **1193**

Don't be afraid to enjoy the stress of a full life nor too naive to think you can do so without some intelligent thinking and planning. Man should not try to avoid stress any more than he would shun food, love, or exercise.   *Newsweek*

Sara Murray Jordan; 1958   **1194**

Every businessman over 50 should have a daily nap and nip—a short nap after lunch and a relaxing highball before dinner. Frying pans should be abolished.... Nobody should smoke cigarettes.   *Reader's Digest*

Vincent Askey; 1960   1195
When it comes to your health, I recommend frequent doses of that rare commodity among Americans—common sense.   *The Land of Hypochondriacs*

René Jules Dubos; 1961   1196
Health...is not a static condition, but rather is manifested in dynamic responses to the stresses and challenges of life. The more complete the human freedom, the greater the likelihood that new stresses will appear—organic and psychic—because man himself continuously changes his environment through technology, and because endlessly he moves into new conditions during his restless search for adventure.
Bulletin of the American College of Physicians

Leroy Robert "Satchel" Paige; 1962   1197
Satchel Paige's Rules for Staying Young: Avoid fried meats which angry up the blood. If your stomach disputes you, lie down and pacify it with cool thoughts. Keep the juices flowing by jangling around gently as you move. Go very light on the vices, such as carrying on in society—the social ramble ain't restful. Avoid running at all times. And don't look back. Something might be gaining on you.   *Maybe I'll Pitch Forever*

René Jules Dubos; 1968   1198
Conditions for mental misery may be compatible with glowing physical health, and happiness may reside in a diseased body.   *Man, Medicine, and Environment*

Henry George Miller; 1971   1199
The normal state of most people is to feel faintly tired, harrassed, and under the weather.... My clinical observations lead me to believe that an abounding sensation of positive health usually presages either a cardiac infarction or incipient hypomania.... The concept of positive health...postulates a state that could apparently be achieved by the careful observation of a set of rules that vary...but which are always inconvenient and uncomfortable and usually eccentric. I question the whole concept of positive health and the validity of the prescriptions claimed to ensure it.
McLachlan G and Mckeown T, Medical History and Medical Care

Earle P. Scarlett; 1972   1200
The word itself, *health*, I find is derived from the Old English *haelth*, the condition of being *hal*—that is, safe and sound.... Essentially, health is another name for human harmony, harmony not only among our several parts, but also between ourselves and our environments.   *Roland CG, In Sickness and in Health*

Earle P. Scarlett; 1972   1201
When I was a student...the presumption was that health, in fact, was the absence of disease—a shabby and negative conception indeed, and one that inevitably kept medicine in blinkers. The more recent advent of the psychosomatic viewpoint in medicine has done a good deal to correct that narrow conception. Man is now seen in relation to his inner self and his outer world, something more than a protagonist struggling against bacterial invaders, organic deterioration and trauma.   *Roland CG, In Sickness and in Health*

Lewis Thomas; 1975   1202
As a people we have become obsessed with health. There is something fundamentally, radically unhealthy about all this. We do not seem to be seeking more exuberance in living as much as staving off failure, putting off dying. We are losing confidence in the human form.   *New England Journal of Medicine*

Lewis Thomas; 1975   1203
The television and radio industry, no small part of the national economy, feeds on health, or more precisely on disease, for a large part of its sustenance.... The food industry plays the role of surrogate physician.... Chewing gum is sold as a tooth cleanser. Vitamins have taken the place of prayer.   *New England Journal of Medicine*

J.P.M. Tizard; 1981   **1204**

[The opening sentence of "Anna Karenina" is,] "All happy families are more or less like one another; every unhappy family is unhappy in its own particular way."... The truth happens to be exactly the other way round.... Health and happiness have infinite variety; disease and unhappiness one sees again and again in stereotypes.

Journal of the Royal Society of Medicine

Norman Cousins; 1989   **1205**

Good health is a serious business. Like life itself, it has to be worked at and it takes on added meaning with effort.   *Head First*

[Anonymous]; 1990   **1206**

"Probably nothing wrong" is the leading cause of health care in America.

Washington Post Magazine

Bashir Qureshi; 1997   **1207**

Many ambitious people spend the first half of their life ruining their health to earn money and the second half spending that money to regain their health.

Journal of the Royal Society of Medicine

Melinda S. Meade, Robert J. Earickson; 2000   **1208**

The only absence of health is death.   *Medical Geography*

Croatian proverb   **1209**

Warm dress, small meals, moderate drinks—long life.   *Proverb*

Croatian proverb   **1210**

If you close windows to the sun, you open them to the disease.   *Proverb*

HEALTH EDUCATION

John Ruskin; 1862   **1211**

There should be training schools for youth, established at Government cost, and under Government discipline, over the whole country... Every child born in the country should, at the parent's wish, be permitted to pass through them... The child should be...imperatively taught...the laws of health, and the exercises enjoined by them; habits of gentleness and justice; and the calling by which he is to live.   *Unto This Last*

Norman Cousins; 1989   **1212**

One of the unfortunate aspects of health education is that it tends to make us more aware of our weaknesses than of our strengths. By focusing our attention and concerns on things that can go wrong, we tend to develop a one-sided view of the human body, regarding it as a ready receiver for all sorts of illnesses.   *Head First*

HEALTH GAPS

Andrew Haines; 1997   **1213**

The polarisation of wealth has become grotesque, and we are seeing the consequences.... Life expectancy among men has declined in some of the countries of eastern and central Europe over the past five years, and in Russia and the Ukraine infant mortality has risen.... Worldwide, around a third of children under 5 show evidence of malnutrition as judged by their weight for age.   *British Medical Journal*

HEALTH POLICY

George Bernard Shaw; 1911   **1214**

The demands of this poor public are not reasonable, but they are quite simple. It dreads disease and desires to be protected against it. But it is poor and wants to be protected cheaply.

The Doctor's Dilemma, Preface

Charles Horace Mayo; 1919   **1215**

It is a poor government that does not realize that the prolonged life, health, and happiness of its people are its greatest asset.   *Journal of the American Medical Association*

Henry George Miller; 1969   **1216**

The physician must...keep the public fully informed about the directions in which medicine is moving, the advances...on so wide a front, and the enormous benefits to health and happiness [that can] so easily be achieved as well as the risks involved. He must also state the cost of such developments clearly and firmly, so that the public can make an intelligent choice as to how much it is prepared to devote to medicine in the widest sense.

Encounter

Rosemary Stevens; 1971   **1217**

There is no blueprint of how a health service system should be constructed. Given the pluralistic nature of American health care institutions, the continually shifting body of technological knowledge, the existence of regional and local differences in health care resources...one ideal system may never be attainable, and is probably undesirable.

American Medicine and the Public Interest

A. Wildavsky; 1977   **1218**

Health policy is pathological because we are neurotic and insist on making our government psychotic. Our neurosis consists in knowing what is required for good health (Mother was right... Don't drink! Don't smoke! Keep clean! And don't worry!) but not being willing to do it. Government's ambivalence consists in paying coming and going: once for telling people how to be healthy and once for paying their bills when they disregard this advice.   *Daedalus*

Charles E. Rosenberg; 1987   **1219**

We will support research and education, we will feel uncomfortable with a medical system that does not provide a plausible (if not exactly equal) level of care to the poor and socially isolated. Health care policy will continue to reflect the special character of our attitudes toward sickness and sobriety.   *The Care of Strangers*

Steven A. Schroeder; 1996   **1220**

A constant feature of health care in the United States is our national willingness to tolerate having large numbers of people without health insurance. This is in stark contrast to the situation in virtually every other developed country, where guaranteed health insurance is provided either by the state or through employers, with government backup for the unemployed.   *New England Journal of Medicine*

Steven A. Schroeder; 1996   **1221**

At present, most of the attention in health care is focused on the many changes resulting from market forces—the mergers and consolidations of hospital systems and the new organizational and ethical questions raised by managed care. But meanwhile, the problem of the uninsured continues to grow quietly; in the long run, its effects will be so pervasive that it is bound to reemerge as a major national issue. If it does not, then we will find ourselves living in a much meaner America than many of us who entered the healing professions ever imagined.   *New England Journal of Medicine*

Uwe E. Reinhardt; 1997   **1222**

As a matter of conscious national policy, the United States always has and still does openly countenance the practice of rationing health care for millions of...children by their parents' ability to procure health insurance for the family or, if the family is uninsured, by their parents' willingness and ability to pay for health care out of their own pocket or, if the family is unable to pay, by the parents' willingness and ability to procure charity care in their role as health care beggars.   *Journal of the American Medical Association*

HEART

Aristotle; [384-322 BC]   **1223**
The heart...is the only one of the viscera, and indeed the only part of the body, that is unable to tolerate any serious injury.   *De Partibus Animalium*

Aretaeus the Cappadocian; [81-138?]   **1224**
In the midst of [the lungs] is seated a hot organ, the heart, which is the origin of life and respiration. It imparts to the lungs the desire of drawing in cold air, for it raises a heat in them; but it is the heart which attracts. If, therefore, the heart suffer primarily, death is not far off.   *On Pneumonia*

Galen; [130-200]   **1225**
Nature never wished to fatigue the heart with useless work, neither bringing anything unnecessarily to it, nor taking anything unecessarily from it. Thus there are four openings, two in each ventricle, on of which leads into the heart, the other out of it.
                                         On the Usefulness of the Parts of the Body

Leonardo da Vinci; 1510   **1226**
[The heart] moves of itself and does not stop unless forever.   *Notebooks*

Andrea Cesalpino (Caesalpinus); 1571   **1227**
The passages of the heart are so arranged...that from the vena cava a flow takes place into the right ventricle, whence the way is open to the lung. From the lung...there is another entrance into the left ventricle of the heart, from which then a way is open into the aorta artery, certain membranes being so placed at the mouths of the vessels that they prevent return. Thus there is a sort of perpetual movement from the vena cava through the heart and lungs into the aorta artery.   *Quaestiones Medicae*

William Harvey; 1628   **1228**
The heart, like the prince in a kingdom, in whose hands lie the chief and highest authority, rules over all; it is the...foundation from which all power is derived, on which all power depends in the animal body.
                     An Anatomical Treatise on the Movement of the Heart and Blood in Animals

William Harvey; 1628   **1229**
Since all living things are warm, all dying things cold, there must be a...seat and fountain, a kind of home and hearth, where the cherisher of nature, the original of the native fire, is stored and preserved; from which heat and life are dispensed to all parts as from a fountain head; from which sustenance may be derived; and upon which concoction and nutrition, and all vegetative energy may depend. Now that the heart is this place, that the heart is the principle of life... I trust no one will deny.
                     An Anatomical Treatise on the Movement of the Heart and Blood in Animals

Ambrose Bierce; 1906   **1230**
Heart, *n.* An automatic, muscular blood-pump. Figuratively, this useful organ is said to be the seat of emotions and sentiments—a very pretty fancy which, however, is nothing but a survival of a once universal belief.   *The Devil's Dictionary*

Thomas Lewis, M.A. Rothschild; 1915   **1231**
That [electrical] activity first reveals itself in the region of the sino-auricular node...has been shown...beyond question. It spreads from this node in every direction, progressing to all the margins of the musculature.   *Philosophical Transactions of the Royal Society*

Ernest Henry Starling; 1918   **1232**
The law of the heart is thus the same as the law of muscular tissue generally, that the energy of contraction, however measured, is a function of the length of the muscle fibre.
                                                                The Law of the Heart

Willis John Potts; 1959   **1233**

The heart is a tough organ: a marvellous mechanism that, mostly without repairs, will give valiant pumping service up to a hundred years.   *The Surgeon and the Child*

HEART BLOCK

Marko Gerbec (Marcus Gerbezius); 1717   **1234**

I observed this in two patients about the pulse: truly that one of them a melancholy hypochondriac indeed had commonly when well a pulse so slow, that before a subsequent pulse followed the preceding one, three pulsations would have certainly passed in another healthy person.... The man at other times was robust, exact in his movements, but is now slow, often seized with dizziness, and from time to time subject to slight epileptic attacks.   *Major RH, Classic Descriptions of Disease*

Giovanni Battista Morgagni; 1769   **1235**

He was in his sixty-eighth year...when he was first seiz'd with the epilepsy, which left behind it the greatest slowness of pulse, and in a like manner a coldness of the body.
                                                                The Seats and Causes of Diseases

Thomas Spens; 1793   **1236**

I was sent for to see...a common laboring mechanic.... I was much surprised, upon examining the state of his pulse, to find, that it beat only twenty-four strokes in a minute.... He informed me, that, about 3 o'clock in the afternoon, he had been suddenly taken ill while standing on the street; that he had fallen to the ground senseless.   *Medical Commentaries*

Robert Adams; 1827   **1237**

What most attracted my attention was...the remarkable slowness of pulse, which generally ranged at the rate of 30 in a minute.... [In his apoplectic attacks] he would...fall down in a state of complete insensibility and was on several occasions hurt by the fall. When they attacked him, his pulse would become even slower than usual.
                                                                       Dublin Hospital Reports

William Stokes; 1846   **1238**

The pulse was varied from twenty-eight to thirty in the minute.... On listening attentively to the heart's action, we perceived that there were occasional semi-beats between the regular contractions, very weak, unattended with impulse, and corresponding to a similar state of the pulse, which thus probably amounts to about 36 in the minute, the evident beats being only 28.   *Dublin Quarterly Journal of Medical Science*

Alfred L. Galabin; 1875   **1239**

Richard B.... had been invalided on account of attacks of... faitness, and it was then noticed that his heart beat very slowly.... A tracing from the patient's heart [disclosed] small irregularities in the long diastolic interval.... Another tracing, taken on the same day, shows a repetition of them so exact that it might almost be supposed a copy of the first.... We have here a heart the auricle of which sometimes contracts twice in the interval between two ventricular pulsations.   *Guy's Hospital Report*

HEART DISEASE

Jean-Nicolas Corvisart des Marest; 1806   **1240**

It is commonly during a hasty walk, or violent exercise, that [the heart disease] exhibits the first sign of its evolution or presence. Thus an individual, being otherwise in health, will from walking or any other exercise, be suddenly stopped by a previous dyspnea, accompanied or followed by palpitations more or less violent; these symptoms will soon disappear, and leave the patient in a state of apparent health, until, in the same circumstances, and often from similar exciting causes, the same symptoms are reproduced.
                                            Organic Diseases and Lesions of the Heart and Great Vessels

HEART FAILURE

Jean-Nicolas Corvisart des Marest; 1806   1241
The inferior extremities swell, especially when the patient is erect, but diminish at night from a horizontal posture.   *Organic Diseases and Lesions of the Heart and Great Vessels*

Jean-Nicolas Corvisart des Marest; 1806   1242
Patients...are generally immoveable; with the body bent forward, or assuming every other forced posture, the face bloated and livid, the lips blackish...respiration being short, interrupted, impossible; continued cough, with spitting of blood or an abundance of mucus; the parieties of the thorax and abdomen distended with the serum; the arms and legs deformed by infiltration.   *Organic Diseases and Lesions of the Heart and Great Vessels*

James Hope; 1839   1243
Amongst the diseases of the heart may be justly reckoned one of the forms of the malady termed in common language *asthma*.... The respiration, always short, becomes hurried and laborious on the slightest exertion or mental emotion. The effort of ascending a staircase is peculiarly distressing.... Incapable of lying down, he is seen for weeks, and even for months together, either reclining in the semi-erect posture supported by pillows, or sitting with the trunk bent forwards.   *A Treatise on the Diseases of the Heart*

William Stokes; 1854   1244
Although these cases are to be met with every day, especially in private practice, we still observe that physicians differ as to their nature. One holds that the liver is the organ in fault; another, that the disease is in the valves of the heart; a third believes that the symptoms are those of hydrothorax, from disease of the kidney; while a fourth sees nothing but misplaced gout. Each of them may be said to be in one sense right, all of them in another sense wrong.   *The Diseases of the Heart and Aorta*

HEART SOUNDS

James Hope; 1839   1245
First Sound. This is a compound, consisting, first, of the click of the auricular valves: secondly, of the sound of muscular extension—a loud, smart sound.... Second Sound. This results from the sudden expansion of the semilunar valves, occasioned by the reflux upon them of the columns of blood in the aorta and pulmonary artery during the ventricular diastole.   *A Treatise on the Diseases of the Heart*

HEART SURGERY

Christian Albert Theodor Billroth; 1881   1246
Anyone who would attempt to operate on the heart should lose the respect of his colleagues.   *Address to the Vienna Medical Society*

Stephen Paget; 1896   1247
Surgery of the heart has probably reached the limits set by Nature to all surgery: no new method and no new discovery, can overcome the natural difficulties that attend a wound of the heart.   *The Surgery of the Chest*

Ludwig Rehn; 1897   1248
I quickly decided to suture the cardiac wound.... After the third suture...the bleeding was completely stopped.... Gentlemen! The feasibility of a cardiac suture should from now on no longer be held in doubt.... I sincerely hope that this case will not remain a curiosity, but that it will provide a stimulus for further work in cardiac surgery.   *Archiv für Klinische Chirurgie*

Luther Leonidas Hill Jr.; 1902   1249
Any operation which reduces the mortality of a given injury from 90 to about 63 per cent is entitled to a permanent place in surgery, and...every wound of the heart should be operated upon immediately.   *Medical Record*

Elliott C. Cutler, Samuel A. Levine; 1923   **1250**

The experience with this case...does show that surgical intervention in cases of mitral stenosis bears no special risk, and should give us further courage and support in our desire to attempt to alleviate a chronic condition, for which there is now not only no treatment, but one which carries a terrible prognosis. A...case of mitral stenosis [in a girl 12 years old] was operated upon with recovery. The method of attack used was one evolved after years of laboratory investigation concerning the surgery of the heart.

Boston Medical and Surgical Journal

Henry Sessions Souttar; 1925   **1251**

I believe that this is the first occasion upon which an attempt has been made to reach the mitral valve by this route in the human being, or to subject the interior of the heart to digital examination.... To hear a murmur is a very different matter from feeling the blood itself pouring back over one's finger. *British Medical Journal*

Alfred Blalock, Helen Brooke Taussig; 1945   **1252**

An operation for increasing the flow of blood through the lungs and thereby reducing the cyanosis in patients with congenital malformations of the heart consists in making an anastomosis between a branch of the aorta and one of the pulmonary arteries; in other words, the creation of an artificial ductus arteriosus. Thus far the procedure has been carried out on only 3 children, each of whom had a severe degree of anoxemia. Clinical evidence of improvement has been striking and includes a pronounced decrease in the intensity of the cyanosis. *Journal of the American Medical Association*

Bernard J. Miller, John Heysham Gibbon Jr., Mary H. Gibbon; 1951   **1253**

1. An improved oxygenator for blood has been developed which consists of six stainless steel scre[e]ns in parallel, suspended from a distributing chamber and inclosed in a clear plastic case. 2. Using this oxygenator in an improved extracorporeal blood circuit the cardiorespiratory functions have be[e]n maintained in 21 dogs during occlusion of the venae cavae. Seven of these dogs survived the experiment. *Annals of Surgery*

Forest Dewey Dodril, Edward Hill, Robert Gerisch; 1952   **1254**

Sixty-five experiments on dogs using the artificial heart have been performed. These include: (a) right-sided substitution, (b) complete extra-corporeal circulation with mechanical oxygenation, and (c) left-sided substitution.... There are profound atriopressor reflexes present on the right side of the heart in dogs which greatly lower the systemic blood pressure, in fact, we have found it necessary to support the blood pressure by large transfusions as well as by the administration of vasoconstrictor drugs. *Journal of Thoracic Surgery*

Robert H. Goetz, Michael Rohman, Jordan D. Haller, and others; 1961   **1255**

A coronary mammary anastomosis between the right mammary artery and right coronary artery, using the tantalum ring, has been successfully performed on a 38-year-old patient at the Van Etten Hospital, Bronx Municipal Hospital Center, New York on May 2, 1960. The patient is doing well and it is intended to report the case in detail in a separate communication. *Journal of Thoracic and Cardiovascular Surgery*

Christiaan Neethling Barnard; 1967   **1256**

On 3 December 1967, a heart from a cadaver was successfully transplanted into a 54-year-old man to replace a heart irreparably damaged by repeated myocardial infarction.

South African Medical Journal

René G. Favaloro; 1968   **1257**

A new operative technique is described to correct severe segmental occlusion of the right dominant coronary artery. A saphenous vein autograft replaces the occluded arterial segment. Fifteen patients were operated upon without mortality. Postoperative angiographic catheterization has demonstrated excellent function of the grafts. Further application of the technique will help to determine the possibilities of its use on the left coronary artery in selected patients who have severe localized obstruction. *Annals of Thoracic Surgery*

H. Edward Garrett, Edward W. Dennis, Michael E. DeBakey; 1973   **1258**

A 42-year-old man had extensive occlusive disease of the coronary artery and angina pectoris. An autogenous saphenous vein bypass from the ascending aorta to the anterior descending coronary artery was performed on Nov 23, 1964.... Seven years after the operation, the graft functions with normal left ventricular hemodynamics.

Journal of the American Medical Association

HEBERDEN NODES

William Heberden; 1802   **1259**

What are those little hard knobs, about the size of a small pea, which are frequently seen upon the fingers, particularly a little below the top, near the joint? They have no connexion with the gout, being found in persons who never had it: they continue for life; and being hardly ever attended with pain, or disposed to become sores, are rather unsightly, than inconvenient, though they must be some little hindrance to the free use of the fingers.

Commentaries on the History and Cure of Diseases

HEMATOLOGY

James de Back; 1653   **1260**

I call the generall doctrine of man Anthropologie, the parts of which , I do ordain to be, according to this division, Psychologie, Somatologie, and Haematologie, into the doctrine of the soul, bodie, and blood.

A Discourse of the Heart

Maxwell M. Wintrobe; 1984   **1261**

One practice I did develop...was to keep paper and pencil beside me when I went to bed because I found that an idea might come to me in the middle of the night. Unless I was able to get it down on paper it might have escaped me by the following morning. The idea of calculating the mean corpuscular volume (MCV), mean corpuscular hemoglobin (MCH), and mean corpuscular hemoglobin concentration (MCHC) came to me in this way.

Weisse AB, Conversations in Medicine

Maxwell M. Wintrobe; 1984   **1262**

I...discovered that there were no reliable normal blood values. What was called "normal" was based on only a few counts that had been made in the nineteenth century. So I proceeded to collect normal blood values. Others elsewhere, also mindful of this deficiency, were beginning to do the same. A major problem, however, was methodology, and this was what led me to devise the hematocrit as a simple and accurate means of quantitating blood.

Weisse AB, Conversations in Medicine

HEMIPLEGIA

[Anonymous]; *circa* 2500 BC   **1263**

[He] walks shuffling with his sole, on the side of him having that injury which is in his skull.... As for: "He walks shuffling with his sole,"...it is not easy for him to walk, when it (the sole) is feeble and turned over, while the tips of his toes are contracted to the ball of his sole, and they (the toes) walk fumbling the ground.   *The Edwin Smith Surgical Papyrus*

HEMODIALYSIS

John Jacob Abel, Leonard. G. Rowntree, B.B. Turner; 1914   **1264**

There are numerous toxic states in which the eliminating organs, more especially the kidneys, are incpabable of removing from the body at an adequate rate, either the autochthonous or the foreign substances whose presence in excessive amount is detrimental to life processes.... We have devised a method by which the blood of a living animal may be submitted to dialysis outside the body... without any alteration which would necessarily be prejudicial to life. The process may be appropriately referred to as *vivi-diffusion*. The apparatus constitutes what has been called an artificial kidney.

Journal of Pharmacology and Experimental Therapeutics

HEMOGLOBIN

Oscar Zinoffsky; 1885　　　　1265

It follows without doubt that for 1 atom of iron haemoglobin contains exactly 2 atoms of sulphur and that haemoglobin is a chemical individual.

Zeitschrift für Physiologische Chemie

HEMOPHILIA

John Conrad Otto; 1803　　　　1266

About seventy or eighty years ago a woman by the name of Smith...transmitted the following idiosyncrasy to her descendants.... If the least scratch is made on the skin of some of them, as mortal a hemorrhage will eventually ensue as if the largest wound is inflicted.... It is a surprising circumstance that the males only are subject to this strange affection, and that not all of them are liable to it.... Although the females are exempt, they are still capable of transmitting it to their male children. *Medical Repository*

HEMORRHOIDS

Hippocrates; [460-375 BC]　　　　1267

If bile or phlegm be determined to the veins in the rectum, it heats the blood in the veins: and these veins becoming heated attract blood from the nearest veins, and being gorged the inside of the gut swells outwardly, and the heads of the veins are raised up, and being at the same time bruised by the faeces passing out, and injured by the blood collected in them, they squirt blood, most frequently along with the faeces, but sometimes without faeces. *On Hemorrhoids*

Cotton Mather; 1724　　　　1268

Tis no rare thing, for the *Haemorrhoidal Veins*, to be distended, and Even Corroded, by the Resort of a *Blood full* of Acrimony thither. A grievous pain accompanies it; with an Inflammation. And oftentimes a Flux of pure *Blood follows*.... The *Seat* of it, in the *Parts of Dishonour*, which can't be mentioned among people of any Breeding without a sort of Blush, seems to oblige the Sufferer unto *Self-Abasement*. *The Angel of Bethesda*

William Heberden; 1802　　　　1269

Women during the state of pregnancy, and just after the menses have finally left them, are particularly subject to the piles. *Commentaries on the History and Cure of Diseases*

HENOCH-SCHÖNLEIN PURPURA

William Heberden; 1802　　　　1270

Some children, without any alteration of their health at the time, or before, or after, have had purple spots come out all over them, exactly the same as are seen in purple fevers. In some places they were no broader than a millet-seed, in others they were as broad as the palm of the hand. In a few days they disappeared without the help of any medicines. It was remarkable, that in one of these the slightest pressure was sufficient to extravasate the blood, and make the part appear as it usually does from a bruise.

Commentaries on the History and Cure of Diseases

Johann Lucas Schönlein; 1837　　　　1271

The patients have either suffered earlier from rheumatism or rheumatic symptoms appear in the same time...in the joints...which are oedematous, swollen and very painful when moved; the characteristic spots...appear in the majority of cases first on the extremities and particularly on the lower ones.... The spots are small, the size of a lentil, a millet seed, bright red, not elevated above the skin, disappearing on pressure of the finger...the eruption comes by fits and starts, often throughout several weeks.

Allgemeine und Specielle Pathologie und Therapie

Eduard Heinrich Henoch; 1882   **1272**
Numerous smaller, and larger, dark red, or bluish, round patches are especially noticed on the legs and feet, while the upper portions of the body are free, or present but a few specks. They are not changed by pressure.... The purpura in these cases was always combined with colic, tenderness of the colon, vomiting, intestinal hemorrhage, and, with one exception, with rheumatic pains, with swelling of the joints being less constant.

Lectures on Diseases of Children

HEPARIN

William Henry Howell, Luther Emmett Holt; 1918   **1273**
Two new substances are described which are connected with the process of coagulation of blood: a. A phosphatid designated as heparin since it is obtained most readily from the liver (dog).... It retards or prevents the coagulation of blood, both in the body and when the blood is shed.... Heparin inhibits clotting mainly by preventing the activation of prothrombin to thrombin. *American Journal of Physiology*

HEPATITIS

Q-L. Choo, G. Kuo, A. J. Weiner, and others; 1989   **1274**
An RNA molecule present in NANBH [non-A, non-B hepatitis] infection... consists of at least 10,000 nucleotides and... is positive-stranded with respect to the encoded NANBH antigen. These data indicate that this clone is derived from the genome of the NANBH agent and are consistent with the agent being similar to the togaviridae or flaviviridae.

Science

HEPATOLENTICULAR DEGENERATION (WILSON DISEASE)

Samuel Alexander Kinnier Wilson; 1912   **1275**
Progressive lenticular degeneration is a disease of the motor nervous system, occurring in young people and very often familial. It is not congenital or hereditary.... The neurological symptoms constitute a syndrome of the corpus striatum.... Although cirrhosis of the liver is constantly found in this affection, and is an essential feature of it, there are no signs of liver disease during life.... The morbid agent is probably of the nature of a toxin.... It is probable that the toxin is associated with the hepatic cirrhosis. *Brain*

John Nathaniel Cumings; 1948   **1276**
Copper and iron estimations have been made in the liver and in various parts of the brain in hepato-lenticular degenerations.... There has been shown to be a considerable retention of copper in these tissues.... The possibility that the condition is a metabolic disorder similar to that of haemochromatosis has been discussed. *Brain*

HERBS

Samuel Stearns; 1801   **1277**
The Author hereby presents you with the first American Herbal, ever compiled in America.... Every man and woman, ought to be their own physician in some measure.... They should know how to shun mineral, vegetable, and animal poisons.... They ought to be thoroughly acquainted with...the qualities of the medicines they exhibit.

The American Herbal

HEREDITARY HEMORRHAGIC TELANGIECTASIA

Henri-Jules-Marie Rendu; 1896   1278

He...had his first nose bleeds at the age of 12 years, and throughout his youth.... Since the age of 35 the hemorrhages have become very frequent, always in the form of epistaxis.... He has had two teeth pulled without having had notable consequent hemorrhages. This is, therefore, no true hemophilia.... Small purple spots...are true cutaneous hemangiomas.... This anatomic disposition is not limited to the skin; it extends also to the mucous membranes.   *Gazette Hôpital*

HERNIAS

Greensville Dowell; 1876   1279

The number of sufferers from hernia is immensely large, and too often the inadequate knowledge of their attending physicians leads them to the nets of the charlatans who advertise trusses and bandages.   *A Treatise on Hernia*

HERNIORRHAPHY

Edoardo Bassini; 1887   1280

This method reconstructs the inguinal canal as it is physiologically, with two rings, one abdominal, the other subcutaneous; and with two walls, one posterior and the other anterior, between which the spermatic cord passes obliquely.   *Attività di Congresso Associazone Medicina di Italia*

HEROIN

[Anonymous]; 1971   1281

King Heroin is my shepherd, I shall always want. He maketh me to lie down in the gutters.... Yea, I shall walk through the valley of poverty and will fear all evil for thou, Heroin, art with me.... Thou strippest the table of groceries in the presence of my family. Thou robbest my head of reason.... Surely heroin addiction shall stalk me all the days of my life and I will dwell in the House of the Damned forever.   *The Psalm of the Addict*

HERPES ZOSTER

William Heberden; 1802   1282

The herpes, or shingles, has begun with a pain which has lasted in some for two or three days before the eruption appeared. It consists of a heap of watery bladders, itching at first, of which there are sometimes so many as nearly to surround the body, whence it has its name of shingles, from *cingulum*.   *Commentaries on the History and Cure of Diseases*

HIGH-ALTITUDE MEDICINE

Too Kim; *circa* 50 BC   1283

On passing the Great Big Headache Mountain, and the Little Headache Mountain, the Red Land and the fever Slope, men's bodies become feverish, they lose colour, and are attacked with headache and vomiting; the asses and cattle being all in like condition.   *Wylie A, Journal of the Royal Anthropological Institute of Great Britain and Ireland*

José de Acosta; 1590   1284

There is in Peru, a high mountaine which they call Pariacaca, and having heard speake of the alteration it bred, I went as well prepared as I could.... When I came to mount the degrees, as they call them, which is the top of this mountaine, I was suddenly surprized with so mortall and strange a payn, that I was ready to fall from the top to the ground.... I was surprised with such pangs of straining and casting, as I thought to cast up my heart too.... In the end I cast up blood, with the straining of my stomacke.   *Historia Natural y Moral de las Indias*

Charles S. Houston; 1960   **1285**

A case of acute pulmonary edema [occurred] in a healthy young athlete with a normal heart.... The condition is attributed to the combined stresses of cold, exertion, and the anoxia occurring at 12,000 feet.... The mechanism...is not known, but the disease... deserves further attention by mountain climbers in particular.

New England Journal of Medicine

HIPPOCRATES

[Anonymous]; *circa* 375 BC   **1286**

Here lieth the Thessalian Hippocrates, by descent a Cosan, spring from the immortal stock of Phoebus. Armed by Health he gained many victories over Disease, and won great glory not by chance, but by Science.   *Epitaph*

Aulus Cornelius Celsus; [25 BC - AD 50]   **1287**

At first the science of healing was held to be part of philosophy.... Hence we find that many who professed philosophy became expert in medicine.... But it was, as some believe, a pupil of [Democritus], Hippocrates of Cos, a man first and foremost worthy to be remembered, notable both for professional skill and for eloquence, who separated this branch of learning from the study of philosophy.   *On Medicine*

Erik H. Erikson; 1964   **1288**

The clinical arts and sciences, while employing the scientific method, are not defined by it or limited by it. The healer is committed to a highest good; rather, he is precommitted to this basic proposition while investigating what can be verified by scientific means. This is...the meaning of the Hippocratic oath, which subordinates all medical methods to a humanist ethic.   *Insight and Responsibility*

Richard Gordon; 1993   **1289**

The "Father of Medicine" was a disastrous ancestor. He left the Hippocratic tradition. That is, shortly: any nondoctor telling a doctor how to do his job is committing outrageous impertinence; any interference with the wherewithal for any doctor's selfless devotion to his patient is shockingly immoral.   *The Alarming History of Medicine*

HIRSCHSPRUNG DISEASE

Harald Hirschsprung; 1888   **1290**

[My first specimen] is a colon, but a colon of such a size that it will no doubt surprise you to learn that it comes from a child only 11 months old when it died.... Only [the] rectum was not dilated, nor indeed subject to any obstruction.   *Jahrbuecher für Kinderheilkunde*

HIRSUTISM

Fuller Albright; 1963   **1291**

Of the many thorns in the side of the endocrinologist the most aggravating is the patient whose life is made miserable by excessive hair growth on the face and elsewhere. In only one case in a hundred can the physician find an endocrine fault.... What is needed more than any other one thing is a razor in disguise, e.g., an electric razor that has been camouflaged with some fancy embellishment and called an "electric depilator."

Annals of Internal Medicine

HISTORY OF MEDICINE

John Warren; 1812   **1292**

In our inquiries into any particular subject of Medicine, our labours will generally be shortened and directed to their proper objects, by a knowledge of preceding discoveries.

Remarks on Angina Pectoris

Christian Albert Theodor Billroth; *circa* 1850   **1293**
Only the man who is familiar with the art and science of the past is competent to aid in its progress in the future.   *Rutkow IM, The History of Surgery in the United States*

William Osler; 1897   **1294**
Of the altruistic instincts veneration is not the most highly developed at the present day, but I hold strongly with the statement that it is the sign of a dry age when the great men of the past are held in light esteem.   *The Functions of a State Faculty*

William Osler; 1901   **1295**
By the historical method alone can many problems in medicine be approached profitably. For example, the student who dates his knowledge of tuberculosis from Koch may have a very correct, but he has a very incomplete, appreciation of the subject. Within a quarter of a century our libraries will have certain alcoves devoted to the historical consideration of the great diseases, which will give to the student that mental perspective which is so valuable an equipment in life. The past is a good nurse, as Lowell remarks, particularly for the weanlings of the fold.   *Books and Men*

William Osler; 1902   **1296**
Modern medicine is a product of the Greek intellect, and had its origin when that wonderful people created positive or rational science.   *Chauvinism in Medicine*

Charles E. Rosenberg; 1992   **1297**
The most fundamental theme—and attraction—of the history of medicine is its potentially integrative quality [and] medicine's necessary integration of theory and practice, of life and death, of family and institutional life, of the historical and the timeless. Medicine has its origins in the social response to unchanging realities: pain, death, childbirth, trauma and disease, the working out of the life cycle in men and women.   *Explaining Epidemics*

Lewis Thomas; 1992   **1298**
One reason why medical history is not much taught in medical schools is that so much of it is an embarrassment.   *The Fragile Species*

Norman Gevitz; 1995   **1299**
The history of medicine can teach students about the structure of medical discovery and how it [affects] the way we think and the way we behave. It explores the fundamental values underlying medical practice and how they evolved. It examines both the experience of being a physician and a patient and brings understanding to the dimensions of suffering and healing. Finally, the history of medicine offers an intellectual challenge for the student.   *University of Chicago Department of Medical Education Bulletin*

Barbara Gottlieb; 1996   **1300**
The history and heritage of medicine are inadequately integrated into the education of physicians and are rarely incorporated into the body of knowledge held by medical practitioners and scholars. But the past establishes the context for the present. Students and practitioners who are not familiar with the past lack the tools with which to analyze the present and make meaningful decisions.   *Doctors of Conscience*

HISTORY-TAKING

Benjamin Franklin; 1748   **1301**
To Friend, Lawyer, Doctor, tell plain your whole Case,
Nor think on bad Matters to put a good Face:
How can they advise, if they see but a part?
'Tis very ill driving black Hogs in the dark.   *Poor Richard's Almanac*

HODGKIN DISEASE

Thomas Hodgkin; 1832   1302

[The lymph glands of the neck] exhibited a firm cartilaginous structure of a light colour and very feeble vascularity, but with no appearance of softening or suppuration. Glands similarly affected accompanied the vessels into the chest, where the bronchial and mediastinal glands were in the same state and greatly enlarged.... The spleen was enlarged to at least four times its natural size...presenting the same structure as the enlarged glands.

Medico-Chirurgical Transactions

Samuel Wilks; 1865   1303

I must call attention to...a disease where the lymphatic glands are increased in size, and associated with a deposit of a morbid kind in the internal viscera, more especially in the spleen.... Dr. Hodgkin...was the first...to call attention to this peculiar form of disease.

Guy's Hospital Reports

Louis Sanford Goodman, Maxwell M. Wintrobe, William Dameshek, and others; 1946   1304

This...preliminary communication presents the...results obtained for 67 patients treated with the nitrogen mustards (halogenated alkyl amine hydrochlorides) for Hodgkin's disease, lymphosarcoma, leukemia, and certain related and miscellaneous diseases.... Salutary results have been obtained particularly in Hodgkin's disease, lymphosarcoma, and chronic leukemia. Indeed, in the first two disorders dramatic improvement has been observed.... In an impressive proportion of terminal and so-called radiation resistant cases...the B-chloroethylamines have produced clinical remissions lasting from weeks to months.   *Journal of the American Medical Association*

Vincent T. DeVita, A.A. Serpick, Paul P. Carbone; 1970   1305

The response rate [with "MOPP" therapy] was superior to that previously reported with the use of single drugs with 35 of 43, or 81% of the patients achieving a complete remission, defined as the complete disappearance of all tumor and return to normal performance status.   *Annals of Internal Medicine*

HOMEOPATHY

Armand Trousseau; 1861   1306

To know how to wait is a great science in our art, prudent waiting often explains successes; it explains, above all, those obtained sometimes by those of the Hahnemann sect.

On Erysipelas

Joseph W. Freer; 1865   1307

It is impossible for a Homeopathic physician to be an educated man, or an educated man to be a Homeopathic physician. To say "Homeopathic physician" is as great a solecism as to say "black white bird."   *Chicago Medical Journal*

Oliver Wendell Holmes; 1891   1308

If you want to be sure *not* to reach threescore and twenty, get a little box of homeopathic pellets and a little book of homeopathic prescriptions. I had a poor friend who fell into that way.... The poor fellow had cultivated symptoms as other people cultivate roses or chrysanthemums. What a luxury of choice his imagination presented to him!   *Over the Teacups*

Ambrose Bierce; 1906   1309

Homeopathist, *n*. The humorist of the medical profession.   *The Devil's Dictionary*

HOMEOSTASIS

Walter Bradford Cannon; 1932   1310

The coordinated physiological processes which maintain most of the steady states in the organism are so complex and so peculiar to living things—involving as they may, the brain and nerves, the heart, lungs, kidneys, and spleen, all working cooperatively—that I have suggested a special designation for these states, homeostasis. The word does not imply something set and immobile, a stagnation. It means a condition—a condition which may vary, but which is relatively constant. *The Wisdom of the Body*

HOMOSEXUALITY

Alfred Charles Kinsey, Wardell B. Pomeroy, Clyde E. Martin; 1948   1311

Of the 40 or 50 percent of the male population which has homosexual experience, certainly a high proportion would not be considered psychopathic personalities on the basis of anything else in their histories. It is argued that an individual who is so obtuse to social reactions as to continue his homosexual activity and make it any material portion of his life, therein evidences some social incapacity.... There is an increasing proportion of the most skilled psychiatrists who make no attempt to re-direct behavior, but who devote their attention to helping an individual accept himself. *Sexual Behavior in the Human Male*

Fuller Albright; 1963   1312

The author has yet to see a homosexual patient in whom the trouble was based on faulty endocrine function or in whom the giving of a hormone influenced the direction of the libido. *Annals of Internal Medicine*

HOPELESS CASES

Eugene G. Laforet; 1963   1313

It must by now be apparent that the term "hopeless case" is a misnomer applied to a patient for whom the physician has little hope. It does not, however, represent the judgment of the patient. For there are no "hopeless" patients, only hopeless doctors. *Archives of Internal Medicine*

HORNER SYNDROME

Johann Friedrich Horner; 1869   1314

The pupil of the right eye is considerably more constricted than that of the left, but reacts to light; the globe has sunk inward very slightly.... Both eyes...have normal visual acuity. During the clinical discussion of the case, the right side of her face became red and warm...while the left side remained pale and cool. The right side seemed turgid and rounded, the left more sunken and angular; the one perfectly dry, the other moist. The boundary of the redness and warmth was exactly in the midline. *Klinische Augenheilkunde*

HOSPITAL STAFFS

Caroline Fenger; *circa* 1880   1315

A position on the [Cook County] Hospital's consulting staff could be obtained for an overcoat and a case of champagne, but a permanent position came at a higher price. *Procedures of the Institute of Medicine of Chicago*

[Anonymous]; 1907   1316

In this age, the church a man attends, his political leanings, or the amount of influence he is able to exert with hospital managers, has as much to do with hospital staff appointments as his especial experience or skill. *National Hospital Record*

[Anonymous]; 1915   1317

We all know, only too well, the great scramble for hospital association.... A physician not in the coterie of a hospital staff pulls every wire to get one.... A crooked politician would blush with shame to be seen in the company of some of our physicians did he know the extent of knavery they have gone to [to] get on a hospital staff. *Starr P, The Social Transformation of American Medicine*

HOSPITALISTS

Robert Wachter, Lee Goldman; 1996   1318

We anticipate the rapid growth of a new breed of physician we call "hospitalist" —specialists in inpatient medicine— who will be responsible for managing the care of hospitalized patients in the same way that primary care physicians are responsible for managing the care of outpatients.   *New England Journal of Medicine*

HOSPITALS

Thomas More; 1516   1319

Every city [in Utopia] has four [hospitals], slightly outside the walls, and spacious enough to appear like little towns. The hospitals are large...so that the sick...will not be packed closely and uncomfortably together, and also so that those who have a contagious disease, such as might pass from one to the other, may be isolated. The hospitals are...supplied with everything needed to cure the patients, who are nursed with tender and watchful care. Highly skilled physicians are in constant attendance.... Hardly anyone in the city...would not rather be treated...at the hospital than at home.   *Utopia*

Jacques Tenon; 1788   1320

There are two dangers to avoid when discharging convalescents from a hospital: compromising their health by keeping them too long, and discharging them before they are strong enough to work.   *Memoirs on Paris Hospitals*

Claude Bernard; 1865   1321

I consider hospitals only as the entrance to scientific medicine. They are the first field of observation which a physician enters, but the true sanctuary of medical science is a laboratory.   *An Introduction to the Study of Experimental Medicine*

Bayard Holmes; 1906   1322

The hospital is essentially part of the armamentarium of medicine.... If we wish to escape the thralldom of commercialism, if we wish to avoid the fate of the tool-less wage worker, we must control the hospital.   *Journal of the American Medical Association*

E.B. White; 1963   1323

And one of the best parts, I thought, was the part about time becoming fluid in a hospital, and the way you float in it. Last summer I spent seven days in Harkness, floating. Nobody came to see me, nothing happened, I didn't eat or drink, I didn't read, it was a private room, my doctor left town, the nurses disappeared one by one into the heat of summer and vacations, and I was alone, truly afloat in time, more alone than I have ever been in my life.   *Letter*

Charles Percy Snow; 1973   1324

The climate of a hospital always has within it some wafts of fear.   *Journal of the American Medical Association*

Philippe Ariès; 1981   1325

The hospital has become the place of solitary death.   *The Hour of Our Death*

Paul Starr; 1982   1326

Few institutions have undergone as radical a metamorphosis as have hospitals in their modern history. In developing from places of dreaded impurity and exiled human wreckage into awesome citadels of science and bureaucratic order, they acquired a new moral identity, as well as new purposes and patients of higher status.   *The Social Transformation of American Medicine*

Arnold S. Relman; 1985   1327

The steps necessary to ensure adequate emergency care of the indigent and uninsured are, unfortunately, at odds with the currently fashionable philosophy in Washington. We cannot expect to see much action until enough policy makers lose their fascination with the view that hospitals are basically businesses.   *New England Journal of Medicine*

Charles E. Rosenberg; 1987   **1328**
The hospital is both more and less than a creature of twentieth-century technology and bureaucracy; it is both alike and fundamentally different from a factory, public school, or corporate headquarters.   *The Care of Strangers*

John L. McClenahan; 1993   **1329**
A modern hospital can provide a CT scan in twenty minutes. An enema may take two days.   *Aphorism*

HUMAN BODY

Lewis Thomas; 1974   **1330**
We are paying too little attention, and respect, to the built-in durability and sheer power of the human organism. Its surest tendency is toward stability and balance. It is a distortion, with something profoundly disloyal about it, to picture the human being as a teetering, fallible contraption, always needing watching and patching, always on the verge of flapping to pieces.   *Lives of a Cell*

HUMANITIES

William Osler; 1897   **1331**
...By the neglect of the study of the humanities, which has been far too general, the profession loses a very precious quality.   *British Medicine in Greater Britain*

HUMANS

Johann Wolfgang von Goethe; [1749-1832]   **1332**
It is not the doctor in the long cloak, who from his lecturing desk teaches down to us; it is the human being, who roves about, pays attention, is amazed, seized with joy and pain and forces the passionate information upon us.   *Nager F, Der Heilkundige Dichter*

Karl Marx; 1844   **1333**
Certainly, eating, drinking, and procreating are...genuinely human functions. But abstractly taken separated from the sphere of all other human activities and turned into sole and ultimate ends, they are animal functions.
Economic and Philosophical Manuscripts of 1844

William Osler; 1904   **1334**
Curious, odd compounds are these fellow-creatures, at whose mercy you will be; full of fads and eccentricities, of whims and fancies; but the more closely we study their little foibles of one sort and another in the inner life which we see, the more surely is the conviction borne in upon us of the likeness of their weaknesses to our own.
Aequanimitas. Aequanimitas

Santiago Ramón y Cajal; 1920   **1335**
What would be man if described by monkeys? Probably an interesting case of apish degeneration caused by his unfortunate habit of talking and thinking.
Chatting over Coffee

René Jules Dubos; 1959   **1336**
To grow in the midst of dangers is the fate of the human race, because it is the law of the spirit.   *Mirage of Health*

Hugo Roesler; 1960   **1337**
Man is born nude, but not equal.   *Temple University Medical Center Bulletin*

René Jules Dubos; 1968   **1338**

In the course of their evolution, the various animal species have developed a high degree of anatomical, physiological, and behavioral specialization; as a result they have become committed to certain habitats and ways of life. Contrastingly, man has remained the great amateur of the living world.... Man is outdone by many animal species in such attributes as speed, physical strength, acuity of sense organs, accuracy of responses, and resistance to stresses. Probably he leads them all in adaptability, precisely because he exhibits so little biological specialization.   *Man, Medicine, and Environment*

Oliver W. Sacks; 1985   **1339**

If we wish to know about a man, we ask "what is his story—his real, inmost story?"—for each of us *is* a biography, a story. Each of us *is* a singular narrative, which is constructed continually, unconsciously, by, through, and in us—through our perceptions, our feelings, our thoughts, and our actions, not least, our discourse, our spoken narrations. Biologically, physiologically, we are not so different from each other; historically, as narratives, we are each of us unique.   *The Man Who Mistook His Wife for a Hat*

Lewis Thomas; 1992   **1340**

I am a member of a fragile species, still new to the earth, the youngest creatures of any scale, here only a few moments as evolutionary time is measured, a juvenile species, a child of a species. We are only tentatively set in place, error-prone, at risk of fumbling, in real danger at the moment of leaving behind only a thin layer of our fossils, radioactive at that.   *The Fragile Species*

HUMOR

Thomas Sydenham; [1624-1689]   **1341**

The arrival in town of a good clown is of more benefit to the people than the arrival of 20 asses laden with medicine.   *Strauss MB, Familiar Medical Quotations*

HUNTER'S SYNDROME

Charles Hunter; 1917   **1342**

The children present an extraordinary appearance. [They] are undersized... ; heads extremely large.... The head is curiously shaped, with a very marked bulging of the squamous portion of the temporal bone and of the frontal bones.... The face is very large,... of deep burnt-red colour.... Very large tongue... very short neck... The chest is broad.... The gait is very clumsy and stiff.... The children are bright and intelligent... though both are hampered by distinct dullness of hearing.   *Proceedings of the Royal Society of Medicine*

HUNTINGTON CHOREA

George Huntington; 1872   **1343**

The hereditary chorea...is confined to...a *few* families, and has been transmitted to them, an heirloom from generations...back in the dim past.... It is attended generally by all the symptoms of common chorea, only in an aggravated degree, hardly ever manifesting itself until *adult* or *middle* life, and then coming on gradually but surely...until the hapless sufferer is but a quivering wreck of his former self.   *Medical and Surgical Reporter*

HYDROCEPHALUS

William Heberden; 1802   **1344**

The heads of children sometimes grow enormously large, the sutures give way, and the membranes of the brain are pushed up with the water within, and make a soft tumor rising above the edges of the sutures.... They daily become more and more stupid, with a pulse not above seventy-two.   *Commentaries on the History and Cure of Diseases*

HYGIENE

Charles V. Chapin; 1917   1345
The introduction, or even the purification, of a municipal water supply may require millions.... To wash the hands before eating and after the toilet costs nothing.

How to Avoid Infection

Jacob Markowitz; 1946   1346
The extent of human commerce in faecal particles is not adequately appreciated. The management of defaecation is not aseptic and seldom clean. Moreover, the expulsion of flatus should be regarded in the same light as the cough of an open case of tuberculosis. This point has not been emphasized enough, obviously on the grounds of indelicacy.

Journal of the Royal Army Medical Corps

Richard A. Kern; 1962   1347
Do not eat anything in tropical climes unless it grows four feet above the ground, has a rind on it, and is known not to be grown in night soil. Boil all water thoroughly before drinking, too. In the Orient, particularly, there is crap everywhere.

Temple University Medical Center Bulletin

HYPERTENSION

Thomas Clifford Allbutt; 1895   1348
In the middle and later stages of life men and women...are liable to a rise of the mean arterial pressure to an abnormal and even high degree [which] cannot be measured by the instruments at our disposal; and the evidence...be that of our unassisted senses. I took many sphygmograms in these cases but they are destroyed, and I am satisfied to ask you to accept my clinical estimate of the state of the pulse.... The rise of pressure is unaccompanied by any clinical evidence...of disease...unless dilatation of the left ventricle...be regarded as a disease.   *Transactions of the Hunterian Society*

James Mackenzie, James Orr; 1926   1349
The systolic pressure represents the maximum force of the heart, while the diastolic pressure measures the resistance the heart has to overcome.... Change in the diastolic pressure is due to more permanent factors, as a rule, such as agencies which increase the peripheral resistance, e.g. thickening of the walls of the arterioles, obliteration of capillaries, etc.

Principles of Diagnosis and Treatment in Heart Affections

Norman Macdonnell Keith, Henry P. Wegener, Nelson W. Barker; 1929   1350
We have considered the usual benign cases [of hypertension] as belonging to Group 1; those of more marked hypertension, presenting few untoward symptoms, without retinitis as belonging to Group 2; those of mild vasospastic retinitis as belonging to Group 3, and those revealing the so-called malignant hypertension as belonging to Group 4.

American Journal of the Medical Sciences

Harry Goldblatt, James Lynch, Ramon Hanzal, Ward Summerville; 1934   1351
These experiments indicate that, in dogs at least, ischemia localized to the kidneys is a sufficient condition for the production of persistently elevated systolic pressure. When the constriction of both main renal arteries is made only modestly severe...the elevation of systolic blood pressure is unaccompanied by signs of materially decreased renal function.... Almost complete constriction of both main renal arteries...results in great elevation of systolic blood pressure which is accompanied by...uremia.   *Journal of Experimental Medicine*

Juan Carlos Fasciolo, Bernardo Alberto Houssay, A.C. Taquini; 1938   1352
The ischaemic kidney secretes directly a vasoconstrictor substance which causes a permanent hypertension. This substance is active in the absence of the adrenals. The healthy kidney is capable of diminishing the action of this blood-pressure raising substance.

Journal of Physiology

Alfred Blalock; 1940   **1353**
The evidence indicates that diminution in the renal blood flow produces peripheral vaso-constriction and hypertension by means of the action of a pressor substance which is formed in the ischemic kidney and which enters the blood stream. The exact nature of the product elaborated by the kidney has not been identified.   *Physiological Reviews*

Eduardo Braun-Menendez, J.C. Fasciolo, L.F. Leloir, J.M. Muñoz; 1940   **1354**
The pressor and vasoconstrictor properties of the venous blood from kidneys in acute ischaemia have been studied. Extracts of this blood contain a pressor substance (hyper-tensin) which is also formed *in vitro* when blood proteins are incubated with renin.
    Journal of Physiology

George White Pickering; 1968   **1355**
The "disease" essential hypertension, representing the consequences of raised pressure with-out evident cause, is... a type of disease not hitherto recognized in medicine in which the defect is one of degree, not of kind; quantitative, not qualitative.   *High Blood Pressure*

George White Pickering; 1968   **1356**
High blood pressure.... is a sign, not a disease.   *High Blood Pressure*

Mary Lou McIlhany, John H. Shaffer, Edgar A. Hines Jr.; 1975   **1357**
Blood pressure in 200 pairs of twins...were measured at basal levels and in response to the cold pressor test. Intraclass correlations were consistently larger...in monozygotic as com-pared to diazygotic pairs.... Sex differences in heritability were somewhat greater for sys-tolic than for diastolic blood pressures.   *Johns Hopkins Medical Journal*

N.O. Borhani, M. Feinleib, R.T. Garrison, and others; 1977   **1358**
For both systolic and diastolic blood pressure there is evidence that in a substantial por-tion of the total population *variability can be attributed to genetic differences*.... We cal-culated the "heritability" index for systolic and diastolic blood pressures.... [The] indices were 0.82 and 0.64 respectively for systolic and diastolic blood pressures.
    Acta Geneticae Medicae Gemellologia

Laryssa N. Kaufman, Mary M. Peterson, Stephen M. Smith; 1991   **1359**
Male Sprague-Dawley rats fed either a high-fat diet or a glucose-enriched diet developed higher blood pressures than rats fed a control diet.... Rats fed the high-fat diet developed hypertension only when they were allowed to overeat and become obese and hyperinsu-linemic. But when their feeding was restricted to prevent obesity... they remained nor-motensive.   *American Journal of Physiology*

HYPERTHYROIDISM

Caleb Hillier Parry; 1825   **1360**
Grace B...became subject to more or less of palpitation of the heart...till my attendance, when it was so vehement, that each systole of the heart shook the whole thorax.... About three months after lying-in,...a lump about the size of a walnut was perceived on the right side of her neck. This continued to enlarge...when it occupied both sides of the neck, so as to have reached an enormous size.... The eyes were protruded from their sockets.
    Enlargement of the Thyroid Gland

Robert James Graves; 1835   **1361**
I have lately seen three cases of violent and long-continued palpitations in females, in each of which the sample peculiarity presented itself—viz., enlargement of the thyroid gland.... A lady, aged twenty, became affected with some symptoms which were supposed to be hysterical.... It was now observed that the eyes assumed a singular appearance, for the eyeballs were apparently enlarged, so that when she slept, or tried to shut her eyes, the lids were incapable of closing.   *Clinical Lectures*

Carl Adolph von Basedow; 1840 1362

After weaning, the menses were very scanty and then...they were entirely suppressed.... Madame F...lost a great deal of weight; at which time the eyeballs began to protrude from the *Orbita*.... She had a very rapid, small pulse...a resounding heart beat, she could not hold her hand still, spoke with striking rapidity.... In the neck there appeared a strumous swelling of the thyroid gland; the area of pulsation of the heart was now broadened.... The eyelids were pushed wide from one another. *Wochenschrift für die Gesamte Heilkunde*

Carl Adolph von Basedow; 1840 1363

Mrs. G. [the first of three cases described] lost weight, suffered from oedema of the legs, general emaciation, amenorrhoea, palpitation of the heart,...shortness of breath, and a sense of depression about the chest. There was a noticeable protrusion of the eyeballs which were otherwise healthy and functioned completely, although she slept with open eyes. She had a frightened look and was known in our whole town as a crazy woman.
Wochenschrift für die Gesamte Heilkunde

Friedrich Wilhelm Ernst Albrecht von Graefe; 1864 1364

The protrusion of the eyeball is one of the most important symptoms of Basedow's disease [but] not enough attention [is] paid to another symptom.... When normal individuals elevate or lower their glance, the upper eyelid makes a corresponding movement. In patients suffering from Basedow's disease this is entirely abolish[ed] or reduced to the minimum.... As the cornea looks down, the upper eyelid does not follow. *Deutsche Klinik*

Edwin Bennett Astwood; 1943 1365

The daily administration of 1 to 2 Gm. of thiourea or of 0.2 to 1 Gm. of thiouracil to hyperthyroid persons resulted in the relief of symptoms and the return to normal of the serum cholesterol and the basal metabolic rate. There were observed a latent period of one to two weeks before these effects occurred, a sustained remission during treatment, and a return of hyperthyroidism when therapy was discontinued.
Journal of the American Medical Association

HYPERTROPHIC OSTEOARTHROPATHY (DIGITAL HIPPOCRATISM)

Pierre Marie; 1890 1366

The volume of all the phalanges of the fingers are increased, but above all in the case of the phalangette. The nail is enlarged; it has the Hippocratic appearance of a parrot's beak.
Revue de Médecine

HYPOCHONDRIA

John Gregory; 1772 1367

There is a numerous class of patients who put a physician's good nature and patience to a severe trial; those I mean who suffer under nervous ailments. Although the fears of these patients are generally groundless, yet their sufferings are real; and the disease is as much seated in the constitution as a rheumatism or dropsy.
Lectures on the Duties and Qualifications of a Physician

William Buchan; 1798 1368

Hypocondriac affections... generally attack the indolent, the luxurious, the unfortunate, and the studious. It becomes daily more common in this country, owing, no doubt to the increase of luxury and sedentary employments.... Men of a melancholy temperament, whose minds are capable of great attention, and whose passions are not easily moved, are in the advanced periods of life, most liable to this disease. It is usually brought on by long and serious attention to abstruse subjects, grief, the suppression of customary evacuations, excess of venery, the repulsion of cutaneous eruptions [and] long-continued evacuations. *Domestic Medicine*

William Heberden; 1802   **1369**

Hypochondriac complaints resemble the gout, and madness, and consumptions, in their not appearing before the age of puberty.   *Commentaries on the History and Cure of Diseases*

William Withey Gull, Edmond Anstey; 1868   **1370**

The most important external feature of hypochondriasis is this—that without any sufficient reason for such conduct, and without any signs of intellectual insanity, the patient is observed to concentrate his attention on some particular organ of his body, and to fancy that it is seriously diseased. This concentration...is often...accompanied by a tendency to depression.... The first duty of the physician is to encourage the hypochondriac to forget his woes; but nothing is more difficult in practice.   *J. Russell Reynolds, A System of Medicine*

Thomas Clifford Allbutt; 1884   **1371**

She is entangled in the net of the gynaecologist, who finds her uterus, like her nose, a little to one side, or again, like that organ, is running a little, or it is as flabby as her biceps, so that the unhappy viscus is impaled on a stem, or perched on a prop, or is painted with carbolic acid every week in the year except during the long vacation when the gynaecologist is grouse shooting.... Arraign the uterus and you fix in the woman the arrow of hypochondria, it may be for life.   *Visceral Neuroses*

Jerome K. Jerome; 1889   **1372**

It is a most extraordinary thing, but I never read a patent medicine advertisement without being impelled to the conclusion that I am suffering from the particular disease therein dealt with in its most virulent form. The diagnosis seems in every case to correspond exactly with all the sensations that I have ever felt.   *Three Men in a Boat*

Ambrose Bierce; 1906   **1373**

Hypochondriasis, *n.* Depression of one's own spirits.   *The Devil's Dictionary*

Robert Hall Babcock; 1914   **1374**

[Cardiac hypochondriacs] may try our patience sorely, but they are to be pitied because they suffer more from their subjective symptoms of palpitation, precordial pain, etc., than does many a patient with veritable organic heart disease.   *New York Medical Journal*

Vincent Askey; 1960   **1375**

We are rapidly becoming a land of hypochondriacs, from the ulcer-and-martini executives in the big city to the patent medicine patrons in the sulfur-and-molasses belt.

The Land of Hypochondriacs

Donald Woods Winnicott; 1966   **1376**

Patients who are always pestering a succession of doctors to examine them very seldom have anything to be discovered by physical test.   *International Journal of Psychoanalysis*

Donald Woods Winnicott; 1966   **1377**

It is the hypochondriacs who fail to get examined when they have cancer of the breast or a hypernephroma, and it is the patients who are physically ill who put themselves forward as needing psycho-analysis or hypnotism.   *International Journal of Psychoanalysis*

[Anonymous]; 1991   **1378**

There must, surely, be a limit to the amount of information one of these things can store. How will they cope with what I call the "Three Volume Novel" patients? You know the sort I mean—three enormous hospital folders, tattered and tied up with string, bearing the names of every consultant on the staff, with a referral letter saying "Is this patient hypochondriacal?" (to which the truthful but tactless answer would be "If not at the start of all of this, then by now, yes"). Will the Three Volume Novel become the Three Compact Disc Album?   *The Lancet*

HYPOGONADISM

Aretaeus the Cappadocian; [81-138?]   **1379**
When the semen is not possessed of its vitality, persons become shrivelled, have a sharp tone of voice, lose their hair and their beard, and become effeminate, as the characteristics of eunuchs prove.   *On Gonorrhoea*

Fuller Albright; 1951   **1380**
A patient who complains of lifelong impotence or lack of libido does not suffer from hormonal lack; a patient with real endocrine insufficiency, e.g., eunuchoidism, has impotence and absent libido, but does not complain of them, but of something more trivial, such as being mistaken for a girl over the telephone.   *Diseases of the Ductless Glands*

HYPOPITUITARISM

Alexander Simpson; 1883   **1381**
Mr Whitehead records his case [of superinvolution of the uterus] as one of "absence of the uterus after repeated pregnancies;" but it is noteworthy that all her labors were complicated with haemorrhage, and most of all after the birth of the last child.
Edinburgh Medical Journal

Morris Simmonds; 1914   **1382**
A previously healthy woman fell ill with a severe puerperal sepsis. She developed a septic necrosis of the pituitary. As a result of the loss of this vital organ there developed severe consequences: menopause, muscle weakness, dizziness and attacks of unconsciousness, anemia, rapid aging—in short: a premature senility. The remaining intact fragments of the gland tended to atrophy in the surrounding fibrotic tissue.The gland becomes completely insufficient and the woman dies in coma. The autopsy reveals as the only cause of death an almost complete dwindling of the hypophysis.   *Deutsche Medizinische Wochenschrift*

Harold Leeming Sheehan; 1937   **1383**
Necrosis of the anterior pituitary is a relatively frequent finding in women dying during the puerperium.... The necrosis begins about the time of delivery.... The thrombosis is usually consequent on the collapse of the patient following severe haemorrhage at delivery.... If the patient survives the puerperium, the lesion heals to a mass of condensed stroma.... This is the stage found in cases of Simmonds's disease which date from a delivery some years earlier.   *Journal of Pathology and Bacteriology*

Harold Leeming Sheehan; 1939   **1384**
In the severest cases [of postpartum necrosis of the anterior pituitary] the ovaries become very atrophic and their functions are completely lost.... The absence of oestrogenic hormone is characterized by complete genital atrophy.... In severe cases there is loss of axillary and pubic hair.... Most of the patients develop a group of somewhat related general symptoms which may be considered together: asthenia, apathy, and undue sensitivity to cold.... A few patients die of other conditions... but the great majority die in coma.
Quarterly Journal of Medicine

HYPOTHESIS

Charles Darwin; 1863   **1385**
How odd it is that anyone should not see that all observations must be for or against some view if it is to be of any service.   *Letter to Henry Fawcett*

HYPOTHYROIDISM

Paracelsus (Theophrastus Bombastus von Hohenheim); [1493-1541]   **1386**
To restore fools, there nothing has been found.... But to speak of these creatures that they perchance also have defects in body, that is they carry growths with them, such as goitres

and the like; this perhaps is not a characteristic of fools, but also of others, however it fits most of them. *De Generatione Stultorum*

Felix Platter; 1602   **1387**
In Valesia Canton Bremis,...many infants are wont to be afflicted: who besides their innate simple mindedness, the head is now and then misformed, the tongue immense and tumid, dumb, a struma often at the throat.... Their eyes wide apart, they show immoderate laughter & wonder at unknown things. *Praxeos Medicae*

Wolfgang Hoefer; 1657   **1388**
There is no denying, that such Hernias of the throat, called Bronchocele or struma, can be contracted by these inhabitants of the Alps themselves, through the drinking of water infected with mercury. *Hercules Medicus sive Locorum Communium Liber*

William Heberden; 1802   **1389**
It is most probably owing to some bad quality of the water, that swellings of the throat are endemial in some parts of England, and notoriously among the inhabitants of the Alps; though I by no means think it owing to the use of snow-water, to which it has been attributed: for I believe on account of its great purity this would be one of the best remedies they could employ. *Commentaries on the History and Cure of Diseases*

Thomas Blizard Curling; 1850   **1390**
In July 1849, Dr. Little invited me to see a case of what he considered cretinism...and to examine some swellings at the sides of the neck...which had been suspected to be enlargements either of the lobes of the thyroid body, or of the lymphatic glands.... The countenance had a marked...idiotic expression. The mouth was large, and the tongue thick and protuberant....The body was examined twenty-four hours after death... The swellings in the neck...were composed of fat.... There was not the slightest trace of a thyroid body. *Medico-Chirurgical Transactions*

William Withey Gull; 1873   **1391**
There had been a distinct change in the mental state. The mind, which had previously been active and inquisitive, assumed a gentle, placid indifference, corresponding to the muscular langour, but the intellect was unimpaired.... The change in the skin is remarkable. The texture being peculiarly smooth and fine, and the complexion fair, at a first hasty glance there might be supposed to be a general slight oedema of it.... The beautiful delicate rose-purple tint on the cheek is entirely different from what one sees in the bloated face of renal anasarca. *Transactions of the Clinical Society of London*

William Withey Gull; 1874   **1392**
Miss B—after the cessation of the catamenial period, became insensibly more and more languid, with general increase of bulk.... Her face altering from oval to round,...the tongue broad and thick, voice guttural, and the pronunciation as if the tongue were too large for the mouth (cretinoid).... In the cretinoid condition in adults which I have seen, the thyroid was not enlarged. *On a Cretinoid State*

Jaques-Louis Reverdin; 1882   **1393**
Can it be that the thyroid body whose functions are still obscure plays a part in hematopoiesis so important that its ablation produces such profound trouble? *Revue Médecine de la Suisse Romande*

Emil Theodor Kocher; 1883   **1394**
We have arrived at the point where we generally recommend the radical operation for goiter as the surest and simplest method of treatment.... Surgeons have simply assumed that the thyroid gland has no function whatever.... Patients with total excision...all show more or less severe disturbances in their general condition.... We cannot fail to recognize [the] relation to idiocy and cretinism.... We see no objection for the time being, to the use of the name *cachexia strumipriva*. *Archiv der Klinische Chirurgie*

E.L. Fox; 1892   1395

She was ordered to take half a thyroid, lightly fried and minced, to be taken with currant jelly once a week. [There were some difficulties in working out the dosage, but within a few months] she considered herself well... Her condition now is in every way satisfactory.

British Medical Journal

George Redmayne Murray; 1920   1396

This patient was thus enabled, by the regular and continued use of thyroid extract, to live in good health for over twenty-eight years after she had reached an advanced stage of myxoedema. During this period she consumed over nine pints of liquid thyroid extract or its equivalent, prepared from the thyroid glands of more than 870 sheep. The results obtained in this case show that: 1. The thyroid is purely an internal secretory gland. 2. The symptoms of myxoedema can be entirely removed.   *British Medical Journal*

HYSTERECTOMY

Walter Burnham; 1854   1397

This is the fourth operation I have performed within the last two years for the removal of ovarian tumours, all successful but one.... [This] operation should be considered as one of the most hazardous which the Surgeon is called upon to perform.... [It] should never be performed in Hospitals where Erysipelas...prevailed.   *Nelson's American Lancet*

John C. Irish; 1878   1398

The operation of laportomy was performed by Dr. Burnham.... This is the first operation for removal of the uterus by abdominal section that resulted in recovery. Though the operation was made on an erroneous diagnosis...the error seems to me...an excusable one, when it is remembered that this happened twenty-five years ago, at a time when very little was known of the pathology of the uterus.   *Transactions of the American Medical Association*

HYSTERIA

William Buchan; 1798   1399

Young ladies who are subject to hysteric fits should not be sent to boarding school, as the disease may be caught by imitation. I have known madness itself to be brought on by sympathy.   *Domestic Medicine*

Robertson Davies; 1994   1400

There are always hysterical people undergoing extraordinary cures.   *The Cunning Man*

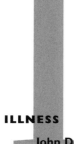

ILLNESS

John Donne; 1624   **1401**

As Sicknesse is the greatest misery, so the greatest misery of sicknes is *solitude*; when the infectiousness of the disease deterrs them who should assist, from comming; even the Phisician *dares* scarse come. *Solitude* is a torment which is not threatned in *hell* it selfe.

Devotions upon Emergent Occasions

Samuel Johnson; 1776   **1402**

Infirmity will come but let us not invite it; Indulgence will allure us, but let us turn resolutely away. Time cannot be always defeated, but let us not yield till we are conquered.

Letter to Edmund Hector

Johann Wolfgang von Goethe; [1749-1832]   **1403**

I have learned much from disease which life could never have taught me anywhere else.

Nager F, Der Heilkundige Dichter

Oliver Wendell Holmes; 1883   **1404**

Nature is a benevolent old hypocrite; she cheats the sick and dying with illusions better than any anodynes.   *The Young Practitioner*

Karl Jaspers; 1963   **1405**

What "sick" in general may mean depends less on a doctor's judgment than on the judgment of the patient and the prevailing conceptions of the contemporary culture.... With psychic illnesses [this] is very much so. The same psychic state will bring the one individual to the psychiatrist as a sick person while it will take another to the confessional as one suffering from sin and guilt.   *General Psychopathology*

Eric J. Cassell; 1976   **1406**

"Illness" [stands] for what the patient feels when he goes to the doctor and "disease" for what he has on the way home from the doctor's office. Disease...is something an organ has; illness is something a man has.   *The Healer's Art*

Anthony R. Moore; 1978   **1407**

The experiences of illness are protean. In some cases disease can dignify, in others it creates heroic capacities. It can lead to self-realization; it can level unequal men; it can be thought of as an agent of retribution.... Even patients who see disease as a despoiler often experience sentiments of greater complexity. They see illness as an ever-present reminder of the unexpected, and of man's fundamental vulnerability. *The Missing Medical Text*

Susan Sontag; 1978 **1408**
Illness is the night-side of life, a more onerous citizenship. Everyone who is born holds dual citizenship, in the kingdom of the well and in the kingdom of the sick. Although we all prefer to use only the good passport, sooner or later each of us is obliged, at least for a spell, to identify ourselves as citizens of that other place. *Illness as Metaphor*

Susan Sontag; 1978 **1409**
Illness expands by means of two hypotheses. The first is that every form of social deviation can be considered an illness... The second is that every illness can be considered psychologically.... As the first seems to relieve guilt, the second reinstates it. Psychological theories of illness are a powerful means of placing the blame on the ill. *Illness as Metaphor*

Norman Cousins; 1979 **1410**
The more serious the illness, the more important it is for you to fight back, mobilizing all your resources—spiritual, emotional, intellectual, physical. *Anatomy of an Illness*

Peter B. Medawar; 1984 **1411**
Twice in my life I very nearly died as a result of cerebral vascular accidents, and I don't look forward a bit to making, in due course, a clean job of it. I neither cursed God for depriving me of the use of two limbs nor thanked and praised Him for sparing me the use of two others. On these two occasions I derived no comfort from religion or from the thought that God was looking after me. *The Limits of Science*

John Wiltshire; 1991 **1412**
Illness has from ancient times been conceived as punishment, as a derivative of sin (with venereal disease providing the obvious paradigm), and even when this nexus is broken or disavowed by the conscious mind, it is always creeping back in less conscious forms...as in the production of "asthmatic" or "cancer prone" personality types. Or it may take another form when a sudden "attack" of disease is connected—to all intents and purposes arbitrarily—with some personal guilt, and thereby given a form of explanation.

Samuel Johnson in the Medical World

O.T. Bonnett; 1996 **1413**
A little illness is truly a wonderful thing to have if you are afraid of life. *Why Healing Happens*

Croatian proverb **1414**
The sooner you lie down in sickness, the quicker you get up in health. *Proverb*

The Bible, The Apocrypha **1415**
My son, if you have an illness, do not neglect it, but pray to the Lord, and he will heal you. Renounce your faults, amend your ways, and cleanse your heart from sin.... Then call in the doctor, for the Lord created him; do not let him leave you, for you need him. There may come a time when your recovery is in their hands; then they too will pray to the Lord to give them success in relieving pain and finding a cure to save their patient's life.

Ecclesiasticus 38:9,10,12-14

IMMUNITY

Paul Ehrlich; 1908 **1416**
The immunity of an animal is...explained as being due to the great energy of the cells of its body, which are able to appropriate nutritious substances for themselves, and in so doing to deprive parasites of them. The opposite condition must be due to a certain disposing influence, and immunity of the parasites must be a condition of the cause of infectivity. The bacterial cells may in the same way be immune against haptine substances, and may withstand the action of the serum. *On Immunity*

IMMUNIZATION

Edward Jenner; 1798   1417

It clearly appears that this disease leaves the constitution in a state of perfect security from the infection of the Smallpox, may we not infer that a mode of Inoculation may be introduced preferable to that at present adopted, especially among those families, which, from previous circumstances we may judge to be predisposed to have the disease unfavourably?   *An Inquiry into the Causes and Effects of the Variolae Vaccinae*

August von Wassermann; 1893   1418

It is definitely possible to protect guinea pigs against the intraperitoneal infection with living cholera bacilli. In order to achieve this, one must inject cholera vibrios or their body substance in such doses that a mild specific illness, a general reaction, follows.   *Zeitschrift für Hygiene und Infektionskrankheit*

IMMUNOLOGY

Rupert Everett Billingham, L. Brent, Peter B. Medawar; 1953   1419

Mice and chickens never develop, or develop to only a limited degree, the power to react immunologically against foreign homologous tissue cells with which they have been inoculated in foetal life. Animals so treated are tolerant not only of the foreign cells of the original inoculum but also of skin grafts freshly transplanted in adult life from the original donor or from a donor of the same antigenic constitution.   *Nature*

IMMUNOSUPPRESSION

Charles G. Craddock; 1978   1420

The hypercorticism of body injury and disease may be designed to protect the body from its own police force, leaving intact the "seasoned, experienced" troops but reducing the number of naive trainees whose commitment to destroy might lack discrimination between self and non-self.   *Annals of Internal Medicine*

IMPOTENCE

Hildegard of Bingen; *circa* 1150   1421

If a male, perhaps due to a natural defect or due to castration, is without [the two testes], then he does not have... virile greenness and this virile wind that erects the stem to its full strength. For that reason the stem cannot become erect to plough woman like soil, because it has lost the wind of its powers that had to strengthen it it for the task of producing offspring. Similarly a plough is unable to dig up soil if it is without a ploughshare.   *Causae et Curae*

William Shakespeare; 1597   1422

Is it not strange that desire should so many years outlive performance?   *Henry IV, Part II, Act II, Scene iv*

Richard A. Kern; 1951   1423

Failure of sexual function is a normal accompaniment of aging.... The attempts to restore potency and libido by measures ranging from the administration of hormones to glandular transplants are of doubtful value. Even if they proved successful, one might still question the wisdom of putting new wine into old bottles.   *Internal Medicine*

INDIGESTION

Ambrose Bierce; 1906   1424

Indigestion, *n.* A disease which the patient and his friends frequently mistake for deep religious conviction and concern for the salvation of mankind. As the simple Red Man of the western wild put it, with, it must be confessed, a certain force: "Plenty well, no pray; big bellyache, heap God."

The Devil's Dictionary

INDUSTRIAL MEDICINE

Alice Hamilton; 1938   1425

Even if we reach a point when all poisons and harmful dust are brought under control, we shall still have to deal with the much more baffling and widespread industrial evil: fatigue of mind, body, and soul.

The American Scholar

INFANTS

Galen; [130-200]   1426

Whoever undertakes the bringing up of infants must be able to guess accurately what is moderate and comfortable and provide this before increasing distress throws the body and mind into excess of activity, and if ever the increasing distress escapes his notice, to try to provide immediately the thing desired or to remove the annoyance either by rocking in the arms or by modulation of the voice, which sagacious nurses are accustomed to employ.

Hygiene

INFECTION

William Shakespeare; 1608   1427

Pursue him to his house, and pluck him thence,
Lest his infection, being of catching nature,
Spread further.

Coriolanus, Act III, Scene i

Ignaz Phillip Semmelweis; 1861   1428

Since the only cause of childbed fever, i.e. a decomposed animal-organic matter, can either be introduced from without, or...formed within the individual, the problem in the prophylaxis of childbed fever consists [in part] in preventing the introduction of the decomposed matter from without.... The decomposed matter is most frequently introduced [from] the examining finger.... I petitioned all administrative authorities for the proclamation of a law[to] prohibit every person employed in the lying-in hospital...from coming in contact with things which might contaminate his hands.

The Etiology, the Concept, and the Prophylaxis of Childbed Fever

Louis Pasteur; 1880   1429

When I began the studies now occupying my attention, I was attempting to extend the germ theory to certain common diseases. I do not know when I can return to that work. Therefore, in my desire to see it carried on by others, I take the liberty of presenting it to the public in its present condition.... It appears certain that every furuncle contains an aerobic microscopic parasite, to which is due the local inflammation and the pus formation that follows.... Under the expression *puerperal fever* are grouped very different diseases, but all appearing to be the result of the growth of common organisms.

Comptes Rendus l'Académie des Sciences

Irving Wilson Voorhees; 1917   1430

Perpetual warfare ought to be waged against those who willfully cough and sneeze into the open without protecting the face with a handkerchief. *American Medicine*

Richard Gordon; 1993   1431

To terrorize us, our unicellular aggressors can evoke powerful allies. Mosquitoes are their airborne divisions. The swift and stealthy rat is their personnel carrier, stuffed with nimble fleas. The savage-clawed lice are their tenacious, mobile armoured vehicles of infection.

The Alarming History of Medicine

INFECTIOUS DISEASE

Fracastorius (Girolamo Fracastoro); 1584   1432

The fundamental differences of all contagions are seen to be three in number: those infecting by contact alone, those only by contact and leaving fomites...and then several things which not only by contact, not only by fomites, but which transfer infection at a distance, such as pestilential fevers, and phthisis and certain ophthalmia and other exanthemata, which are called variola and the like.   *Complete Works*

Athanasius Kircher; 1658   1433

That this living effluvia is composed of invisible living corpuscula, is obvious from the innumerable worms which abound in such bodies, some of which grow large enough to be visible, while others remain of a size which is invisible.... Clothing and household goods infected...when carried somewhere else, in a short time produce tragic catastrophes; indeed not only whole cities are attacked by the sudden and unexpected contagion but also provinces and entire kingdoms.

Scrutinium Physico-medicum Contagiosae Luis Quae Pestis Dicitur

Charles Darwin; 1868   1434

A particle of small-pox matter, so minute as to be borne by the wind, must multiply itself many thousandfold in a person thus inoculated; and so with the contagious matter of scarlet fever.... A minute portion of the mucous discharge from an animal infected with rinderpest, if placed in the blood of a healthy ox, increases so fast that in a short space of time the whole mass of blood, weighing many pounds, is infected, and every small particle of that blood contains enough poison to give, within less than forty-eight hours, the disease to another animal.   *The Variation of Animals and Plants Under Domestication*

Hans Zinsser; 1934   1435

But however secure and well-regulated civilized life may become, bacteria, Protozoa, viruses, infected fleas, lice, ticks, mosquitoes, and bedbugs will always lurk in the shadows ready to pounce when neglect, poverty, famine, or war lets down the defenses.

Rats, Lice, and History

Hans Zinsser; 1934   1436

Infectious disease is one of the few genuine adventures left in the world.

Rats, Lice, and History

INFECTIOUS MONONUCLEOSIS

Emil Pfeiffer; 1889   1437

[This] is a disease which appears very frequently in children.... The medical literature...say nothing whatsoever concerning it.... The fever is marked—between 39 and 40?C.... Over the neck there is a great tenderness...and...we find numerous swollen and painful lymph glands around the entire neck.... After a few days, the glands have all gone down.... The chronic cases give rise to more errors.... The course of the disease is always favorable.... Clinical experience characterizes this disease...as an infectious disease.

Jahrbuch für Kinderheilkunde und Physische Erziehung

INFERTILITY

Samuel Weissell Gross; 1881   1438

The importance of examining the husband before subjecting the wife to operation will be appreciated when I state that he is, as a rule, at fault in at least one instance in every six.

A Practical Treatise on Impotence

Seale Harris; 1950   1439

Particularly distressing to the sensibilities of certain critics was [the] account of the way [J. Marion Sims] had found it necessary in some instances to visit sterile married couples in their bedrooms and to apply there various measures (including, occasionally, etherization of the wife) to overcome the obstacles preventing conception.

Woman's Surgeon: The Life Story of J. Marion Sims

INFLAMMATION

John Hunter; 1794   1440

This operation of the body, termed inflammation, requires our greatest attention, for it is one of the most common and most extensive in its causes, and it becomes itself the cause of many local effects, both salutary and diseased.   *A Treatise on the Blood*

Joseph Lister; 1858   1441

The morbid process designated by the term Inflammation, being one to which every organ and probably every tissue of the body is liable, and comprehending as it does in its progress and consequences by far the greater number of the ills to which flesh is heir, possesses a deeper interest for the physician or surgeon than any other material subject which could be named.   *Philosophical Transactions of the Royal Society*

INFLUENZA

Gabriel Andral; 1838   1442

The influenza, like all epidemics, was not always accompanied by all its symptoms: some individuals were but slightly affected by it, or presented but an isolated symptom,...the autopsical characteristics may be wanting. The influenza is, therefore, a general affection, the nature and cause of which are unknown, as are those of the greater part of epidemics which appear at irregular epochs.   *Medical and Surgical Monographs*

Maurice Jacobs; 1918   1443

In Hull it began on a glorious summer's day[in] 1918 with the suddenness of some great catastrophe of nature.... My first intimation of something amiss was the inordinate length of my visiting lists.... I set off on my round, and...began to suspect...the opening phase of a major tragedy. Robust young men and women who had been to work only a day or two before were stricken low. The symptoms...were those of a profound toxaemia, as if from an overwhelming onslaught of some infective agency. Many were already in a state of coma and at the point of death.   *Reflections of a General Practitioner*

Henry Louis Mencken; 1956   1444

The influenza epidemic of 1919, though it had an enormous mortality in the United States and was, in fact, the worst epidemic since the Middle Ages, is seldom mentioned, and most Americans have apparently forgotten it. This is not surprising. The human mind always tries to expunge the intolerable from memory, just as it tries to conceal it while current.

Minority Report: H. L. Mencken's Notebooks

INFORMED CONSENT

Herbert George Wells; 1922   1445

It is not reasonable that those who gamble with men's lives should not stake their own.

The Salvaging of Civilization

Nuremberg Code; 1947   1446

The Nuremberg Code—The voluntary consent of the human subject [for an experiment] is absolutely essential. This means that the person involved should have legal capacity to give consent; should be so situated as to be able to exercise free power of choice, without the intervention of any element of force, fraud, deceit, duress, overreaching, or other ulterior form of constraint or coercion; and should have sufficient knowledge and comprehension of the elements of the subject matter involved as to enable him to make an understanding and enlightened decision.   *Annas GJ and Grodin MA, The Nazi Doctors and the Nuremberg Code*

Billy F. Andrews; 1968   **1447**

That the personhood of each child be fully appreciated and that each be informed of all matters including health as they grow in intellect and in capability; and that they learn to be involved, as maturity allows, and to participate in all decisions concerning their well-being.   *The Children's Bill of Rights*

Rosalyn S. Yalow; 1977   **1448**

In our laboratory, we always used ourselves because we are the only ones who can give truly informed consent.   *Altman LK, Who Goes First?*

High Court of Australia; 1992   **1449**

Except in... an emergency or where disclosure would prove damaging to the patient, a medical practitioner has a duty to warn the patient of a material risk inherent in proposed treatment. A risk is material if... a reasonable person in the patient's position would be likely to attach significance to it or if the medical practitioner is or should reasonably be aware that the particular patient, if warned of the risk, would be likely to attach significance to it.... That a body of reputable medical practitioners would have given the same advice... does not preclude a finding of negligence.   *High Court of Australia*

INNOVATION

Wilfred Batten Lewis Trotter; 1941   **1450**

If mankind is to profit freely from the small and sporadic crop of the heroically gifted it produces, it will have to cultivate the delicate art of handling ideas. Psychology is now able to tell us with reasonable assurance that the most influential obstacle to freedom of thought and to new ideas is fear; and fear which can with inimitable art disguise itself as caution, or sanity, or reasoned scepticism, or on occasion even as courage.

British Medical Journal

INSANITY

William Heberden; 1802   **1451**

Great anxiety of mind, whatever may have been its origin, is a principal cause of insanity, that is, a disordered understanding with a quiet pulse and without any acute illness. It has been the consequence of some diseases, particularly of worms, and epileptic fits, and of many affections of the head, as dropsies of the ventricles of the brain, and scirrhous tumors, and also of blows.   *Commentaries on the History and Cure of Diseases*

Daniel R. Brower; 1879   **1452**

The plea of impulsive insanity, as from time to time presented in our courts...has no foundation in scientific observation. It is simply the cunning device of astute lawyers and so-called experts, who either have badly digested views on the subject, or else are impelled to their opinion by motives other than love of science.   *Chicago Medical Examiner*

Ambrose Bierce; 1906   **1453**

Mad, *adj.* Affected with a high degree of intellectual independence; not conforming to standards of thought, speech and action derived by the conformants from study of themselves; at odds with the majority; in short, unusual.   *The Devil's Dictionary*

INSOMNIA

Gustav Monod; 1926   **1454**

A lady suffered from intractable insomnia—one of those who "do not sleep a wink"—was ordered to take a spoonful of [the] famous water every half hour during the night. The nurse had no difficulty with the first two or three doses. But when the fourth was presented, the indignant lady insisted on being allowed to sleep in peace.   *The Lancet*

Thomas Merton; 1953   **1455**
Insomnia can become a form of contemplation. You just lie there, inert, helpless, alone, in the dark, and let yourself be crushed by the inscrutable tyranny of time.

The Sign of Jonas: The Journal of Thomas Merton

INSULIN

Frederick Grant Banting; 1920   **1456**
Diabetes. Ligate pancreatic ducts of dog. Keep dogs alive till acini degenerate leaving Islets. Try to isolate the internal secretion of these to relieve glycosuria.

Banting's Notebook

Frederick Grant Banting; 1922   **1457**
This case was one of severe juvenile diabetes with ketosis. Previous to admission, he had been starved without evident benefit. During the first month of his stay in hospital, careful dietetic regulation failed to influence the course of the disease.... Daily injections of the extract [of pancreas] were made from January 23rd to February 4th.... This resulted in immediate improvement. The excretion of sugar...became much less.... The acetone bodies disappeared from the urine. The boy became brighter, more active, looked better, and said he felt stronger.   *Canadian Medical Association Journal*

Frederick Grant Banting; 1922   **1458**
A neutral or faintly acid extract of the degenerated gland [following ligation of the major pancreatic ducts of dogs] injected intravenously or subcutaneously invariably caused marked reduction of the percentage of sugar in the blood and the amount of sugar excreted in the urine.   *American Journal of Physiology*

Frederick Grant Banting; 1923   **1459**
I feel very badly that Mr. Charles Best was not mentioned in the Nobel award. I am very anxious that it should be known that Mr. Best had an intimate part in the discovery of insulin. I am sure that Mr. Best will feel it too. I am of course going to share the award with him in every way and want everyone to know the part he played.

Hemingway E, The Toronto Star

Oskar Minkowski; 1923   **1460**
This...is the first insulin to reach our country. It has been sent to me by Dr. Banting and Dr. Best, of Toronto, who have discovered it. It was once my hope that I would be the father of insulin. Now I am happy to accept the designation as its grandfather, which the Toronto scientists have conferred on me so kindly.   *Lecture*

INTELLIGENCE

Santiago Ramón y Cajal; 1920   **1461**
Grey matter abounds in countries with grey skies.   *Chatting over Coffee*

INTERNAL MEDICINE

William Bennett Bean; 1982   **1462**
The term [*Innere Medizin*] became common in Germany only in the 1880s. The first written use of it I have found was in the transactions of the Congress of Internal Medicine held in Wiesbaden in 1882. [The term] was introduced in an effort to correct the misconception that certain physicians were dealing only with matters that were purely clinical.   *New England Journal of Medicine*

Lynn O. Langdon, Phillip P. Toskes, Harry R. Kimball; 1996   **1463**
Internal medicine demands both the intellectual pursuit of scientific knowledge and the compassionate provision of high-quality patient care. The training of subspecialist basic

scientists and clinical investigators must be protected and nurtured to ensure continued discovery and scholarly application of new knowledge to future patient care.

Annals of Internal Medicine

INTERNISTS

Thomas Findley; 1944   **1464**

Accustomed to legerdemain and quick results[the surgeon] is apt to regard the diagnosis and treatment of a headache, for example, as a trivial matter, forgetting that the internist may require hours of probing before discovering that what the patient needs is not a new pair of glasses but a different mother-in-law.   *Surgery*

Thomas Findley; 1944   **1465**

An internist has been defined as a man who is totally unable to answer either yes or no to any question.... If there is such a thing as a typical internist, he is a sedentary individual, curious, skeptical, reflective. He is accustomed to look at the patient as a unit rather than as a collection of separate organs and, if he had the fundamental scientific training he should have had, he is eager to distinguish between a fact and someone's opinion.

Surgery

INTERNSHIP

Mary Elizabeth Bates; *circa* 1880   **1466**

The first six months were hell; the second six months were purgatory; the third six months were heaven; and when it came time for me to leave, I wept bitter tears.

Medical Women's Journal

INTESTINAL LIPODYSTROPHY (WHIPPLE DISEASE)

George Hoyt Whipple; 1907   **1467**

[This] case was characterized clinically by a gradual loss of weight and strength, stools consisting chiefly of neutral fat and fatty acids, indefinite abdominal signs, and a peculiar multiple arthritis.... [At autopsy] the intestinal mucosa showed enlarged villi due to deposits of large masses of neutral fats and fatty acids in the lymph spaces.... The mesenteric glands...showed the same deposits in even greater amounts.

Johns Hopkins Hospital Bulletin

Kenneth H. Wilson, Rhonda Blitchington, Richard Frothingham, Joanne A.P. Wilson; 1991   **1468**

Nucleotide sequencing and amplification by the polymerase chain reaction was done in the bacterial 16 S ribosome DNA present in a small-bowel biopsy specimen taken from a patient with Whipple's disease. A search by computer for similar rRNA sequences filed in databases showed the Whipple's-associated organism to be most similar to the bacteria of the *Rhodococcus*, *Streptomyces*, and *Arthrobacter* genera, and more weakly related to mycobacteria.... The probable aetological agent for our patient's illness has not been identified previously in a patient with Whipple's disease.   *The Lancet*

INTESTINES

William Maddock Bayliss, Ernest Henry Starling; 1899   **1469**

One of the most important [among the factors governing intestinal movement] is the fact that the muscular coat of the intestines is subject to inhibitory and augmentor impulses dependent, in the first place, on the condition of neighbouring parts of the gut, through the intermediation of the local nervous system (Auerbach's and Meissner's plexus), and secondly, on impulses ascending to the central nervous system from the intestine, abdominal wall, or other parts of the body, and affecting the intestines reflexly.   *Journal of Physiology*

William M. Bayliss, Ernest Henry Starling; 1899   1470
Local stimulation of the gut produces excitation above and inhibition below the excited spot. These effects are dependent on the activity of the local [i.e., the autonomic] nervous mechanism.   *Journal of Physiology*

INTUBATION

Frank E. Waxham; 1888   1471
Intubation has now become so thoroughly recognized as a practical and successful operation, that I believe it to be a duty the medical profession at large owe to the public, that at least one physician in every village, town and city throughout this great country, should possess the necessary instruments, pluck and skill to successfully perform this operation.
                                                                       Intubation of the Larynx

IRON-DEFICIENCY ANEMIA

Cotton Mather; 1724   1472
There is a Malady which is called, *The White Jaundice*, as well as, *The Green Sickness....Yea, Hearken, O Daughter, and Consider!* And *beholding thy Natural Face in a glass*; beholding how pale, how wan, how like a ghost it looks.   *The Angel of Bethesda*

J

JAUNDICE

Cotton Mather; 1724   1473

There is a Disease, which has been called, Morbus Regius, or, The Royal Disease; because it brings with it the Colour of Gold unto them that have it. But so poor a Recommendation will not make the Jaundice to be wished for.... The Excretion of the Bile into the Intestines, meets with some Obstruction, and so it Regurgitates and is Carried with the Blood all over the Body, whereby all the Parts, both the Solid and the Fluid, come to be tinged with a Yellow.   *The Angel of Bethesda*

Albert Abraham Hymans van den Bergh, J. Snapper; 1913   1474

It was suspected that bilirubin passes into the urine, as soon as the bilirubin content passes a threshold value.... Now the question is, at what content of bilirubin is this threshold?

Deutsch Archiv der Klinische Medizin

JUDGMENT

Robert H. Brook; 1989   1475

Because the scientific basis on which medical decisions are made will always be incomplete, we must determine how we can validly combine what is contained in the medical literature with expert judgment to arrive at a judgment of appropriateness.

Journal of the American Medical Association

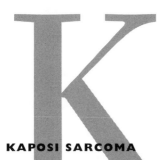

KAPOSI SARCOMA

Moriz Kaposi (Kohn); 1872   **1476**

I have seen sixteen cases, all in men, and others have been reported by various writers. It always begins upon both feet and hands, and advances by separate growths along the legs and arms, until, at the end of two to three years, it appears upon the face and trunk. We find reddish-brown, later bluish-red, round, moderately firm nodules.... Fever, bloody diarrhea, haemoptysis, and marasmus soon set in at this stage, and are followed by death.... Histologically we find a round-cell sarcoma.   *Pathology and Treatment of Diseases of the Skin*

Yuan Chang, Ethel Cesarman, Melissa S. Pessin, and others; 1994   **1477**

Unique sequences present in more than 90 percent of Kaposi's sarcoma tissues obtained from patients with acquired immunodeficiency syndrome... are homologous to, but distinct from, capsule and tegument protein genes of the gamma-Herpesviridae, herpesvirus saimiri and Epstein-Barr virus. These K-S associated herpesvirus-like sequences appear to define a new human herpesvirus.   *Science*

KIDNEY

Aretaeus the Cappadocian; [81-138?]   **1478**

The kidneys are of a glandular nature, but redder in colour, like the liver, rather than like the mammae and testicles; for they, too, are glands, but of a whiter colour.... Their cavities are small and like sieves, for the percolation of the urine; and these have attached to each of them nervous canals, like reeds, which are inserted into the shoulders of the bladder on each side; and the passage of the urine from each of the kidneys to the bladder is equal.   *On the Affections About the Kidneys*

Marcello Malpighi; 1666   **1479**

The glands [i.e., the glomeruli] that have been discovered in the kidney...contribute a special service in the excretion of the urine.... They appear...spherical, precisely like fish eggs: and when a dark fluid is perfused through the arteries they grow dark.

Hayman JM Jr., Annals of Medical History

Friedrich Gustave Jacob Henle; 1862   **1480**

In examining the anatomical characteristics of the medulla of the kidney we discovered a new type of canaliculi which do not enter the open urinary tubules but end at the cortex.... Each pair of tubules forms a horseshoe loop which penetrates deep into the medulla from the cortex. *Akademische Wissenschaft*

Joseph Treloar Wearn, Alfred Newton Richards; 1924   **1481**
A technique has been devised for simultaneous collection of glomerular and bladder urine in frogs.... The glomerular fluid is free from protein when blood flow through the glomerular capillaries is rapid. *American Journal of Physiology*

Alfred Newton Richards; 1925   **1482**
These experiments [on the frog] revealed by direct tests the absence of protein and the presence of chloride and of sugar in the fluid leaving the blood stream flowing through the glomerular capillaries, and are completely in accord, in so far as they go, with the demands of the filtration theory. They contain incontestable proof of the reality of reabsorption within the tubules, and provide the basis for further argumentative support of the view that the glomerular function is a physical rather than a "vital" or "secretory" one. *American Journal of the Medical Sciences*

Homer William Smith; 1939   **1483**
It is no exaggeration to say that the composition of the blood is determined not by what the mouth ingests but by what the kidneys keep; they are the master chemists of our internal environment, which, so to speak, they synthesize in reverse.
Lectures on the Kidney

Arthur M. Walker, Phyllis A. Bott, Jean Oliver, M.C. McDowell; 1941   **1484**
Occasional glomeruli, in guinea pigs, and certain portions of the proximal and distal tubules in a variety of mammals, are accessible to observation on the kidney surface during life.... Glomerular fluid, entirely or nearly free of protein, contains reducing substances and creatinine in concentrations similar to those existing in plasma water. Within the proximal convolution, all of the reducing substances and at least two-thirds of the fluid are reabsorbed. *American Journal of Physiology*

Homer William Smith; 1943   **1485**
All we know for certain about the kidney, is that it makes urine.   *Lectures on the Kidney*

Homer William Smith; 1959   **1486**
Bones can break, muscles can atrophy, glands can loaf, even the brain can go to sleep, and endanger our survival; but should the kidneys fail in their task neither bone, muscle, gland nor brain could carry on. *From Fish to Philosopher*

KIDNEY, ARTIFICIAL

Willem Johan Kolff, H.T.J. Berk; 1944   **1487**
The artificial kidney is a dialysing-apparatus with a small blood volume and a dialysing area of about 20,000 sq. cms., in which the blood of a patient is cleared of retention products. With one patient...35 grams of urea could be dialysed out in...6 hours.... Other retention products [also] were removed.... We believe to be able to keep patients suffering from uremia and anuria alive so long as blood vessels for punction are available.... In the case of acute uremia the possibility exists for the kidneys to regenerate in the meantime. *Acta Medica Scandinavia*

Willem Johan Kolff; 1950   **1488**
Vivo dialysis can replace all known excretory functions of the kidney. Moreover it can regulate the electrolyte pattern of the blood plasma water inasmuch as it approaches the composition of the rinsing fluid. Clinical improvement has been convincing in cases of acute or chronic uremia. In experienced hands treatment with the artificial kidney imposes little risk. It may be an effective adjunct to other methods of treatment.
Cleveland Clinic Quarterly

KIDNEY DISEASE

Gulielmus de Saliceto (Salicetti; William of Salicet); 1476   **1489**
The signs of hardness in the kidneys are that the quantity of the urine is diminished, that there is heaviness of the kidneys, and of the spine with some pain: and the belly begins to swell up after a time and dropsy is produced the second day.   *Liber in Scientia Medicinali*

Richard Bright; 1827   **1490**
I have often found the dropsy connected with the secretion of albuminous urine, more or less coagulable on the application of heat.... I have never yet examined the body of a patient dying with dropsy attended with coagulable urine, in whom some obvious derangement was not discovered in the kidneys.... During some part of the progress of these cases of anasarca, I have...found a great tendency to throw off the red particles of the blood by the kidneys, betrayed by various degrees of haematuria.   *Reports of Medical Cases*

Paul Kimmelstiel, Clifford Wilson; 1936   **1491**
Cases...show a striking hyaline thickening of the intercapillary connective tissue of the glomerulus. Evidence is presented which...suggests that arteriosclerosis and diabetes may play a part in its causation.... The characteristic clinical features are a previous history of diabetes, severe and widespread edema of the nephrotic type and gross albuminuria. Hypertension is frequently present.   *American Journal of Pathology*

KIDNEY FUNCTION

William Heberden; 1802   **1492**
A total suppression [of urine] has lasted seven days, and yet the patient has recovered. It has been fatal so early as on the fourth day. But in general those patients, who could not be cured, have sunk under their malady on the sixth or seventh day.
   Commentaries on the History and Cure of Diseases

William Bowman; 1842   **1493**
It occurred to me that as the tubes and their plexus of capillaries were probably...the parts concerned in the secretion of that portion of the urine to which its characteristic properties are due (the urea, lithic acid, etc.), the Malpighian bodies might be an apparatus destined to separate from the blood the watery portion.   *Philosophical Transactions of the Royal Society*

Carl Friedrich Wilhelm Ludwig; 1844   **1494**
[The glomerular filtrate] is driven...into the urinary vessels and thereby comes in contact with the blood which is flowing in the narrow vessels...and...has originated from the glomerulus [and] would draw water from the urinary canals into the blood vessels whereby the urine would become concentrated.   *Handwörter der Physiologie*

Ernest Henry Starling, E.B. Verney; 1924   **1495**
It is clear...that the formation of the urine cannot be explained on the basis of filtration and reabsorption of a fluid of constant and invariable composition. Selective reabsorption or secretion, or both, must be called into play.   *Proceedings of the Royal Society*

Poul Brandt Rehberg; 1926   **1496**
The amount of creatinine present in the urine of man after ingestion of this substance is so large that it requires a filtration of up to 200 cc. per min. to explain it.... The result is taken to be in favour of the filtration theory.   *Biochemical Journal*

Eggert Hugo Heiberg Möller, J.F. McIntosh,
Donald Dexter Van Slyke; 1928   **1497**
When the urine volume output is at any point *above the augmentation limit*, urea excretion proceeds at maximum speed, and the output per minute represents the urea content of a maximum blood volume. This blood volume, averaging in normal men about 75 cc. per minute, we...term the *maximum blood urea clearance*.   *Journal of Clinical Investigation*

Homer William Smith; 1937   1498

A substance suitable for measuring the glomerular clearance...must be completely filterable at the glomerulus...and it must not be reabsorbed, excreted or synthesized by the tubules.... We began our examination of the excretion of non-metabolized carbohydrates...in normal and phlorizined animals, in relation to the simultaneous excretion of urea, creatinine, etc.... The evidence is now fairly convincing that the polysaccharide, inulin, fulfills the specifications for measuring glomerular filtration in all vertebrates. *The Physiology of the Kidney*

Alf S. Alving, Benjamin F. Miller; 1940   1499

It is now possible to make precise measurements of the glomerular filtration rate, the effective renal blood flow and the capacity of the tubular cells to reabsorb or excrete certain compounds. Many of these measurements are too difficult at present for clinical purposes, but...one can measure the glomerular filtration rate rather simply with both normal and diseased persons by employing a simplified inulin clearance test.

Archives of Internal Medicine

Homer William Smith; 1943   1500

As Van Slyke sat on the train seeking a solution of how to dispense with mathematics for the benefit of the medical profession, it occurred to him that all that the equation for high urine flows said was that in effect some constant volume of blood was being "cleared" of urea in each minute's time. *Lectures on the Kidney*

Carl W. Gottschalk, Margaret Mylle; 1959   1501

Fluid from the bends of loops of Henle, and from collecting ducts and vasa recta at the same level were equally hyperosmotic, consistent with the hypothesis that the mammalian nephron functions as a countercurrent multiplier system.

American Journal of Physiology

KIDNEY SURGERY

Gustav Simon; 1870   1502

In some English and French journals I find communications about the extirpation of a kidney which I carried out in a surgical clinic of this country. Our operation had not previously been undertaken in a human.... I wish to discuss the suitability of the use of nephrotomy in our case. [First successful planned nephrectomy for urinary tract fistula]

Deutsche Klinik

KIDNEY TRANSPLANTATION

Johann Wolfgang von Goethe; [1749-1832]   1503

If only God would present me with one of the kidneys of the Russians fallen at Austerlitz.

Nager F, Der Heilkundige Dichter

Alexis Carrel; 1908   1504

An animal which has undergone a double nephrectomy and grafting of both kidneys from another animal can secrete almost normal urine with his new organs, and live in good health for at least a few weeks. *Journal of Experimental Medicine*

John Putnam Merrill, Joseph E. Murray, J. Hartwell Harrison, Warren R. Guild; 1956   1505

A patient whose illness had begun with edema and hypertension was found to have suffered extreme atrophy of both kidneys.... Transplantation of one kidney from the patient's healthy identical twin brother was undertaken.... The hypertension persisted until the patient's diseased kidneys were both removed. The homograft has survived for 11 months, and the marked clinical improvement...has included disappearance of the signs of malignant hypertension. *Journal of the American Medical Association*

KLINEFELTER SYNDROME

Harry Fitch Klinefelter, Edward C. Reifenstein Jr., Fuller Albright; 1942   **1506**
Nine cases are presented of a syndrome characterized by gynecomastia, and small testes with aspermatogenesis but without a-leydigism. The follicle-stimulating hormone (FSH) excretion in the urine is increased to a degree comparable to that found in castrates.... These studies support the point of view that the testis produces two hormones; *a)* androgen from the Leydig cells, and *b)* X-hormone (inhibin) from the tubules. Inhibin is analogous and probably very similar to estrin.   *Journal of Clinical Endocrinology*

KNOWLEDGE

Oliver Wendell Holmes; 1867   **1507**
This is an inquisitive age, and if we insist on piling up beyond a certain height knowledge which is in itself mere trash and lumber to a man whose life is to be one long fight with death and disease, there will be some sharp questions asked by and by.
Scholastic and Bedside Teaching

Oliver Wendell Holmes; 1891   **1508**
The air we breathe is made up of four elements, at least: oxygen, nitrogen, carbonic acid gas, and knowledge.   *Over the Teacups*

KORSAKOV PSYCHOSIS

Sergei Sergeivich Korsakov; 1890   **1509**
I have described a special form of *psychic disorder* which occurs *in conjunction with multiple neuritis*.... In many instances, after the first days of agitation a considerable confusion appears: the patient begins to mix words, he cannot speak coherently, and confuses facts. Day after day the confusion increases. The patient begins to tell implausible stories about himself...confuses old recollections with recent events, is unaware of where he is and who are the people around him.   *Allgemein Zeitschrift für Psychiatrie*

L

LANGUAGE

George White Pickering; 1961   **1510**

We may... ask why people, especially doctors and scientists, like to use these strange words which other men do not or cannot understand. I am quite sure that usually it is no more than a bad habit which most acquire unwittingly. But its underlying basis is more than that. Its purpose is to advance the standing of its user; its method is deception: deception of others, and ultimately self-deception.   *The Lancet*

Jerome Groopman; 2000   **1511**

Language is as vital to the physician's art as the stethoscope or the scalpel. A doctor begins by examining the words of his patient to determine their clinical significance. He then translates the words into medical language, describing how the condition came to be, what it means, and how it may evolve. Of all the words the doctor uses, the name he gives the illness has the greatest weight. It forms the foundation of all subsequent discussion, not only between doctor and patient but also between doctor and doctor and between patient and patient.   *The New Yorker*

LARYNGOSCOPE

Benjamin Guy Babington; 1829   **1512**

Dr. Benjamin Babington submitted to the meeting an ingenious instrument for the examination of parts within the fauces not admitting of inspection by unaided sight.... The epiglottis and upper part of the larynx become visible.... The doctor proposed to call it the *glottiscope*.   *Hunterian Society, London Medical Gazette*

W. Hale-Wight; 1924   **1513**

Hodgkin suggested the term "laryngiscope" for the "glothiscope" which his colleague Babington had invented.   *Guy's Hospital Reports*

LAXATIVES

[Anonymous]; *circa* 1550 BC   **1514**

Another for the purging (*wekha*) of the belly and to drive out suffering from the belly of a man. Fruits/seeds (*peret*) of ricinus (*degem*), chewed (*wesha*) and swallowed with beer so that everything which is in his belly comes forth. *Ebers Papyrus*

LEAD POISONING

Paul of Aegina (Paulus Aegineta); [625-690]   1515
I consider moreover a colicky affection...which took its origin from regions in Italy.... Wherefore in many cases it passed into epilepsy, to some there came loss of motion, with sensation unhurt, to many both, and of those who fell victims to the epilepsy, very many die. Of those indeed who were paralised, not a few recovered.

The Seven Books of Paulus Aegineta

François Citois (Citesius); 1616   1516
A new painful Colic appeared called Bilious from the most severe pains due to the bile so it is believed, and it still rages. Those whose bodies it attacks, sink down as if struck, suddenly he changes his posture, a pallor spreads over his face, his extremities shiver, his strength languishes, his mind is disturbed, his body is troubled, constant wakefulness, fainting spells, or severe frequent stomach pains, loss of appetite, perpetual nausea.... The motion of his elbows and hands, legs and feet is lost, sensation however is intact.... And in many several epileptic convulsions preceded this paralysis.

De Novo et Populari apud Pictones Dolore Colico Bilioso Diatriba

Theodore Tronchin; 1757   1517
No less fortunate are those who drink water impregnated with lead. Houses roofed with lead sheets, where rain-water only is drunk, collected in cisterns or preserved in leaden vessels, produces commonly this very bad and frequent disease: and this is the reason why the painful colic formerly rare, now rages in Amsterdam.... I have seen the malady rage in whole families. Eleven in one house at one time down in bed, convulsed with horrible torments, with their extremities flaccid; the roof changed, the water renewed, they recover.

De Colica Pictonum

John Huxham; 1759   1518
This Disease began its Attack by an excessively tormenting Pain in the Stomach, and epigastric Region.... Some...totally lost the Use of their Hands, the Power of Feeling only remaining; Palsy for Pain, a miserable Exchange.... Some, but very few, after having been long and greatly afflicted with this Disease, were seized with Epileptic-Fits and died of it.

Observations on the Air and Epidemic Diseases

George Baker; 1767   1519
In a plentiful year of apples, I knew a farmer who, wanting casks, filled a large leaden cistern with new cyder, and kept it there, till he could procure hogsheads sufficient to contain the liquor. The consequence was, that all, who drank of it, were affected by it as leadworkers usually are. We had eleven of them, at one time, in our infirmary.

An Essay Concerning the Cause of the Endemial Colic of Devonshire

Henry Burton; 1840   1520
In the total number of fifty patients who were examined whilst under the influence of lead, a peculiar discoloration was observed on their gums, which I could not discern on the gums of several hundred patients, who were not under the influence of lead.... The edges of the gums...were distinctly bordered by a narrow leaden-blue line, about the one-twentieth part of an inch in width. *Medico-Chirurgical Transactions*

Gabriel Andral; 1843   1521
When the influence of lead has acted for a long time upon the human constitution, there may result from it the production of a cachectic condition... I have found that, in this condition, the globules of the blood suffer as great a diminution as in spontaneous anaemia, and, as in this latter, the fibrine and other elements of the blood preserve their normal quantity. *Essai d'Hématologie Pathologique*

LEARNING

Samuel Bard; 1769   1522

Do not therefore imagine, that from this Time [i.e., on receipt of the MD degree] your Studies are to cease; so far from it, you are to be considered as but just entering upon them; and unless your whole Lives, are one continued Series of Application and Improvement, you will fall short of your duty.   *A Discourse on the Duties of a Physician*

James Paget; 1869   1523

All my recollections would lead me to tell that every student may draw from his daily life a very likely forecast of his life in practice, for it will depend upon himself a hundredfold more than on circumstances. The time and the place, the work to be done, and its responsibilities, will change; but the man will be the same, except in so far as he may change himself.   *St. Bartholomew Hospital Reports*

Jacob M. Da Costa; 1874   1524

All that goes on in medicine is to be the chief matter of interest to you. Hence you must be busy readers; and, as habits form, you will learn to look to medical journals with avidity, and new publications will be examined with keen relish. But to become distinguished, nay, to become even respectable in your profession, you must be something more than readers, you must become active thinkers and sifters of knowledge, learn, as Bacon counsels, to weigh and consider books.   *Manning PR and DeBakey L, Medicine: Preserving the Passion*

William Osler; 1894   1525

Experience in the true sense of the term does not come to all with years, or with increasing opportunities. Growth in the acquisition of facts is not necessarily associated with development. Many grow through life as the crystal, by simple accretion, and at fifty possess, to vary the figure, the unicellular mental blastoderm with which they started.   *The Army Surgeon*

William Osler; *circa* 1900   1526

The hardest conviction to get into the mind of a beginner is that the education upon which he is engaged is not a college course, not a medical course, but a life course.   *Aphorisms*

Eugene A. Stead Jr.; 1968   1527

One learns by asking one's self questions, then going out and finding the answers.   *Annals of Internal Medicine*

Peter Richards; 1985   1528

There is no royal road to learning medicine. The path is long, the demands heavy, and the sacrifices real. Learning never stops: it starts when the student is a spectator but sinks deep only when learning is through service. All doctors must continue to learn, and not only about new advances but to appreciate the limitations of all knowledge. They also need to learn humility, in the face of their own imperfect understanding and their patients' courage.   *Learning Medicine*

Norman Cousins; 1989   1529

In the years after medical school, much of what had been regarded as "hard" turned out to be frail or faulty, and much of what had been regarded as "soft" turned out to be durable and essential.   *Head First*

LEECHES

William Buchan; 1798   1530

I have been accustomed for some time past, to apply leeches to the inflamed testicle, which practice has always been followed with most happy effects.   *Domestic Medicine*

William Heath Byford; 1865   **1531**
A common glass speculum, introduced so as to include and isolate the cervix, is what I have been in the habit of using. The leeches are thrown down to the bottom of the speculum after the parts are cleaned of mucus, and the leeches are watched until they seize the part. Three are about as many as can conveniently be used in the speculum at one time.
The Practice of Medicine and Surgery Applied to Women

LEGIONNAIRES DISEASE

Joseph E. McDade, Charles C. Shepard, David W. Fraser, and others; 1977   **1532**
From the lungs of four of six patients we isolated a gram-negative, non-acid-fast bacillus in guinea pigs.... When compared to controls[serum] specimens from 101 of 111 patients meeting clinical criteria of Legionnaires' disease showed diagnostic increases in antibody titers.
New England Journal of Medicine

LEUKEMIA

John Hughes Bennett; 1845   **1533**
He noticed a tumour in the left side of the abdomen, which has greatly increased in size till four months since.... Several other small tumours have appeared in his neck, axillae, and groins.... The blood...was seen to have separated into a red or inferior, and a yellow or superior portion.... The *spleen* also enormously enlarged from simple hypertrophy.... The *lympatic glands* were every where much enlarged.   *Edinburgh Medical and Surgical Journey*

Rudolf Ludwig Karl Virchow; 1845   **1534**
On admission there was...marked enlargement and moderate tenderness of the spleen.... As I examine [at autopsy] the further course of the blood-vessels; there was everywhere in them a pus-like mass.... Spleen enormously hypertrophied...very heavy, dark brownish red.... Except for a very few red blood corpuscles, the greater part [of the loose coagulum] was composed of colorless or white corpuscles.   *Neue Notizen Gebiete Natur- und Heilkunde*

LIBIDO

Pierre-Charles-Alexandre Louis; 1844   **1535**
I have, in several instances, made inquiry of phthisical [i.e., tuberculous] patients respecting the state of their amative propensities, and in every instance these have appeared to me to have failed in proportion to the loss of strength, the general uneasiness, and the other symptoms, very much in the same manner as in individuals affected with any other kind of chronic ailment and enfeebled to a similar amount.   *Researches on Phthisis*

LIFE

Buddha (Siddhartha Gautama); [563?-483? BC]   **1536**
Birth is suffering; Decay is suffering; Death is suffering; Sorrow, Lamentation, Pain, Grief and Despair are suffering.   *Saying*

Thomas Browne; 1643   **1537**
For the World, I count it not an Inn, but an Hospital; and a place not to live, but to dye in. The world that I regard is my self; it is the Microcosm of my own frame. *Religio Medici*

Oliver Wendell Holmes; 1858   **1538**
The more we study the body and the mind, the more we find both to be governed, not *by*, but *according to*, laws, such as we observe in the larger universe.
The Autocrat of the Breakfast Table

Charles Darwin; 1859   **1539**
There is grandeur in this view of life, with its several powers, having been originally breathed by the Creator into a few forms or into one; and that, whilst this planet has gone cycling on according to the fixed law of gravity, from so simple a beginning endless forms most beautiful and most wonderful have been, and are being, evolved.   *The Origin of Species*

Claude Bernard; 1870   **1540**
The vital force directs phenomena that it does not produce; the physical agents produce phenomena they do not direct.
Lessons on the Phenomena of Life common to Animals and Vegetables

Ernest Fenollosa; 1893   **1541**
Flesh is a flower
That blooms for an hour.   *The Separated East*

Ambrose Bierce; 1906   **1542**
Life, *n*. A spiritual pickle preserving the body from decay. We live in daily apprehension of its loss; yet when lost it is not missed. The question, "Is life worth living?" has been much discussed; particularly by those who think it is not, many of whom have written at great length in support of their view and by careful observance of the laws of health enjoyed for long terms of years the honors of successful controversy.   *The Devil's Dictionary*

Lawrence Joseph Henderson; 1913   **1543**
No other environment consisting of primarily constituents made up of other known elements, or lacking water and carbonic acid, could possess a like number of fit characteristics or such highly fit characteristics, or in any manner such great fitness to promote complexity, durability, and active metabolism in the organic mechanism we call life.
The Fitness of the Environment

Lawrence Joseph Henderson; 1928   **1544**
The phenomena of life is a particular kind of physico-chemical system.... There are...grounds for objecting to this statement. Some will say that the elementary condition of the phenomena of life is the cell. Others will prefer a metaphysical definition. To the latter objectors it may be replied that the physiologist is seeking his own ends; to the former that this is but a question of means to those ends, and that for the present rational, mathematical, and physico-chemical studies of equilibria and stationary states in living organisms are fruitful of the results that he seeks.   *Blood: A Study in General Physiology*

Carl Gustav Jung; 1952   **1545**
Once more we are appalled by the incongruous attitude of the world creator towards his creatures, who to his chagrin never behave according to his expectations. It is as if someone started a bacterial culture which turned out to be a failure. He might curse his luck, but he would never seek the reason for the failure in the bacilli and want to punish them morally for it. Rather, he would select a more suitable culture medium.   *Answer to Job*

Lionel Trilling; 1955   **1546**
Death and suffering, when we read, are our only means of conceiving of the actuality of life.   *The Opposing Self. Wordsworth and the Rabbis*

Louis Lasagna; 1962   **1547**
It would seem important to devote more of the energies of man toward improving the quality of life, so that it may be joyous or noble or creative. Otherwise, existence is nothing but the bored molecular unwinding of a dismal biological clock.   *The Doctors' Dilemmas*

Isaac Bashevis Singer; 1964   **1548**
Once you have been planted in the womb, the nine months that follow are not painful.... Coming out of the womb will be a shock, but childhood is often pleasant. You will begin to study the lore of death, clothed in a fresh, plaint body, and soon will dread the end of your exile.   *Jachid and Jechidah*

LIFE STYLE

Hippocrates; [460-375 BC]   1549

[The physician] must consider.... the mode of life also of the inhabitants that is pleasing to them, whether they are heavy drinkers, taking lunch, and inactive, or athletic, industrious, eating much and drinking little.   *On Airs, Waters, and Places*

Thomas Percival; 1803   1550

Whoever reflects on the variety of diseases to which the human body is incident, will find that a considerable part of them are derived from immoderate passions and vicious indulgences. Sloth, intemperance, and irregular desires are the greatest sources of those evils, which contract the duration, and embitter the enjoyment, of life.   *Medical Ethics*

J.S. Mills; 1972   1551

Millions of our citizens live emotionally undisciplined lives with disastrous consequences to their health and life expectancy. Few of these health problems are particularly affected by the availability of physicians, hospitals, clinics, or nursing homes. No program of national health insurance will protect people from the consequences of their behaviour.
Annals of Internal Medicine

Margaret C. Heagarty; 1976   1552

We eat too much, drink too much, smoke too much, drive too fast, and walk too little.
Pediatrics

LISTER, JOSEPH

H. Charles Cameron; 1948   1553

Once a small urchin in the wards, as his eyes followed Lister's movements, confided to a bystander, "It's us wee yins he likes best, and next it's the auld women."
Recollections of Lister

LITERATURE

William Osler; 1899   1554

While medicine is to be your vocation, or calling, see to it that you have also an avocation—some intellectual pastime which may serve to keep you in touch with the world of art, of science, or of letters. Begin at once the cultivation of some interest other than the purely professional. The difficulty is in a selection and the choice will be different according to your tastes and training. No matter what it is—but have an outside hobby. For the hard working medical student it is perhaps easiest to keep up an interest in literature.
After Twenty-five Years

William Williams Keen; 1900   1555

Make it a point not to let your intellectual life atrophy through non-use. Be familiar with the classics of English literature in prose and verse; read the lives of the great men of the past, and keep pace with modern thought in books of travel, history, fiction, science. A varied intellectual life will give zest to your medical studies.... Let music and art shed their radiance upon your too often weary life and find in the sweet cadences of sound or the rich emotions of form and color a refinement which adds polish to the scientific man.
Journal of the American Medical Association

William Osler; 1919   1556

[Recommended literary works for medical students:] 1) Old and New Testament, 2) Shakespeare, 3) Montaigne, 4) Plutarch's "Lives", 5) Marcus Aurelius, 6) Epictetus, 7) *Religio Medici*, 8) *Don Quixote*, 9) Emerson, 10) Oliver Wendell Holmes' "Breakfast Table" series.   *Johns Hopkins Hospital Bulletin*

Enid Rhodes Peschel; 1980   **1557**

The dialogue between medicine and literature is, essentially, a continuing interchange between the flesh and the word; between man's body and his spirit. Both medicine and literature probe, although from radically different perspectives, the same subject: the truths are revealed—concealed—in man.   *Medicine and Literature*

LITIGATION

Henry George Miller; 1961   **1558**

The exploitation of his injury represents one of the few weapons available to the unskilled worker to acquire a larger share—or indeed a share of any kind—in the national capital. Its possible yield may not bear comparison with the weekly recurring fantasy of a win in the pools, but it is more clearly within his grasp, and it may yet endow him with a capital sum such as he could never have saved during a lifetime of unremitting labour. The employer or his representative, the insurance company, is fair game.

British Medical Journal

LIVER

Francis Glisson; 1654   **1559**

Moreover, peculiar swellings are found in the biliary tract; in which it may happen that its tunic [Glisson capsule] appears...thicker than normal.   *Anatomia Hepatis*

Ambrose Bierce; 1906   **1560**

Liver, *n.* A large red organ thoughtfully provided by nature to be bilious with.... The liver is heaven's best gift to the goose; without it that bird would be unable to supply us with the Strasbourg paté.   *The Devil's Dictionary*

Richard Selzer; 1976   **1561**

The liver,...that great maroon snail.... No wave of emotion sweeps it. Neither music nor mathematics gives it pause in its appointed tasks.   *Mortal Lessons. Liver*

LIVER DISEASE

René-Théophile-Hyacinthe Laennec; 1826   **1562**

This type of growth [of the liver] belongs to the group of those which are confused under the name of *scirrhus*. I believe we ought to designate it with the name of *cirrhosis*, because of its color. Its development in the liver is one of the most common causes of ascites, and has the peculiarity that...the tissue of the liver is absorbed, and it ends often...by disappearing entirely.   *Traité de l'Auscultation Médiate*

Richard Bright; 1836   **1563**

In cases of jaundice from inflammatory action, the condition of the liver after death differs according to the period at which the disease has proved fatal; but, in general, the size of the organ is not materially increased; though, on the contrary, it is not unfrequently perceptibly diminished.   *Guy's Hospital Report*

LIVER TRANSPLANTATION

T.E. Starzl, T.L. Marchioro, K.N. von Kaulla, and others; 1963   **1564**

An ideal treatment for several kinds of liver disease would be removal of the diseased organ and orthotopic replacement with a hepatic homograft.

Surgery, Gynecology, and Obstetrics

LIVING

Hippocrates; [460-375 BC]   **1565**
Neither a surfeit of food, nor of fasting is good, nor anything else which exceeds the measure of nature.   *Lloyd GER, Hippocratic Writings*

[Anonymous]; 1490   **1566**
Wine, women, Baths, by Art or Nature warme,
Us'd abus'd do men much good or harme.   *The School of Salernum*

Michel de Montaigne; 1580   **1567**
The utility of living consists not in the length of days, but in the use of time; a man may
have lived long, and yet lived but a little.   *Essays. That to Philosophize is to Learn How to Die*

Benjamin Franklin; 1735   **1568**
Early to bed and early to rise, makes a man healthy wealthy and wise.
                                                                    Poor Richard's Almanac

William Osler; 1905   **1569**
It is more particularly on the younger men that I would urge the advantages of an early
devotion to a peripatetic philosophy of life. Just so soon as you have your second teeth
think of a change; get away from the nurse, cut the apron strings of your old teachers, seek
new ties in a fresh environment, if possible, where you can have a certain measure of freedom and independence.   *Journal of the American Medical Association*

William Osler; 1905   **1570**
Nothing will sustain you more potently than the power to recognize in your humdrum
routine, as perhaps it may be thought, the true poetry of life—the poetry of the commonplace, of the ordinary man, of the plain, toil-worn woman, with their loves and their
joys, their sorrows and their griefs.   *The Student Life*

William Osler; 1913   **1571**
Now the way of life that I preach is a habit to be acquired gradually by long and steady repetition. It is the practice of living for the day only, and for the day's work.   *A Way of Life*

Warfield T. Longcope; 1932   **1572**
As I grow older, I have less and less sympathy with the conscientious efforts merely to
extend life in old age....It is the duty of the doctor to preserve, not only health and life,
but joy of living, and if most of us had to make our choice we would take the latter. Why
ward off death if in the attempt we kill living?   *Johns Hopkins Hospital Bulletin*

Albert Camus; 1942   **1573**
What counts is not the best living but the most living.   *The Myth of Sisyphus*

Viktor E. Frankl; 1962   **1574**
One should not search for an abstract meaning of life. Everyone has his own specific vocation or mission in life to carry out a concrete assignment which demands fulfillment.
Therein he cannot be replaced, nor can his life be repeated. Thus, everyone's task is as
unique as is his specific opportunity to implement it.   *Man's Search for Meaning*

Elisabeth Kübler-Ross; 1970   **1575**
Few of us live beyond our three score and ten years and yet in that brief time most of us
create and live a unique biography and weave ourselves into the fabric of human history.
                                                                      On Death and Dying

Norman Cousins; 1979   **1576**
Your heaviest artillery will be your will to live. Keep the big gun going.
                                                                    Anatomy of an Illness

Matko Marusic; 1982   **1577**

It is easy to die; living is difficult.   *Personal communication*

Norman Cousins; 1989   **1578**

Death is not the ultimate tragedy in life. The ultimate tragedy is to die without discovering the possibilities of full growth. The approach of death need not be denial of that growth.   *Head First*

Sherwin B. Nuland; 1994   **1579**

The greatest dignity to be found in death is the dignity of the life that preceded it. This is a form of hope we can all achieve, and it is the most abiding of all. Hope resides in the meaning of what our lives have been.   *How We Die*

Michael Rose; 1996   **1580**

You spend all your life learning how to do things, learning what it all means, and then you die.   *Gladwell M, The New Yorker*

LONGEVITY

Benjamin Franklin; 1733   **1581**

To lengthen thy Life, lessen thy Meals.   *Poor Richard's Almanac*

George Bernard Shaw; 1911   **1582**

Do not try to live for ever. You will not succeed.   *The Doctor's Dilemma, Preface*

Richard Asher; 1959   **1583**

I would like to see our patients and our public cease their vain strivings after longevity, and to realise it is better to live for seventy years without fussing, than to achieve the age of eighty with elaborate, painstaking care.   *The Medical Education of the Patient and the Public*

Richard A. Kern; 1962   **1584**

When asked his secret of youth, a 70 year-old said: "That's easy. Meet this gentleman, my father, he's 95."   *Temple University Medical Center Bulletin*

LOVE

Margaret Sanger; 1928   **1585**

Pregnancy... usually interrupts the normal development of the growing love between husband and wife. Psychic adjustment and the establishment of an enduring harmony between the two personalities is seldom based on a sound foundation. Romantic love is one thing; procreation is another. As long as the two are entangled together in an inextricable and inexplicable mess, it is not likely that any great success can be made of either.   *Motherhood in Bondage*

Karl Menninger, Martin Mayman, Paul Pruyser; 1963   **1586**

It is surely little wonder that, with the start they receive in childhood and adolescence, many people reach adult life without the faintest conception of what [love] is, or what it might be for them. Companionship, group membership, infatuation, exhibitionistic dominance or submisssion, and especially unselective sexual desire are all commonly mistaken for and called "love."   *The Vital Balance*

LUNG

Michael Servetus (Villanovanus); 1553   **1587**

It is in the lungs, consequently, that the mixture (of the inspired air with the blood) takes place, and it is in the lungs also, not in the heart, that the crimson colour of the blood is acquired.   *Christianismi Restitutio*

John Scott Haldane, Claude G. Douglas, Yandell Henderson, Edward C. Schneider; 1913   **1588**

The raising of arterial oxygen pressure [with high-altitude acclimatisation] is attributable to secretory activity of the cells lining the lung alveoli.... On breathing air rich in oxygen the secretory activity was rapidly diminished.   *Philosophical Transactions of the Royal Society*

Joseph Barcroft; 1923   **1589**

A number of tests were made for the purpose of discovering whether the pressure of oxygen in the blood was or was not higher than that in the alveolar air. In all cases they were so nearly the same that we attribute the passage of gas through the pulmonary epithelium to diffusion.   *Philosophical Transactions of the Royal Society*

LUNG DISEASE

René-Théophile-Hyacinthe Laennec; 1819   **1590**

The crepitous rhonchus is the pathognomonic sign of the first stage of peripneumony.... It conveys the notion of very small equal-sized bubbles.... The further we remove the cylinder from the point affected, the rhonchus becomes more obscure.... When the hepatization is near the surface...bronchophony becomes then almost like pectoriloquy.... Hepatization...is always further accompanied by a dull sound on percussion, over the affected parts.... When the pus...collects into one spot, a very strong mucous or cavernous rhonchus, with large bubbles, is perceived over the site of the abscess.

Traité de l'Auscultation Médiate

William Osler; 1903   **1591**

Pneumonia is the captain of the men of death and tuberculosis is the handmaid.

Aphorisms

LUPUS ERYTHEMATOSUS

William Osler; 1895   **1592**

By exudative erythema is understood a disease of unknown etiology with polymorphic skin lesions—hyperaemia, oedema, and hemorrhage—arthritis occasionally, and a variable number of visceral manifestations, of which the most important are gastro-intestinal crises, endocarditis, pericarditis, acute nephritis, and hemorrhage from the mucous surfaces. Recurrence is a special feature...and attacks may come on...even throughout a long period of years.   *American Journal of the Medical Sciences*

Malcolm M. Hargraves, Helen Robinson, Robert Morton; 1948   **1593**

We have been observing a phenomenon in our bone marrow preparations which, to our kniowledge, has never been described in the literature.... The first cell we have called a "tart" cell.... The second cell... has been called an "L.E." cell... because of its frequent appearance in the bone marrow in cases of acute disseminated lupus erythematosus.... To date... we have found [the LE cell] only in the bone marrow in certain cases of acute disseminated lupus erythematosus.   *Proceedings of the Staff Meeting of the Mayo Clinic*

John R. Haserick, Lena A. Lewis, Donald W. Bortz; 1950   **1594**

The gamma globulin of acute disseminated lupus erythematosus contains the factor which is responsible for inducing rosettes of leukocytes and formation of the LE cell in mixtures of normal bone marrow preparations and LE plasma.... The LE factor disappears from the blood during remissions, and reappears during relapses.

American Journal of the Medical Sciences

LYME DISEASE

Allen C. Steere, Stephen E. Malawista, David R. Syndman, and others; 1977   **1595**

Thirty-nine children and 12 adults in three contiguous Connecticut communities were found to have an apparently similar type of arthritis. It was characterized by usually short but recurrent attacks of pain and swelling in a few large joints, often the knee, with longer intervening periods of complete remission and with, as yet, no permanent joint deformity.... The authors believe that the arthritis described here is a previously unrecognized clinical entity and have named it "Lyme arthritis" after the community where it was first studied. *Arthritis and Rheumatism*

Willy Burgdorfer, Alan G. Barbour, Stanley F. Hayes, and others; 1982   **1596**

That the *I. dammini* spirochete is antigenically related to the etiologic agent of Lyme disease was suggested by the positive reactions [1:80 to 1:1280] we obtained when we examined serum samples from nine patients with clinically diagnosed Lyme disease by means of indirect immunofluorescence.... In contrast, serum samples from four people from New York and ten from Montana with no history of the disease did not react with the spirochete in titers higher than 1:20. *Science*

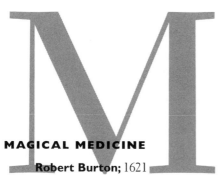

MAGICAL MEDICINE

Robert Burton; 1621   1597

Cunning men, wizards, and white witches, as they call them, in every village, which, if
they be sought unto, will help almost all infirmities of body and mind.

The Anatomy of Melancholy

Croatian proverb   1598

Believing a village healer prolongs the disease.   *Proverb*

MALARIA

Marcus Terentius Varro; 27 BC   1599

If you must build on the bank of a river, take care that you do not let the steading face
the river, for it will be very cold in winter and unhealthy in summer. Like precautions must
be taken against swampy places for the same reasons and particularly because as they dry,
swamps breed certain animalculae which cannot be seen with the eyes and which we
breathe through the nose and mouth into the body where they cause grave maladies.

Rerum Rusticarum

Aulus Cornelius Celsus; [25 BC - AD 50]   1600

Now there follows the treatment of fevers, a class of disease which both affects the body
as a whole, and is exceedingly common. Of fevers, one is quotidian, another tertian, a
third quartan.   *On Medicine*

John Evelyn; 1658   1601

After six fitts of a Quartan Ague it pleased God to visite my deare Child Dick with fitts
so extreame, especiale one of his sides, that after the rigor was over and he in his hot fitt,
he fell into so greate and intollerable a sweate, that being surpriz'd with the abundance
of vapours ascending to his head, he fell into...fatal Symptoms.... He plainely expird, to
our unexpressable griefe and affliction.   *Diary*

Robert Talbor; 1682   1602

Amongst the Authors whom I have named, there are some who endeavoring to explain
the properties of *Quinquina* or the *Jesuits Powder*...think it enough to say that it is hot and

dry.... That we may give the World somewhat more satisfactory as to that point, we must in the first place, (with *Willis*), take our measures from *Experience*, and allow with him, That all things which are actually bitter, have great virtue in sifting preternatural fermentations.   *The English Remedy*

Frances Trollope; 1832   **1603**
Whenever we found out a picturesque nook, where turf, and moss, and deep shade, and a crystal stream, and fallen trees...tempted us to sit down...and be happy, we invariably found that spot lay under the imputation of malaria.   *Domestic Manners of the Americans*

Alphonse Laveran; 1881   **1604**
Attacks of malaria are produced by the introduction into the blood of parasites which appear in the various forms herewith described; it is because quinine kills these parasites that it cures malaria.   *Comptes Rendus l'Académie des Sciences*

Albert Freeman Africanus King; 1883   **1605**
Viewed in the light of our modern "germ theory" of disease, the punctures of proboscidian insects, like those of Pasteur's needles, deserve consideration, as probable means by which bacteria and other germs may be inoculated into human bodies, so as to infect the blood and give rise to special fevers.... I now propose to present a series of facts...with regard to the so-called "malarial poison" and to show how they may be explicable by the supposition that the mosquito is the real source of disease, rather than the inhalation of cutaneous absorption of a marsh-vapor.   *Popular Science Monthly*

Ronald Ross; 1897   **1606**
The method adopted has been to feed mosquitoes, bred in bottles from the larva, on patients having crescents in the blood, and then to examine their tissues for parasites similar to the haemamoeba in man.... I succeeded in finding in two of them certain remarkable and suspicious cells containing pigment identical in appearance to that of the parasite of malaria.   *British Medical Journal*

Richard A. Kern; 1962   **1607**
In patients with blackwater fever, primaquine may convert claret to champagne.
                                                                                      Temple University Medical Center Bulletin

MALINGERING

Gustav Monod; 1926   **1608**
He [Dr. David Gruby] was called to a paralysed patient. He found her immobilised in her armchair. "What oil do you use in your kitchen? Can I see it?" When the bottle was produced Gruby uncorked it and calmly began emptying it on the carpet. The patient jumped up: "Here, that's a Persian rug." The rug was ruined—the lady cured.
                                                                                                                                                  The Lancet

Richard Asher; 1945   **1609**
Three Golden Rules for Malingering:
1. You must make the impression you hate to be ill.
2. Make up your mind for one disease and stick to it.
3. Don't tell the doctor too much.   *Richard Asher Talking Sense*

Richard Asher; 1958   **1610**
The pride of a doctor who has caught a malingerer is akin to that of a fisherman who has landed an enormous fish; and his stories (like those of fishermen) may become somewhat exaggerated in the telling.   *Richard Asher Talking Sense*

MALPRACTICE

Hippocrates; [460-375 BC]   **1611**

When bad physicians.... meet with a severe, violent, and dangerous illness, then it is that their errors and want of skill are manifest to all. The punishment... is not postponed, but follows speedily.   *On Ancient Medicine*

Matthew Prior; 1714   **1612**

Cur'd yesterday of my Disease,
I died last night of my Physician.   *The Remedy Worse Than the Disease*

George Bernard Shaw; 1911   **1613**

No doctor dare accuse another of malpractice. He is not sure enough of his own opinion to ruin another man by it. He knows that if such conduct were tolerated in his profession no doctor's livelihood or reputation would be worth a year's purchase. I do not blame him: I should do the same myself. But the effect of this state of things is to make the medical profession a conspiracy to hide its own shortcomings.   *The Doctor's Dilemma, Preface*

Nathan P. Couch, Nicholas L. Tilney, Francis D. Moore; 1978   **1614**

It would be a tragic irony if the current epidemic of malpractice lawsuits brought quiet concealment of unfavorable results, so that medical progress is impeded rather than promoted.   *American Journal of Surgery*

Joseph E. Hardison; 1979   **1615**

The malpractice excuse: "If we don't order this test, we might get sued." As if the ordering of the test protects against a malpractice suit or the threat of the suit actually increases the incidence of pathologic findings in the patient!   *New England Journal of Medicine*

George A. Annas; 1985   **1616**

The more things doctors are able to do, the more likely that at least a few doctors won't do them. And the result will be more people suing for negligence.   *The Wall Street Journal*

Sara C. Charles; 1985   **1617**

I think it's an enormously complex issue. It is not a battle between doctors and lawyers. And if you perceive it that way, you're misreading the whole thing. It is not a purely economic issue. Because if you see it that way that's a very limited vision of what's really going on. It's a cultural problem.   *Realities of Medicine*

Edward Shorter; 1991   **1618**

Some authorities feel that the disintegration of the doctor-patient relationship is the cause, and blame the patients for losing their former willingness to trust. But we must bear in mind that malpractice suits are an *effect* of the disintegration of this relationship as well as a cause of it. The doctor's very own behaviour is one of the wedges driving them apart from the patients.   *Doctors and Their Patients*

MAMMOGRAPHY

Jacob Gershon-Cohen, Mortimer B. Hermel, Simon M. Berger; 1961   **1619**

Periodic x-ray examination at 6-month intervals among 1,312 women for 5 years uncovered 23 cancers, at a case finding rate of 17.5 per 1,000.... *Axillary metastasis was absent in 70%.* In 6 patients the tumor was not palpable and the operation was undertaken *on the x-ray findings alone.*   *Journal of the American Medical Association*

MANAGED CARE

Christine K. Cassel; 1996   **1620**

Managed care is not the problem; profit is the problem.   *Annals of Internal Medicine*

Mack Lipkin Jr.; 1996   **1621**

With the increasing corporatization of medicine, are physicians becoming Sisyphean drudges toiling futilely, forced to roll the stone uphill faster and faster, losing patients, pride in quality care, autonomy, and their own health?   *Annals of Internal Medicine*

Daniel J. Baxter; 1997   **1622**

As managed care organizations rotate patients from one doctor to another, the inevitable increase in impersonal care will risk further patient alienation and inability to face illness and even death.   *The Least of These My Brethren*

David Loxterkamp; 1997   **1623**

Yea, though we walk through the valley of managed care and our business (if not our soul) is traded on the floor of the New York Stock Exchange, we are lucky to be here, doing what we do, still students of medicine, tending to the afflictions and infirmities of those who call us doctor.   *New England Journal of Medicine*

Clif Cleaveland; 1998   **1624**

Increasingly, I deal with anonymous voices at toll-free numbers to determine what procedures and consultations can be approved for my patients. Sometimes these judgments are simply wrong-headed and unjust.   *Sacred Space*

Jerome P. Kassirer; 1998   **1625**

When patients are sick and vulnerable, they expect their physicians to be their advocates for optimal care, not for some minimalist standard. Benefits vary substantially between [managed care] plans.... There is already considerable injustice in the distribution of care, but why should physicians collude to exacerbate the problem?
                                          New England Journal of Medicine

Robert Kuttner; 1998   **1626**

Managed care sneaked up on physicians; by the time they fully grasped the implications, it was a *fait accompli*. Physicians are now caught between patients anxious about the availability and reliability of care and payers demanding further cost control through often perverse financial pressure on doctors.   *New England Journal of Medicine*

MANIC-DEPRESSIVE ILLNESS

Thomas Willis; [1621-1675]   **1627**

After Melancholy, it remains for us to treat of Madness, which is so far ally'd to the other, that these affects often change turns, and each passes into the other; for a melancholy disposition growing worse brings a Fury, and a Fury coming to abate, often ends in a melancholy disposition.   *The Practice of Physick*

Philippe Pinel; 1801   **1628**

The nervous excitement, which characterises the greatest number of cases, affects not the system physically by increasing muscular power and action only, but likewise the mind, by exciting a consciousness of supreme importance and irresistible strength.
                                          Treatise on Insanity

Jean-Ètienne-Dominique Esquirol; 1838   **1629**

It would be difficult not to concede a hereditary transmission of mania, when one recalls that everywhere some members of certain families are struck in several successive generations.   *Des Maladies Mentales*

MARFAN SYNDROME

Antoine Marfan; 1896   **1630**

Gabrielle P..., a young girl age five and a half years.... suffers from a congenital deformation of her four limbs, more pronounced in their extremities, characterized by elongation of the bones with a degree of thinning. One could perhaps name this deformation *dolichostenomelia*.... The muscles are slender but react normally to electrical stimulation.

Bulletin of the Medical Society of Paris

MARIJUANA

Jacques Joseph Moreau; 1845   **1631**

One of the effects of hashish that struck me most forcibly and which generally gets the most attention is that manic excitement always accompanied by a feeling of gaiety and joy inconceivable to those who have not experienced it.   *Hashish and Mental Illness*

Jacques Joseph Moreau; 1845   **1632**

I challenge the right of anyone to discuss the effects of hashish if he is not speaking for himself and if he has not been in a position to evaluate them in light of sufficient repeated use.   *Hashish and Mental Illness*

Institute of Medicine; 1999   **1633**

Scientific data indicate the potential therapeutic value of cannabiniod drugs, primarily [tetrahydrocannabinol], for pain relief, control of nausea and vomiting, and appetite stimulation; smoked marijuana, however, is a crude...delivery system that also delivers harmful substances.... The psychological effects of cannabinoids, such as anxiety reduction, sedation, and euphoria can influence their potential therapeutic value.

Marijuana and Medicine

MARRIAGE

Tertullian (Quintus Septimius Tertullianus); *circa* 197   **1634**

Look at women now. Every limb is weighed down with gold; because of wine, no kiss is freely given. Yes, and now it is divorce which is prayed for, as though that were the natural issue of marriage.   *Apologetical Works*

Cherubino da Siena; *circa* 1450   **1635**

The devil knows how to do so much between husband and wife. He makes them touch and kiss not only the honest parts but the dishonest ones as well. Even just to think about it, I am overwhelmed by horror, fright and bewilderment.... You call this holy matrimony?

Regole della Vita Matrimoniale

Benjamin Disraeli; 1831   **1636**

It destroys one's nerves to be amiable every day to the same human being.

The Young Duke

Sydney Smith; [1771-1845]   **1637**

Marriage resembles a pair of shears, so joined that they can not be separated; often moving in opposite directions, yet always punishing anyone who comes between them.

Lady Holland, Memoir of Sydney Smith

Gilbert Keith Chesterton; 1911   **1638**

Marriage rests upon the fact that you cannot have your cake and eat it; that you cannot lose your heart and have it.   *Preface to Dickens, David Copperfield*

Th. H. Van de Velde; 1926   **1639**

Marriage is the permanent form of monogamous erotic relationships.   *Ideal Marriage*

Th. H. Van de Velde; 1926   **1640**

Let there be love, let there be attachment, let there be mutual partnership in things of the mind; but, with all the utmost possible sympathy in word and deed—leave each other enough leisure, enough space, enough repose! Respect each other's personality and privacy! Learn when and how to leave each other alone!   *Ideal Marriage*

Pius XI; 1930 1641
Now, alas, not secretly nor under cover, but openly, with all sense of shame put aside, now by word again by writings, by theatrical productions of every kind, by romantic fiction, by amorous and frivolous novels, by cinematographs portraying in vivid scene, in addresses broadcast by radio telephony, in short by all the inventions of modern science, the sanctity of marriage is trampled upon and derided. *Casti Connubi*

MASTECTOMY

Fanny Burney; 1811 1642
When the dreadful steel was plunged into the breast—cutting through veins—arteries—flesh—nerves—I needed no more injunctions not to restrain my cries. I began a scream that lasted unintermittingly during the whole time of the incision—& I almost marvel that it rings not in my Ears still! so excruciating was the agony. *Letter to Esther Burney*

MASTURBATION

Samuel Auguste David Tissot; 1760 1643
All the intellectual faculties are enfeebled...and sometimes the patients become slightly deranged.... Their sleep, if they get any, is disturbed with frightful dreams.... The powers of the body fail entirely.... Pimples not only appear on the face... Pustules are also seen...in different parts of the body.... Finally, the impossibility of coition, or the vitiation of the semen, render sterile almost all those addicted to this vice. *A Treatise on the Diseases Produced by Onanism*

Marc Colombat (d'Isere); 1838 1644
[The young girl at a boarding school] soon contracts improper habits, and constantly tormented by an amorous melancholy, becomes sad, dreamy, sentimental and languishing.... The desire for happiness and love, so sweet and attractive in their native truth, are in her converted into a devouring flame, and onanism, that execrable and fatal evil, soon destroys her health and conducts her almost always to a premature grave.
Traité des Maladies des Femmes et de l'Hygiène Spéciale de leur Sexe

MEASLES

Thomas Sydenham; 1676 1645
The measles generally attack children. On the first day they have chills and shivers, and are hot and cold in turns. On the second they have the fever in full.... The nose and eyes run continually; and this is the surest sign of measles.... The symptoms increase till the fourth day. Then—or sometimes on the fifth—there appear on the face and forehead small red spots, very like the bites of fleas.... The spots take hold the face first; from which they spread to the chest and belly, and afterwards to the legs and ankles.
Observationes Medicae

Henry Koplik; 1896 1646
If we look in the mouth at [the first twenty-four to forty-eight hours of the invasion] we see a redness of the fauces; perhaps, not in all cases, a few spots on the soft palate. On the buccal mucous membrane and the inside of the lips, we invariably see...small irregular spots, of a bright red color. In the centre of each spot, there is noted, in strong daylight, a minute bluish white speck. These...are absolutely pathognomonic of beginning measles.
Archives of Pediatrics

MECKEL DIVERTICULUM

Johann Friedrich Meckel; 1809 1647
It appears at a specific site in the ileum and the wall contains each of the several layers of

the intestinal tract.... The proof that the diverticulum is a residuum of the communication between the intestinal canal and the umbilical stalk rests in the findings which I have observed in three stillborn, full-term fetuses.   *Archives of Physiology*

MEDICAL AUDIT

Ernest Amory Codman; 1916   1648
The Trustees of Hospitals should see to it that an effort is made to follow up each patient they treat, long enough to determine whether the treatment given has permanently relieved the condition or symptom complained of.... A layman could not enter authoritatively into the details...but he could insist that the End Results System should be used.
A Study in Hospital Efficiency

MEDICAL BOOKS

Henry Ingersoll Bowditch; 1867   1649
Modern science does not let any book remain long useful.   *Letter to Olivia Bowditch*

MEDICAL CARE

Hippocrates; [460-375 BC]   1650
Practice two things in your dealings with disease: either help or do not harm the patient.
Hippocratic Writings

Hippocrates; [460-375 BC]   1651
The physician must be experienced in many things, but most assuredly in rubbing.
Collinge W, The Complete Guide to Alternative Medicine

Hippocrates; [460-375 BC]   1652
Where there is love of man, there is also love of the art.   *Precepts*

Galen; [130-200]   1653
The physician is Nature's assistant.   *On the Humour*

Robert Burton; 1621   1654
The body's mischiefs, as Plato proves, proceed from the soul: and if the mind be not first satisfied, the body can never be cured.   *The Anatomy of Melancholy*

Giovanni Battista Morgagni; 1761   1655
In the treatment of disease, oftentimes to do nothing is to do everything.
The Seats and Causes of Diseases

William Heberden; 1802   1656
Lastly, where there is no room for anything else, there it is the duty of a physician to exert himself as much as possible in supporting the powers of life, by strengthening the appetite and digestion, and by providing that the stools, and sleep, and every other article of health, shall approach as nearly as may be to its natural state.
Commentaries on the History and Cure of Diseases

William Heberden; 1802   1657
Though the recovery of the patient be the grand aim of their profession, yet where that cannot be attained, they should try to disarm death of some of its terrors, and if they cannot make him quit his prey, and the life must be lost, they may still prevail to have it taken away in the most merciful manner.   *Commentaries on the History and Cure of Diseases*

Thomas Percival; 1803   1658
At the close of every interesting and important case, especially when it hath terminated fatally, a physician should trace back, in calm reflection, all the steps which he had taken in the treatment of it.   *Medical Ethics*

Samuel Taylor Coleridge; [1772-1834]   **1659**
He is the best physician who is the most ingenious inspirer of hope.   *Table Talk*

Charles Darwin; 1871   **1660**
Our medical men exert their utmost skill to save the life of everyone to the last moment.... Thus the weak members of civilized societies propagate their kind. No one who has attended to the breeding of domestic animals will doubt that this must be highly injurious to the race of man.   *The Descent of Man*

Oliver Wendell Holmes; 1871   **1661**
The young man knows the rules, but the old man knows the exceptions.
                                                          The Young Practitioner

Arthur Conan Doyle; 1894   **1662**
Someone described our condition as that of a blind man with a club, who swung it at random. Sometimes he hit the disease and sometimes the patient.
                                        Round the Red Lamp. The Romance of Medicine

William Osler; 1895   **1663**
Can anything be more doleful than a procession of four or five doctors into the sick man's room?   *Ephemerides*

William Osler; 1899   **1664**
Care more particularly for the individual patient than for the special features of the disease.   *Aphorisms*

Stephen Paget; 1909   **1665**
"Talk of the patience of Job," said a hospital nurse, "Job was never on night-duty."
                                                          Confessio Medici

Abraham Flexner; 1910   **1666**
The physician's function is fast becoming social and preventative, rather than individual and curative.   *Medical Education in the United States and Canada*

Charles Horace Mayo; 1919   **1667**
The government has dabbled in medical affairs at enormous expense for what has been accomplished.   *Journal of the American Medical Association*

Francis W. Peabody; 1927   **1668**
The most common criticism made at present by older practitioners is that young graduates have been taught a great deal about the mechanism of disease, but very little about the practice of medicine—or, to put it more bluntly, they are too "scientific" and do not know how to take care of patients.   *Journal of the American Medical Association*

Francis W. Peabody; 1927   **1669**
The treatment of a disease may be entirely impersonal; the care of a patient must be completely personal.   *Journal of the American Medical Association*

L.P. Gaertner; 1929   **1670**
I have always contended that our present day system provides for millionaires and paupers, but does not properly consider the self-respecting wage earner.
                                                          Letter to Louis E. Schmidt

Wilfred Batten Lewis Trotter; 1932   **1671**
The ordinary patient goes to his doctor because he is in pain or some other discomfort and wants to be comfortable again; he is not in pursuit of the ideal of health in any direct sense. The doctor on the other hand wants to discover the pathological condition and control it if he can. The two are thus to some degree at cross purposes from the first, and

unless the affair is brought to an early and happy conclusion this divergence of aims is likely to become more and more serious as the case goes on.   *Art and Science in Medicine*

James Edgar Paullin; 1947   **1672**
Frequently, more is accomplished by treating the person rather than the disease the patient has.   *The Georgia Review*

Herman L. Kretschmer; [1879-1951]   **1673**
Gentle, Doctor, it makes lots of difference which end of that thing you're on.
Instructions on the Use of the Cystoscope

William Boyd; 1961   **1674**
Medicine can never be purely a science; it contains too many immeasurables. The patient with heart disease is not just an internal combustion engine with a leaking valve but a sensitive human being with a diseased heart.... It may be the man or woman rather than the disease that needs to be treated.   *A Textbook of Pathology*

Lawrence L. Weed; 1964   **1675**
The present illness should be a statement of... a problem or series of problems. Each... should be discussed separately. All the... information concerning a... problem should be presented, whether it came from the patient, a relative, a friend, an old chart, a laboratory data book, a pathology slide cabinet, or the files in an x-ray department.... Enslavement to the conventional format of the medical history can make a problem almost incomprehensible by separating the... facts, putting some in the past history, some under laboratory data and some in the systems review.... Each problem should have its own plan.
Irish Journal of Medical Science

Douglas Arthur Kilgour Black; 1968   **1676**
For the patient, Medicine should mean simply help in sickness—help which comes promptly, is given willingly, which is manifestly efficient, and which does not cripple him financially.   *The Logic of Medicine*

Eugene A. Stead Jr.; 1968   **1677**
Take care of people, not illnesses.   *Annals of Internal Medicine*

Macfarlane Burnet; 1968   **1678**
In the twenty-first century there will...be a complete separation of the two essential functions of the present-day doctor. I [pictured] first the "doctor of first contact" and second, the hospital. The doctor of first contact...will have as his most important function to decide how best the needs of the patient before him can be met.... I pictured him as a wise counsellor with a training fitting him to understand the whole predicament of the patient...to help him bring any patient not needing hospital care back to full effectiveness in the community.   *Changing Patterns*

René Jules Dubos; 1968   **1679**
Medical advances create an atmosphere of rising expectations; human beings are no longer willing to tolerate even the mild physical disabilities to which all flesh is heir once they become aware that pain and discomfort can be mollified.
Man, Medicine, and Environment

A.E. Clark-Kennedy; 1970   **1680**
Science tells us the nature of disease. Applied science tells us how to treat it, but only human judgment tells us whether or not to apply our science in a particular case. And all the most difficult decisions in medical practice today are of this human kind. We must

not keep people alive, just because we can. Technical achievement must not become our God. *Journal of the Royal College of Physicians*

Henry George Miller; 1971   **1681**
Those of us who have spent our lives in academic clinical medicine have averted our gaze from the major causes of public ill-health: ...the problems of psychiatry,...the care of the mentally subnormal,...chronic illness of all kinds—including the neglected area of terminal care, and...the care of the elderly, the most rapidly growing and most neglected section of our population. *Then and Now*

Rosemary Stevens; 1971   **1682**
The problems [in medical care] lie not in the lack of achievements but in the widening gap between what *can* be done for an individual under optimal conditions and what *is* being done...under average and minimal conditions. The crisis is in the delivery, not in the potential, of care. *American Medicine and the Public Interest*

Thomas McKeown; 1971   **1683**
Since most major diseases and disabilities are likely to prove relatively intractable if they cannot be prevented, the role of therapeutic medicine should be modified to include as the major commitment the concept of care. *Medical History and Medical Care*

Lewis Thomas; 1975   **1684**
If people are educated to believe that they are fundamentally fragile, always on the verge of mortal disease, perpetually in need of support by health-care professionals at every side, always dependent on an imagined discipline of "preventive medicine," there can be no limit to the numbers of doctors' offices, clinics, and hospitals required to meet the demand. In the end, we would all become doctors, spending our days screening each other for disease. *New England Journal of Medicine*

Alvan Barach; 1977   **1685**
Remember to cure the patient as well as the disease.
Simpson JB, Simpson's Contemporary Quotations

Michael Rose; 1977   **1686**
The trail we follow...has nothing to do with the patient's subjective trouble. It is neither a crime nor is it stupid to follow this trail. It is not easy, and it is often impossible, to know that it is a false trail until one is told, when flushed with victory, that the finishing post is still a long way off, perhaps further off than it was when you started. Often when we've done our best, it's not easy to accept that it has all added up to nothing to the fellow or lady on the other side of the consulting table. *The Lancet*

Albert R. Jonsen; 1978   **1687**
To possess medical skills is to be able to care for the sick.... Caring means being "troubled by another's trouble." *Annals of Internal Medicine*

Samuel Shem; 1978   **1688**
The delivery of medical care is to do as much nothing as possible. *The House of God*

Joseph E. Hardison; 1979   **1689**
The "If it were my mother or father, I'd want it done" excuse. To argue against this excuse is unpatriotic and blasphemous, akin to belittling apple pie or baseball. *New England Journal of Medicine*

Norman Cousins; 1981   **1690**
The science of medicine and the art of medicine come together when three things are achieved. The first is the accuracy of the diagnosis. The second is the proportionate nature of the treatment. The thid is the full mobilization and release of a patient's heal-

ing resources in which robust expectations of full recovery play an important part. If the physician can orchestrate these three elements, he will be doing what he is supposed to.

Human Options

Paul Starr; 1982   **1691**
The development of medical care, like other institutions, takes place within larger fields of power and social structure. These external forces are particularly visible in conflicts over the politics and economics of health and medical care.

The Social Transformation of American Medicine

Paul Starr; 1982   **1692**
In its commitment to the preservation of life, medical care ironically has come to symbolize a prototypically modern form of torture, combining benevolence, indifference, and technical wizardry.   *The Social Transformation of American Medicine*

House of Lords; 1985   **1693**
The Bolam principle may be formulated as a rule that a doctor is not negligent if he acts in accordance with a practice accepted at the time as proper by a responsible body of medical opinion even though other doctors adopt a different practice. In short, the law imposes the duty of care: but the standard of care is a matter of medical judgement.

Law Reports

Dr. Seuss (Theodore Geisel); 1986   **1694**
When at last we are sure
you've been properly pilled,
then a few paper forms
must be properly filled
so that you and your heirs
may be properly billed.   *You're Only Old Once*

Charles E. Rosenberg; 1987   **1695**
Scientific medicine has raised expectations and costs, but has failed to confront the social consequences of its own success. We are still wedded to acute care and episodic, specialized contacts with physicians.   *The Care of Strangers*

Norman Cousins; 1989   **1696**
People go to doctors out of fear and hope—fear that something may be wrong but hope that it can be set right. If these emotional needs don't figure in the physician's approach, he may be treating half the patient. The question is not now—any more than it has ever been—whether physicians should attach less importance to their scientific training than to their relationships with patients, but rather whether enough importance is being attached to everything involved in effective patient care.   *Head First*

Robert H. Brook; 1989   **1697**
Methods for judging appropriateness have almost always been applied to people who received a procedure as opposed to people who have a complaint or symptom. Thus, the literature can be used to say something about the potential overuse of services, but it does not contain information on detecting underuse.   *Journal of the American Medical Association*

Patrick O'Brien; 1991   **1698**
One of the miseries of medical life is that on the one hand you know what shocking things can happen to the human body and on the other you know how very little we can really do about most of them. You are therefore denied the comfort of faith.

The Nutmeg of Consolation

Anatole Broyard; 1992   **1699**
In learning to talk to his patients, the doctor may talk himself back into loving his work.

Intoxicated by My Illness. The Patient Examines the Doctor

Robert Buckman; 1992   **1700**

Breaking bad news is not an optional add-on to a professional's specialist abilities; it is a mandatory part of his or her basic skills. The public expects it and is vociferous when it is not done well.   *How to Break Bad News*

Joseph Bernardin; 1995   **1701**

In addition to societal changes, there are causes specific to the medical enterprise that contribute to medicine's disconnection from its underlying moral foundation. For example, advances in medical science and technology have improved the prospect of cure but has de-emphasized medicine's traditional caring function. Other contributions include the commercialization of medical practice, the growing preoccupation of some physicians with monetary concerns, and the loss of the sense of humility and humanity by certain practitioners.   *Address to the AMA House of Delegates*

Christine K. Cassel; 1996   **1702**

We must understand that we have a responsibility to use medical resources wisely precisely because health care is a public good. As our power to heal grows, the cost of care increases, thus increasing the importance of prudent purchasing. But the reason to contain cost must be to grant expanded access to the vulnerable and the needy and not to enrich ourselves or investors.   *Annals of Internal Medicine*

Morris Barer, N.P. Roos; 1996   **1703**

Death is ultimately very democratic, but the deferral of death seems to be a privilege that is related to rank and status.   *Prairie Medical Journal*

Daniel J. Baxter; 1997   **1704**

Pious lip service notwithstanding, pastoral care is frequently deemed a frill. Emotional support is not easily quantified on a hospital's computer printouts or quality-assurance reviews.   *The Least of These My Brethren*

Clif Cleaveland; 1998   **1705**

[In his painting, "The Doctor"] Fildes...defines a sacred space, or circle of caring, whose center is a terribly sick or injured fellow mortal. The caregiver...and the beloved ones occupy the space.... The space speaks of caring, of quiet, of compassion.... There is candor and inquiry, but overarching all are love and respect for human life.... Issues of race, gender, religious creed, or economic circumstance should in no way lessen the care given in this space. Profit motives and bureaucratic regulation are alien to it.   *Sacred Space*

Sherwin B. Nuland; 1998   **1706**

It is judgement that lies at the heart of diagnosis, of therapy, and of all that is gathered under the umbrella called case management.... Clinical decision making must always be accomplished in the face of incomplete and largely ambiguous information. The process is one of sifting, weighing, and judging.... To accept [uncertainty] is the essence of wisdom; to enjoy it is the essence of the enrichment of a doctor's soul.   *The American Scholar*

Brahmanic saying   **1707**

In illness the physician is a father; in convalescence, a friend; when health is restored, he is a guardian.   *Brahmanic Saying*

MEDICAL ECONOMICS

John Ruskin; 1862   **1708**

The difference...between one physician's opinion and another's...is far greater, as respects the qualities of mind involved, and far more important in result to you personally, than the difference between good and bad laying of bricks.... Yet you pay with equal fee, contentedly, the...good and bad workmen upon your body.   *Unto This Last*

[Anonymous]; 1921   **1709**
[Is] the family practitioner...being replaced by a corporation?
Journal of the American Medical Association

American Medical Association, Bureau of Medical Economics; 1935   **1710**
Where physicians become employees and permit their services to be peddled as com-
modities, the medical services usually deteriorate, and the public which purchases such
services is injured.   *Economics and the Ethics of Medicine*

William Bennett Bean; 1954   **1711**
The cynic has too well said that hereabouts [in a rural setting] ragweed would have been
eradicated long ago if hogs had hay fever.   *Journal of Medical Education*

Archibald Leman Cochrane; 1972   **1712**
I hope clinicians in the future will abandon the pursuit of the "margin of the impossible"
and settle for "reasonable probability." There is a whole rational health service to gain.
Effectiveness and Efficiency

Archibald Leman Cochrane; 1972   **1713**
If we are ever going to get the "optimum" results from our national expenditure on the NHS
[National Health Service] we must finally be able to express the results in the form of the
benefit and the cost to the population of a particular type of activity, and the increased benefit that could be obtained if more money were made available.   *Effectiveness and Efficiency*

Arnold S. Relman; 1980   **1714**
The new medical-industrial complex is now a fact of American life. It is still growing and
is likely to be with us for a long time. Any conclusions about its ultimate impact on our
health-care system would be premature, but it is safe to say that the effect will be profound.... We should not allow the medical-industrial complex to distort our health-care
system to its own entrepreneurial ends.   *New England Journal of Medicine*

Paul Starr; 1982   **1715**
Whoever provides medical care or pays the costs of illness stands to gain the gratitude and
good will of the sick and their families. The prospect of these good-will returns to investment in health care creates a powerful motive for governments and other institutions to
intervene in the economics of medicine.   *The Social Transformation of American Medicine*

Paul Starr; 1982   **1716**
Some services, like cataract surgery, are financial "winners" because they pay much more
than they cost to produce, while other services, like talking to a patient, are "losers"
because they pay less than they cost.   *The Social Transformation of American Medicine*

Paul Starr; 1982   **1717**
The difficulty in controlling costs in health insurance arises because sickness is not always
a well-defined condition and many of the costs of treatment are within the control of the
insured.   *The Social Transformation of American Medicine*

Arnold S. Relman; 1985   **1718**
Health care is being converted from a social service to an economic commodity, sold in the
market place and distributed on the basis of who can afford to pay for it.
The New York Times

Charles E. Rosenberg; 1987   **1719**
There are many equities to be maximized in the hospital, many interests to be served, but
the collective interest does not always have effective advocates. The discipline of the marketplace will not necessarily speak to that interest; the most vulnerable will inevitably suffer.
The Care of Strangers

Charles E. Rosenberg; 1987   **1720**
Like the U.S. Defense Department, the hospital system has grown in response to per-

ceived social need—in comparison with which normal budgetary constraints and compromises have come to seem niggling and inappropriate. *The Care of Strangers*

Charles E. Rosenberg; 1987 **1721**
The increasing ability of physicians to disentangle specific disease entities...was an intellectual achievement of the first magnitude and not unrelated to the increasingly scientific and prestigious public image of the medical profession. Yet, we have seen a complex and inexorably bureaucratic reimbursement system grow up around these diagnostic entities; disease does not exist if it cannot be coded. *The Care of Strangers*

Norman Cousins; 1989 **1722**
Doctors don't get paid for talking to patients. In a medical economy dominated by third-party paymasters—insurance companies, the government, health plans, etc.—the harsh reality is that doctors get paid mostly for tests and procedures. It is not surprising, therefore, that patients should be subjected to a multitude of encounters with expensive medical technology, not all of which is essential or without risk.... Even more serious, of course, is the reduced time for the careful questioning by the physician that has held such a high place in medical tradition. *Head First*

Mark Siegler; 1993 **1723**
The steeply rising health-care costs remind me of what Jack Kent Cooke, the owner of the Washington Redskins, supposedly said when he was asked why he fired George Allen as his football coach: Cooke is quoted as saying, "I gave Allen an unlimited budget and he exceeded it." *Mayo Clinic Procedures*

Steven A. Schroeder; 1996 **1724**
The problem of the uninsured continues to grow quietly; in the long run, its effects will be so pervasive that it is bound to re-emerge as a major national issue. If it does not, then we will find ourselves living in a much meaner America than many of us who entered the healing professions ever imagined. *New England Journal of Medicine*

Sydney Walker III; 1996 **1725**
HMOs and PPOs are the latest development in a trend that is changing medicine from a noble calling into a commodity market. *A Dose of Sanity*

Frank Davidoff; 1997 **1726**
The sad truth is that our trillion-dollar medical care system seems to feel that time spent with patients is a luxury it simply can't afford. *Annals of Internal Medicine*

Jerome Lowenstein; 1997 **1727**
The current hospital reimbursement system, which categorizes all illnesses into disease-related groups (DRGs), encourages the practice of viewing patients as "examples of disease." *The Midnight Meal and Other Essays*

Jerome P. Kassirer; 1997 **1728**
Many acknowledge their deep concern about the system privately but publicly remain silent. Compromising care to control cost is a vexing social issue in which the integrity of the profession is at stake, and medicine must have a clear, strong voice in these public decisions. Before we face far more odious choices, we must come to grips with these difficult trade-offs. So far...the air is filled with a strained silence. *New England Journal of Medicine*

International Anti-Euthanasia Task Force; 1998 **1729**
The cost effectiveness of hastened death is as undeniable as gravity. The earlier a patient dies, the less costly is his or her care.
Emanuel EJ and Battin MP, New England Journal of Medicine

Jerome P. Kassirer; 1998 **1730**
A system in which there is no equity is, in fact, already unethical. We gave up the idea of

having an equitable system when we decided several years ago to give up on a proposed national health system with consistent coverage for the entire population. Although the chance of rekindling such a proposal seems remote now, we should not stop trying.

New England Journal of Medicine

Roy Porter, G.S. Rousseau; 1998   **1731**
There are strong reasons to be apprehensive that modern medical imperialism may, albeit inadvertently, multiply costs without enhancing health.   *Gout: The Patrician Malady*

George Soros; 1999   **1732**
Health care companies are not in business to heal people or save lives; they provide health care to make profits. In effect, in the necessary effort to control health care costs through the market mechanism, power has shifted from physicians and patients to insurance companies and other purchasers of services.   *Ramirez A, The New York Times*

John Kitzhaber; 2000   **1733**
The legislature is clearly accountable not just for what is funded in the health care budget, but for what is not funded. Accountability is inescapable.   *Speech*

Wendell Berry; 2000   **1734**
Such nominally altruistic sciences as medicine and plant-breeding have now become so deeply interpenetrated with economics and politics that their motives are at best mixed with, and at worst replaced by, the motives of corporations and governments.... One can only assume that pure science now needs to move fast (and beg hard) to keep its skirts from being lifted by the ever randy and handy corporate giants.   *Life is a Miracle*

MEDICAL EDUCATION

Hippocrates; [460-375 BC]   **1735**
Instruction in medicine is like the culture of the productions of the earth. For our natural disposition is, as it were, the soil; the tenets of our teacher are, as it were, the seed; instruction in youth is like the planting of the seed in the ground at the proper season; the place where the instruction is communicated is like the food imparted to vegetables by the atmosphere; diligent study is like the cultivation of the fields; and it is time which imparts strength to all things and brings them to maturity.   *The Law*

Galen; [130-200]   **1736**
Even a trained student should attend to every detail, if he wishes to master with assurance and speed each aspect of his profession which he has already learned by the general method.   *On the Affected Parts*

Isidore of Seville; [570-636]   **1737**
The physician ought to know literature...to be able to understand or to explain what he reads. Likewise also rhetoric, that he may delineate in true arguments the things which he discusses; dialectic also so that he may study the causes and cures of infirmities in the light of reason.   *Sharpe WD, Transactions of the American Philosophical Society*

John Ward; *circa* 1660   **1738**
Physick, says Sydenham, is not to be learned by going to universities, but he is for taking apprentices; and says one had as good send a man to Oxford to learn shoemaking as practicing physick.   *Dewhurst K, Dr. Thomas Sydenham*

Thomas Sydenham; 1669   **1739**
This is all very fine, but it won't do—anatomy, botany. Nonsense, Sir! I know an old woman in Covent Garden who understands botany better, and as for anatomy, my butcher can dissect a joint full as well. No, young man, all this is stuff: you must go to the bedside, it is there alone you can learn disease.   *De Arte Medica*

Thomas Sydenham; [1624-1689]   **1740**
The art of medicine was to be properly learned only from its practice and its exercise.
Works

John Morgan; 1765   **1741**
It will not be improper however to observe here, that young men ought to come well prepared for the study of Medicine; by having their minds enriched with all the aids they can
receive from the languages, and the liberal arts.
A Discourse upon the Institution of Medical Schools in America

Philippe Pinel; 1793   **1742**
The true method to teach medicine is the one appropriate to all the natural sciences:
focus the student's attention on concrete situations, impart high standards of accuracy
for their perceptions and observations, warn them against hasty judgments and fanciful
reasoning; choose readings that confirm their taste for rigor—in a word train their judgment rather than their memory and inspire them with that noble enthusiasm for the healing art that masters all difficulties.   *The Clinical Training of Doctors*

Philippe Pinel; 1793   **1743**
The healing art should be taught only in hospitals: this assertion needs no proof. Only in
the hospital can one follow the evolution and progress of several illnesses at the same time
and study variations of the same disease in a number of patients. This is the only way to
understand the true history of diseases.   *The Clinical Training of Doctors*

John Rollo; 1801   **1744**
[Life is too short for a conscientious physician] to acquire—even with the most suitable
education, unremitting observation, accurate investigation, and unwearied reading—...
satisfactory confidence in the unreserved treatment of the sick committed to his charge.
A Short Account of the Royal Artillery Hospita at Woolwich

Johann Wolfgang von Goethe; [1749-1832]   **1745**
Everything...in our sciences has become too multilayered.... The number of real innovations is small, particularly if one considers them in their context over a period of some
centuries. Most of what is now being pursued is only a repetition of what this or that
famous predecessor has said. One can hardly speak of independent knowledge. The young
people are being herded in flocks into rooms and lecture rooms and one feeds
them...words. Concepts and perceptions frequently lacking in the teacher himself, the
students may afterwards acquire themselves.   *Nager F, Der Heilkundige Dichter*

Peter Mere Latham; 1864   **1746**
Have a very great care, then, of your medical student, and how you guide him at starting.
Now especially is the time for good advice, if you have any to give. Take him now into the
wards of the hospital at once; fit or unfit, as people reckon fitness, thither take him.... As
soon as you have become his masters, thither take him, and there let him remain and
make it for the present his sole field of observation and thought, or curiosity.
A Word or Two on Medical Education

John Stuart Mill; 1867   **1747**
Men are men before they are lawyers, or physicians...and if you make them capable and sensible men, they will make themselves sensible lawyers or physicians.   *Inaugural address*

Thomas Clifford Allbutt; 1870   **1748**
The student of medicine must now educate himself in the methods of the exact sciences,
of optics, hydraulics, electricity, heat, of chemistry also, and of experimental physiology,
so that he brings to the mystery of life that habit of mind which will lead him...to regard
it as an "orderly mystery," and that method which will require him to weigh, measure, and
co-ordinate its phenomena, which method alone can produce results of lasting value.
British and Foreign Medico-Chirurgical Review

George Murray Humphry; 1879   **1749**
The knowledge of the facts of anatomy [is] essential to the practice of surgery, and to an appreciation of physiology; and the correct learning of them promotes the habit of attention, and of accuracy which is the associate of attention. Still it may be questioned whether...the result is proportionate to the time and labour expended.... Certainly there is no subject which men exhibit so much proneness to forget.... The knowledge, painfully acquired, is strainingly held and cheerfully let go.   *British Medical Journal*

Thomas Henry Huxley; 1881   **1750**
How is medical education to be arranged so that, without entangling the student in those details of the systematist which are valueless to him, he may be enabled to obtain a firm grasp of the great truths respecting animal and vegetable life, without which, notwithstanding all the progress of scientific medicine, he will still find himself an empiric?
                                                                      Science and Culture

George Frank Lydston; 1893   **1751**
My personal opinion is that no man is competent to pass an instrument upon a patient until he has practiced the maneuver upon himself a few times.   *Stricture of the Urethra*

Jacob M. Da Costa; 1893   **1752**
I have often asked myself why it is that medical education is so discussed by the profession, why this never-ceasing upheaval. We do not see the education in law, we do not see the education in theology, a matter of constant dispute and agitation. And I have concluded that the keen interest, the deep feeling, which it engenders is really due to the state of medicine itself. The agitation is but a sign of the unrest in medicine we see everywhere.   *Address to the Harvard Medical Alumni Association*

Arthur Conan Doyle; 1894   **1753**
The moral training to keep a confidence inviolate, to act promptly on a sudden call, to keep your head in critical moments, to be kind and yet strong—where can you, outside medicine, get such training as that?   *Round the Red Lamp. The Romance of Medicine*

Arthur Conan Doyle; 1894   **1754**
The healthy scepticism which medical training induces, the desire to prove every fact, and only reason from such proved facts—these are the finest foundation for all thought.
                                          Round the Red Lamp. The Romance of Medicine

William Osler; 1899   **1755**
Perfect happiness for student and teacher will come with the abolition of examinations, which are stumbling blocks and rocks of offence in the pathway of the true student.
                                                                      After Twenty-five Years

Denslow Lewis; 1900   **1756**
It is but justice for me to pay this tribute [to my teacher] and yet, when I graduated, I had never seen a pregnant woman. I knew about Baudelocque, Naegele and Simpson. I had learned the Prague method, Deventer's method and Kristeller's method, but I had never seen a woman in labor.   *Obstetric Clinic*

Francis R. Packard; 1900   **1757**
The first man to receive a medical diploma in North America was Daniel Turner, who was awarded an honorary degree of Doctor of Medicine in 1720 from Yale College. Turner had given much money to the College.... Those of humorous turn of mind are said to have interpreted M.D. as signifying Multum Donavit.
                          Transactions and Studies of the College of Physicians of Philadelphia

William Osler; 1903   **1758**
The training of the medical school gives a man his direction, points him the way, and furnishes him with a chart, fairly incomplete, for the voyage, but nothing more.   *Aphorisms*

William Osler; 1903   **1759**

The student begins with the patient, continues with the patient, and ends his studies with the patient, using books and lectures as tools, as means to an end.

The Hospital as a College

William Osler; 1903   **1760**

The best teaching is that taught by the patient himself.   *Medical News*

Thomas Clifford Allbutt; 1906   **1761**

No teacher reaches his best till middle life. Not till then does he gather the fruits of experience, or attain to a rich and vital sense of our ignorance; not till then does he wholly escape from formulae and routine; not till then does he learn what to leave unsaid; then it is that erudition and experience mellow into wisdom.   *On Professional Education*

Abraham Flexner; 1910   **1762**

It follows that in other respects, too, the clinical professors will be on the common university basis: salaried, as other professors are. Of course, their salaries will be inadequate, i.e., less than they can earn outside—all academic salaries paid to the right men are. But there is no inherent reason why a professor of medicine should not make something of the financial sacrifice that the professor of physics makes; both give up something—less and less, let us hope, as time goes on—in order to teach and to investigate.

Medical Education in the United States and Canada

Abraham Flexner; 1910   **1763**

The development...suggested for medical education is conditioned largely upon three factors: first, upon the creation of a public opinion which shall discriminate between the ill trained and the rightly trained physician, and which will also insist upon the enactment of such laws as will require all practitioners...to ground themselves in the fundamentals upon which medical science rests; secondly, upon the universities and their attitude towards medical standards and medical support; finally, upon the attitude of the...medical profession towards the standards of their own practice and upon their sense of honor with respect to their own profession.   *Medical Education in the United States and Canada*

Abraham Flexner; 1910   **1764**

The country needs fewer and better doctors; and...the way to get them better is to produce fewer.   *Medical Education in the United States and Canada*

Abraham Flexner; 1910   **1765**

Teachers of modern medicine, clinical as well as scientific, must, then, be men of active, progressive temper, with definite ideals, exacting habits in thought and work, and with still some margin for growth.   *Medical Education in the United States and Canada*

Abraham Flexner; 1910   **1766**

Low standards give the medical schools access to a large clientele open to successful exploitation by commercial methods. The crude boy or the jaded clerk who goes into medicine at this level has not been moved by a significant prompting from within; nor has he as a rule shown any forethought in the matter of making himself ready.

Medical Education in the United States and Canada

Abraham Flexner; 1910   **1767**

In methods of instruction there is...nothing to distinguish medical from other sciences. Out-and-out didactic treatment is hopelessly antequated; it belongs to an age of accepted dogma or supposedly complete information, when the professor "knew" and the students "learned." The lecture indeed continues of limited use. It may be employed in beginning a subject to orient the student, to indicate relations, to forecast a line of study in its practical bearings; from time to time, too, a lecture may profitably sum up, interpret, and relate results experimentally ascertained.

Medical Education in the United States and Canada

Abraham Flexner; 1910   **1768**

Clinical teaching...was first didactic: the student was told what he would find and what he should do when he found it. It was next demonstrative: things were pointed out in the amphitheater or the wards.... Latterly it has become scientific: the student brings his own faculties into play at close range—gathering his own data, making his own construction, proposing his own course, and taking the consequences when the instructor who has worked through exactly the same process calls him to account.

Medical Education in the United States and Canada

Abraham Flexner; 1910   **1769**

Anatomy and physiology are ultimately biological sciences. Do the professional purposes of the medical school modify the strict biological point of view? Should their teaching...be affected by the fact that these subjects are parts of a medical curriculum? Or ought they be presented exactly as they would be presented to students of biology not intending to be physicians?   *Medical Education in the United States and Canada*

Abraham Flexner; 1910   **1770**

A hospital under complete educational control is as necessary to a medical school as is a laboratory of chemistry or pathology. High grade teaching within a hospital introduces a most wholesome and beneficial influence into its routine. Trustees of hospitals, public and private, should therefore go to the limit of their authority in opening hospital wards to teaching, provided only that the universities secure sufficient funds on their side to employ as teachers men who are devoted to clinical science.

Medical Education in the United States and Canada

Abraham Flexner; 1910   **1771**

It will never happen that every professor in either the medical school or the university faculty is a genuinely productive scientist. There is room for men of another type—the non-productive, assimilative teacher of wide learning, continuous receptivity, critical sense, and responsive interest. Not infrequently these men, Catholic in their sympathies, scholarly in spirit and method, prove the purveyors and distributors through whom new ideas are harmonized and made current. They preserve balance and make connections.

Medical Education in the United States and Canada

Abraham Flexner; 1910   **1772**

Over-production of ill trained men is due in the main to the existence of a very large number of commercial schools, sustained in many cases by advertising methods through which a mass of unprepared youth is drawn out of industrial occupations into the study of medicine.   *Medical Education in the United States and Canada*

Albert V. Harmon; 1911   **1773**

While theoretically the better class of medical colleges were founded solely for the advancement of science, it is none the less true that self-aggrandizement has been the pedestal on which most of our disinterested giants in the teaching arena have stood and are standing.   *Large Fees and How to Get Them*

William Osler; 1911   **1774**

No bubble is so iridescent or floats longer than that blown by the successful teacher.

Cushing H, The Life of Sir William Osler

John Benjamin Murphy; 1913   **1775**

In our plan of teaching...the purpose is to get the student *to think*, and to think not only when he is in his seat but also when he is on his feet, which is a much more difficult proposition. When I press him for words and for answers, remember it is always impersonal.... We know he will not answer as well at that time as he is capable of answering on the benches. We ask him questions for the purpose of fixing the attention of the others who are in the seats.   *The Surgical Clinics*

James Mackenzie; 1919   **1776**
One special function of a consultant is to foretell, what is going to happen to a patient if treated, or if left untreated. To obtain this knowledge it is necessary to see patients through the various stages of disease, and this can only be done by the individual who has the opportunity.   *Willius FA and Dry TJ, A History of the Heart and the Circulation*

Abraham Flexner; 1925   **1777**
Medical education is a technical or professional discipline; it calls for the possession of certain portions of many sciences arranged and organized with a distinct practical purpose in view. That is what makes it a "profession." The point of view is not that of any one of the sciences as such.   *Medical Education: A Comparative Study*

Abraham Flexner; 1925   **1778**
The student is to collect and evaluate facts. The facts are locked up in the patient. To the patient, therefore, he must go. Waiving the personal factor, always important, that method of clinical teaching will be excellent which brings the student into close and active relation with the patient: close, by removing all hindrance to immediate investigation; active, in the sense, not merely of offering opportunities, but of imposing responsibilities.   *Medical Education: A Comparative Study*

William J. Mayo; 1933   **1779**
One of the chief defects in our plan of education in this country is that we give too much attention to developing the memory and too little to developing the mind; we lay too much stress on acquiring knowledge and too little on the wide application of knowledge.   *Collected Papers of the Mayo Clinic and Mayo Foundation*

Foster Kennedy; 1939   **1780**
Much of the present school curriculum is no more than a vestigial remnant of the past. One is asked to learn to breathe intellectually through gill slits handed to one on a Renaissance platter by a medieval ecclesiastic.   *A Critique of Trends in Medical Education*

Foster Kennedy; 1939   **1781**
My observations on tendencies in the present medical educational system are prompted by my feelings of distress at the advanced age, the wrinkled brows and the sere-and-withered-leaf appearance of those completing their medical undergraduate careers, and at the infantilism imposed through their prolonged sojourn in the nurseries of the profession.   *A Critique of Trends in Medical Education*

Michel Foucault; 1963   **1782**
Since disease can be cured only if others intervene with their knowledge, their resources, their pity, since a patient can be cured only in society, it is just that the illnesses of some should be transformed into the experience of others; and that pain should be enabled to manifest itself.   *Rothman DJ et al., Medicine and Western Civilization*

[Anonymous]; 1965   **1783**
The preclinicians have almost always had the idea that the clinicians are robber barons; now they feel that anyone really interested in clinical work bears watching, that he is an anachronism.   *Kendall PL, The Relationship Between Medical Educators and Medical Practitioners*

Eugene A. Stead Jr.; 1968   **1784**
Learning is an active process and each of us learns more when we teach than when we are taught.   *Annals of Internal Medicine*

W. Bryan Jennett; 1969   **1785**
The encounter between senior clinician and patient is part of the educational experience.... Students should see the clinician himself recognizing and acting on the various diagnostic clues which the patient offers...and see the experienced clinician deal with difficult situa-

tions: the patient who asks whether he has cancer, whether he really needs an operation or whether he should change his job. *Proceedings of the Royal Society of Medicine*

Mark D. Altschule; 1970   **1786**
Medicine can be learned, but it cannot really be taught. *Medical Counterpoint*

[Anonymous]; 1971   **1787**
No books, no tapes, no audio-visual aids, no seminars, no avant-garde philosophy will ever be substitutes for the discipline of the bedside medicine—the one-to-one situation where tradition, humanity, art and science are blended. *Medical Journal of Australia*

Edmund D. Pellegrino; 1971   **1788**
How much basic science information do capable clinicians actually use in making prudent decisions? Is the assumption correct that the basic and laboratory sciences impart the qualities of clear and critical thinking? Is it appropriate to think of intensive training in the biochemical sciences for some physicians, the social sciences for others, and management and information science for still others? *Journal of Medical Education*

Eugene A. Stead Jr.; 1973   **1789**
The basic science faculties in the medical schools are not interested in admitting students who will do family practice. They are interested in students who will do well in their courses. The entire intake into medicine is thus controlled by persons who will never practice medicine. These admissions policies produce excellent specialists and bioscientists. They do not produce many doctors who want to give primary medical care. *Family Practice*

George E. Miller; 1978   **1790**
We say we want sensitive, thoughtful, analytical independent scholars, then treat them like Belgian geese being stuffed for pâte de fois gras. We reward them for compliance, rather than independence, for giving the answers we taught them rather than for challenging the conclusions we have reached; for admiring the brilliance of purely scientific advances rather than developing greater sensitivity to the inequities in health care we have too long ignored.... We have our medical students in jail in order that they shall learn to become free men. *Medical Education*

Lewis Thomas; 1979   **1791**
The influence of the modern medical school on liberal arts education in this country over the last decade has been baleful and malign, nothing less. The admission policies of the medical schools are at the root of the trouble. *The Medusa and the Snail*

Franz J. Ingelfinger; 1980   **1792**
One might suggest, of course, that only those who have been hospitalized during their adolescent or adult years be admitted to medical school. Such a practice would not only increase the number of empathic doctors; it would also permit the whole elaborate system of medical-school admissions to be jettisoned. *New England Journal of Medicine*

Eric J. Cassell; 1984   **1793**
Almost no department ever voluntarily surrenders curriculum time—spouses and all earthly possessions may be relinquished, but curricular time, never.
The Place of the Humanities in Medicine

Peter Richards; 1985   **1794**
Few would accept personal experience of illness as the sole qualification for entry to medical school but as a supplementary qualification it has much to recommend it.
Learning Medicine

Clarence J. Berne; 1987   **1795**
The most important function of a medical school is to make the student a self-educator.
Manning PR and DeBakey L, Medicine: Preserving the Passion

Robert G. Petersdorf; 1987   **1796**

Pre-clinical curricula are stuffed with too many courses, too many lectures, and too many faculty hobby horses that leave students at the end of two years exhausted, disgruntled, and, what is worse, cynical about the educational process.   *Medical Education*

Norman Cousins; 1989   **1797**

It is a serious error to suppose that either admissions policy or curriculum policy are fashioned entirely outside the arena of public consensus and consent. If medical school officials are encouraged by the public to search actively for the young men and women who are capable of bringing a certain artistry to the science of medicine, then the stage may be set for wide reforms and great benefits.   *Head First*

Howard Spiro; 1992   **1798**

During medical education, we first teach the students science, and then we teach them detachment. To these barriers to human understanding, they later add the armor of pride and the fortress of a desk between themselves and their patients.... College students start out with much empathy and genuine love.... In medical school, however, they learn to mask their feelings, or worse, to deny them...to focus not on patients, but on diseases.
Annals of Internal Medicine

Thomas Clark Chalmers; 1993   **1799**

I don't think anybody in his right mind thinks for one minute that you can learn how patients should be treated by observing how doctors are treating them.
Annals of the New York Academy of Science

James A. Knight; 1995   **1800**

The inner and outer pressures to be competent are so great, that...students may convert themselves into knowledge machines, robots, and encyclopedias and neglect other essential qualities.... They can risk losing their capacity for compassion.... Competence and compassion should develop hand in hand, and there is no sound reason for one to be accomplished to the neglect of the other.   *Theoretical Medicine*

Norman Gevitz; 1995   **1801**

Medical education needs to be broadly conceived, with an appreciation of the person who will go through our educational system and enter practice. We need to consider the intellectual breadths as well as the scientific depth of our physicians-in-training. We need to encourage students to think reflexively about the meaning of the medical enterprise.
University of Chicago Department of Medical Education Bulletin

Lofty L. Basta; 1996   **1802**

Medical students and the medical community at large must be better educated in how to discuss issues of life and death. They must be trained in communicating with patients and families under the dire circumstances of an imminent death.   *A Graceful Exit*

Paul Rodenhauser; 1996   **1803**

Medical education requires and reinforces compulsive behavior. Not only do medical schools select from an applicant pool of mostly orderly, competitive, perfectionistic overachievers, the process of medical education only intensifies these characteristics. The need to memorize massive amounts of information, to learn to succeed on multiple-choice examinations, to master methods and procedures with precision—without error—understandably requires and reinforces perfectionistic behavior.   *The Pharos*

Jerome Lowenstein; 1997   **1804**

I have come to believe that the time and place to teach compassion are the time and place in which all of the rest of medicine is taught.   *The Midnight Meal and Other Essays*

Roy Porter; 1997   **1805**

I am well aware that in these days, when a student must be converted into a physiologist, a physicist, a chemist, a biologist, a pharmacologist, and an electrician, there is no time to make a physician of him. This consummation can only come after he has gone out into the world of sickness and suffering, unless indeed his mind is so bemused by the long process of education in those sciences, that he is forever excluded from the art of medicine...and is destined for the laboratory, the professor's chair, or the consultant's office.

The Greatest Benefit to Mankind

Daniel F. Duffy; 1998   1806

Although taking a medical history, performing a physical examination, and carrying out procedures are considered "learnable" skills, expressing empathy and listening to patients and their families are thought of as "personality traits." This suggests that...the latter are enduring characteristics not influenced by education.... [There is] growing evidence to the contrary; that...these "traits" can be changed through education.

Annals of Internal Medicine

Sherwin B. Nuland; 1999   1807

All the vastness and chaotic intellectual ferment of the modern academic medical center have grown out of attempts to teach individual students how to care for the sick. Yet more often than not, the pedagogical mission of our schools has been lost in the thicket of the undertakings that now consume the faculty and staff.

American Scholar

MEDICAL EPISTEMOLOGY

Jean-Martin Charcot; 1892   1808

Theory is good, but it doesn't prevent things from existing.   *Tuesday's Lessons*

MEDICAL ERROR

Washington Lemuel Atlee; 1873   1809

Mistakes teach most valuable lessons, and, when discovered, are not likely to be repeated. Hence, in medicine, they should be recorded for the benefit both of science and of humanity.   *General and Differential Diagnosis of Ovarian Tumors*

William Osler; 1905   1810

Pirogoff's comment...has always appealed to me very strongly: "There are in everyone's practice moments in which his vision is holden so that even an experienced man cannot see what is nevertheless perfectly clear. At least, I have noticed this in my own case. An overweening self-confidence, a preconceived opinion, vanity, and weariness are the causes of these astounding mistakes."   *The Lancet*

Norman Cousins; 1989   1811

Medical science has made enormous progress. Even so, it is constantly coping with error—not only of theory but of practice. But mistakes have a way of concealing themselves or, indeed, of becoming institutionalized.   *Head First*

MEDICAL ETHICS

Hippocrates; [460-375 BC]   1812

I will keep this Oath and this stipulation—To reckon him who taught me this Art equally dear to me as my parents...and to teach...this art...without fee or stipulation.... Into whatever houses I enter, I will go into them for the benefit of the sick, and will abstain from every voluntary act of mischief and corruption...from the seduction of females or males, of freemen and slaves. Whatever, in connexion with my professional practice, or not in connexion with it, I see or hear, in the life of men... I will not divulge.

The Hippocratic Oath

Charaka; *circa* 250 BC   1813

Day and night, however thou mayest be engaged, thou shalt endeavour for the relief of patients with all thy heart and soul. Thou shalt not desert or injure thy patient even for the sake of thy life or thy living.... Thy behaviour must be in consideration of time and place and heedful of past experience. Thou shalt act always with a view to the acquisition of knowledge.... There is no limit at all to the Science of Life, Medicine. So thou shouldst apply thyself to it with diligence. *Medical Student Oath*

Charaka; *circa* 50   **1814**
Not for the self, not for the fulfillment of any worldly desire or gain, but solely for the good of suffering humanity, I will treat my patients and excel all. *Medical Student Oath*

Chen Shih-kung; 1618   **1815**
Physicians should be ever ready to respond to any calls of patients, high or low, rich or poor. They should treat them equally and care not for financial reward.... A physician or surgeon must first know the principles of the learned. He must study all the... standard medical books... day and night and understand them thoroughly.... A physician should not be arrogant and insult other physicians.... Medicine should be given free to the poor.... The physician should improve his knowledge by studying medical books... and reading current publications. *An Orthodox Manual of Surgery*

Francis Bacon; [1561-1626]   **1816**
I hold every man a debtor to his profession; from which as men of course do seek to receive countenance and profit, so ought they of duty to endeavour themselves, by way of amends, to be a help and ornament thereunto. This is performed, in some degree, by the honest and liberal practice of a profession; where men shall carry a respect not to descend into any course that is corrupt and unworthy thereof, and preserve themselves free from the abuses wherewith the same profession is noted to be infected. *Maxims of the Law, Preface*

Asaf Judaeus; *circa* 1650   **1817**
Do not administer to an adulterous wife an abortifacient drug. Let not the beauty of woman arouse in thee the passion of adultery. Do not divulge any secret entrusted to thee and do no act of injury or harm for any price. Do not close thy heart to mercy toward the poor and the needy. *Friedenwald H, The Jews and Medicine*

Nicholas Culpeper; *circa* 1660   **1818**
I did by all persons as I would they should do by me. I was always just in my practice; I never gave my patient two medicines when one would serve the turn.
Chance B, Annals of Medical History

Benjamin Rush; 1782   **1819**
Avoid intimacies with your patients if possible, and visit them only in sickness.
Letter to Dr. William Claypoole

Johann Peter Frank; 1790   **1820**
[The professor] will teach everybody the necessity of keeping an inviolable silence on all the depositions of their patients and he will invite the greatest discretion toward those who must confide in them their defects both physical and moral. *Plan d'Ecole Clinique*

Benjamin Rush; 1801   **1821**
The most important contract that can be made, is that which takes place between a sick man and his doctor. The subject of it is human life. The breach of this contract, by willful negligence, when followed by death, is murder; and it is because our penal laws are imperfect, that the punishment of that crime is not inflicted upon physicians who are guilty of it. *The Vices and Virtues of Physicians*

Thomas Percival; 1803   **1822**
Whenever cases occur, attended with circumstances not heretofore observed, or in which the ordinary modes of practice have been attempted without success, it is for the public good, and in an especial degree advantageous to the poor...that new remedies and new methods of chirurgical treatment should be devised. But...the faculty should be scrupulously and conscientiously governed by sound reason, just analogy, or well authenticated

facts. And no such trials should be instituted, without a previous consultation of the physicians or surgeons. *Medical Ethics*

Thomas Percival; 1803 **1823**
It is the characteristic of a wise man to act on determinate principles.... The relations in which a physician stands to his patients, to his brethren, and to the public, are complicated, and multifarious; involving much knowledge of human nature, and extensive moral duties. The study of professional Ethics, therefore, cannot fail to invigorate and enlarge your understanding. *Medical Ethics*

James Jackson; 1855 **1824**
We do not resemble each other in temperament, and cannot see all things alike. From this cause, and not always looking at objects from the same point of view, we often differed in opinion. But we have always agreed to differ. We have not often disputed, and never have quarrelled on account of this difference of opinion, nor on any other account. In our intercourse with the sick, each has given the other credit for what was good in him, instead of studying and publishing the other's faults.
Letters to a Young Physician Just Entering upon Practice. Dedication

John Hughes Bennett; 1858 **1825**
The first piece of advice [is] always to cherish a feeling of deep responsibility.... [Let] me... impress upon you the importance of practising the art and cultivating the science of medicine, in a spirit of sincerity and of truth.... You ought to be strongly imbued with a sense of duty and of moral obligation. *Clinical Lectures on the Principles and Practice of Medicine*

John Ruskin; 1862 **1826**
What ever [the physician's] science, we should shrink from him in horror if we found him regard his patients as subjects to experiment upon. *Unto This Last*

Claude Bernard; 1865 **1827**
Experiments...may be performed on man, but within what limits? It is our duty and our right to perform an experiment on man whenever it can save his life, cure him or gain him some personal benefit. The principle of medical and surgical morality, therefore, consists in never performing on man an experiment which might be harmful to him to any extent, even though the result might be highly advantageous to science, i.e., to the health of others.
An Introduction to the Study of Experimental Medicine

William Stokes; [1804-1878] **1828**
Never originate discussion on medical topics in conversation. As regards conduct toward the profession, consider first the patient, second your professional brother, lastly yourself. Be reticent, lest by a casual word upon the previous treatment of the case, you inflict a stab in the dark on your brother's reputation. *William Stokes: His Life and Work*

Elizabeth Blackwell; 1889 **1829**
The arbitrary distinction between the physician of the body and the physician of the soul—doctor and priest—tends to disappear as science advances. Every branch of medicine involves moral considerations, both as regards the practitioner and the patient. Even the amputation of a limb, the care of a case of fever, the birth of a child, all contain a moral element which is evident to the clear understanding, and which cannot be neglected without injury to the doctor, to the individual, and to society.
The Influence of Women in the Profession of Medicine

George Bernard Shaw; 1911 **1830**
Nobody supposes that doctors are less virtuous than judges; but a judge whose salary and reputation depended on whether the verdict was for plaintiff or defendant, prosecutor or

prisoner, would be as little trusted as a general in the pay of the enemy.... It is simply unscientific to allege or believe that doctors do not under existing circumstances perform unnecessary operations and manufacture and prolong lucrative illnesses.

The Doctor's Dilemma, Preface

William Osler; [1849-1919]   **1831**
Do not judge your confreres by the reports of patients, well meaning, perhaps, but often strangely and sadly misrepresenting.   *Aphorisms*

William Osler; [1849-1919]   **1832**
Never let your tongue say a slighting word of a colleague.   *Aphorisms*

Bertrand Russell; 1925   **1833**
What distinguishes ethics from science is not any special kind of knowledge but merely desire. The knowledge required in ethics is exactly like the knowledge elsewhere; what is peculiar is that certain ends are desired, and that right conduct is what conduces to them.

What I Believe

World Medical Association; 1949   **1834**
I solemnly pledge myself to consecrate my life to the service of humanity.... I will practice my profession with conscience and dignity; The health of my patient will be my first consideration; I will respect the secrets which are confided in me.... I will maintain the utmost respect for human life, from the time of conception.   *Declaration of Geneva*

Henry Louis Mencken; 1956   **1835**
One of the chief objects of medicine is to save us from the natural consequences of our vices and follies. The moment it becomes moral it becomes quackery. A scientific physician should have no opinion about the ethical standards and deserts of his patient.

Minority Report: H. L. Mencken's Notebooks

Austin Bradford Hill; 1963   **1836**
The ethical obligation always and entirely outweighs the experimental.

British Medical Journal

World Medical Association; 1964   **1837**
It is the mission of the physician to safeguard the health of the people. His or her knowledge and conscience are dedicated to the fulfillment of this mission.... Medical progress is based on research which ultimately must rest in part on experimentation involving human subjects.... The physician can combine medical research with professional care...only to the extent that medical research is justified by its potential diagnostic or therapeutic value for the patient.... In research on man, the interest of science and society should never take precedence over considerations related to the well-being of the subject.   *Journal of the American Medical Association*

Jean Hamburger; 1966   **1838**
The ethical training of a doctor cannot be limited...to the teaching of a few ready-made rules; it should also encourage a lucid inner understanding of the relationship between doctor and patient, of the dignity of the latter, and of the extent of the services which the former can offer. In this way will be developed, more surely than by a code, the deep sense of personal responsibility essential for every doctor.

Wolstenholme GEW and O'Connor M, Ethics in Medical Progress

J. Russell Elkinton; 1968   **1839**
We do not want to apply a double ethical standard: one for the unconscious patient with a head injury who is not being considered as a possible donor of an organ and another for the same kind of patient who is.   *Annals of Internal Medicine*

René Jules Dubos; 1968   **1840**
The welfare of the individual patient is often incompatible with the general interest.

Since deciding between what is right and what is wrong involves value judgements, the relation of medical ethics to the public weal is by necessity ill-defined. Most medical situations are socially and ethically complex, and for this reason it is desirable that judges of professional conduct be persons experienced both in the law and in the art of medicine.

Man, Medicine, and Environment

Paul Ramsey; 1970   **1841**

A man of serious conscience means to say in raising urgent ethical questions that there may be some things that men should never do. The good things that men do can be made complete only by the things they refuse to do. *Fabricated Man*

John Noble Wilford; 1972   **1842**

Custom prevents the medicine man from amassing great wealth. If he does, he may be accused of causing illness to collect fees, which could lead to his ostracism.

The New York Times

David P. Byar; 1976   **1843**

A physician treating a patient in a manner that he does not believe is best for that patient is unethical.... This definition leads to a paradoxical situation in which a poorly informed physician who treats his patient in a way he believes is in the patient's best interest, despite the fact that it may cause great harm to the patient, is ethically equivalent to a well-informed...physician who might treat the patient quite differently.... It is not enough that one do what one believes is best; one must do what is in accord with sound medical evidence. *New England Journal of Medicine*

Willem Johan Kolff; 1984   **1844**

If a patient needs help to save his life, you give that help and don't ask whether or not he is a National Socialist or anything else. In regard to the selection of patients for the dialysis program, they originally set up these life-and-death committees, which I always fought tooth and nail and will continue to fight. *Weisse AB, Conversations in Medicine*

Frederick Lowy; 1988   **1845**

Protecting our ethical heritage is not an abstract, pious counsel of perfection. It is the key to our profession's survival. *Canadian Medical Association Journal*

Ralph Crawshaw, David E. Rogers, Edward D. Pellegrino, and others; 1995   **1846**

Medicine is, at its center, a moral enterprise grounded in a covenant of trust. This covenant obliges physicians to be competent and to use their competence in the patient's best interests. Physicians, therefore, are both intellectually and morally obliged to act as advocate for the sick whenever their welfare is threatened and for their health at all times.

Journal of the American Medical Association

Raymond Tallis; 1998   **1847**

The gap between the discourses of professional ethicists...and the decision-making processes in the real mess of the real world of everday medical practice probably explains why few doctors I know actually read books on medical ethics. Even fewer consult such books to resolve specific ethical dilemmas.... Clinical medicine will never be an exact science like bridge building, though it will advance by tightening the meshes within which legitimate practice is defined. *Times Literary Supplement*

Jacques Jouanna; 1999   **1848**

The roots of modern medical ethics, embodied in law, are to be found on the [Hippocratic] Oath, whether it is a matter of technical secrets or of respect for human life. The absolute prohibitions of the Hippocratic code are qualified by contemporary law only in the case of abortion, which is now permitted under certain conditions.

Hippocrates

M. Gregg Bloche; 1999   **1849**

Understandings of the duties implied by clinical fidelity [to the patient] are bound to differ and to change over time. But at the core lies faithfulness to persons, not adherence to disembodied principles. Assessment of the social costs and benefits of breaches of fidelity should be done from a perspective sympathetic to the experiences of trust and betrayal.

Journal of the American Medical Association

MEDICAL EVIDENCE

James Lind; 1753   1850

As it is no easy matter to root our prejudices,...it became...requisite...to exhibit a full and impartial view of what had hitherto been published on the scurvy, and that in a chronological order, by which the sources of these mistakes may be detected. Indeed, before this subject could be set in a clear and proper light, it was necessary to remove a great deal of rubbish.

A Treatise on the Scurvy

John Gregory; 1772   1851

Every physician must rest on his own judgment, which appeals for its rectitude to nature and experience alone. Among the infinite variety of facts and theories with which his memory has been filled in the course of a liberal education, it is his business to make a judicious separation between those founded in nature and experience, and those which owe their birth to ignorance, fraud, or the capricious systems of a heated and deluded imagination.

Lectures on the Duties and Qualifications of a Physician

Gilbert Blane; 1819   1852

The proper object of this work... is to enumerate and elucidate the various causes which have most materially obstructed the improvement of medicine.... 1) The fallacy and danger of hypothetical or theoretical reasoning. 2) The diversity of constitutions. 3) The difficulty of appreciating the efforts of nature, and of discriminating them from the operations of art. 4) Superstition. 5) The ambiguity of language. 6) The fallacy of testimony [and] excessive deference to authority and fashion.

Elements of Medical Logic

Oliver Wendell Holmes; 1860   1853

A Pseudo-science consists of a *nomenclature*, with a self-adjusting arrangement, by which all positive evidence, or such as favors its doctrines, is admitted, and all negative evidence, or such as tells against it, is excluded. It is invariably connected with some lucrative practical application.

The Professor at the Breakfast Table

Arthur Conan Doyle; 1892   1854

I have no data yet. It is a capital mistake to theorise before one has data. Insensibly one begins to twist facts to suit theories, instead of theories to suit facts.

The Adventures of Sherlock Holmes. A Scandal in Bohemia

Abraham Flexner; 1910   1855

The laity has...more to fear from credulous doctors than from advertisements themselves: for a nostrum containing dangerous drugs is doubly dangerous if introduced into the household by the prescription of a physician who knows nothing of its composition and is misled as to its effect. Experimental physiology and pharmacology must train the student both to doubt unwarranted claims and to be open to really authoritative suggestion.

Medical Education in the United States and Canada

Archibald Leman Cochrane; 1972   1856

The oldest, and probably still the commonest, form of evidence proffered [for the value of a treatment] is clinical opinion.... Its value must be rated low, because there is no quantitative measurement, no attempt to discover what would have happened if the patients had had no treatment, and every possibility of bias affecting the assessment of the result. It could be described as the simplest (and worst) type of observational evidence.

Effectiveness and Efficiency

George V. Mann; 1977   1857

Avoid using therapies where proof of efficacy is lacking—even if the treatment is a hun-

Paul H. Wood; 1950   1880

The best history-taker is he who can best interpret the answer to a leading question.

Diseases of the Heart and Circulation

George White Pickering; 1961   1881

To receive, to record, and to transmit information accurately and succinctly is a skill that is basic to the practice of every branch of medicine. The patient's history at its best and its most useful is a narrative which can and should have form and beauty in the same way as any other literary composition can and should have.   *The Lancet*

Carl Gustav Jung; 1963   1882

In psychiatry, the patient who comes to us has a story that is not told, and which as a rule no one knows of.... Therapy only really begins after the investigation of that wholly personal story. It is the patient's secret, the rock against which he is shattered. If I know his secret story, I have a key to the treatment. The doctor's task is to find out how to gain that knowledge.... The problem is always the whole person, never the symptom alone.

Memories, Dreams, Reflections

Arthur W. Frank; 1965   1883

Survival does not include any particular responsibility other than continuing to survive. Becoming a witness assumes a responsibility for telling what happened. The witness offers testimony to a truth that is generally unrecognized or suppressed. People who tell stories in illness are witnesses, turning illness into moral responsibility.   *The Wounded Story Teller*

Oliver W. Sacks; 1972   1884

There is only one cardinal rule: one must always *listen* to the patient.   *Migraine*

Brian Bird; 1973   1885

Of all the technical aids which increase the doctor's power of observation, none comes even close in value to the skillful use of spoken words—the words of doctor and the words of the patient.   *Talking with Patients*

Walter C. Alvarez; 1976   1886

Blessed is the physician who takes a good history, looks keenly at his patient and thinks a bit.   *Scott DH, American Man of Medicine*

Kathryn Montgomery Hunter; 1991   1887

Anecdotes represent and preserve the recognition of this intractable particularity of the individual in medicine. They are a reminder of the fundamental nature of the object of medicine's study: the workings of an abstraction called disease in the individual human being. As the irreducible knot at the center of medicine as a discipline of human knowledge—the problem of a scientific discipline applied to particular cases—anecdotes are an emblem of the human science of medicine.   *Doctor's Stories*

Howard Spiro; 1992   1888

Physicians need rhetoric as much as knowledge, and they need stories as much as journals if they are to be more empathetic than computers.   *Annals of Internal Medicine*

J. Willis Hurst; 1995   1889

Pretending must never be a part of doctoring. The physician who listens to a patient describe his or her symptoms but hears no clues to the presence of a disease is pretending.

Essays from the Heart

Sydney Walker III; 1996   1890

Most of the details learned in the course of questioning are irrelevant, but the doctor who sifts through them carefully almost always finds a few diagnostics gems.   *A Dose of Sanity*

Sydney Walker III; 1996   1891

Patients are gold mines of information to a doctor who's willing to listen.   *A Dose of Sanity*

Lewis Mehl-Madrona; 1997   **1892**

I wondered what he [a patient] might have told us about his illness and his recovery if we had only listened more and measured less. *Coyote Medicine*

Sherwin B. Nuland; 2001   **1893**

A medical case history... is a story in which the altering of a few apparently small details may have a significant effect on the judgments to be made or the lessons to be drawn. The finest distinctions of fact, or the most intimate characteristics of a patient, may carry clues to the entire point of the story   *The American Scholar*

MEDICAL ILLUSTRATION

William Hunter; 1774   **1894**

The art of engraving supplies us, upon many occasions, with what has been the great desideratum of the lovers of science, a universal language. Nay, it conveys clearer ideas of most natural objects than words can express; makes stronger impressions upon the mind; and to every person conversant with the subject gives an immediate comprehension of what it represents.   *The Anatomy of the Human Gravid Uterus*

MEDICAL JOURNALS

Thomas Wakley; 1823   **1895**

The "Lancet" was devised to disseminate medical information primarily, and incidentally to make war upon the family intrigue and foolish nepotism that swayed the election to lucrative posts in the metropolitan hospitals and medical corporations.

Sprigge SS, The Life and Times of Thomas Walkey

William Williams Keen; 1864   **1896**

Papers vary greatly in their merit and importance, and it would seem to me that to the trustees and the editor of the *Journal [of the American Medical Association]* should be confided the entire responsibility of selecting the more important papers for publication in full, and of presenting the less important in longer or shorter abstracts. The example of the *British Medical Journal* may well guide us in this matter.

Journal of the American Medical Association

John Hamilcar Hollister; 1889   **1897**

There never was a time when medical journalism was so enterprising as now, nor its pages so filled with valuable instruction, and there never was a time when a physician could so soon fall behind and be lost sight of as now.   *Journal of the American Medical Association*

John Hamilcar Hollister; 1893   **1898**

A man without his medical journals in this age is not far from the end of his professional race.   *North American Practitioner*

Rudolf Ludwig Karl Virchow; [1821-1902]   **1899**

In my journal, anyone can make a fool of himself.   *Minerva*

George Frank Lydston; 1904   **1900**

I cannot believe that my own cases are the only ones in which disappointments and disagreeable results occasionally occur, and I am free to say that in my experience prostatectomy, like all other fields of surgical endeavor, is not always smooth sailing. The tendency to reporting only ideal cases or, what is worse, omitting the disagreeable features of cases and reporting them as ideal, is far more general in the profession than it should be, and can only work injury to surgical science.   *New York Medical Journal*

George Bernard Shaw; 1906   **1901**

I've never opened a book since I was qualified thirty years ago. I used to read the medical papers at first; but you know how soon a man drops that; besides, I can't afford them; and what are they after all but trade papers, full of advertisements?... Bedside experience is the main thing, isn't it? *The Doctor's Dilemma, Act I*

[Anonymous]; 1967 **1902**
Those who can, write. Those who cannot, edit. Those who cannot edit, set editorial policy. *New England Journal of Medicine*

[Anonymous]; 1971 **1903**
As far as journals are concerned, the medical profession can be roughly divided into three main groups: the readers, the scanners and the shirkers. *South African Medical Journal*

Peter Ustinov; 1978 **1904**
I played...the depressing doctor in that superb piece of far-flung Empire kitsch, *White Cargo*.... I had to make an appeal for medical magazines from Blighty so that I might keep up with the latest trends in Vienna, Harley Street, and the Mayo Clinic in spite of the sweat, heat, and filth of tropical existence. A copy of *Lancet* arrived at the stage door, with a letter from the editor, saying that he had been so moved by my appeal that he had dispatched the latest copy forthwith. *Dear Me*

[Anonymous]; 1981 **1905**
The articles in some journals seem to be written by the same writers, using different aliases and apparently working in different hospitals or institutions. The names and titles may be the only non-conventional part of the article. *The Lancet*

Alistair Cooke; 1986 **1906**
I know that most of you have not the time to say in two hundred words what the *Journal of the American Medical Association* manages to say in two thousand.
The Patient Has the Floor

John Maddox; 1991 **1907**
Too much of what passes for the scientific literature is not literature at all but a way of stringing code words together in such a way that the perpetrators can enjoy the warm glow of knowing that a piece of research has been written up and given a prominent place on library shelves throughout the world. *Journal of the Royal College of Physicians*

MEDICAL LICENSURE

N.P. Colwell; 1914 **1908**
The medical profession approves the system which requires the same general professional education of all of its members. The specialist upon the eye and the specialist upon the throat, the physician and the surgeon, must each undergo the same training and must pass the same State examination.... What the State requires for one body of practitioners it should not abate in favor of another. *Medical Education*

MEDICAL MARRIAGES

W.U. McClenahan; 1974 **1909**
It is sad to see a doctor and a nurse drawn together in a flash by one acute, intense interest in medicine, and then discover, too late, that it is the only thing they have in common. Perhaps the hardest thing of all on medical marriages is success, a sweet poison.
G.P.

MEDICAL OPPOSITION

Robert Kuttner; 1998 **1910**
Whereas organized medicine once opposed group health as socialistic, medical societies now resist excessive corporate meddling by non clinicians running HMOs.
New England Journal of Medicine

MEDICAL PRACTICE

Hippocrates; [460-375 BC]   **1911**
The physician takes care, nature heals.   *Reichert HG, Latin Proverbs*

Hippocrates; [460-375 BC]   **1912**
Life is short, and the Art long; the occasion fleeting; experience fallacious, and judgment difficult. The physician must not only be prepared to do what is right himself, but also to make the patient, the attendants, and externals co-operate.   *Aphorisms*

Hippocrates; [460-375 BC]   **1913**
The physician must be able to tell the antecedents, know the present, and foretell the future—must mediate these things, and have two special objects in view with regard to diseases, namely, to do good or to do no harm. The art consists in three things—the disease, the patient, and the physician. The physician is the servant of the art, and the patient must combat the disease along with the physician.   *Of the Epidemics*

Hippocrates; [460-375 BC]   **1914**
Where there is love of man, there is also love of the art.   *Precepts*

Hippocrates; [460-375 BC]   **1915**
The medical man sees terrible sights, touches unpleasant things, and the misfortunes of others bring a harvest of sorrows that are peculiarly his.   *Breaths*

Plato; [427-347 BC]   **1916**
The reason why many diseases are unknown to the Greek physicians is because they are ignorant of the whole, to which attention ought to be paid, for the part can never be well unless the whole is well.   *Dialogues. Charmides*

John Locke; 1693   **1917**
What we know of the Works of Nature, especially in the Constitution of Health, and the Operations of our own Bodies, is only by the sensible Effects, but not by any Certainty we can have of the Tools she uses, or the Way she works by. So there is nothing left for a Physician to do, but to observe well, and so by analogy argue the like Cases, and thence make to himself Rules of Practice.   *Letter to Richard Morton*

Philip Dormer Stanhope, Lord Chesterfield; 1751   **1918**
It seems to me that your doctor [Tronchin] is more of a philosopher than a physician. As for me, I much prefer a doctor who is an optimist and who gives me remedies that will improve my health. Philosophical consolations are, after all, useless against real ailments. I know only two kinds of sickness—physical and moral: all the others are purely in the imagination.   *Letter to Baton De Kruenigen*

William Douglass; 1755   **1919**
Experience and sedulous observation are too much neglected by the indolent practitioners of our colonies; they chuse to practice from authorities, wherease authorities must always give way to experience; the nature of medical affairs allow of no other demonstration than that of good observation.   *The Present State of the British Settlements of North America*

William Small; 1770   **1920**
Physic exhausts my whole faculties and pays but indifferently.
                    Journal of the Royal Society of Medicine

William Small; 1773   **1921**
The Practice of Medicine is worse than a Jail.   *Journal of the Royal Society of Medicine*

Peter Mere Latham; 1836   **1922**
Physiology, pathology, and practice, often part company just where an intelligent looker on would make sure of their becoming sociable and cooperative. The practice of medicine is a perpetual compromise between what we know and what we can do, between our knowledge and our power.   *Aphorisms*

Peter Mere Latham; 1836   **1923**

This body must be your study, and your continual care—your active, willing, earnest care. Nothing must make you shrink from it. In its weakness and infirmities, in the dishonours of its corruption, you must still value it—still stay by it—to mark its hunger and thirst, its sleeping and waking, its heat and its cold; to hear its complaints, to register its groans.

Collected Works

Peter Mere Latham; 1845   **1924**

The practice of physic is jostled by quacks on one side, and by science on the other.

Aphorisms

Ivan Turgenev; 1852   **1925**

Meantime a fellow creature's dying and another doctor would have saved him. "We must have a consultation," you say, "I will not take the responsibility on myself." And what a fool you look at such times! Well, in time you learn to bear it; it's nothing to you. A man has died—but it's not your fault; you treated him by the rules. But what's still more torture to you is to see blind faith in you, and to feel yourself that you are not able to be of use. *A Sportsman's Sketches. The District Doctor*

Jacob Bigelow; 1854   **1926**

He is a great physician who, above other men, understands diagnosis. It is not he who promises to cure all maladies, who has a remedy ready for every symptom...who boasts that success never fails him, when his daily history gives the lie to such assertion. It is rather he who, with just discrimination, looks at a case in all its difficulties; ...who looks at the necessary results of inevitable causes; who promptly does what man may do of good, and carefully avoids what he may do of evil. *Nature in Disease*

John Hughes Bennett; 1858   **1927**

The object of science is to discover facts and determine laws; the object of art is to accomplish an end, and determine the means of effecting it.

Clinical Lectures on the Principles and Practice of Medicine

Richard F. Burton; 1858   **1928**

Here, there is no such royal road to medical fame. You must begin by sitting with the porter, who is sure to have blear eyes, into which you drop a little nitrate of silver, whilst you instill in his ear the pleasing intelligence that you will never take a fee from the poor. He recovers; his report of you spreads far and wide, crowding your doors with paupers.... When the mob has raised you to fame, patients of a better class will slowly appear on the scene.

A Pilgrimage to El-Madinah and Meccah

D.W. Cathell; 1882   **1929**

Though money is not the chief object in the practice of medicine, it ever has been and ever must be one of the objects. *The Physician Himself*

Sarah Orne Jewett; 1884   **1930**

The practical medical men are the juries who settle all the theories of the hour, as they meet emergencies day after day. *A Country Doctor*

Silas Weir Mitchell; 1892   **1931**

We now use as many instruments as a mechanic.

The Early History of Instrumental Precision in Medicine

Denslow Lewis; 1896   **1932**

Too often it is forgotten that the science of medicine finds expression only in the application of the art. *Journal of the American Medical Association*

William Osler; 1901   **1933**

It is astonishing with how little reading a doctor can practise medicine, but it is not astonishing how badly he may do it.   *Books and Men*

[Anonymous]; 1902   **1934**

Life is short, patients fastidious, and the brethren deceptive.

Medical Ethics and Cognate Subjects

William Osler; 1902   **1935**

But there is a still greater sacrifice which many of us make, heedlessly and thoughtlessly forgetting that "Man does not live by bread alone." One cannot practice medicine alone and practice it early and late, as so many of us have to do, and hope to escape the malign influences of a routine life. The incessant concentration of thought upon one subject, however interesting, tethers a man's mind in a narrow field. The practitioner needs culture as well as learning.   *Chauvinism in Medicine*

William Osler; 1903   **1936**

The practice of medicine is an art, not a trade, a calling, not a business, a calling in which your heart will be exercised equally with your head.   *The Master-Word in Medicine*

William Osler; 1903   **1937**

The problems of disease are more complicated and difficult than any others with which the trained mind has to grapple; the conditions in any given case may be unlike those in any other; each case, indeed, may have its own problem.   *Boston Medical and Surgical Journal*

Rudyard Kipling; 1908   **1938**

The world has long ago decided that you have no working hours that anyone is bound to respect, and nothing except extreme bodily illness will excuse you in its eyes from refusing to help a man who thinks he may need your help at any hour of the day or night. Nobody will care whether you are in your bed or in your bath, on your holiday or at the theatre.   *A Book of Words. A Doctor's Work*

George Bernard Shaw; 1911   **1939**

Doctoring is not even the art of keeping people in health (no doctor seems able to advise you what to eat any better than his grandmother or the nearest quack): it is the art of curing illnesses.   *The Doctor's Dilemma, Preface*

William Osler; 1919   **1940**

The art of the practice of medicine is to be learned only by experience; 'tis not an inheritance; it cannot be revealed.   *Thayer LS, Johns Hopkins Hospital Bulletin*

Abraham Flexner; 1925   **1941**

The fact that disease is only in part accurately known does not invalidate the scientific method in practice. In the twilight region probabilities are substituted for certainties. There the physician may indeed only surmise, but, most important of all, he knows that he surmises.... Investigation and practice are thus one in spirit, method, and object.

Medical Education: A Comparative Study

Francis W. Peabody; 1927   **1942**

The application of the principles of science to the diagnosis and treatment of disease is only one limited aspect of medical practice. The practice of medicine...includes the whole relationship of the physician with his patient. It is an art, based to an increasing extent on the medical sciences, but comprising much that still remains outside the realm of any science. The art of medicine and the science of medicine are not antagonistic but supplementary to each other. There is no more contradiction between the science of medicine and the art of medicine than between the science of aeronautics and the art of flying.

Journal of the American Medical Association

Charles Horace Mayo; 1928   **1943**

Medicine is about as big or as little in any community, large or small, as the physicians make it.   *University of Toronto Medical Journal*

George Newman; 1931   **1944**

There are four questions which in some form or other every patient asks of his doctor:
(a) What is the matter with me? This is *diagnosis.*
(b) Can you put me right? This is *treatment* and *prognosis.*
(c) How did I get it? This is *causation.*
(d) How can I avoid it in future? This is *prevention....*
He may not be called upon to attempt a full answer to his patient, but he must give a fair working answer to himself.   *The Lancet*

Robert Hutchison; 1935   **1945**

From inability to let well alone; from too much zeal for what is new and contempt for what is old; from putting knowledge before wisdom, science before art, and cleverness before common sense, from treating patients as cases, and from making the cure of the disease more grievous than the endurance of the same, Good Lord, deliver us!
                                                                    British Medical Journal

Arthur Hall; 1941   **1946**

Medicine...must always remain an "applied science," and one differing from all the rest in that the application is to man himself. Were there no sick persons there would be no need for Medicine, either the Science or the Art.... The application of its Science...must be made in such a way that it will produce the maximum of relief to the sick man. This calls for certain qualities in the practising physician which differ entirely from anything required in the practice of other applied sciences. Herein lies the Art of Medicine.
                                                                    Coope R, The Quiet Art

Wilfred Batten Lewis Trotter; 1941   **1947**

The first [quality] to be named must always be the power of attention, of giving one's whole mind to the patient without the interposition of anything of oneself. It sounds simple but only the very greatest doctors ever fully attain it.... The second thing to be striven for is intuition. This sounds an impossibility, for who can control that small quiet monitor? But intuition is only inference from experience stored and not actively recalled....The last aptitude I shall mention that must be attained by the good physician is that of handling the sick man's mind.   *Collected Papers*

James Spence; 1949   **1948**

The essential unit of medical practice is the occasion when, in the intimacy of the consulting room or sick room, a person who is ill, or believes himself to be ill, seeks the advice of a doctor whom he trusts. This is a consultation and all else in the practice of medicine derives from it.   *The Need for Understanding the Individual*

Robert Hutchison; 1953   **1949**

From inability to let well enough alone; from too much zeal for the new and contempt for what is old; from putting knowledge before wisdom, science before art, and cleverness before common sense, from treating patients as cases, and from making the cure of the disease more grievous than the endurance of the same, Good Lord, deliver us.
                                                                    British Medical Journal

Russell Brain; 1953   **1950**

Medicine alone takes as its province the whole man.... With man in all the complexity of his body and mind from his conception to his last breath; and its concern extends increasingly beyond his sicknesses, to the conditions which make it possible for him to lead a healthy and a happy life. We speak of medicine as both a science and an art, and surely these two aspects are complementary. Science is analytic,...art is intuitive, and sees in the whole something more than can be explained as the sum of its parts.   *The Lancet*

John L. McClenahan; 1961   **1951**

It is because we have begun to act like merchants, and in many instances to observe the same hours, that the public expects us to be regulated by the same restraints.

X-ray Technician

John Romano; 1961   **1952**

Is the clinician a biochemist, a biophysicist, a biologist, a pathologist, a psychologist, a psychiatrist, a social scientist, a statistician? In my view, he is none of these and at the same time he must be something of all of them. *Journal of the American Medical Association*

René Jules Dubos; 1968   **1953**

The art of medicine consists to a large extent in the ability of medical men to devise practical measures best suited to the human beings involved. Usually, physicians must deal with problems they cannot fully comprehend and conditions that they cannot entirely control. *Man, Medicine, and Environment*

René Jules Dubos; 1968   **1954**

To approach the ideal, precise scientific knowledge of the body machine must be supplemented with a more empirical attitude in the practice of medicine.

Man, Medicine, and Environment

N. Henry Moss; 1973   **1955**

Patients are now being bounced from one specialist or superspecialty to another, and this ping-pong referral system results in a multiple of prescribed medications and escalating costs. *Medical Affairs*

Arthur Lytton Sells; 1974   **1956**

A prescription which he [Oliver Goldsmith] wrote for a Mrs. Sidebotham was declared by the apothecary to be unsafe, and the lady took fright. Goldsmith then said he would prescribe no more for his friends. Beauclerk agreed with him: "My dear doctor, whenever you undertake to kill, let it be only your enemies. *Oliver Goldsmith: His Life and Works*

W.U. McClenahan; 1974   **1957**

Today, most American doctors are successful men...as chemists or geneticists, but they are no man's servant. They function with a bleak matter-of-factness. They bleed statistics. One of them put to me beautifully. "Please don't think of me as a practitioner; I'm a *diagnostician.*" The question is, What happens after the diagnosis? *G.P.*

Edmond A. Murphy; 1975   **1958**

There is a caricature of the pure mathematician who sees a house burning beside a lake, recognizes that a solution exists—there is water in the lake and water extinguishes fire— and decides that nothing further has to be done. We flatter ourselves that medicine is a profession much more responsibly practical, but it would be hard to defend before a cosmic tribunal the thesis that we do very well in the delivery of what we do know.

New England Journal of Medicine

Charles D. Aring; 1979   **1959**

Many of the most difficult medical decisions depend mainly on character, the slowly matured power of judgment, and a grasp of fundamental principle, and detailed knowledge and technical skill are not as helpful as we sometimes would like to think. In making such decisions, statistics are useful but secondary. They save us from having ignorance foisted on us. But they are relegated to a position below empathy and compassion aided and abetted by experience. *Journal of the American Medical Association*

Douglas Arthur Kilgour Black; 1981   **1960**

Good medical practice requires a high level of professional knowledge, personal dedication, the ability to communicate, and—most of all—the ability to make time. It also demands a difficult balance between self-confidence and self-questioning. Too much of the former leads to arrogance, too much of the latter to indecision.

McLachlan G, Reviewing Practice in Medical Care

Derek Bok; 1985   **1961**

Rising quantities of knowledge not only place heavier demands on human memory but create new difficulties in analyzing problems. Scientific progress constantly expands the range of alternative diagnoses to be considered and the number of tests that can be given to test the clinician's hypotheses. Keeping these possibilities in mind, assessing the risks of harmful side effects from a growing number of tests and drugs, calculating the meaning to be derived from larger quantities of data—all are tasks that burden the most sophisticated minds. *The Realities of Medicine*

Ann Lennarson Greer; 1987   **1962**

The first step in conceptualizing the relationship between science and practice should be to reject the idea that practitioners are merely slow scientists. Just as science is not practice, practice is not merely applied science.... The goal of biomedical research is the advancement of knowledge.... In contrast, the goal of practice is healing; it is particular and local in its nature. *Journal of the American Medical Association*

Howard Brody; 1987   **1963**

We rarely encounter a physician as insightful as a surgeon of my acquaintance who has been heard to remark that the major reward in being a physician is having the opportunity to sit in an office all day while one patient after another comes in to tell him his or her life story in full, frank, and intimate detail. *Stories of Sickness*

Robertson Davies; 1994   **1964**

Mine is a profession of compassion, and when compassion does not arise naturally it must be faked. *The Cunning Man*

James Cleary, Paul B. Carbone; 1995   **1965**

I often tell medical students and young physicians that if they are going into medicine with cure as their major goal, they should consider obstetrics—a specialty in which cures are achieved regularly. The rest of us spend much of our time trying to control the symptoms of illness. *Hospital Practice*

Joseph Bernardin; 1995   **1966**

More and more members of the community of medicine no longer agree on the universal moral principles of medicine or on the appropriate means to realize those principles. Conscientious practitioners are often perplexed as to how they should act when they are caught up in a web of economics, politics, business practice, and social responsibility.... The practice of medicine no longer has the surety of an accurate compass to guide it through these challenging and difficult times.... Medicine, along with other professions including my own (the clergy), is in need of a moral renewal.

Address to the AMA House of Delegates

Louis de Bernières; 1995   **1967**

Dr. Iannis had enjoyed a satisfactory day in which none of his patients had died or got any worse. He had attended a surprisingly easy calving, lanced one abscess, extracted a molar, dosed one lady of easy virtue with Salvarsan, performed an unpleasant but spectacularly fruitful enema, and had produced a miracle by a feat of medical prestidigitation.

Corelli's Mandolin

Lofty L. Basta; 1996   **1968**

It takes a real professional to advise against more intrusive treatment; it merely takes a technician to undertake one more procedure. *A Graceful Exit*

Robert G. Petersdorf; 1996   **1969**

I sometimes say that...residents...go through inordinate mental gyrations over differential diagnosis and overtreatment—spending a lot of time and money on things that are unlikely to pay off. My definition of excellence is knowing how to take shortcuts and how to become efficient. If you can practice more effectively, you may miss one diagnosis in

1,000. That is not really sacrificing excellence. But internal medicine is still enmeshed in exceptional detail. *The Internist*

Eugene A. Stead Jr.; 1997 **1970**
We understand only about 10 percent of what patients complain of. Ninety percent of what they report you have to handle empirically. In that 90 percent of your practice, you will be practicing like a quack. You will not know what you are doing.
Hughes SG et al., The Pharos

Eugene A. Stead Jr.; 1997 **1971**
An error commonly made by young people in medicine is to tell a patient that he must lose weight, he must stop smoking, he must take medicines, have a regular schedule.... In the end, they fail because they try to change too much of the brain at one time. They don't appreciate the basis of the patient's behavior. *Hughes SG et al., The Pharos*

Eugene A. Stead Jr.; 1997 **1972**
Taking care of patients is different from taking care of disease.
Hughes SG et al., The Pharos

Nuala P. Kenny; 1997 **1973**
Science...and clinical practice move in opposite directions. Science moves from individual observations to generalizable theories and laws. Clinical practice brings this generalized body of knowledge to bear to benefit an individual. Science has a unique and essential role in clinical practice. Clinical practice is not a science but an endeavour that uses science. Good science is necessary but insufficient for good practice.
Canadian Medical Association Journal

MEDICAL PROFESSION

Moses Maimonides; [1135-1204] **1974**
Preserve my strength, that I may be able to restore the strength of the rich and the poor, the good and the bad, the friend and the foe. Let me see in the sufferer the man alone.
Daily Prayer of a Physician

Moses Maimonides; [1135-1204] **1975**
If physicians more learned then I wish to guide and counsel me, inspire me with confidence in, obedience toward recognition of them, for the study of the science is great. It is not given to one man alone to see what others see.... O, God, Thou has appointed me to watch over the health of Thy creatures; here am I ready for my vocation.
Minkin JS, The World of Moses Maimonides

François Rabelais; 1532 **1976**
[Pantagruel] went then to Montpellier, where he met with the good wives of Mirevaux, and good jovial company withal, and thought to have set himself to the study of physic; but he considered that the calling was too troublesome and melancholic, and that physicians did smell of glisters like old devils. *Gargantua and Pantagruel*

Thomas Browne; 1643 **1977**
To speak more generally, these three Noble Professions which all civil Commonwealths do honour, are raised upon the fall of Adam, and are not any way exempt from their infirmities; there are not only diseases incurable in Physick, but cases indissolvable in Law, Vices incorrigible in Divinity. *Religio Medici*

Thomas Sydenham; [1624-1689] **1978**
Whoever takes up medicine should seriously consider the following points: firstly, that he must one day render to the Supreme Judge an account of the lives of those sick men who have been intrusted to his care. Secondly, that such skill and science as, by the blessing of

Almighty God, he has attained, are to be specially directed towards the honour of his Maker, and the welfare of his fellow-creatures. *Works*

John Gregory; 1772 **1979**

The dignity of [the] profession.... is to be maintained by the superior learning and abilities of those who profess it, by the liberal manners of gentlemen, and by that openness and candour, which disdain all artifice, which invite to a free inquiry, and thus boldly bid defiance to all that illiberal ridicule and abuse to which medicine has been so much and so long exposed. *Lectures on the Duties and Qualifications of a Physician*

Adam Smith; 1776 **1980**

We trust our health to the physician: our fortune and sometimes our life and reputation to the lawyer and attorney. Such confidence could not safely be reposed in people of a very mean or low condition. Their reward must be such, therefore, as may give them that rank in the society which so important a trust requires. The long time and the great expense which must be laid out in their education, when combined with this circumstance, necessarily enhance still further the price of their labour. *The Wealth of Nations*

John Hamilcar Hollister; 1844 **1981**

I wasn't good enough to be a preacher, nor pugnacious enough to be a lawyer. I had not means to set myself up in business, nor money enough to buy a farm. The question narrowed itself down to this: "Shall I be a pedagogue or a doctor?" *Memories of Eighty Years*

Peter Mere Latham; 1845 **1982**

The powers of art must be brought to overrule the operations of nature by force. To know these powers and how to wield them to such a purpose is an affair beyond all trick and all skill of practicing upon the fancies of mankind. It can only proceed from a faithful and candid search after truth by each of us for himself according to his opportunities, and for a ready communication of what we believe to be the truth by all of us among one another, and from a comparison of their experiences and conclusions among the best minds.

Aphorisms

John Call Dalton Jr.; *circa* 1855 **1983**

Whatever be said of the practice of medicine by the disappointed or over-sensitive, all will agree that its study, as a worthy pursuit for vigorous and cultivated minds, has no superior in the whole field of knowledge, open to human investigation.

Address to the College of Physicians and Surgeons

Oliver Wendell Holmes; 1860 **1984**

If every drug from the vegetable, animal, and mineral kingdom were to disappear from the market, a body of enlightened men, organized as a distinct profession, would be required just as much as now, whose province should be to guard against the causes of disease, to eliminate them if possible when still present...and to give those predictions of the course of disease which only experience can warrant.

Currents and Counter-Currents in Medical Science

John Ruskin; 1862 **1985**

Five great intellectual professions, relating to the daily necessities of life, have hitherto existed...in every civilized nation:
The Soldier's profession is to *defend* it.
The Pastor's to *teach* it.
The Physician's to *keep it in health*.
The Lawyer's to *enforce justice* in it.
The Merchant's to *provide* for it.
And the duty of all these men is, on due occasion, to *die* for it.
"On due occasion," namely...
The Physician, rather than leave his post in plague. *Unto This Last*

George Eliot; 1871   **1986**

I might have got into some stupid draught-horse work or other, and lived always in blinkers. I should never have been happy in any profession that did not call forth the highest intellectual strain, and yet kept me in a good warm contact with my neighbors. There is nothing like the medical profession for that: one can have the exclusive scientific life that touches the distance and befriend the old fogies in the parish too.   *Middlemarch*

Anton Chekhov; 1888   **1987**

You advise me not to chase after two hares at once and to forget about practicing medicine.... I feel more alert and more satisfied with myself when I think of myself as having two occupations instead of one. Medicine is my lawful wedded wife, and literature my mistress. When one gets on my nerves, I spend the night with the other...Neither one loses anything by my duplicity.   *Letter to A.S. Suvorin*

Elizabeth Blackwell; 1889   **1988**

There is no career nobler than that of the physician. The progress and welfare of society is more intimately bound up with the prevailing tone and influence of the medical profession than with the status of any other class of men.   *The Influence of Women in the Profession of Medicine*

Arthur Conan Doyle; 1894   **1989**

How can a man spend his whole life in seeing suffering bravely borne and yet remain a hard or a vicious man? It is a noble, generous, kindly profession, and you youngsters have got to see that it remains so.   *Round the Red Lamp. The Surgeon Talks*

Arthur Conan Doyle; 1894   **1990**

A doctor has much to be thankful for.... It is such a pleasure to do a little good that a man should pay for the privilege instead of being paid for it.... He goes from house to house, and his step and his voice are loved and welcomed in each. What could a man ask for more than that? and besides, he is forced to be a good man. It is impossible for him to be anything else.... It is a noble, generous, kindly profession.   *Round the Red Lamp. The Surgeon Talks*

Daniel R. Brower; 1902   **1991**

We belong to a profession that has been in all ages characterized by a most self-sacrificing spirit. With one breath we ask our Maker to give us our daily bread, and with the very next breath we teach the people preventive medicine.   *Bulletin of the American Academy of Medicine*

William Osler; 1902   **1992**

A rare and precious gift is the Art of Detachment, by which a man may so separate himself from a life-long environment as to take a panoramic view of the conditions under which he has lived and moved: it frees him from Plato's den long enough to see the realities as they are, the shadows as they appear. Could a physician attain to such an art he would find in the state of his profession a theme calling as well for the exercise of the highest faculties of description and imagination as for the deepest philosophic insight.   *Chauvinism in Medicine*

William Osler; 1903   **1993**

From the day you begin practice never under any circumstances listen to a tale told to the detriment of a brother practitioner. And when any dispute or trouble does arise, go frankly, ere sunset, and talk the matter over, in which way you may gain a brother and a friend.   *The Master-word in Medicine*

William Osler; 1903   **1994**

Think not to light a light to shine before men that they may see your good works; contrariwise, you belong to the great army of quiet workers, physicians and priests, sisters and nurses, all over the world, the members of which strive not neither do they cry, nor are their voices heard in the streets, but to them is given the ministry of consolation in sorrow, need, and sickness. *The Master-word in Medicine*

Samuel Hopkins Adams; 1905 **1995**
With the exception of lawyers, there is no profession which considers itself above the law so widely as the medical profession. *The Great American Fraud*

William Edward Quine; 1905 **1996**
I know of no better way to uphold the honor and dignity of my profession than to uphold my own honor and dignity as a man. *Illinois Medical Journal*

William Osler; 1905 **1997**
I have had three personal ideals. One to do the day's work well and not to bother about tomorrow.... The second ideal has been to act the Golden Rule, as far as in me lay, towards my professional brethren and towards the patients committed to my care. And the third has been to cultivate such a measure of equanimity as would enable me to bear success with humility, the affection of my friends without pride and to be ready when the day of sorrow and grief came to meet it with the courage befitting a man. *L'Envoi*

Abraham Flexner; 1910 **1998**
By professional patriotism amongst medical men I mean that sort of regard for the honor of the profession and that sense of responsibility for its efficiency which will enable a member of that profession to rise above the consideration of personal or of professional gain. *Medical Education in the United States and Canada*

George Bernard Shaw; 1911 **1999**
All professions [are] conspiracies against the laity; and I do not suggest that the medical conspiracy is either better or worse than the military conspiracy, the legal conspiracy, the sacerdotal conspiracy, the pedagogic conspiracy, the royal and aristocratic conspiracy, the literary and artistic conspiracy, and the innumerable industrial, commercial, and financial conspiracies, from the trade unions to the great exchanges, which make up the huge conflict which we call society. But it is less suspected. *The Doctor's Dilemma, Preface*

George Bernard Shaw; 1911 **2000**
Unless a man is led to medicine or surgery through a very exceptional aptitude, or because doctoring is a family tradition, or because he regards it unintelligently as a lucrative and gentlemanly profession, his motives in choosing the career of a healer are clearly generous. However actual practice may disillusion and corrupt him, his selection in the first instance is not a selection of a base character. *The Doctor's Dilemma, Preface*

George Bernard Shaw; 1911 **2001**
Until the medical profession becomes a body of men trained and paid by the country to keep the country in health it will remain what it is at present: a conspiracy to exploit popular credulity and human suffering. *The Doctor's Dilemma, Preface*

James Bryce; 1914 **2002**
Medicine [is] the only profession that labours incessantly to destroy the reason for its own existence. *Speech*

John Chalmers Da Costa; 1915 **2003**
Sometimes when a doctor gets too lazy to work, he becomes a politician. *New York Medical Journal*

W. Somerset Maugham; 1915 **2004**
The medical profession is the only one which a man may enter at any age with some chance of making a living. *Of Human Bondage*

Henry Louis Mencken; 1927 **2005**
A certain section of medical opinion, in late years, has succumbed to the messianic delu-

sion. Its spokesmen are not content to deal with the patients who come to them for advice; they conceive it to be their duty to force advice upon everyone, including especially those who don't want it.... A physician, however learned, has no more right to intrude his advice upon persons who prefer the advice of a Christian Scientist, a chiropractor, or a pow-wow doctor than he has to intrude upon persons who prefer the advice of some other physician.   *A Mencken Chrestomathy*

William J. Mayo; 1927   **2006**

These heroic men whose life work marked epochs in medicine we think of as individuals, but what they accomplished singly was perhaps of less importance than the inspiration they gave to the group of men who followed them.   *Canadian Medical Association Journal*

Harvey Cushing; 1936   **2007**

The practising neurologist, finding his activities encroached upon in several directions, tends more and more to turn to psychotherapy for his livelihood.... Medicine has always been like this, with ever-changing realignments. There must be some...principle constantly at work, and I suspect it has much to do with those native qualities that distinguish thinkers from doers.... Why one chooses to solve his problems in his study, like psychiatrists, we may say, while another, like the surgeon or laboratory worker, instinctively prefers somehow to work them out with his hands.   *Neurological Biographies and Addresses*

Archibald Joseph Cronin; 1937   **2008**

We're not nearly liberal enough. If we go on trying to make out that everything's wrong outside the profession and everything is right within, it means the death of scientific progress. We'll just turn into a tight little trade protection society. It's high time we started putting our own house in order, and I don't mean the superficial things either.

      The Citadel

Ogden Nash; 1940   **2009**

Professional men, they have no cares;
Whatever happens, they get theirs.   *I Yield to My Learned Brother*

Herrman L. Blumgart; 1964   **2010**

The profession of medicine is a "house of many mansions." It embraces numerous professions within itself, requiring diverse capabilities and different types of persons.

      New England Journal of Medicine

John H. Knowles; 1966   **2011**

The expert-specialist position of learned ignoramus...lies at the very roots of the modern doctor's dilemma.... Perhaps it is time the medical profession developed what Max Weber called the three cardinal qualities of the politician, namely a feeling of responsibility, a sense of proportion, and finally, passion...passionate commitment to the solution of public problems in medical care and not passionate commitment to one's guild or one's own expert interest.   *Connecticut Medicine*

Paul Starr; 1982   **2012**

Doctors and other professionals...claim authority, not as individuals, but as members of a community that has objectively validated their competence. The professional offers judgments and advice, not as a personal act based on privately revealed or idiosyncratic criteria, but as a representative of a community of shared standards. The basis of those standards in the modern professions is presumed to be rational inquiry and empirical evidence. Professional authority also presumes an orientation to specific, substantive values—in the case of medicine, the value of health.

      The Social Transformation of American Medicine

Peter Richards; 1985   **2013**

Medicine is no career for the faint hearted, nor for the weak in health, nor for complainers or clock watchers. Yet for all its demands it offers the opportunity of a deeply satisfying lifetime of service to those prepared to give themselves to it.   *Learning Medicine*

Peter Richards; 1985   **2014**

Why should so many school leavers, some of those finishing another degree course, and even those already established in a different career consider becoming doctors? A desire to help people is often given as a reason. But do not policemen, porters, and plumbers of sympathetic disposition do that? It surely is not necessary to become a doctor to help people. If more pastoral care is in mind why not become a priest, a social worker, or a school teacher? If a curing edge on caring is the attraction remember that doctors do not always cure.   *Learning Medicine*

Billy F. Andrews; 1991   **2015**

Medicine, then is more than a profession.
Medicine is a worthy calling, a true avocation.
Medicine is a most magnificent obsession.
Medicine requires all the abilities in one's possession.
Its influence on life and death's progression
Makes medicine more than a profession.   *Southern Medical Journal*

Sherwin B. Nuland; 1994   **2016**

Of all the professions, medicine is one most likely to attract people with high personal anxieties about dying. We become doctors because our ability to cure gives us power over the death of which we are so afraid, and loss of that power poses such a significant threat that we must turn away from it, and therefore from the patient who personifies our weakness.   *How We Die*

Charles B. Strozier; 1995   **2017**

The medical profession has never been a haven for social and political activism.
    The American Scholar

Jerome P. Kassirer; 1998   **2018**

If we capitulate to an ethic of the group rather than the individual, and if we allow market forces to distort our ethical standards, we risk becoming economic agents instead of health care professionals. Inevitably, patients will suffer, and so will a noble profession.
    New England Journal of Medicine

Ruzha Cleaveland; 1999   **2019**

I wish my husband were no longer practicing medicine. [He] no longer has a profession; he has a job.   *New England Journal of Medicine*

MEDICAL PROGRESS

William Heberden; 1802   **2020**

No aphorism of Hippocrates holds truer to this day, than that in which he laments the length of time necessary to establish medical truths, and the danger, unless the utmost caution be used, of our being misled even by experience.
    Commentaries on the History and Cure of Diseases

William Osler; 1902   **2021**

The philosophies of one age have become the absurdities of the next, and the foolishness of yesterday has become the wisdom of tomorrow.   *Chauvinism in Medicine*

John Chalmers Da Costa; 1907   **2022**

Enthusiasm is the motive force of progress. No really great deed was ever done in arts or arms, in literature or science, that was not the product of enthusiasm.... May we feel it; may we realize it; may we be animated by this immortal principle; may we be driven by this divine fire!   *Address*

MEDICAL RECORDS

Ian R. Mackay; 1987   2023

An impeccably constructed record should be educational for both the recorder and the users of the record, should encourage preservation of basic clinical skills, and should be a model for medical students.   *Manning PR and DeBakey L, Medicine: Preserving the Passion*

MEDICAL RESEARCH

John Hunter; 1775   2024

But why think, why not try the experiment?   *Letter to Edward Jenner*

Friedrich Theodor von Frerichs; 1860   2025

The main part of the science of disease is of a purely descriptive character; a scientific interpretation of facts and a clear insight into the intimate connection subsisting between different phenomena, which may precede all attempts at a rational method of cure, having been attained in a few instances only.... Therapeutic researchers must be regulated in the same manner as pathological.... The more careful tracing of the progress of morbid processes, and the insight into their modes of origin and retrogression, enable us to determine the principles of treatment with greater clearness than formerly.

A Clinical Treatise on Diseases of the Liver

Claude Bernard; 1865   2026

The first requirement...in practising experimental medicine, is to be an observing physician and to start from pure and simple observations of patients made as completely as possible.   *An Introduction to the Study of Experimental Medicine*

Louis Pasteur; 1888   2027

Put forward nothing that cannot be proved simply and conclusively. Venerate the critical spirit.... Without it all else is nothing. It always has the last word.

Remarks at the dedication of the Pasteur Institute of Paris

Thomas Clifford Allbutt; [1836-1925]   2028

The use of hypotheses lies not in the display of ingenuity, but in the labour of verification.

Asher R, A Sense of Asher

Ronald Aylmer Fisher; 1926   2029

A physician observing a number of patients to sicken and die in similar though not identical conditions, and with similar though not identical symptoms, would surely make an initial error if he did not seek for a single common cause of the disorder.

Eugenics Review

Theobold Smith; 1934   2030

To those who have the urge to do research and who are prepared to give up most things in life eagerly pursued by the man in the street, discovery should come as an adventure rather than as the result of a logical process of thought. Sharp, prolonged thinking is necessary that we may keep on the chosen road but it does not itself necessarily lead to discovery. The investigator must be ready and on the spot when the light comes from whatever direction.   *Journal of Bacteriology*

Henry E. Sigerist; 1944   2031

Not every physician will become a researcher, but as a student every doctor has spent a number of years at the very source of medical research, in daily contact with a group of men who have devoted their life to the advancement of science, who have permitted him to enter their sanctum, to breathe its atmosphere and to share the joys and sorrows of the researcher. This is a great privilege that imposes upon every medical man the obligation to keep in close touch with science and to make his experience available for the advancement of medicine.   *Classics of Medicine*

René Jules Dubos; 1968   **2032**

Medical research could in theory find a scientific solution for most of the disease problems of our times. There are not, and cannot be, enough resources or scientific skills to attack all the problems that cry out for solution or to apply all the theoretical knowledge that has been developed. The question will be what of all the things that could be done should be done. In all cases these decisions will involve criteria that transcend scientific knowledge and judgement. They will have to be made on the basis of social and ethical values.   *Man, Medicine, and Environment*

MEDICAL SCHOOLS

William Henry Welch; 1907   **2033**

The...proper home of the medical school is the university, of which it should be an integral part coordinate with the other faculties.... Two reforms are especially needed in most of our medical schools. The first is that the heads of the principal clinical departments, particularly the medical and surgical, should devote their main energies and time to their hospital work and to teaching and investigating without the necessity of seeking their livelihood in a busy outside practice.... The other reform is the introduction of the system of practical training of students in the hospital.   *Medicine and the University*

Abraham Flexner; 1910   **2034**

Where any criticism is attempted of inadequate methods or inadequate facilities, no reply is more common than this: "Our institution cannot be judged from its financial support. It depends upon the enthusiasm and the devotion of its teachers and its supporters, and such devotion cannot be measured by financial standards."

Medical Education in the United States and Canada

Abraham Flexner; 1910   **2035**

The existence of many of these unnecessary and inadequate medical schools has been defended by the argument that a poor medical school is justified in the interest of the poor boy. It is clear that the poor boy has no right to go into any profession for which he is not willing to obtain adequate preparation; but...this argument is insincere, and that the excuse which has hitherto been put forward in the name of the poor boy is in reality an argument in behalf of the poor medical school.

Medical Education in the United States and Canada

Abraham Flexner; 1910   **2036**

Practically the medical school is a public service corporation.

Medical Education in the United States and Canada

Abraham Flexner; 1910   **2037**

Educational institutions, particularly those which are connected with a college or a university, are peculiarly sensitive to outside criticism, and particularly to any statement of the circumstances of their own conduct or equipment which seems to them unfavorable in comparison with that of other institutions.   *Medical Education in the United States and Canada*

William Carlos Williams; [1883-1963]   **2038**

Look, you're not out on a four-year picnic at that medical school, so stop talking like a disappointed lover. You signed up for a spell of training and they're dishing it out to you, and all you can do is take everything they've got, everything they hand to you, and tell yourself how lucky you are to be on the receiving end—so you can be a doctor, and that's no bad price to pay for the worry, the exhaustion.   *Letter to Dr. Coles*

Rosemary Stevens; 1971   **2039**

The medical school became [from the 1950s] a scientific and research complex which, both ideologically and financially, was largely independent of the university which sheltered it.   *American Medicine and the Public Interest*

Rosemary Stevens; 1971   **2040**
The problems of medical schools...are the products not of a failure in medicine but of releasing the potentials of the technological successes of the previous 30 years in a medical system which has been developing for over 300 years, and which could not easily bend to change. At issue now is how the pieces are to be linked together.
American Medicine and the Public Interest

Rosemary Stevens; 1971   **2041**
Today's medical school, with its sprawling complex of departments, teaching programs, research units and service facilities, its sheer size, its dependence on public support, bears little resemblance to the schools which emerged from World War II, whose mission was primarily to educate physicians.   *American Medicine and the Public Interest*

Howard Spiro; 1992   **2042**
Occasions for spontaneous collegiality have diminished under the pressure of research grants or diagnostic machinery. My medical school has no faculty club, nor even a doctors' dining room.... Elegant centers exist for study and an ever increasing number of laboratories are provided for molecular research, but these are structures only for scientific collaboration and cooperation. Meeting our colleagues in an unstructured way, as people, has become much more difficult.   *Annals of Internal Medicine*

MEDICAL SCIENCE

James Parkinson; 1817   **2043**
The advantages which have been derived from the caution with which hypothetical statements are admitted, are in no instance more obvious than in those sciences which more particularly belong to the healing art.   *Essay on the Shaking Palsy*

Claude Bernard; 1865   **2044**
In the present state of biological science, no one can presume to explain pathology by physiology alone; we must move in that direction because it is the scientific path, but we must shun belief in the illusion that our problem is solved. For the moment, therefore, the prudent and reasonable thing to do is to explain all that we can explain in a disease by physiology and leave what is still inexplicable to the future progress of biological science.   *An Introduction to the Study of Experimental Medicine*

Claude Bernard; 1865   **2045**
If based on statistics, medicine can never be anything but a conjectural science; only by basing itself on experimental determinism can it become a true science.
An Introduction to the Study of Experimental Medicine

Ivan Petrovich Pavlov; 1897   **2046**
It is only by an active interchange of opinion, between the physiologist and the physician, that the common goal of physiological science and of medical art will be most quickly and securely reached.   *The Work of the Digestive Glands*

William Osler; *circa* 1900   **2047**
Modern science has made to almost everyone of you the present of a few years.
Aphorisms

Ernest Henry Starling; 1918   **2048**
In physiology, as in all other sciences, no discovery is useless, no curiosity misplaced or too ambitious, and we may be certain that every advance achieved in the quest of pure knowledge will sooner or later play its part in the service of man.
The Linacre Lecture on the Law of the Heart

Wilfred Batten Lewis Trotter; 1933   **2049**

The fundamental activity of medical science is to determine the ultimate causation of disease.   *The Lancet*

Edmund D. Pellegrino, David C. Thomasma; 1981   **2050**

La Mettrie and then Claude Bernard[developed] the concept of a quantifiable, experimental, and mechanistic reductionist enterprise.... The modern positivistic and reductionistic bias of medicine, and the believers in medicine as high technology are their linear descendants.... Ethics...places its greatest emphasis on competence, scientific certitude, and the advancement of knowledge and clinical experiment. It tends to depreciate caring and in its most severe form would assign the non scientific aspects of care to others—not to physicians.   *A Philosophical Basis of Medical Practice*

MEDICAL SERVICES

Benjamin Rush; 1801   **2051**

Humanity in physicians manifests itself in gratuitous services to the poor.

The Vice and Virtues of Physicians

George Bernard Shaw; 1911   **2052**

Make up your mind how many doctors the community needs to keep it well. Do not register more or less than this number; and let registration constitute the doctor a civil servant with a dignified living wage paid out of public funds.   *The Doctor's Dilemma, Preface*

Walton H. Hamilton; 1932   **2053**

In this country, up until near the turn of the century, the professional outlook and professional values [in medicine] were dominant. The "family doctor" was an institution: his trade was to him a sacred calling.... If there has been a change, the physician is not primarily to blame. On the contrary, it is a tribute to the profession that the older idealism has exhibited such persistence in an unfavorable environment. The fault—if fault there be—is that the profession has now to be practiced in an industrial world dominated by business.   *Realities of Medicine*

Henry E. Sigerist; 1958   **2054**

Group medicine is a superior form of service. The best way to make full use of the present technology of medicine is to organize medical groups, teams that will practice in health centers. These must be close to the people, in industrial centers, residential neighborhoods, or farms.   *Falk LA, Journal of the History of Medicine and Allied Sciences*

René Jules Dubos; 1968   **2055**

A continually increasing demand for medical care can thus be expected to create eventually a debilitating drain on financial and technical resources, even in wealthy countries. Important in this regard, the practices of modern therapeutic medicine depend increasingly upon highly skilled persons with long, expensive, and specialized training, men who must constantly undergo further education in order to keep in step with scientific advances. A scarcity of adequately trained personnel, rather than a shortage of funds, is likely to constitute the Achilles' heel of disease control in the future.

Man, Medicine, and Environment

Roy Porter; 1997   **2056**

An expanding medical establishment, faced with a healthier population, is driven to medicalizing normal events like menopause, converting risks into diseases, and treating trivial complaints with fancy procedures. Doctors and "consumers" are becoming locked within a fantasy that *everyone* has *something* wrong with them, everyone and everything can be cured.   *The Greatest Benefit to Mankind*

MEDICAL SINS

Richard Asher; 1948   2057

There is an unlimited number of medical sins, but I am going to catalogue and comment on seven of them in the hope that those students who wish to avoid them may do so and those who wish to indulge in them may enlarge their repertoire or refine their technique. The seven sins are obscurity, cruelty, bad manners, over-specialisation, love of the rare, stupidity, and sloth. *The Lancet*

MEDICAL SOCIETIES

William Osler; 1894   2058

You cannot afford to stand aloof from your professional colleagues in any place. Join their associations, mingle in their meetings, giving of the best of your talents, gathering here, scattering there; but everywhere showing that you are at all times faithful students, as willing to teach as to be taught. *The Army Surgeon*

MEDICAL STUDENTS

Charles Dickens; 1837   2059

"They're Medical Students, I suppose?" said Mr. Pickwick.... "I am glad of it.... They are...very fine fellows, with judgements matured by observation and reflection; tastes refined by reading and study.... Overflowing with kindly feelings and animal spirits. Just what I like to see!"

"One of em's got his legs on the table, and is drinkin' brandy neat, vile the t'other one—him in the barnacles—has got a barrel o' oysters atween his knees...and as fast as he eats 'em, he takes a aim with the shells at young dropsy, who's a sittin' down fast asleep, in the chimbley corner."

"Eccentricities of genius, Sam." *The Pickwick Papers*

William Osler; 1905   2060

The student often resembles the poet—he is born, not made. *The Student Life*

Abraham Flexner; 1910   2061

The student...does not have to be a passive learner, just because it is too early for him to be an original explorer. He can actively master and securely fix scientific technique and method in the process of acquiring the already known.... The undergraduate student of medicine will for the most part acquire the methods, standards, and habits of science by working over territory which has been traversed before, in an atmosphere freshened by the search for truth. *Medical Education in the United States and Canada*

Earle P. Scarlett; 1972   2062

Their lot has always been much the same. Hard work, long hours, poor accommodation for the majority, a sharp meeting with reality at a relatively young age, a long grind of years—these have prevailed in every generation. *Roland CG, In Sickness and in Health*

MEDICAL SUPERSTITIONS

Oliver Wendell Holmes; 1871   2063

You cannot and need not expect to disturb the public in the possession of its medical superstitions. A man's ignorance is as much his private property, and as precious in his own eyes, as his family Bible. *The Young Practitioner*

MEDICAL TECHNOLOGY

Lewis Thomas; 1983   **2064**

If I were a medical student or an intern, just getting ready to begin...I would be apprehensive that my real job, caring for sick people, might soon be taken away, leaving me with the quite different occupation of looking after machines.   *The Youngest Science*

Lofty L. Basta; 1996   **2065**

The medical community has displayed total ethical paralysis on how to handle [the] horrible consequences of advanced medical technology. Health-care professionals may think they have mastered this medical technology, but by ignoring or avoiding the ethical context in which this technology should be enacted, the technology has in effect mastered them.   *A Graceful Exit*

MEDICAL TESTIMONY

William Edward Quine; 1894   **2066**

I concur...in the opinion of the essayist that the status of expert testimony is the scandal and disgrace of the medical profession. The so-called expert is employed not because he is an expert physician, not because he is an expert diagnostician or an expert therapeutist, but because he is an expert swearer.   *Transactions of the Illinois State Medical Society*

MEDICAL WORKFORCE

Abraham Flexner; 1910   **2067**

In a society constituted as are our modern states, the interests of the social order will be served best when the number of men entering a given profession reaches and does not exceed a certain ratio.... When...six or eight ill trained physicians undertake to gain a living in a town which can support only two, the whole plane of professional conduct is lowered in the struggle which ensues, each man becomes intent upon his own practice, public health and sanitation are neglected, and the ideals and standards of the profession tend to demoralization.   *Medical Education in the United States and Canada*

Abraham Flexner; 1910   **2068**

Even long-continued over-production of cheaply made doctors cannot force distribution beyond a well marked point.... There is, then, no reason to fear an unheeded call or a too tardy response, if urban communities support one doctor for every 2000 inhabitants. On that showing, the towns have now four or more doctors for every one that they actually require—something worse than waste, for the superfluous doctor is usually a poor doctor.
Medical Education in the United States and Canada

MEDICALIZATION OF LIFE

Lewis Thomas; 1975   **2069**

We keep telling each other this sort of thing, and back it comes on television or in the weekly newsmagazines, confirming all the fears, instructing us...to "seek professional help." Get a checkup. Go on a diet. Meditate. Jog.... Take two tablets, with water. Spring water. If pain persists, if anomie persists, if boredom persists, see your doctor.
New England Journal of Medicine

Roy Porter; 1997   **2070**

What has been styled, particularly by critics, the "medicalization of life" cannot be understood purely or primarily as some kind of professional ramp. What has occurred is not a conspiracy by medical elites to push professional dominance into domains traditionally outside medicine's province, but rather the destabilization of the boundaries of lay and professional competence in an age of democracy.   *The Greatest Benefit to Mankind*

MEDICARE

Rosemary Stevens; 1971   **2071**
With Medicare, the public emerged as the dominant decision maker.... The passage of
Medicare marked the beginning of a new era.   *American Medicine and the Public Interest*

Marcia Angell; 1997   **2072**
The Medicare system is imbedded in a fragmented, profit-driven health care system,
which it increasingly subsidizes through payments to HMOs and teaching hospitals....
Nevertheless, there is too much waste and profiteering, and that needs to be controlled.
When the baby-boom generation reaches retirement age...it is unlikely that even an efficient, streamlined Medicare system will be able to cover all beneficiaries. What happens
then? A decent society cares for its most vulnerable members, including children and the
elderly. As our society ages, it may be necessary to increase our spending to honor that
commitment.   *New England Journal of Medicine*

MEDICINE

Hippocrates; [460-375 BC]   **2073**
For the art of Medicine would not have been invented at first, nor would it have been
made a subject of investigation (for there would have been no need of it), if when men
are indisposed, the same food and other articles of regimen which they eat and drink
when in good health were proper for them, and if no others were preferable to these. But
now necessity itself made medicine to be sought out and discovered by men.
                                                                    On Ancient Medicine

Hippocrates; [460-375 BC]   **2074**
Let us inquire then regarding what is admitted to be Medicine; namely, that which was
invented for the sake of the sick, which possesses a name and practitioners.
                                                                    On Ancient Medicine

Hippocrates; [460-375 BC]   **2075**
Medicine is of all the Arts the most noble; but, owing to the ignorance of those who practice it, and of those who, inconsiderately, form a judgment of them, it is at present far
behind all the other arts. Their mistake appears to me to arise principally from this, that
in the cities there is no punishment connected with the practice of medicine (and with
it alone).... Physicians are many in title but very few in reality.   *The Law*

Plato; [427-347 BC]   **2076**
In a community where licentiousness and disease are rife, law courts and dispensaries
have their doors constantly open. Law and medicine begin to give themselves airs, when
even among free men, large numbers take too keen an interest in them.   *The Republic*

Cicero; [106-43 BC]   **2077**
The art of medicine is valuable to us because it is conducive to health, not because of its
scientific interest.   *De finibus*

Tertullian (Quintus Septimius Tertullianus); *circa* 160   **2078**
Medicine is the sister of philosophy.   *Reichert HG, Latin Proverbs*

Galen; [130-200]   **2079**
The aim of the art of medicine is health, but its end is the possession of health. Doctors
have to know by which means to bring about health, when it is absent, and by which
means to preserve it, when it is present.   *On the Sects for Beginners*

Galen; [130-200]   **2080**
The method...which proceeds by means of reason admonishes us to study the nature of
the body which one tries to heal and the forces of all the causes which the body encounters daily. For it is as a result of these that it becomes healthier or sicker than it was before.
                                                              On the Sects for Beginners

Avicenna (Abu- Ali al-Husayn ibn Abdallah ibn Sina); [981-1037]   **2081**
Medicine is the science of which we learn the various states of the human body, in health, when not in health, the means by which health is likely to be lost, and when lost, is likely to be restored to health.   *Gruner OC, A Treatise on the Canon of Medicine of Avicenna*

Petrarch (Franceso Petrarca); 1370   **2082**
When we see how doctors themselves live, how their slight illnesses turn to tragic ends, we may well suspect that this thing called medicine, whatever it may be in itself, is yet among men a certain art of deception, invented to men's peril, to enrich a few and endanger many. Or we may think it a true art, contrived for useful ends, but little understood by men of our time. Or perhaps better, it may be understood , but hardly applicable to men's natures, in their infinite and incredible variety.   *Letter to Giovanni Dondi*

Desiderius Erasmus; 1518   **2083**
The special glory of the healing arts is self-sufficient and recommends itself to mankind by its value and utility.   *In Praise of the Healing Arts*

Paracelsus (Theophrastus Bombastus von Hohenheim); 1536   **2084**
The art of medicine cannot be inherited nor can it be copied from books.
        Das Zweite Buch der Grossen Wundarznei

Francis Bacon; 1605   **2085**
The poets did well to conjoin music and medicine in Apollo, because the office of medicine is but to tune this curious harp of man's body and to reduce it to harmony.
        The Advancement of Learning

William Shakespeare; 1606   **2086**
Throw physic to the dogs; I'll none of it.   *Macbeth, Act V, Scene iii*

René Descartes; 1637   **2087**
The mind is so intimately dependent upon the condition and relation of the organs of the body, that if any means can ever be found to render men wiser and more ingenious than hitherto, I believe that it is in medicine they must be sought for.   *A Discourse on Method*

Thomas Sydenham; [1624-1689]   **2088**
Inasmuch as the structure of the human frame has been so set together by Nature, that it is unable, from the continuous flux of particles, to remain unchanged; whilst, from the action of external causes, it is subjected to influences beyond its own: and since, for these reasons, a numerous train of diseases has pressed upon the earth since the beginning of time; so without doubt the necessity of investigations into the Art of Healing has exercised the wit of mankind for many ages.   *Works*

Samuel Garth; 1699   **2089**
Now sick'ning Physick hangs her pensive head
And what was once a Science, now's a Trade.
Her Son's ne'er rifle her Mysterious Store,
But study Nature less, and Lucre more.   *The Dispensary*

Duro Armeno Bagliavi; [1668-1707]   **2090**
The foundations of medicine are reason and observation.   *Dubrovnik Archives*

Jonathan Swift; 1711   **2091**
Apollo was held the God of Physick, and Sender of Diseases: Both were originally the same Trade, and still continue.   *Thoughts on Various Subjects*

John Morgan; 1765   **2092**
As the most precious metals in a state of ore are mixed with dross, so the choice truths of Medicine are frequently blended with a heap of rubbish.
        A Discourse upon the Institution of Medical Schools in America

John Gregory; 1772   **2093**

People may dispute, whether physick, on the whole, does more good or harm to mankind; just as they may dispute, whether the faculty of reason, considering how it is often perverted, really contributes to make human life more or less happy.

Lectures on the Duties and Qualifications of a Physician

Theodore Tronchin; [1709-1781]   **2094**

In medicine, sins of commission are mortal, sins of omission venial.

Garrison FH. Bulletin of the New York Academy of Medicine

Thomas Jefferson; 1799   **2095**

The state of medicine is worse than that of total ignorance.... From Hippocrates to Brown we have had nothing but a succession of hypothetical systems each having its day of vogue, like the fashions and fancies of caps and gowns, and yielding in turn to the next caprice. Yet the human frame, which is to be the subject of suffering and torture under these learned modes, does not change.   *Letter to William Green Munford*

Elisha Bartlett; 1844   **2096**

The hold which medicine has so long held upon the popular mind is loosened; there is a wide-spread skepticism as to the power of its curing diseases, and men are everywhere to be found who deny its pretensions as a science, and reject the benefits and blessings which it proffers them as an art.   *Essay on the Philosophy of Medical Science*

Reveille Parisé; 1851   **2097**

Medicine is the most noble profession and the most depressing occupation.

La Gazette Médicale

Jacob Bigelow; 1854   **2098**

Most men form an exaggerated estimate of the powers of medicine, founded on the common acception of the name, that medicine is the art of curing diseases. That this is a false definition is evident from the fact that many diseases are incurable, and that one such disease must at last happen to every living man. A far more just definition would be that medicine is the art of understanding diseases, and of curing or relieving them when possible.

Nature in Disease

Oliver Wendell Holmes; 1860   **2099**

The truth is that medicine, professedly founded on observation, is as sensitive to outside influences, political, religious, philosophical, imaginative, as is the barometer to the changes of atmospheric density. Theoretically it ought to go on its own straightforward inductive path, without regard to changes of government or, tofluctuations of public opinion. [But, there is] a closer relation between the Medical Sciences and the conditions of Society and the general thought of the time, than would at first be suspected.

Currents and Counter-Currents in Medical Science

Claude Bernard; 1865   **2100**

To conserve health and to cure disease: Medicine is still pursuing a scientific solution of this problem, which has confronted it from the first.

An Introduction to the Study of Experimental Medicine

Thomas Henry Huxley; 1881   **2101**

Medicine not merely denotes a kind of knowledge, but it comprehends the various applications of that knowledge to the alleviation of the sufferings, the repair of the injuries, and the conservation of health, of living beings.   *Science and Culture*

Alfred Stillé; 1884   **2102**

It behooves us to remember that medicine is, above all else humane... ; that its beginning, middle, and end is to relieve suffering, and that whatever is outside this may indeed be science... , but certainly is not medicine.   *Address*

William Withey Gull; 1896   **2103**

The study of Medicine is an object lesson; the object, man's body in health and disease.
                                                    A Collection of the Published Writings

Samuel Gee; 1902   **2104**

Physiology owes more to medicine than medicine to physiology. Nature in disease performs vivisections for us. The greater and better part of what we know concerning the functions of the many organs of the body is derived from pathological observation and not from physiological experiment.   *Medical Lectures and Aphorisms*

William Osler; 1902   **2105**

The critical sense and sceptical attitude of the Hippocratic school laid the foundations of modern medicine on broad lines, and we owe *first*, the emancipation of medicine from the shackles of priestcraft and of caste; *secondly*, the conception of medicine as an art based on accurate observation, and as a science, an integral part of the science of man and of nature; *thirdly*, the high moral ideals, expressed in that most "memorable of human documents" (Gomprez), the Hippocratic oath; and *fourthly*, the conception and realization of medicine as the profession of a cultivated gentleman.   *Chauvinism in Medicine*

Denslow Lewis; 1906   **2106**

It is a happy sign of the times when medical men understand that they must study sociology, that they must appreciate economic conditions, that they must face the facts and know life as it is, and not as their wishes would have it to be.   *Buffalo Medical Journal*

William Osler; 1907   **2107**

The old art cannot possibly be replaced by, but must be absorbed in, the new science.
                                                          St. Mary's Hospital Gazette

Charles Horace Mayo; 1909   **2108**

While medicine is a science, in many particulars it cannot be exact, so baffling are the varying results of varying conditions of human life.
                                  Collected Papers of the Mayo Clinic and Mayo Foundation

Abraham Flexner; 1910   **2109**

Medicine is a discipline, in which the effort is made to use knowledge procured in various ways in order to effect certain practical ends.... It harbors no preconceptions as to diseases or their cure.... It has progressively become less cocksure and more modest. It distrusts general propositions, *a priori* explanations, grandiose and comforting generalizations. It needs theories only as convenient summaries in which a number of ascertained facts may be used tentatively to define a course of action. It makes no effort to use its discoveries to substantiate a principle formulated before the facts were even suspected.
                                  Medical Education in the United States and Canada

George Bernard Shaw; 1911   **2110**

The notion that therapeutics or hygiene or surgery is any more or less scientific than making or cleaning boots is entertained only by people to whom a man of science is still a magician who can cure diseases, transmute metals, and enable us to live forever.
                                                          The Doctor's Dilemma, Preface

Marcel Proust; 1920   **2111**

Medicine being a compendium of the successive and contradictory mistakes of medical practitioners, when we summon the wisest of them to our aid, the chances are that we may be relying on a scientific truth the error of which will be recognized in a few years' time.   *Remembrance of Things Past. The Guermantes Way*

Bertrand Russell; 1925   **2112**

An able physician is more useful to a patient than the most devoted friend, and progress in medical knowledge does more for the health of the community than ill-informed philanthropy.   *What I Believe*

William J. Mayo; 1928   **2113**

The aim of medicine is to prevent disease and prolong life; the ideal of medicine is to eliminate the need of a physician.   *Proceedings of the National Education Association*

William J. Mayo; 1931   **2114**

The church and the law deal with the yesterdays of life; medicine deals with the tomorrows.   *Collected Papers of the Mayo Clinic and Mayo Foundation*

Walton H. Hamilton; 1932   **2115**

The ways and means for putting medicine in order must take account of the conditions of life and work among the people whom it must serve.   *Realities of Medicine*

Walter L. Palmer; 1947   **2116**

We are all weary of discussions of state medicine, of the high cost of medical care, of the adequacy of medical care for the indigent, of the shortage of hospital beds for those who can pay, of the shortage of nurses, and so on. But these are, in part, our problems; if their solution is to be to our liking, we must be active in them.... Unless we ourselves reorganize the practice of medicine, it will be reorganized for us.   *Gastroenterology*

William Carlos Williams; 1951   **2117**

My "medicine" was the thing that gained me entrance to these secret gardens of the self. It lay there, another world, in the self. I was permitted by my medical badge to follow the poor, defeated body into these gulfs and grottos.

Rosenthal ML, The William Carlos Williams Reader

Russell Brain; 1953   **2118**

Medicine alone takes as its province the whole man.... It is concerned with...man in all the complexity of his body and mind from his conception to his last breath; and its concerns extend increasingly beyond his sicknesses, to the conditions which make it possible for him to lead a healthy and a happy life.   *The Lancet*

Henry Louis Mencken; 1956   **2119**

It would be brutal to inflict scientific medicine upon the generality of American morons, for they never turn to it when they have clear choice. They always prefer patient medicine, chiropractic, faith healing or something worse. If the Federal bureaucracy ever really takes over the job of looking at their tongues, it should choose as its agents, not graduates of Class A medical schools, but such Hippocrateses of the folk as the heirs and assigns of Lydia Pinkham, Dr. Munyon, Brinkley (the great gland man), and Mary Baker G. Eddy.   *Minority Report: H. L. Mencken's Notebooks*

George White Pickering; 1965   **2120**

Medicine is perhaps the oldest of the technologies. It represents a skill based on a body of knowledge daily growing in extent and in exactitude, and applied to the limited end of alleviating human suffering.   *The Lancet*

George White Pickering; 1968   **2121**

It is apparently difficult for doctors to understand [hypertension as a quantitative, not qualitative disease] because it is a departure from the ordinary process of binary thought to which they are brought up. Is it normal or abnormal, physiological or pathological, health or disease, good or bad? Quantity is not an idea that is as yet allowed to intrude. Medicine in its present state can count up to two but not beyond.   *High Blood Pressure*

René Jules Dubos; 1968   **2122**
Throughout history, and whatever the level of civilization, the structure of medicine has been determined not only by the state of science but also by religious and philosophical beliefs. This is just as true of the most evolved urban and industrialized societies as it is of the most primitive populations. Like his Stone Age ancestors, modern man lives by myths.   *Man, Medicine, and Environment*

E. Mumford; 1970   **2123**
Medicine is the science of uncertainty and an art of probability.
From Students to Physicians

Rosemary Stevens; 1971   **2124**
In the bad old days when medicine was barely or rarely efficacious, it was possible to consider questions of purely professional development in a context dissociated from social welfare politics.... With the remarkable changes in the context and potential of medicine...the professional and political aspects of medicine have become inextricably intertwined.
American Medicine and the Public Interest

Oliver W. Sacks; 1973   **2125**
We rationalize, we dissimilate, we pretend: we pretend that modern medicine is a rational science, all facts, no nonsense, and just what it seems. But we have only to tap its glossy veneer for it to split wide open, and reveal to us its roots and foundations, its old dark heart of metaphysics, mysticism, magic and myth.   *Awakenings*

Thomas McKeown; 1976   **2126**
To assist us to come safely into the world and comfortably out of it, and during life to protect the well and care for the sick and disabled.
The Role of Medicine: Dream, Mirage, or Nemesis?

Lewis Thomas; 1979   **2127**
There is within medicine, somewhere beneath the pessimism and discouragement resulting from the disarray of the health-care system and its stupendous cost, an undercurrent of almost outrageous optimism about what may lie ahead for the treatment of human disease if we can only keep learning.   *The Medusa and the Snail*

Lewis Thomas; 1979   **2128**
For century after century, all the way into the remote millennia of its origins, medicine got along by sheer guesswork and the crudest sort of empiricism. It is hard to conceive of a less scientific enterprise among human endeavors. Virtually anything that could be thought up for the treatment of disease was tried out at one time or another, and, once tried, lasted decades or even centuries before being given up. It was, in retrospect, the most frivolous and irresponsible kind of human experimentation, based on nothing but trial and error, and usually resulting in precisely that sequence.   *The Medusa and the Snail*

Paul Starr; 1982   **2129**
The organizational culture of medicine used to be dominated by the ideals of professionalism and volunteerism which softened the underlying acquisitive activity. The restraint exercised by these ideals now grows weaker, the health center of one era is the profit center of the next.   *The Social Transformation of American Medicine*

Paul Starr; 1982   **2130**
From a relatively weak, traditional profession of minor economic significance, medicine has become a sprawling system of hospitals, clinics, health plans, insurance companies, and myriad other organizations employing a vast labor force.
The Social Transformation of American Medicine

Paul Starr; 1982   2131

Modern medicine is one of those extraordinary works of reason: an elaborate system of specialized knowledge, technical procedures, and rules of behavior. By no means are these all purely rational: our conceptions of disease and responses to it unquestionably show the imprint of our particular culture, especially its individualist and activist therapeutic mentality.... Few cultural relativists, suffering from a bad fever or a broken arm, would go so far to prove a point as to trade a modern physician for a traditional healer. They recognize, in behavior if not always in argument, that in medicine the dream of reason has partially come true.   *The Social Transformation of American Medicine*

Paul Zimmer; 1983   2132

When asked, I used to say,
"I want to be a doctor."
Which is the same thing
As a child saying,
"I want to be a priest,"
Or
"I want to be a magician,"
Which is the laying on
Of hands, the vibrations,
The rabbit in the hat
Or the body in the cup,
The curing of the sick
And the raising of the dead....   *What Zimmer Would Be*

Edward Janavel Huth; 1986   2133

Two functions are central to medicine: caring and knowing.... To survive we need to be able to read the world around us, to deduce what may harm us, to deduce what may help us. This is knowing. When we ask physicians to care for us, we expect them to know what they need to know to help us survive. They need a special knowledge of the world.
                                                                        The Pharos

Edward Shorter; 1991   2134

Can the profession recognize that, although its organic advances are of enormous value, they must be combined with concern for individuals' well-being—a well-being that provides psychological comfort and therefore promotes healing? Will doctors return to training students in the nearly abandoned "art of curing"? If not, despite brilliant new chemical and diagnostic knowledge, the medical profession will continue on its path of crisis and frustration. But if medicine can stretch sufficiently to be both an advanced science *and* a healing art, it will successfully fulfill its ancient aspirations in unprecedented ways.
                                                                  Doctors and Their Patients

Richard Gordon; 1993   2135

The history of medicine is not the testament of idealistic seekers after health and life.... The history of medicine is largely the substitution of ignorance by fallacies.
                                                              The Alarming History of Medicine

H. Jack Geiger; 1996   2136

Medicine must bring about change in the social order.   *A Life in Social Medicine*

Roy Porter; 1997   2137

Medicine has become the prisoner of its success. Having conquered many grave diseases and provided relief from suffering, its mandate has become muddled. What are its aims? Where is it to stop? Is its prime duty to keep people alive as long as possible, willy-nilly, whatever the circumstances? Is its charge to make people lead healthy lives? Or is it but a service industry, on tap to fulfil whatever fantasies its clients may frame for their bodies?

The Greatest Benefit to Mankind

Roy Porter; 1997   **2138**

Medicine is a notoriously messy mix of laboratory research and clinical crisis, the itch for knowledge and the need to act. Different experts contribute diverse skills, and the whole has been likened to a jigsaw [puzzle] being pieced together by total strangers, each of whom is only guessing at the picture.   *The New York Times*

MEDICINES

Benjamin Franklin; 1734   **2139**

Many dishes, many diseases; many medicines, few cures.   *Poor Richard's Almanac*

Thomas Jefferson; 1807   **2140**

The patient, treated on the fashionable theory, sometimes gets well in spite of the medicine.   *Letter to Dr. Caspar Wistar*

[Anonymous]; *circa* 1850   **2141**

"Six of the patients have died, sir," said the hospital nurse to the physician, as he went his rounds. "Why, I wrote medicine for seven," mused the doctor, passing to another ward. "Yes, but one of them wouldn't take his," was the naïve reply.

Dana CL, Proceedings of the Charaka Club

Josh Billings (Henry Wheeler Shaw); 1874   **2142**

There is no medicine like a good joke; it is a silver-coated pill that frolicks and phisicks on the run.   *Everybody's Friend*

Josh Billings (Henry Wheeler Shaw); 1874   **2143**

Phun is the best phisick i kno ov; it iz both cheap and durable.   *Everybody's Friend*

Robertson Davies; 1984   **2144**

When I was a boy[the] doctor...examined me gravely, asked questions that were searching [and] retired.... [He] emerged with a bottle from which he instructed me to drink three times a day.... I regarded the doctor as a magician.... My adult life my various doctors have given me medicine—it tends to be in pill form nowadays—which plainly comes from a pharmaceutical company, and I leave his office thinking of him as a middleman between me and a large pill works. He has lost his magic.

The Merry Heart. Can a Doctor Be a Humorist?

MEN

Lewis Thomas; 1983   **2145**

Childhood lasts considerably longer in the males of our species than in the females.

The Youngest Science

MENIÈRE SYNDROME

Prosper Menière; 1861   **2146**

These disturbances of function which have their origin in the internal auditory apparatus can give rise to attacks reputedly of cerebral origin, such as vertigo, dizziness, uncertain gait, staggering and falling, and are furthermore accompanied by nausea, vomiting and syncope.   *Gazette de Médecine*

MENOPAUSE

Hildegard of Bingen; *circa* 1150   **2147**
From her fiftieth, or sometimes from her sixtieth year, a woman feels some irritation and dries out around the windowlike sites of her body... Menstruation ceases and the uterus begins to shrink.
Causae et Curae

MENSTRUATION

Soranus of Ephesus; *circa* 150   **2148**
Menstruation, in most cases, first appears around the fourteenth year, at the time of puberty and swelling of the breasts.... The amount of secretion increases and after remaining the same for some time, it diminishes again and so it finally comes to an end, usually not earlier than forty, nor later than fifty years.... In some women menstruation continues till sixty.
Gynecology

Hildegard of Bingen; *circa* 1150   **2149**
For women, the rivulet of menstruation indicates her greenness and flowering that blooms in her offspring.
Causae et Curae

Mary Putnam Jacobi; 1877   **2150**
The habitual modesty of American speech often enforces silence...but from time to time the silence is broken, and it is plumply asserted that "during the temporary insanity of menstruation" female judgment is unreliable, even unsafe, because no form of mental action can be adequately carried on at that time.
The Question of Rest for Women During Menstruation

Mary Putnam Jacobi; 1877   **2151**
If it be said, "It is necessary that women rest during menstruation" we must ask necessary for what purpose? The preservation of life? Evidently not, since the most superficial observation shows thousands of women of all races and ages engaged in work of various degrees of severity without attempting to secure repose at the menstrual epoch.
The Question of Rest for Women During Menstruation

John Chalmers Da Costa; 1910   **2152**
Female suicide is most common at a menstrual period, as are acts of criminal violence and attacks of insanity.
Address to the American Philosophical Society

Edgar Allen; 1927   **2153**
Menstruation is a catabolic process due to the temporary absence of [ovarian follicular hormone] or its decrease below a subliminal amount after its anabolic influence has induced the growth of a certain amount of genital tissue.
Contributions to Embryology

Marge Piercy; 1983   **2154**
Some lesser number
of women in other bedrooms and bathrooms
See that red banner unfurl and mourn!
Another month, another chance missed.
The Watch

Katha Pollitt; 2001   **2155**
As Simone de Beauvoir noted, menstruation functions, misleadingly, as a bright line dividing the asexual child from the sexual female: parents treat their daughters differently once they get their periods, allowing them to dress more alluringly and to date boys; and girls, too, see their bodies differently.
London Review of Books

MENTAL HOSPITALS

Philippe Pinel; 1801   **2156**

Public asylums for maniacs have been regarded as places of confinement for such of its members as are become dangerous to the peace of society. The managers of those institutions, who are frequently men of little knowledge and less humanity, have been permitted to exercise towards their innocent prisoners a most arbitrary system of cruelty and violence; while experience affords ample and daily proofs of the happier effects of a mild, conciliating treatment, rendered effective by steady and dispassionate firmness.

Treatise on Insanity

MESSENGER RIBONUCLEIC ACID (MRNA)

François Jacob, Jacques Monod; 1961   **2157**

[The] system of regulation [of the rate of protein synthesis] appears to operate directly at the level of the synthesis by the gene of a short-lived intermediary, or messenger, which becomes associated with the ribosomes where protein synthesis takes place.

Journal of Molecular Biology

Sydney Brenner, François Jacob, Matthew Meselson; 1961   **2158**

The hypothesis put forward by Jacob and Monod [is] that the ribosomal RNA is not the intermediate carrier of information from gene to protein, but rather that ribosomes are non-specialized structures which receive genetic information from the gene in the form of an unstable intermediate or "messenger." We present here the results of experiments on phage-infected bacteria which give direct support to this hypothesis.   *Nature*

METABOLISM

Galen; [130-200]   **2159**

Since the substances of all animals are in perpetual flux, the whole body will be thus destroyed and dispersed, unless other similar substances be supplied to replace what has flowed away.   *Hygiene*

Gabriel Andral, Louis-Dominique-Jules Gavarret; 1843   **2160**

In the two sexes and at all ages, the quantity of carbonic acid exhaled by the lung is greater as the constitution is stronger and the muscular system more developed.

Annales de Chimie et de Physique

MICRO-ORGANISMS

Athanasius Kircher; 1658   **2161**

It is certain that the air, water and earth are filled with innumerable small animals; and furthermore that they can be demonstrated. It has been moreover known to everyone that worms grow from putrefying corpses; but since that admirable invention the microscope, it is known that everything putrid is filled with innumerable worms, invisible to the naked eye; which moreover I would not have believed had I not proved it by the experiments of many years.   *Scrutinium Pestis*

MICROSCOPE

Anton van Leeuwenhoek; 1676   **2162**

I have oft-times been besought, by divers gentlemen, to set down on paper what I have beheld through my newly invented *Microscopia*: but I have generally declined: first, because I have no style, or pen, wherewith to express my thoughts properly; secondly, because I have not been brought up to languages or arts, but only to business; and in the third place, because I do not gladly suffer contradiction or censure from others.

Philosophical Transactions of the Royal Society

MIGRAINE

Aretaeus the Cappadocian; [81-138?]   2163
If the head be suddenly seized with pain from a temporary cause... the disease is called Cephalalgia... In certain cases... the pain... remains in the half of the head. This is called Heterocrania.... If at any time it sets in acuity, it occasions unseemingly and dreadful symptoms... spasm and distortion of the countenance... nausea... vomiting.... [Patients] flee the light; the darkness soothes their disease... the patients wish to die.   *On Cephalaea*

Hildegard of Bingen; *circa* 1150   2164
Migraine stems from black bile and from all the other bad humors that are in a person. It strikes the middle of the head and not the entire head, so that it is sometimes located on the right side and sometimes on the left.... Migraine has such a force within itself that, if it occupied the entire head all at once, a person could not withstand it.   *Causae et Curae*

William Shakespeare; 1594   2165
Lord, how my head aches! what a head have I!
It beats as it would fall in twenty pieces.   *Romeo and Juliet, Act II, Scene v*

Alexander Pope; 1714   2166
And screen'd in Shades from Day's detested Glare,
She sighs for ever on her pensive Bed,
Pain at her Side, and Megrin at her Head.   *The Rape of the Lock*

John Fothergill; 1778   2167
There is a singular kind of glimmering in the sight,...then headache over one eye, or over both, sometimes over one parietal bone.... Sickness succeeds, in some cases only nausea.... Such an attack in a young person may last two or three hours; as the years pass on it is apt to continue longer, twenty-four hours or more, and the patients suffer with a violence scarcely to be endured, the least light or noise seems to throw them on the rack.   *Medical Observations and Inquiries*

William Heberden; 1802   2168
There is a dimness of sight in which dark spots float before the eyes, or only half, or some part of all objects appear, which continues for twenty or thirty minutes, and then is succeeded by a head-ach lasting for several hours, and joined sometimes with sickness.   *Commentaries on the History and Cure of Diseases*

William Heberden; 1802   2169
The hemicrania, or pain of one half of the head, was very early distinguished by medical writers from the other species of head-achs: but we have not yet advanced much in knowing how this differs from other pains of the head.   *Commentaries on the History and Cure of Diseases*

Leo M. Davidoff; 1952   2170
When the operation is over...all hell breaks loose. The pain seems to tear away from its moorings like a torpedo, and great swollen, humming pulses of pain streak through my temples and the base of the head. My face assumes a greenish pallor; I break out into a cold perspiration.... Even a dim light in the room sends additional shafts of pain through my eyes. I wish that I could vomit but usually cannot, and the thought of food is a revulsion and a mockery.... The underlying causes, I am convinced, are anxiety and tension.   *Pinner M and Miller BF, When Doctors Are Patients*

Oliver W. Sacks; 1972   2171
If migraine patients have a common and legitimate second complaint beside their migraines, it is that they have not been listened to by physicians. Looked at, investigated, drugged, charged: but not listened to.   *Migraine*

Joan Didion; 1979   2172

That no one dies of migraine seems, to someone deep into an attack, an ambiguous blessing.   *The White Album*

Seymour Diamond; 1979   2173

Patients with migraines know precisely when and how often and how long their headaches
strike. They often come in with long lists. When you have a patient with lists, you have
a patient with migraine.   *The New York Times*

Joseph Russell Elkinton, John R. Graham; 1985   2174

The symptoms of an attack were protean and distressing...usually one-sided and more frequently on the left...the periodicity varied between 10 and 21 days... That psychic factors
of anxiety and stress, as well as genetic factors, played a causative role in my migraine was
attested by its complete disappearance within six months after retirement, at the age of
62, from a hectic professional life in urban America to an unpressured life in rural
England. This was a dramatic and welcome escape from this almost life-long *bête noire*
that had afflicted this compulsive perfectionist personality.   *Cephalalgia*

MILIEU INTÉRIEUR

Claude Bernard; 1870   2175

There is a true interior environment [in the body] that serves as an intermediary between
the external world and life itself.... It is the internal environment that provides the physical needs for life.   *Lessons on the Phenomena of Life common to Animals and Vegetables*

MILITARY MEDICINE

Homer; *circa* 700 BC   2176

A man who can cut out shafts and dress our wounds—a good healer is worth a troop of
other men.   *The Iliad*

Raymund Mindererus; 1620   2177

An able and dextrous Chirurgion is a great Treasure in an Army, and cannot be enough
valued, especially if he consult in all dangerous cases with an understanding Physitian.
These two, Physitians and Chirurgions, are to be intimate friends together, assisting one
another without envy and pride, for the better relief and the greater safety of their
Patients.   *Medicina Militaris*

James Tilton; 1813   2178

Cleanliness is essential in all conditions of life, but especially to soldiers. Without the
necessary cautions on this score, an army is literally poisoned, and dwindles into insignif-
icance.   *Economical Considerations on Military Hospitals*

Dominique Jean Larrey; 1814   2179

My proposition [to provide rapid evacuation of the wounded from the field of battle] was
accepted, and I was authorized to construct a carriage, which I called the *flying ambulance*.   *Memoirs of Military Surgery*

James McGrigor; 1861   2180

It is not only in the sense of humanity, but in that of a sound policy and real economy,
that the state should provide able medical and surgical advice for the soldier when sick or
wounded.   *Autobiography and Services*

MILITARY SURGERY

Edmund Andrews; 1863   2181

In western warfare, the constant occurrence of battles in the forest, gives predominance
to the operations of skirmishers, who deliver their fire usually from the right hand side of

the trees that shelter them; in consequence of this, the right hand, arm, and shoulder, and the right thigh, knee, and leg, receive many more wounds than the left.

Chicago Medical Examiner

Edmund Andrews; 1863   2182

The enormous statistics of almost all our great battles [have] been lost to the profession, and the vast and costly experience of so much blood and death [have] been rendered worthless for the settlement of the many questions in practical surgery.

Chicago Medical Examiner

MILLER-ABBOTT TUBE

T. Grier Miller, W. Osler Abbott; 1934   2183

A new apparatus, involving the use of a newly developed double-lumened tube, for intubation of the human small intestine, and the technique for its employment are described.... The distal part of the apparatus will usually reach the upper ileum within about 6 hours.... The apparatus may be used to secure intestinal contents from, or to inject substances into, any area within the upper half of the intestinal tract or to secure records of pressure changes.   *American Journal of Medical Sciences*

MIND

Tobias Smollett; 1771   2184

I find my spirits and my health affect each other reciprocally—that is to say, everything that decomposes my mind produces a correspondent disorder in my body; and my bodily complaints are remarkably mitigated by those considerations that dissipate the clouds of mental chagrin.   *Humphry Clinker*

Ambrose Bierce; 1906   2185

Mind, *n*. A mysterious form of matter secreted by the brain. Its chief activity consists in the endeavor to ascertain its own nature, the futility of the attempt being due to the fact that it has nothing but itself to know itself with.   *The Devil's Dictionary*

MIRACLES

David Hume; 1748   2186

No testimony is sufficient to establish a miracle, unless the testimony be of such a kind that its falsehood would be more miraculous than the fact which it endeavors to establish.

An Enquiry Concerning Human Understanding. Of Miracles

Alexander Solzhenitsyn; 1968   2187

Whether they admit it as much or denied it, they all without exception in the depths of their hearts believed that there was a doctor, or a herbalist, or some old witch of a woman somewhere, whom you only had to find and get that medicine...to be saved.... It just wasn't possible that their lives were already doomed. However much we laugh at miracles when we are strong, healthy and prosperous, if life becomes so hedged and cramped that only a miracle can save us, then we clutch at this unique, exceptional miracle and—believe in it!   *Cancer Ward*

MITRAL REGURGITATION

James Hope; 1839   2188

When the mitral orifice is permanently patescent, so that, at each ventricular contraction, blood regurgitates into the auricle, this cavity suffers in a remarkable degree: for it is not only gorged with blood which it cannot transmit but, in addition, sustains the pressure of the ventricular contraction. Permanent patescence of the mitral orifice, therefore, constitutes an obstruction on the left side of the heart, and the effect of this, as of contraction of the orifice, may be propagated backwards to the right side.   *A Treatise on the Diseases of the Heart*

MITRAL STENOSIS

Raymond Vieussens; 1715   2189

The entrance of the left ventricle (mitral opening) being so contracted and its margin having lost all its natural suppleness, the blood could not freely and in adequate amount flow into the cavity of the left ventricle.... The trunk of the pulmonary vein began to dilate and the blood was blocked up in the lung.... Air could not freely enter or leave, which caused on the one hand the difficulty in breathing...and on the other the gradual seeping through of some of the serous fluid and its accumulation in the cavity of the chest.

Herrick J, A Short History of Cardiology

Jean-Nicolas Corvisart; 1806   2190

Of the preceding number of symptoms is a peculiar rushing like water, difficult to be described, sensible to the hand applied over the precordial region, a rushing which proceeds, apparently, from the embarrassment which the blood undergoes in passing through an opening which is no longer proportioned to the quantity of fluid which it ought to discharge.

Organic Diseases and Lesions of the Heart

René-Théophile-Hyacinthe Laennec; 1819   2191

The symptoms of ossification of the mitral valve are little different from those attending the same affection of the sigmoid.... According to M. Corvisart the principal sign of the former lesion is "a peculiar rustling sensation (bruissement) perceived on the application of the hand to the region of the heart."... When the purring-thrill co-exists with this—we may be assured that the left auriculo-ventricular orifice is contracted. This contraction is more frequently owing to ossification of the mitral valves than to any other cause.

Traité de l'Auscultation Médiate

René-Joseph-Hyacinthe Bertin; 1824   2192

When the disease affects the auriculo-ventricular orifice, we hear, during the contraction of the auricles, which continues longer than in the natural state, a very distinct sound, which resembles the sound of a blow given by a file on wood, or that of a bellows quickly pressed.

Treatise on the Disease of the Heart

Sulpice Antoine Fauvel; 1843   2193

I conclude from the facts presented in this communication, that an abnormal pre-systolic murmur, localized towards the apex of the heart...is the most probable stethoscopic sign of a stenosis of the left auriculo-ventricular orifice.

Archives de Médecine Général

Paul Louis Duroziez; 1877   2194

Approximately 50% of the patients admit a history of acute rheumatic fever.... *Pure mitral stenosis* causes embolism more often than do other lesions. The blood stagnates in the left atrium and creates conditions for embolism. This is one of the greatest dangers of *pure mitral stenosis*.... It may readily escape detection.... The lesion predisposes the patient...to aphasia and right hemiparesis. It is more common in women than in men.

Archives de Médecine Général

MITRAL-VALVE SURGERY

Charles P. Bailey; 1984   2195

When you talk about either me, or Dwight Harken, or Russell Brock, you really have to talk about the other two as well because, within a three-month period, entirely independently, each of us came out with the same ideas,...for mitral valve disease.... If any two of us had died the remaining one would have kept right on and would have brought out exactly the same final product. I just happened to be lucky enough to do the first operation on June 10, 1948.

Weisse AB, Conversations in Medicine

MOLECULAR BIOLOGY

Carl Friedrich Wilhelm Ludwig; 1858   2196
Whenever the body of an animal is subdivided to its ultimate parts, one always finally arrives at a limited number of chemical atoms.... One draws the conclusion in harmony with this observation, that all forms of activity arising in the animal body must be a result of the simple attractions and repulsions which would be observed in the coming together of those elementary objects.   *Quarterly Review*

MORTALITY

Lionel Trilling; 1950   2197
To a man who is aware of man's mortality, the world becomes significant and precious.
The Liberal Imagination. The Immortality Ode

Robert Buckman; 1992   2198
Despite all the best interventions of modern medicine, the death rate will always remain the same—precisely one per person.   *How To Break Bad News*

MOTHER AND CHILD

Galen; [130-200]   2199
I order all women who are nursing babies to abstain completely from sex relations. For menstruation is provoked by intercourse, and the milk no longer remains sweet. Moreover some women become pregnant, than which nothing could be worse for the suckling infant. For in this case the best of the blood goes to the foetus. For the latter, which has in it the intrinsic principle of life, is governed thereby, and constantly draws its proper nourishment, as if immovably rooted to the uterus night and day.   *Hygiene*

MULTIPLE MYELOMA

William MacIntyre; 1850   2200
Mr. M___ placed himself under my care on the 30th of October, 1845. He was then confined to the house by excruciating pains of the chest, back and loins.... [In] the post-mortem examination.... all the ribs... were soft and brittle.... Their interior was charged with a soft gelatinous substance of a blood-red colour.... The [spinal column] had the same morbid... structure which was discovered in the ribs and sternum.... Dr. Bence Jones.... succeeded in separating from the urine... a substance displaying... the peculiar reaction with nitric acid.   *Medico-Chemical Society Transactions*

MULTIPLE SCLEROSIS

Jean-Martin Charcot; 1880   2201
The trembling...does not show itself except on the occasion of intentional movements.... Nystagmus is a symptom of great diagnostic importance.... There are cases in which the nystagmus is wanting so long as the look remains vague, without precise direction; but it manifests itself suddenly, in a manner more or less marked so soon as the patients are requested to fix their attention on an object. A symptom more frequent still than nystagmus...is a peculiar difficulty in articulation.... The speech is slow, drawling, and now and again almost unintelligible.   *Clinical Lectures on Diseases of the Nervous System*

Wilhelm Nero Pilatus Barbellion (Bruce Frederick Cummings); 1919   2202
I am over 6 feet high and as thin as a skeleton; every bone in my body, even the neck vertebrae, creak at odd intervals when I move. So that I am not only a skeleton but a badly articulated one to boot. If to this is coupled the fact of the creeping paralysis, you have the complete horror. Even as I sit and write, millions of bacteria are gnawing away my pre-

cious spinal cord, and if you put your ear to my back the sound of the gnawing I dare say could be heard.   *The Journal of a Disappointed Man*

MUMPS

Hippocrates; [460-375 BC]   2203
Swellings appeared about the ears.... In all cases they disappeared without giving trouble, neither did any of them come to suppuration, as is common in swellings from other causes. They were of a lax, large, diffused character, without inflammation or pain... In some instances earlier, and in others later, inflammations with pain seized sometimes one of the testicles, and sometimes both.   *Of the Epidemics*

MUNCHAUSEN SYNDROME

Richard Asher; 1951   2204
Here is described a common syndrome... about which little has been written. Like the famous Baron von Munchausen, the persons affected have always travelled widely; and their stories, like those attributed to him [by Raspe] are both dramatic and untruthful. Accordingly the syndrome is respectfully dedicated to the baron and named after him. The patient... is admitted... with apparent acute illness.... Usually his story is largely made up of falsehoods.   *The Lancet*

Richard Asher; 1959   2205
Munchausen's syndrome: three main types.
A. Laparotomophilia migrans
With mainly abdominal symptoms.
B. Haemorrhagica histrionica.
C. Neurologica diabolica
Specialising in faints, fits, stupor.   *Transactions of the Medical Society of London*

MURMURS

René-Théophile-Hyacinthe Laennec; 1823   2206
[There are] many varieties [of murmurs]: file, grate, bellows, saw [they] indicate spasm only. I used to believe they indicated a[n] obstacle [to blood flow], but [it is] obvious from exper[ience or experiment?] that [this is] not so.   *Musée Laennec*

Peter Mere Latham; 1845   2207
Murmurs are to be caught quickly, and distinguished surely, and turned to a ready use, only by practice.   *Collected Works*

Peter Mere Latham; 1845   2208
The sounds, which naturally accompany the movements of the healthy heart, can only be learnt by the practice of listening to them. It is useless to describe them.   *Collected Works*

Austin Flint; 1860   2209
We have not yet done with the murmurs incident to anaemia. What is called the venous hum... is highly characteristic. This murmur is the continuous humming sound, sometimes musical, which the French writers call *bruit de diable*.... Reference... is had, not to his satanic majesty, but to the spinning top. The murmur often closely resembles that produced by this toy, which in France is known as *le diable*.   *Lecture*

R.D. Rudolph; 1905   2210
We all are too apt to conclude that the heart is organically diseased because murmurs are present...and it may be added, that we too easily assume that the heart is organically sound because murmurs happen to be absent. Either error leads to bad prognosis and treatment.   *International Clinics*

MUSCLE

William Croone; 1667   2211

The motion of a Muscle, is performed only by the Carnous Fibres, and... each Carnous
Fibre had a power of Contracting itself; I [offer] an Hypothesis of the Structure of one
Carnous Fibre, since the force of the whole Muscle is but an aggregate of the
Contractions of each particular Fibre.   *On the Reason of the Movement of the Muscles*

MYASTHENIA GRAVIS

Mary B. Walker; 1934   2212

The abnormal fatiguability in myasthenia gravis has been thought to be due to curare-like
poisoning of the motor nerve-endings.... It occurred to me... that it would be worthwhile
to try the effect of physostigmine, a partial antagonist to curare, on a case of myasthenia
gravis... in the hope that it would counteract the effect of the unknown substance which
might be exerting a curare-like effect.... Hypodermic injections of physostigmine did have
a striking though temporary effect.... It may be significant that physostigmine inhibits the
action of the esterase which destroys acetylcholine.   *The Lancet*

MYOSITIS OSSIFICANS

John Freke; 1740   2213

There came a boy...to ask of us...what should be done to cure him of many large Swellings
on his Back, which began about 3 years since, and have continued to grow as large on
many Parts as a Penny-loaf.... They arise from all the vertebre of the Neck, and reach down
to the Os sacrum.... Joining together in all Parts of his Back, as the Ramifications of Coral
do, they make, as it were, a fixed bony Pair of Bodice.

Philosophical Transactions of the Royal Society

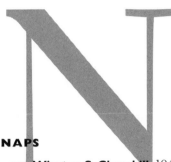

NAPS

Winston S. Churchill; 1948   **2214**

Nature had not intended mankind to work from eight in the morning until midnight
without that refreshment of blessed oblivion which, even if it lasts only twenty minutes,
is sufficient to renew all the vital forces.   *The Gathering Storm*

NARCOLEPSY

Thomas Willis; [1621-1675]   **2215**

They eat and drink well, go abroad, take care indifferently of their household affairs, but
in speaking, or walking, or eating, yea their mouthes being full of meat, they now and
then nod, and unless they are stirred up by others, they are presently overwhelmed with
Sleep.   *The Practice of Physick*

NARCOTICS

Samuel Johnson; 1770   **2216**

One night between the pain and the spasms in my stomach I was insupportably distressed. On the next night, I think, I laid a blister to my back and took opium, my night
was tolerable, and from that time the spasms in my stomach which disturbed me for
many years, and for two past harrassed almost to distraction have nearly ceased. I suppose
the breast is relaxed by the opium.   *Diary*

Ambrose Bierce; 1906   **2217**

Opiate, *n.* An unlocked door in the prison of Identity. It leads into the jail yard.
                                                                        The Devil's Dictionary

NATIONALISM

William Osler; 1902   **2218**

Breathes there a man with soul so dead that it does not glow at the thought of what the
men of his blood have done and suffered to make his country what it is? There is room,
plenty of room, for proper pride of land and birth. What I inveigh against is a cursed spirit of intolerance, conceived in distrust and bred in ignorance, that makes the mental atti-

tude perennially antagonistic, even bitterly antagonistic, to everything foreign, that subordinates everywhere the race to the nation, forgetting the higher claims of human brotherhood.   *Chauvinism in Medicine*

NATIVE AMERICAN MEDICINE

John Noble Wilford; 1972   2219
Some white man's hospitals don't cure the Navajos. They treat the illness, not the person. After an operation, a Navajo often goes to his medicine man to be purified, to be treated psychologically as well as physically.   *The New York Times*

Lewis Mehl-Madrona; 1997   2220
The patient must do seventy percent of the work of getting well. The Creator does twenty percent, and I do ten, which is barely worth mentioning.   *Coyote Medicine*

Lewis Mehl-Madrona; 1997   2221
We weren't used to people who were unwilling to sit in silence, who sought constant eye contact, who had a general lack of respect for illness, death, and dying.   *Coyote Medicine*

NATURE

Pliny the Elder; [23-79]   2222
It is far from easy to determine whether Nature has proved to man a kind parent or a merciless stepmother.   *Natural History*

Richard Selzer; 1984   2223
I stand in front of the hospital with its cargo of patients, doctors, nurses, and orderlies and let it filter through me to the blank page. Such a subject is, I have been told, not for the squeamish. Nor is it for those who cannot see that the truth is at least as accessible in ugliness as it is in beauty.... Nature makes no mistakes. Everything, beautiful or ugly, has its cause and purpose.   *Speech to the University of Dallas*

T.L. Dormandy; 1988   2224
The survival of complex organisms depends on a staggeringly fast turnover of its constituent units. Only under exceptional circumstances does Nature favour repair: anything remotely shop soiled or outworn is discarded and replaced. Theoretically this extravagance could be controlled from the production end, the rate of disposal of old cells being governed by the rate of production of new ones. For reasons unknown this is not what happens. In reality it is the rate of wastage that determines the rate of replacement. This implies a "self-destruct" programme built into every cell and a sensitive feedback.
The Lancet

NECROBIOSIS LIPOIDICA DIABETICORUM

Erich Urbach; 1932   2225
We are dealing with a severe degeneration of tissue below the cutis which leads to necrosis and an alteration of the vessels. The necrotic masses are enclosed by a fatlike substance and contain phosphates and calcium carbonate.   *Archives of Dermatolgy and Syphilis*

NEEDLE ASPIRATION

Samuel Shem; 1978   2226
There is no body cavity that cannot be reached with a #14 needle and a good strong arm.
The House of God

NEPHROBLASTOMA (WILMS TUMOR)

Max Wilms; 1899   **2227**

The patient was a 3-year old girl with a kidney tumor which had grown to immense proportions in a short time. The child, anemic and emaciated, was admitted with an enormous mass in the right abdomen and with definite ascites. After nephrectomy, the little child recovered uneventfully. A few months later, however, a recurring abdominal mass was again palpable and shortly afterward the child died. *Die Mischgeschwulste*

NERVES

Galen; [130-200]   **2228**

In all nerves there are both faculties, by which I mean the faculty of perception and the faculty of motion. *On Nerves, Veins, and Arteries*

Charles Bell; 1821   **2229**

The two sets of nerves distributed to the face have distinct functions.... If we have to plan an incision on the face, we must take especial care to avoid cutting the branches of the seventh nerve, for if it be divided, there will be paralysis of the muscles supplied by that nerve. Whereas, if we divide the fifth nerve, though there may be more pain during the operation, and a defect of sensibility following it, no unseemingly distortion will be produced. *Philosophical Transactions of the Royal Society*

François Magendie; 1822   **2230**

In a few moments I had cut all the pairs [of anterior roots] which I wished to divide... I made the section on one side only, in order to have a point of comparison. It may be conceived with what curiosity I observed the effects of this section: ...the member was completely immovable and flaccid, at the same time preserving an unequivocal sensibility. Finally, that nothing be neglected, I cut the anterior and posterior roots at the same time; there ensued absolute loss both of sensibility and of motion.

Journal de Physiologie et Experimentale Pathologie

Henry Pickering Bowditch; 1885   **2231**

It was found that stimulation of the nerve lasting from 1 1/2 to 4 hours...did not exhaust the nerve. Physiologists have long been in the habit of comparing nerves to telegraph wires, since they seem to be indifferent conductors transmitting impulses equally well in both directions. It would appear from these experiments that the absence of fatigue in consequence of activity is another very interesting point of resemblance. *Journal of Physiology*

NERVOUS SYSTEM

Hippocrates; [460-375 BC]   **2232**

And, for the most part, convulsions seize the other side of the body; for, if the wound be situated on the left side, the convulsions will seize the right side of the body; or if the wound be on the right side of the head, the convulsion attacks the left side of the body.

On Injuries of the Head

Aretaeus the Cappadocian; [81-138?]   **2233**

If...the commencement of the affection be below the head, such as the membrane of the spinal marrow, the parts which are homonymous and connected with it are paralysed: the right on the right side, and the left on the left side. But if the head be primarily affected on the right side, the left side of the body will be paralysed; and the right, if on the left side. *On Paralysis*

Thomas Willis; 1670   **2234**

We shall conclude... that the animal Spirits being brought from the Head by the passage of the Nerves to every Muscle (and it is very likely), received from the membranaceous fibrils, are carried by their passage into the tendinous fibres, as they are naturally nimble and elastick... and are permitted, expanding themselves, leap into the fleshy fibres.

Treatise on Hysteria and Hypochondria

Luigi Galvani; 1791   **2235**

From the things that have been ascertained and investigated thus far, I believe it has been sufficiently well established that there is present in animals an electricity which we... are wont to designate with the general term "animals".... It is seen most clearly in the muscles and nerves.   *Commentary on the Effects of Electricity on Muscular Motion*

William Heberden; 1802   **2236**

The power of moving in every part of the body by means of the muscles which obey the will, or by means of others the actions of which are involuntary; the various perceptions by the five external senses; and lastly those mental powers named memory, imagination, attention, and judgment, together with the passions of the mind; all these seem to be exercised by the ministry of the nerves; and are impaired, disturbed, or destroyed, in proportion to any injury done to the brain, the spinal marrow, and nerves, not only by their peculiar diseases, of which we know little, but by contusions, wounds, ulcers, and distortions, and by many poisons of the intoxicating kind.   *Commentaries on the History and Cure of Diseases*

Charles Bell; 1811   **2237**

In laying bare the roots of the spinal nerves [by vivisection in an experimental animal], I found that I could cut across the posterior fasciculus of nerves, which took its origin from the posterior portion of the spinal marrow without convulsing the muscles of the back; but that on touching the anterior fasciculus with the point of the knife, the muscles of the back were immediately convulsed.   *The Idea of a New Anatomy of the Brain*

Charles Bell; 1811   **2238**

I have to offer reasons for believing.... That the nerves of sense, the nerves of motion, and the vital nerves, are distinct through their whole course, though they seem sometimes united in one bundle; and that they depend for their attributes on the organs of the brain to which they are severally attached.   *The Idea of a New Anatomy of the Brain*

Marshall Hall; 1833   **2239**

The reflex function exists in the medulla independently of the brain; in the medulla oblongata independentaly of the medulla spinalis; and in the spinal marrow of the anterior extremities, of the posterior extremities, and of the tail, independently of that of each other of these parts, respectively.   *Philosophical Transactions of the Royal Society*

Johannes Müller; 1834   **2240**

Sensation... consists in the communication to the sensorium, not of the quality or state of the external body, but of the condition of the nerves themselves, excited by the external cause.   *Elements of Physiology*

John Hughlings Jackson; 1889   **2241**

Neural organization is dependent on, but distinct from, anatomical structure.

Croonian Lecture

Henry Hallett Dale; 1933   **2242**

We seem to need new words which will briefly indicate action by two kinds of chemical transmission, due in the one case to some substance like adrenaline, in the other case to a substance like acetylcholine, so that we may distinguish between chemical function and anatomical origin. I suggest the words "adrenergic" and "cholinergic," respectively, for use in this sense.   *Journal of Physiology*

Edgar Douglas Adrian; 1935   **2243**

If these records give a true measure of the activity in the sensory nerve fires it is clear that they transmit their messages to the central nervous system in a very simple way. The message consists merely of a series of brief impulses.... In any one fibre the waves are all of the same form.... In fact, the sensory messages are scarcely more complex than a succession of dots in the Morse code. *The Mechanism of Nervous Action*

NEURASTHENIA

E.H. Van Deusen; 1869 **2244**

As to the term "neurasthenia," it is an old term, taken from the medical vocabulary, and used simply because it seemed more nearly than any other to express the character of the disorder, and more definite, perhaps, than the usual term "nervous prostration." *American Journal of Insanity*

George Miller Beard; 1869 **2245**

I have for some time been in the habit of employing the term "neurasthenia" to express the morbid state that is commonly indicated by the indefinite phrase nervous exhaustion.... The diagnosis of the neurasthenic condition is sometimes entirely clear, and again is quite difficult. The diagnosis is obtained partly by the positive symptoms, and partly by exclusion. *Boston Medical and Surgical Journal*

Silas Weir Mitchell; 1877 **2246**

The woman grows pale and thin, eats little, or if she eats, does not profit by it. Everything wearies her—to sew, to write, to read, to walk—and by and by the sofa or the bed is her only comfort. Every effort is paid for dearly, and she describes herself as aching and sore. *Fat and Blood and How To Make Them*

William Osler; 1903 **2247**

A patient with a written list of symptoms—neurasthenia. *Aphorisms*

Edward Shorter; 1997 **2248**

Neurasthenia, like its grandchildren chronic fatigue syndrome and multiple chemical sensitivities a hundred years later, served as a bridge between supposedly organic causes and symptoms involving mood and cognition. *A History of Psychiatry*

NEUROFIBROMATOSIS

Friedrich von Recklinghausen; 1882 **2249**

The skin of the face...particularly the sides of the cheeks, which had little beard, was covered with small flat tumors averaging half the size of a pea.... On the crown of the head there was an especially large, firm nodule, the size of a cherry, with a partial stalk.... On the neck and trunk the nodules...were most numerous on the loins and sides.... My interest turned understandably to the externally palpable peripheral nerve trunks. *Multiple Fibromas of the Skin and Multiple Neuromas*

NEUROLOGY

Thomas Willis; 1664 **2250**

To describe all the several pairs of the spinal Nerves, and to rehearse all their branchings, and to unfold the uses and actions of them, would be a work of an immense labour and trouble: and as this Neurologie cannot be learned nor understood without an exact knowledge of the Muscles, we may justly here forbear entering upon its particular institution. *The Anatomy of the Brain and Nerves*

Thomas Willis; 1664 **2251**

Neurologie, the doctrine of the nerves. *The Anatomy of the Brain and Nerves*

Henry George Miller; 1974 **2252**

The peculiar charm of neurology lies in fact in the satisfaction implicit in its logical structure, and perhaps even more in the essentially clinical nature of the discipline.... The physical signs of a neurological disorder are for the most part unequivocal: the pathognomonic significance of the extensor plantar response is inevitably more clear-cut than that of the basal rale or the suspicion of ankle oedema. *British Clinical Journal*

NEUROTRANSMISSION

Alan Lloyd Hodgkin, A.F. Huxley; 1939   2253
We have recently succeeded in inserting micro-electrodes into the giant axons of squids.... A small action potential was recorded from the upper end of the axon and this gradually increased as the electrode was lowered, until it reached a constant amplitude of 80-95 mv.... The axon appeared to be in a completely normal condition, for it survived and transmitted impulses for several hours.... These results...prove that the action potential arises at the surface. *Nature*

NOMENCLATURE

Richard Lower; 1672   2254
Call your Catarrh a Rheum whene'er it flows
Towards the chest; if it to the throat it goes,
A Cough; and a Coryza, if to th' nose. *De Catarrhis*

Joseph Dalton Hooker; 1865   2255
What the devil is this "suppressed gout" upon which doctors fasten every ill they cannot name? If it is suppressed, how do they know it is gout? If it is apparent, why the devil do they call it suppressed? I hate the use of cant terms to cloak ignorance.
Letter to Charles Darwin

Edmund Andrews; 1868   2256
It is doubtful whether Prof. Bigelow is justified in coining this new name [litholapaxy] for a mere modification of lithotrity. It is best to be very slow to inflict new technical terms upon the memory of students. *Chicago Medical Examiner*

Oliver Wendell Holmes; 1871   2257
I have known the term "spinal irritation" [to] serve well on such occasions, but I think nothing on the whole has covered so much ground, and meant so little, and given such profound satisfaction to all parties, as the magnificent phrase "congestion of the portal system." *The Young Practitioner*

Thomas Lewis; 1944   2258
Diagnosis is a system of more or less accurate guessing, in which the end-point achieved is a name. These names applied to disease come to assume the importance of specific entities, whereas they are for the most part no more than insecure and therefore temporary conceptions. *The Lancet*

Martin H. Fisher; [1879-1962]   2259
When there is no explanation, they give it a name, which immediately explains everything. *Fred HL, Southern Medical Journal*

Sherwin B. Nuland; 1994   2260
To call a natural process by the name of a disease is the first step in the attempt to cure it and thereby thwart it. *How We Die*

NON-COMPLIANCE

Hippocrates; [460-375 BC]   2261
Keep a watch... on the faults of the patients, which often make them lie about the taking of things prescribed. For through not taking disagreeable drinks, purgative or other, they sometimes die. *Decorum*

NOSOCOMIAL INFECTION

Thomas Percival; 1803   2262
The inbred disease of hospitals will almost invariably creep, in some degree, upon one who continues a long time in them, but will rarely attack one whose stay is short.

Medical Ethics

NOSOLOGY

Percival Pott; 1765   2263
Clear and precise definitions of disease, and the application of such names to them as are expressive of their true and real nature, are of more consequence than they are generally imagined to be; untrue or imperfect ones occasion false ideas, and false ideas are generally followed by erroneous practice.   *Remarks on the Disease Commonly Called a Fistula-in-Ano*

John Moore; 1794   2264
To lay hold of the occasional symptoms which arise from the differences of constitution and other circumstances, and erect them into new diseases with terrifying names, burthens the memory, and tends to darken rather than elucidate.   *Medical Sketches*

NUCLEAR WAR

World Health Organization; 1984   2265
The only approach to the treatment of health effects of nuclear explosions is primary prevention of such explosions, that is, the prevention of atomic war.

Effects of Nuclear War on Health and Health Services

Lachlan Forrow, Bruce G. Blair, I. Helfland, and others; 1998   2266
Until the abolition of nuclear weapons reduces the annual probability to zero, our immediate goal must be to reduce the probability of a nuclear accident to as low a level as possible. Given the mass of casualties that would result from such an accident, achieving this must be among the most urgent of all global public health priorities.

New England Journal of Medicine

NURSES

[Anonymous]; 1857   2267
Lectured by Committees, preached at by chaplains, scowled on by treasurers and stewards, scolded by matrons, sworn at by surgeons, bullied by dressers, grumbled at and abused by patients, insulted if old and ill-favored, talked flippantly to if middle-aged and good humoured, seduced if young—they are what any woman would be under the same circumstances.   *Clendening L, Source Book of Medical History*

William Osler; *circa* 1900   2268
The trained nurse has become one of the great blessings of humanity, taking a place beside the physician and the priest, and not inferior to either in her mission.

Nurse and Patient

Peter Finley Dunne; 1901   2269
If th' Christyan Scientists had some science an' th' doctors more Christyanity, it wudden't make anny difference which ye called in—if ye had a good nurse.   *Mr. Dooley's Opinions*

Lewis Thomas; 1983   2270
The doctors worry that nurses are trying to move away from their historical responsibilities to medicine (meaning, really, to the doctors' orders). The nurses assert that they are their own profession, responsible for their own standards, co-equal colleagues with physicians.... The doctors claim that what the nurses really want is to become substitute psychiatrists. The nurses reply that they have unavoidable responsibilities for the mental

health and well-being of their patients, and that these are different from the doctors' tasks.... The arguments will work themselves out...but...some [intelligent agreement] will have to be found to preserve and strengthen the traditional and highly personal nurse-patient relationship.   *The Youngest Science*

NURSING

Florence Nightingale; 1859   2271

The most important practical lesson that can be given to nurses is to teach them what to observe—how to observe—what symptoms indicate improvement—what the reverse—which are of importance—which are of none—which are the evidence of neglect—and of what kind of neglect.   *Notes on Nursing*

Florence Nightingale; 1859   2272

In watching disease, both in private houses and in public hospitals, the thing which strikes the experienced observer most forcibly is this, that the symptoms or the sufferings generally considered to be inevitable and incident to the disease are very often not symptoms of the disease at all, but of something quite different—of the want of fresh air, or of light, or of warmth, or of quiet, or of cleanliness, or of punctuality and care in the administration of diet, of each or of all of these. And this quite as much in private as in hospital nursing.   *Notes on Nursing*

Florence Nightingale; 1859   2273

I use the word nursing for want of a better. It has been limited to signify little more than the administration of medicines and the application of poultices. It ought to signify the proper use of fresh air, light, warmth, cleanliness, quiet, and the proper selection and administration of diet—all at the least expense of vital power to the patient. It has been said and written scores of times, that every woman makes a good nurse. I believe, on the contrary, that the very elements of nursing are all but unknown.   *Notes on Nursing*

George Frank Lydston; 1904   2274

How absurd the situation! It is demanded that a woman should slave for three years and go through what would be a fair medical course, were it conscientiously given, for the privilege of finally earning a salary which, were she constantly employed—which, by the way, she never is—would just equal that of a good stenographer.   *New York Medical Journal*

NUTRITION

Claude Bernard; 1865   2275

We may, of course, strike a balance between what a living organism takes in as nourishment and what it gives out in excretions; but the results would be mere statistics incapable of throwing light on the inmost phenomena of nutrition in living beings. According to a Dutch chemist's phrase, this would be like trying to tell what happens inside a house by watching what goes in by the door and what comes out by the chimney.

An Introduction to the Study of Experimental Medicine

Oliver Wendell Holmes; 1891   2276

The pleasures of the palate are among the last gratifications allowed...and I suppose, if the second childhood could return to the food of the first, it might prove a wholesome diet.

Over the Teacups

Robert Hall Babcock; 1901   2277

We [now] devote more attention to the patient's diet and habits, and more often send him away with good advice than with hastily-written prescriptions.

Transactions of the American Clinical and Climatological Association

Croatian proverb   2278

Don't give the same food to the sick and the healthy.   *Proverb*

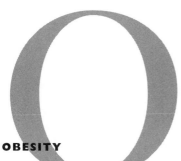

OBESITY

Hippocrates; [460-375 BC]   **2279**
Persons who are naturally very fat are apt to die earlier than those who are slender.

Aphorisms

Cotton Mather; 1724   **2280**
For Extreme Fatness...it may be a Diet of Milk, with *Dry Bread*, under due (progressive)
Limitations [that] may do the Business. After all; There [is] nothing like an *Obstinate
Abstinence* from all Sorts of Liquors; from *Drink* of all Kinds.   *The Angel of Bethesda*

Ernst von Leyden; 1882   **2281**
The concept "fatty heart" refers to cardiac symptoms in obese individuals in whom it is
assumed that they develop as a consequence of obesity.... The diagnosis between arteriosclerosis and a true fatty accumulation with weakening of the heart muscle is not
always possible and is based usually on the age of the patient and the condition of the
peripheral arteries.   *Zeitschrift für Klinische Medizin*

Cyril Connolly; 1945   **2282**
Obesity is a mental state, a disease brought on by boredom and disappointment.

The Unquiet Grave

Robert William Service; 1949   **2283**
This year an ocean trip I took, and as I am a Scot
And like to get my money's worth I never missed a meal
In spite of Neptune's nastiness I ate an awful lot,
Yet felt as fit as if we sailed upon an even keel.
But now that I am home again I'm stricken with disgust;
How many pounds of fat I've gained I'd rather not divulge:
Well, anyway, I mean to take this tummy down or bust,
So here I'm suet-strafing in the Battle of the Bulge.   *The Battle of the Bulge*

Richard A. Kern; 1951   **2284**
Obesity is the commonest disease in the United States. The aged are particularly prone
to it, when one by one other physical pleasures have been outlived or denied, and there
remains only the joys of the table.   *The Care of the Aged*

OBSTETRICS

Denslow Lewis; 1900   2285
There must be no maudlin sentimentality in these matters. The mother's life is the more important. Her interests are pre-eminent. Give her the benefit of the doubt. If there arises a question as to the relative value of the two lives, there can, it seems to me, be no difficulty in arriving at a decision.   *Clinical Review*

Denslow Lewis; 1900   2286
Fortunate is the obstetrician whose hand is small, but it is of greater importance that his hand be skilled.   *Clinical Review*

William Dock; 1968   2287
The proper training for obstetricians consists of nine months of internal medicine, about twenty minutes of obstetrics for multiparous births or two hours for primiparous, a dash of surgery for the occasional caesarean, and forty minutes of pediatrics.   *Medical Grand Rounds*

OCCUPATIONAL MEDICINE

Bernardino Ramazzini; 1713   2288
Not only in antiquity but in our own times also laws have been passed...to secure good conditions for the workers; so it is only right that the art of medicine should contribute its portion for the benefit and relief of those for whom the law has shown such foresight.... [We] ought to show peculiar zeal...in taking precautions for their safety. I for one have done all that lay in my power, and have not thought it beneath me to step into workshops of the meaner sort now and again and study the obscure operations of mechanical arts.   *De Moribus Artificum Diatriba*

Bernardino Ramazzini; 1713   2289
When a doctor arrives to attend some patient of the working class...let him condescend to sit down...if not on a gilded chair...on a three-legged stool.... He should question the patient carefully.... So says Hippocrates in his work "Affections." I may venture to add one more question: What occupation does he follow?   *De Moribus Artificum Diatriba*

OEDIPUS COMPLEX

Sigmund Freud; 1900   2290
Being in love with the one parent and hating the other form part of the permanent stock of psychic impulses which arise in early childhood and are of such importance as the material of the subsequent neurosis.... Antiquity has furnished us with legendary matter which corroborates this belief, and the profound and universal validity is explicable only by an equally universal reality of [this] hypothesis of infantile psychology. I am referring to the legend of King Oedipus and the *Oedipus Rex* of Sophocles.   *The Interpretation of Dreams*

ONCOGENES

Robert Joseph Huebner, G.J. Todaro; 1969   2291
Our hypothesis suggests that the cells of most or all vertebrate species have C-type RNA virus genomes that are vertically transmitted from parent to offspring. Depending on the host genotype and various modifying environment factors, either virus production or tumor formation or both may develop at some time in these animals and/or in their cells grown in culture. This hypothesis implies that the occurrence of most cancer is a natural biological event determined by spontaneous and/or induced derepression of an endogenous specific viral oncogene(s).   *Proceedings of the National Academy of Sciences*

OPHTHALMOSCOPY

Hermann von Helmholtz; 1851   2292

I have chosen the name Augen-spiegel for this [instrument].... The [optic nerve] is distinguished from the rest of the background of the eye by its whiteness.... Usually, the arteries and veins of the retina arise from the medial portion.... I have no doubt that it will be possible to diagnose all the pathologic conditions of the retina by visual observation.   *Beschreibung Eines Augen-Spiegels*

Hermann von Helmholtz; 1851   2293

The present treatise contains the description of an optical instrument, by which it is possible in the living to see and recognize exactly the retina itself and the images of the luminous objects which are cast upon it.   *Description of an Ophthalmoscope*

[Anonymous]; 1976   2294

An honest neurologist would admit that the most useful function of an ophthalmoscope is to provide a quiet time in the consultation, during which he may dwell upon the implications of the history just obtained. On a few occasions each year his ruminations will be interrupted by the appearance of gross papilloedema in a patient who appears otherwise surprisingly well.   *The Lancet*

ORTHOPAEDICS

Nicolas Andry de Bois-Regard; 1741   2295

As it is not within the reach of every Reader to understand the Title of Orthopaedia, which is affixed to this Book, I shall begin with explaining it.... I have formed it of two Greek Words, viz. *orthos*, which signifies streight, free from Deformity, and *paido*, a Child. Out of these two words I have compounded *Orthopaedia*, to express in one Term the Design I propose, which is to teach the different Methods of preventing and correcting the Deformities of Children.   *Orthopaedia*

ORTHOPNEA

Aretaeus the Cappadocian; [81-138?]   2296

The disease Orthopnoea is also called Asthma, for in the paroxysms the patients also pant for breath. The disease is called Orthopnoea, because it is only when in an erect position that they breathe freely; for when reclined there is a sense of suffocation. From the confinement in the breathing, the name Orthopnoea is derived. For the patient sits erect on account of the breathing; and, if reclined, there is danger of being suffocated.   *On Asthma*

OSLER, WILLIAM

Harvey Cushing; 1920   2297

[Osler] was pre-eminently the physician to physicians and their families, and would go out of his way unsolicited and unsparingly to help them when he learned that they were ill or in distress of any kind.   *William Osler, the Man*

Frederick Taylor Gates; 1928   2298

Osler's *Principles and Practice of Medicine* is one of the few scientific books possessed of literary attraction. There was a fascination about the style itself that lead me on and, having once started, I found a hook in my nose that pulled me from page to page, and chapter to chapter, until the whole of about a thousand closely printed pages brought me to the end.   *Chapters in My Life*

OSTEOMALACIA

Thomas Cadwalader; 1745   2299

[The patient] was seized...with a Diabetes, and the usual Symptoms...great Pains in her Shoulders, Back, and Limbs.... About the Beginning of Winter, 1740, she had such a Weakness and Pain in her Limbs as to confine her to Bed altogether; and in a few Months afterwards the Bones in her Legs and Arms felt somewhat soft to the Touch, and were so pliable, as to be bent into a Curve. *An Essay on the West-India Dry-Gripes*

Louis Arthur Milkman; 1933   2300

A New Skeletal disease, which is progressive, fails to respond to medication and may end fatally.... The characteristics of this disease are the disturbance in gait, pains in the back, and peculiar multiple symmetrical involvement of the skeleton.... The characteristic roentgenographic appearance is bands or zones of increased transparency seen throughout the involved bones of the skeleton. They are multiple and symmetrical.
Multiple Spontaneous Idiopathic Symmetrical Fractures

OSTEOPOROSIS

Ernst Ziegler; 1881   2301

If the compact osseous tissue becomes porous from the widening of the Haversian canals, the condition is termed *osteoporosis*.... In the vertebrae and in the bones of the extremities, both concentric and eccentric atrophy take place, the bony trabeculae being thereby in places thinner or even entirely absorbed. *A Text-Book of Special Pathological Anatomy*

C.A. Pfeiffer, W.V. Gardner; 1938   2302

Injection of estrogen into pigeons was followed by a rise in the serum calcium level and hypercalcification of the bone.... Most of the new bone was endosteal.... Osseous spicules extended into the marrow and interlaced to form spongy bone which occupied most of the former marrow space. *Endocrinology*

Fuller Albright, E. Bloomberg, P.H. Smith; 1940   2303

It is our belief that idiopathic osteoporosis is post-menopausal osteoporosis. Bones of male doves are osteoporotic as compared with those of female doves. Estrin therapy in male doves produces a marked increase in the density of the bone by stimulating the osteoblasts. Therefore, it was decided to try estrin therapy on patients with menopausal osteoporosis.... Estrin therapy has a very marked ability to put patients with post-menopausal osteoporosis into a positive calcium and phosphorus balance. Whether the effect of estrin...is sufficient to make its administration of practical value, it is as yet too soon to say.
Transactions of the Association of American Physicians

Fuller Albright; 1947   2304

Osteoporosis is defined as that category of decreased bone mass where the disturbance is a failure of the osteoblasts to lay down bone matrix.... Three factors which influence osteoblastic activity are.... steroidal hormones, mechanical stresses and strains, and nitrogenous building blocks. *Annals of Internal Medicine*

Stanley Wallach, Philip H. Henneman; 1959   2305

A 25-year retrospective study of the results of prolonged estrogen therapy in 292 postmenopausal women showed...excellent results...in the treatment of postmenopausal osteoporosis. *Journal of the American Medical Association*

Silvia Meema, Manzer Bunker, H. Erik Meema; 1975   2306

Eighty-two postmenopausal women.... were subdivided into four groups depending on the type of menopause (artificial or natural) and estrogen administration (treated or untreated).... The change in bone mineral mass per year in the estrogen-treated subjects... differed significantly from that in the untreated subjects.... The findings suggested that postmenopausal osteoporosis could be prevented by estrogen treatment.
Archives of Internal Medicine

OVARIES

Nicholas Culpeper; 1660   2307

The Stones of Women (for they have such kind of toys as well as men) differ from the Stones of men...for they are within the Belly in Women, but without in men.... The use of the Stones in Women, is the same that they are in Men, viz. To concoct seed.

A Directory for Midwives

Regner de Graaf; 1672   2308

The general function of the female testicles is to generate the ova, to nourish them, and to bring them to maturity, so that they serve the same purpose in women as the ovaries of birds. Hence, they should rather be called ovaries than testes because they show no similarity, either in form or contents, with the male testes.   *On the Female Testes or Ovaries*

Karl Ernst von Baer; 1827   2309

Examining the ovaries before making any incision I saw plainly in almost every follicle a yellowish-white point.... I opened one of the follicles and took up the minute object on the point of my knife, finding that I could see it very distinctly and that it was surrounded by mucus. When I placed it under the microscope, I was utterly astonished, for I saw an ovule just as I had already seen in the tubes, and so clearly that a blind man could hardly deny it.   *On the Genesis of the Ovum*

OXYGEN THERAPY

John Scott Haldane; 1917   2310

An ordinary 20-foot oxygen cylinder is fitted with a pressure gauge and adjustable governor of the type employed in mine-rescue apparatus. By means of the governor the delivery of oxygen can be varied at will from nothing to 10 litres a minute.... Where prolonged administration of oxygen seems desirable, the minimum quantity of oxygen which will remove the cyanosis should be carefully ascertained by observation of the patient, and the governor adjusted to give this minimum quantity, which is likely to be anything from 1 to 3 litres per minute.   *British Medical Journal*

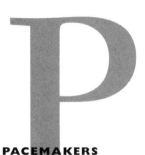

PACEMAKERS

Paul Maurice Zoll; 1952   2311

Effective ventricular beats were regularly produced in 2 patients with ventricular standstill after complete heart block by the application of electric stimuli from an artificial external pacemaker by way of subcutaneous needle electrodes. The heart was kept beating for twenty-five minutes in 1 patient, who finally died of cardiac tamponade, and for five days in the other, who recovered and ultimately resumed spontaneous idioventricular beats. In [this] patient...it was also possible to interrupt a slow idioventricular rhythm with a more rapid and effective, externally controlled rhythm.   *New England Journal of Medicine*

PAGET DISEASE OF BONE (OSTEITIS DEFORMANS)

James Paget; 1877   2312

Soon after the beginning of her pain [in the back and lower limbs] her daughters thought that she was losing in height, and that the shape of her head was changing [and] she had been becoming less tall.... Her head was certainly enlarged.... The femora were exceedingly curved outwards and forwards.... Similarly the tibae were curved forwards and were very large in their whole length.   *Medico-Chirurgical Transactions*

James Paget; 1877   2313

Altogether, the attitude in standing [of a middle-aged man Paget had observed for years] looked simian, strangely in contrast with the large head and handsome features.... [At necropsy] the contents of the Haversian canals were seen to consist generally of a homogeneous or granular basis, containing cells of round or oval form.... The presence of new bone was most evident in the periosteum of the tibia, external to the ordinary compact layer of the shaft.   *Medico-Chirurgical Transactions*

PAGET DISEASE OF THE NIPPLE

James Paget; 1874   2314

I believe it has not yet been published that certain chronic affections of the skin of the nipple and areola are very often succeeded by the formation of scirrhous cancer in the mammary gland.... In the majority [the affection] had the appearance of a florid, intensely red, raw surface...like the surface of very acute diffuse eczema.   *St. Bartholomew's Hospital Reports*

PAIN

Hippocrates; [460-375 BC]   **2315**
Let him shout during the cautery [for hemorrhoids] for that makes the anus stick out
more.   *On Hemorrhoids*

Cotton Mather; 1724   **2316**
WHAT is *Pain*? Tis a Sensation produced on the *Tension* of a *Nerve*.
                                                                     The Angel of Bethesda

Bernard Mandeville; 1729   **2317**
Hor. What an unspeakable and infinitely excruciating torment must it be, to be torn to
pieces, and ate alive by a savage beast!
Cleo. Not greater...than are daily occasioned by the gout in the stomach, and the stone in
the bladder.   *The Fable of the Bees*

Emily Dickinson; 1862   **2318**
Pain...cannot recollect
When it begun—or if there were
A time when it was not—
It has no future—but itself....   *Pain - Has an Element of Blank -*

John Hilton; 1863   **2319**
Pain the monitor, and Rest the cure, are starting points for contemplation which should
ever be present to the mind of the surgeon in reference to his treatment.   *Rest and Pain*

John Hilton; 1863   **2320**
Every pain has its distinct and pregnant signification, if we will but carefully search for it.
                                                                     Rest and Pain

Alphonse Daudet; *circa* 1895   **2321**
Pain is always new to the sufferer, but loses its originality for those around him.
                                                                     In the Land of Pain

Silas Weir Mitchell; 1896   **2322**
The Birth of Pain! Let centuries roll away;
Come back with me to nature's primal day.
What mightly forces pledged the dust to life!
What awful will decreed its silent strife,
Till through vast ages rose on hill and plain
Life's saddest voice, the birthright wail of pain.   *The Birth and Death of Pain*

Ambrose Bierce; 1906   **2323**
Pain, *n.* An uncomfortable frame of mind that may have a physical basis in something
that is being done to the body, or may be purely mental, caused by the good fortune of
another.   *The Devil's Dictionary*

Charles Horace Mayo; 1931   **2324**
Of all the symptoms for which physicians are consulted, pain in one form or another is
the most common and often the most urgent. Properly assessed, it stands pre-eminent
among sensory phenomena of disease as a guide to diagnosis.
                                Procedures of the Interstate Postgraduate Medical Association of North America

George Orwell (Eric Blair); 1934   **2325**
It is devilish to suffer from a pain that is all but nameless. Blessed are they who are strick-
en only with classifiable diseases! Blessed are the poor, the sick, the crossed in love, for at
least other people know what is the matter with them and will listen to their belly-achings
with sympathy.   *Burmese Days*

Dobrisa Cesaric; 1953   **2326**

Some walk with their pain
like an open wound for all to see.
The others crush it into themselves
and do not let it turn into tears and words.   *Poems*

Jean Stafford; 1953   **2327**

He had now to penetrate regions that were not anesthetized.... He began.... It was as if a tangle of tiny nerves were being cut dexterously, one by one.... The pain was a pyramid made of a diamond; it was an intense light; it was the hottest fire, the coldest chill, the highest peak, the fastest force, the furthest reach, the newest time.   *Children Are Bored on Sunday*

Henry George Miller; 1968   **2328**

A curiously moralistic attitude—probably Scottish in origin—makes tractotomy morally acceptable and heroin morally wrong for the treatment of intractable pain in carcinoma.
World Neurology

Isaac Asimov; [1920-1992]   **2329**

No decent human being would allow an animal to suffer without putting it out of its misery. It is only to human beings that human beings are so cruel as to allow them to live on in pain, in hopelessness, in living death, without moving a muscle to help them.
Basta LL, A Graceful Exit

PANCREATITIS

Reginald Heber Fitz; 1889   **2330**

Acute inflammation of the pancreas is both a well-characterized disease, and one which is much more frequent than is generally thought.... It has been repeatedly confounded with acute intestinal obstruction, and has thus led, in several instances, to an ineffective laparotomy; an operation which, in the early stages of this disease, is extremely hazardous.
Boston Medical and Surgical Journal

Reginald Heber Fitz; 1889   **2331**

We learn that pain was an early symptom in nearly one-half of the cases; that it was usually severe, and might be intense, and was to be found in the abdomen or lower chest.... The appearances found after death are conspicuously the hemorrhage within and near the pancreas.... It is evident that all treatment, at the onset, can be nothing but palliative.
Boston Medical and Surgical Journal

PAPANICOLAOU (PAP) SMEAR

George Nicholas Papanicolaou, Herbert Frederick Traut; 1941   **2332**

During the past two years we have collected and studied many hundreds of vaginal smears from normal women and those suffering from gynecologic diseases, and we feel that cells pathognomonic of cervical and fundal carcinoma can be definitely recognized. We are not yet in a position to offer a statistical proof of the reliability of this method of diagnosis, but we can say that in our experience it yields a high percentage of correct diagnoses when checked by tissue biopsies. There is evidence that a positive diagnosis may also be obtained in some cases of early disease.   *American Journal of Obstetrics and Gynecology*

PARADOXICAL PULSE

Adolf Kussmaul; 1873   **2333**

The pulsations of all arteries become smaller or disappear completely in regular intervals and return with expiration; this may be approached during normal heart action. I propose to call this pulse action paradoxical, partly on account of the great discrepancy between heart action and arterial pulse, partly because the pulse, although apparently irregular, is in reality waning and waxing in regular motion.   *Wiener Klinische Wochenschrift*

PARASITOLOGY

Nicolas Andry de Bois-Regard; 1700   2334
What I set myself to do here is to give a full treatise on worms, to explain how they reproduce in us, to describe the symptoms, the effects, the prognoses, to indicate the best treatments for this disease.   *An Account of the Breeding of Worms in the Human Body*

PARATHYROID GLANDS

Ivar Victor Sandström; 1879   2335
About three years ago I found on the thyroid gland...a small organ, hardly as big as a hemp seed, which was enclosed in the same connective tissue capsule as the thyroid, but could be distinguished therefrom by a lighter color. A superficial examination revealed an organ of a totally different structure from that of the thyroid, and with a very rich vascularity.... [I] suggest the use of the name *Glandulae parathyreoideae*; a name in which the characteristic of being bye-glands to the thyroid is expressed.
Uppsala Lakareforenings Forhandlingar

William George MacCallum, Carl Voegtlin; 1909   2336
The parathyroid secretion in some way controls the calcium exchange in the body.... The mechanism of the parathyroid action is not determined, but the result, the impoverishment of the tissues with respect to calcium and the consequent development of...tetany is proven. Only the restoration of calcium to the tissues can prevent this.
Journal of Experimental Medicine

James Bertram Collip; 1925   2337
An extract has been made from the parathyroid glands of oxen by the use of which parathyroid tetany in dogs can be prevented or controlled. The active principle in this extract produces its effect by causing the calcium content of the blood serum to be restored within normal limits.... Overdosage effects have been observed and the blood findings...invariably show hyperalcemia. The symptoms...are anorexia, vomiting, apathy, drowsiness verging into coma, and a failing circulation.   *Journal of Biological Chemistry*

Fuller Albright, Walter Bauer, Marian Ropes, Joseph C. Aub; 1929   2338
The calcium level in the blood is markedly but gradually elevated by parathormone injections.... Parathormone administration *abruptly* increases the urinary phosphorus excretion without affecting the fecal excretion. Following cessation of parathormone administration, the urinary phosphorus excretion rapidly falls to a level below that found before the administration.... These observations on the effect of parathormone suggest that an increased phosphorus excretion is the primary effect. The excreted phosphorus is partly derived from body fluids.   *Journal of Clinical Investigation*

PARKINSONISM

James Parkinson; 1817   2339
The patient can [rarely] form any recollection of the precise period of its commencement. The first symptoms perceived are, a slight sense of weakness, with a proneness to trembling in some particular part; sometimes in the head, but most commonly in one of the hands and arms.... The propensity to lean forward becomes invincible.... As the debility increases and the influence of the will over the muscles fades away, the tremulous agitation becomes more vehement.   *Essay on the Shaking Palsy*

James Parkinson; 1817   2340
Involuntary tremulous motion, with lessened muscular power, in parts not in action and even when supported; with a propensity to bend the trunk forwards, and to pass from a walking to a running pace: the senses and intellects being uninjured.
Essay on the Shaking Palsy

James Parkinson; 1817   2341

As...the influence of the will over the muscles fades away, the tremulous agitation becomes more vehement.... The motion becomes so violent as not only to shake the bed hangings, but even the floor and sashes of the room. The chin is now almost immovably bent down upon the sternum. The slops with which he is attempted to be fed, with the saliva, are continually trickling from the mouth. The power of articulation is lost. The urine and faeces are passed involuntarily; and at the last, constant sleepiness...announce the wished-for release.   *Essay on the Shaking Palsy*

George C. Cotzias, Melvin H. Van Woert, Lewis M. Schiffer; 1967   2342

Although small doses of [L-dopa] can reduce rigidity, the larger amounts used [in this study] are necessary to eliminate both rigidity and tremor. Some of the most striking results were obtained in patients who had advanced disease for which they had been subjected to intensive conventional, medical or surgical therapy before this study.... The sum of the evidence presented indicates that [L-dopa] is an effective agent for certain cases of Parkinson's disease and worthy of further investigation.   *New England Journal of Medicine*

PAROXYSMAL HEMOGLOBINURIA

George Harley; 1865   2343

The urine...assumed the colour of blood, a symptom which greatly alarmed him, as it recurred about three times a week during the whole of that winter.... The almost total absence of blood-corpuscles, notwithstanding the haemorrhagic appearance of the urine, stamps the case as being entirely different from ordinary haematuria...and leads to the conclusion [that it was] haemoglobin itself, which was extracted by the kidneys.   *Medico-Chirurgical Transactions*

William Howship Dickinson; 1865   2344

One morning he was seized with shivering, nausea, and pain in the loins; and when he passed urine, he found it was black and apparently bloody.... From the beginning of the disorder these [attacks] had always been of the same character. They owned no other cause but exposure to cold.... The urine was black and turbid; no blood-globules had ever been found.   *The Lancet*

PAROXYSMAL TACHYCARDIA

William Stokes; 1854   2345

The patient...was for some years the subject of long-continued attacks of violent and extraordinary palpitations, during which the action of the heart became greatly excited, extremely irregular, and attended by a loud bellows murmur.... I saw her again in about ten days; the heart's action was perfectly tranquil, the pulse natural, and every trace of murmur had disappeared.   *The Diseases of the Heart and Aorta*

Richard Payne Cotton; 1867   2346

I was consulted by a tradesman—a tailor, aged 42—on account of shortness of breathing, with a sense of general distress, which had lasted several days. It was the first attack of the kind he had had. The pulse was too rapid to be counted; the respirations were forty; and the *pulsations of the heart two hundred and thirty, in a minute*.... In about three weeks...the patient entirely recovered; the action of the heart becoming *suddenly* in every respect natural, and the pulse eighty in the minute.   *British Medical Journal*

Léon Bouveret; 1889   2347

I propose to give to this affection the name of essential paroxysmal tachycardia (tachycardie essentielle paroxystique).... Each paroxysm begins and ends suddenly in a few seconds.... The acceleration of the heart-beats is very extreme: in one attack 300 beats were counted.... The second observation shows us a very long and severe attack, accompanied by alarming disturbances of the pulmonary and of the system circulation, and which, after a duration of about three weeks, terminated in a fatal collapse.   *Revue de Médecine*

Léon Bouveret; 1889   **2348**

Each paroxysm begins and ends suddenly, in a few seconds. These sudden transitions from normal rhythm to a tachycardial rhythm and vice versa are accompanied sometimes by peculiar sensations in the head or in the precordial region. During the attack, the patient often feels a painful sensation of thoracic constriction with a little numbness of the left arm.   *Revue de Médecine*

PATCH TEST

Josef Jadassohn; 1896   **2349**

A robust young man consulted me last year for extensive dermatitis, the result of an inunction with gray ointment, which had been prescribed for pediculi pubis.... I applied a piece of gray plaster...on the upper part of the left arm. The following day the epidermis under the plaster was raised in a blister, the spot was surrounded by a redness resembling that of scarlatina.... There was very little fever, but serious subjective troubles. The eruption disappeared after a few days.   *Verhandlungen der Deutschen Gesellschaft für Dermatologie*

PATENTS

Henry Jacob Bigelow; 1847   **2350**

Discoveries in medical science, whose domain approaches so nearly to that of philanthropy, have been generally ranked with them; and many will assent with reluctance to the propriety of restricting by letters patent the use of an agent capable of mitigating human suffering.   *Boston Medical and Surgical Journal*

PATHOGENESIS

Galen; [130-200]   **2351**

Every activity of the living organism is connected with a separate part of the body whence it arises. Therefore, an activity is necessarily damaged when the part which produces it is affected.   *On the Affected Parts*

PATHOGNOMONIC EVIDENCE

William Osler; *circa* 1903   **2352**

One swallow does not make a summer, but one tophus makes gout and one crescent malaria.   *Aphorisms*

PATHOLOGY

René-Théophile-Hyacinthe Laennec; 1805   **2353**

If medicine has lost something with the destruction of the old companies known under the names of Faculties and Colleges, it has in a certain way made amends for the loss with the advantages for the advancement of science offered by the new organization of studies [in pathological anatomy].   *Journal de Médecine Vendemiaire*

René-Théophile-Hyacinthe Laennec; *circa* 1813   **2354**

[Pathology,] the painful career.   *Letter to his father*

René-Théophile-Hyacinthe Laennec; 1819   **2355**

Pathological anatomy is without doubt the most certain light to guide the physician...but...it is not easy to appreciate that which is healthy and that which is sick, that which is cause of the disease and that which is merely its effect.

Traité de l'Auscultation Médiate

Samuel David Gross; 1887   **2356**

It was from these dissections, from an elaborate course of reading, and from numerous visits to the pork and slaughter houses of Cincinnati, that I derived the knowledge upon which I founded my work on Pathological Anatomy.   *Autobiography*

[Anonymous]; 1958   **2357**

Apart from teaching, my job in life has centered round the examination of the body after death and the lesson which I am continually learning from post-mortem examinations is the versatility and courage, the ingenuity and determination with which the body strives to keep our house from tumbling about our ears.   *Coope R, The Quiet Art*

PATHOPHYSIOLOGY

Thomas Addison; 1855   **2358**

If Pathology be to disease what Physiology is to health, it appears reasonable to conclude, that in any given structure or organ, the laws of the former will be as fixed and significant as those of the latter; and that the peculiar characters of any structure or organ may be as certainly recognized in the phenomena of disease as in the phenomena of health.   *On the Constitutional and Local Effects of Disease of the Supra-Renal Capsules*

Berkeley George Andrew Moynihan; 1910   **2359**

No recognition has been accorded to the truth that in almost every particular the value of evidence obtained from the living out-weighs that which is disclosed upon the post-mortem table. It is not alone in respect of the pathological changes discovered in the conduct of an abdominal operation that a new knowledge is growing up, but also in reference to the clinical manifestations that are attached to these structural changes.   *The Pathology of the Living and Other Essays*

PATIENT-NURSE RELATIONS

W.U. McClenahan; 1974   **2360**

The bonds that hold patients together today spring chiefly from the detachment of doctors. Julia and the other nurses never asked me how I felt. They knew. They smiled occasionally, stayed close by and listened very well.   *G.P.*

PATIENT-PHYSICIAN RELATIONS

Hippocrates; [460-375 BC]   **2361**

The physician must have at his command a certain ready wit, as dourness is repulsive both to the healthy and to the sick.   *Decorum*

Hippocrates; [460-375 BC]   **2362**

For some patients, though conscious that their condition is perilous, recover their health simply through their contentment with the goodness of the physician.   *Precepts*

Plato; [427-347 BC]   **2363**

One who advises a sick man, living in a way to injure his health, must first effect a reform in his way of living, must he not? And if the patient consents to such a reform, then he may admonish him on other points? If...the patient refuses...it would be the act of a real man and a good physician to keep clear of advising such a man—the act of a poltroon and a quack...to advise him further on those terms.   *Dialogues. Letter VII*

Cicero; 45 BC   **2364**

Although physicians frequently know their patients will die of a given disease, they never tell them so. To warn of an evil is justified only if, along with the warning, there is a way of escape.   *De Divinatione*

Aulus Cornelius Celsus; [25 BC - AD 50]   **2365**

A practitioner of experience does not seize the patient's forearm with his hand, as soon as he comes, but first sits down and with a cheerful countenance asks how the patient finds himself; and if the patient has any fear, he calms him with entertaining talk, and only after that moves his hand to touch the patient.   *On Medicine*

Charaka; *circa* 78   **2366**

No other gift is greater than the gift of life! The patient may doubt his relatives, his sons and even his parents, but he has full faith in his physician. He gives himself up in the doctor's hands and has no misgivings about him. Therefore, it is the physician's duty to look after him as his own.   *Singh M, National Medical Journal of India*

Aretaeus the Cappadocian; [81-138?]   **2367**

Of chronic diseases the pain is great, the period of wasting long, and the recovery uncertain.... And if there also be the suffering from a painful system of cure,...the patients resile as truly preferring even death itself. Hence, indeed, is developed the talent of the medical man, his perseverance, his skill in diversifying the treatment, and conceding such pleasant things as will do no harm, and in giving encouragement. But the patient also ought to be courageous, and co-operate with the physician against the disease.

The Prooemium

Saint Augustine; 401   **2368**

The man who has tried a bad doctor is afraid to trust even a good one.   *Confessions IV*

Rhazes (Abu Bakr Muhammad Ibn Zakariya al-Razi); [864-930]   **2369**

When the disease is stronger than the patient, the physician will not be able to help at all, and the strength of the patient is greater than the strength of the disease, he does not need a physician at all. But when both are equal, then one needs a physician who will support the patient's strength and help him against the disease.

Maimonides M, The Preservation of Youth

Knights Hospitallers of St. John of Jerusalem; 1301   **2370**

We make a promise which no other people make, promising to be the serf and slave of our lords, the sick.   *Hume E, The Medical Works of the Knights*

Henri de Mondeville; [1260-1320]   **2371**

Keep up your patient's spirits by music of viols and ten-stringed psaltery, or by forged letters describing the death of his enemies, or by telling him that he has been elected to a bishopric, if a churchman.   *Garrison FH, An Introduction to the History of Medicine*

Albert de Zancariis; 1325   **2372**

The physician shows the patient three faces: divine, diabolical, and human. Divine when the patient is suffering from his illness and begs his physician to return him to health; diabolical when, recovered, the erstwhile patient flees his unpaid physician like the devil himself; and human when the patient has finally paid his bill and can acknowledge him as his master and friend.   *McVaugh MR, Bulletin of the History of Medicine*

John Donne; 1624   **2373**

I observe the *Phisician*, with the same diligence, as hee the *disease*; I see hee *feares*, and I feare with him: I overtake him, I overrun him in his *feare*, and I go the faster, because he makes his pace slow; I feare the more, because he disguises his fear, and I see it with the more sharpnesse, because hee would not have me see it. He knowes that his feare shall not disorder the practise, and exercise of his *Art*, but he knows that my *fear* may disorder the effect, and working of his practise.   *Devotions upon Emergent Occasions*

[Anonymous]; 1688   **2374**

In explaining a disease, when the case is thoroughly understood, one should announce the diagnosis like unfurling a banner from the rooftop of your house, or blowing a conch. But when the situation is confused, one should talk ambiguously, like a snake with a forked tongue.   *Tibetan Medical Thangas of the Four Medical Tantras*

Thomas Sydenham; [1624-1689]   **2375**

[The physician] must remember that he himself hath no exemption from the common lot, but that he is bound by the same laws of mortality, and liable to the same ailments and afflictions with his fellows. For these and like reasons let him strive to render aid to the distressed with the greater care...the kindlier spirit, and...the stronger fellow-feeling.   *Works*

Jean de la Bruyère; [1645-1696]   **2376**

As long as man is sick and wants to live, he will employ physicians and abuse them.

Dana CL, Proceedings of the Charaka Club

Bernardino Ramazzini; 1713   **2377**

When a doctor arrives to attend some patient of the working class, he ought not to feel his pulse the moment he enters, as is nearly always done without regard to the circumstances of the man who lies sick; he should not remain standing while he considers what he ought to do, as though the fate of a human being were a mere trifle; rather let him condescend to sit down for awhile.   *De Moribus Artificum Diatriba*

Benjamin Rush; 1782   **2378**

Never resent an affront offered to you by a sick man.... Never make light [to a patient] of any case.   *Letter to Dr. William Claypoole*

Samuel Johnson; 1784   **2379**

If the virtue of medicine could be enforced by the benevolence of the prescriber, how soon I should be well.   *Letter to Dr. Richard Brocklesby*

Benjamin Rush; 1789   **2380**

Let me advise you, in your visits to the sick, never appear in a hurry, nor to talk of indifferent matters, before you have made the necessary inquiries into the symptoms of your patient's disease.   *Duties of a Physician*

Benjamin Rush; 1789   **2381**

Do not condemn, or oppose, unnecessarily, the simple prescriptions of your patients. Yield to them in matters of little consequence, but maintain an inflexible authority over them in matters that are essential to life.   *Duties of a Physician*

William Buchan; 1798   **2382**

As matters stand at present, it is easier to cheat a man out of his life than a shilling, and almost impossible to either detect or punish the offender. Not withstanding this, people still shut their eyes, and take everything upon trust that is administered by any Pretender to Medicine, without daring to ask him a reason for any part of his conduct. Implicit faith, every where else the object of ridicule, is still sacred here.   *Domestic Medicine*

Thomas Percival; 1803   **2383**

Hospital physicians and surgeons should minister to the sick...reflecting that the ease, the health, and the lives of those committed to their charge depend on their skill, attention, and fidelity. They should study...in their deportment, so to unite tenderness with steadiness, and condescension with authority, as to inspire the minds of their patients with gratitude, respect, and confidence.   *Medical Ethics*

Thomas Percival; 1803   **2384**

The feelings and emotions of the patients, under critical circumstances, require to be known and to be attended to, no less than the symptoms of their diseases. Thus, extreme timidity, with respect to venaesection, contraindicates its use, in certain cases and constitutions. Even the prejudices of the sick are not to be condemned, or opposed with harshness. For though silenced by authority, they will operate secretly and forcibly on the mind, creating fear, anxiety, and watchfulness.   *Medical Ethics*

Samuel Taylor Coleridge; 1831   **2385**
He is the best physician who is the best inspirer of hope.   *Table Talk*

Peter Mere Latham; 1845   **2386**
I told them, however, what I knew of such cases, and made my little experience go as far as it would in the way of encouragement.   *Aphorisms*

Oliver Wendell Holmes; 1860   **2387**
Not one of these [physicians] was famous in the great world; some were almost unknown beyond their own immediate circle. But they have left behind them that loving remembrance which is better than fame, and if their epitaphs are chiselled briefly in stone, they are written at full length on living tablets in a thousand homes to which they carried their ever-welcome aid and sympathy.   *Currents and Counter-Currents in Medical Science*

Claude Bernard; 1865   **2388**
A physician...is by no means physician to living beings in general, not even physician to the human race, but rather, physician to a human individual in certain morbid conditions peculiar to himself and forming what is called his idiosyncrasy.
                              An Introduction to the Study of Experimental Medicine

Christian Albert Theodor Billroth; 1876   **2389**
The patient longs for the doctor's daily visit; it is the event upon which all his thoughts and emotions turn. The physician can do all he has to do with speed and precision, but he must never appear to be in a hurry, and never absent-minded.
                                     The Medical Sciences in the German Universities

Christian Albert Theodor Billroth; 1876   **2390**
A person may have learned a very great deal and still be an exceedingly unskillful physician, who awakens little confidence in his powers.... The manner of dealing with patients, of winning their confidence, the art of listening to them (the patient is always more anxious to talk than to listen), of soothing and consoling them, or of drawing their attention to serious matters—all this cannot be learned from books.
                                     The Medical Sciences in the German Universities

William Stokes; [1804-1878]   **2391**
Never hold that you have any property in a patient; be tolerant with the sick in their restless desire to seek other advice; preserve your independence; eschew servility.
                                                  William Stokes: His Life and Work

Daniel Webster Cathell; 1882   **2392**
The public love to see a doctor appear to know things intuitively, and you must study and practice to be quick in diagnosis, and ever ready in the treatment of the ordinary cares.... Remember this: Every one likes to believe that the doctor is treating him by a regular plan rather than firing at random.   *The Physician Himself*

William Osler; 1889   **2393**
Imperturbability.... It is the quality which is most appreciated by the laity though often misunderstood by them; and the physician who has the misfortune to be without it, who betrays indecision and worry, and who shows that he is flustered and flurried in ordinary emergencies, loses rapidly the confidence of his patients.   *Aequanimitas. Aequanimitas*

Jean-Martin Charcot; [1825-1893]   **2394**
Mme. Daudet was moved to anger by the brutal way [Charcot] told her husband that he was "incurable". He once said to a patient: "You're in the position of a man sitting in shit

with a sabre flashing above his head: either dive in or have your head cut off." If he was being tactful, he might announce bad news in Latin. *Daudet A, In the Land of Pain*

Sigmund Freud; 1895 **2395**

I wish to call your attention to a well-known fact, namely, that certain maladies and particularly the psycho-neuroses, are more accessible to psychic influences than to any other remedies. It is no[t] modern talk, but a dictum of old physicians, that these diseases are not cured by the drug, but by the doctor—to wit, by the personality of the physician in so far as he exerts a psychic influence. *Studies on Hysteria*

William Withey Gull; 1896 **2396**

Never forget that it is not a pneumonia, but a pneumonic man who is your patient. Not a typhoid fever, but a typhoid man. *Memoir*

William Osler; *circa* 1900 **2397**

Taking a lady's hand gives her confidence in her physician. *Aphorisms*

Silas Weir Mitchell; 1901 **2398**

I was inclined to gloomy prognostications, and this weakened my capacity to do good. And yet I was a conscientious man, and eager to do what was right. I have, however, observed that sanguine men, or men who deliberately and constantly predict relief or cure, are best. If failure comes, it explains itself, or may be explained. I knew once a foxy old country doctor, who said to me, "Hide your indecisions; tell folks they will get well; tell their friends your doubts afterwards." This may be one way of practicing a profession; it was not mine. *Circumstance*

[Anonymous]; 1902 **2399**

Modesty, simplicity, truthfulness!—cleansing virtues, everywhere but the bedside; there simplicity is construed as hesitation, modesty as want of confidence, truth as impoliteness. *Sprague JS, Medical Ethics and Cognate Subjects*

Richard C. Cabot; 1903 **2400**

A straight answer does not mean for me what is often called the "blunt truth," the "naked truth," the dry cold facts. The truth that I mean is a true *impression*, a fully drawn and properly shaded account such as is, as I well know, very difficult to give.... But better than either a misleading half truth or a pleasing lie, is an attempt to answer the patient's question that he shall see not only what he can't do and can't hope for, but what he can do and what there is to *work* for hopefully. *American Medicine*

George Frank Lydston; 1904 **2401**

Changing doctors is with some people a far less serious matter than a change of shirts. *New York Medical Journal*

William Osler; 1905 **2402**

To many of a somber and sour disposition it is hard to maintain good spirits amid the trials and tribulations of the day, and yet it is an unpardonable mistake to go about among patients with a long face. *The Student Life*

George Bernard Shaw; 1914 **2403**

Optimistic lies have such immense therapeutic value that a doctor who cannot tell them convincingly has mistaken his profession. *Misalliance, Preface*

John Chalmers da Costa; 1915 **2404**

The first patient I ever had stole my only umbrella. In those days I regarded my sign as a coffin plate on a stillborn business. *New York Medical Journal*

Robert Tuttle Morris; 1915 **2405**

It is the human touch after all that counts for most in our relation with our patients. *Doctors Versus Folks*

Franz Kafka; 1919   **2406**

To write prescriptions is easy, but to come to an understanding with people is hard.

A Country Doctor

Thomas Clifford Allbutt; 1922   **2407**

A successful physician once told me that he never left a house without giving a favourable prognosis; a counsel which had perhaps a colour of worldly wisdom about it; but this far he was right—that we cannot foresee what benediction words of hope may bestow.

Coope R, The Quiet Art

Francis W. Peabody; 1927   **2408**

The good physician knows his patients through and through, and his knowledge is bought dearly. Time, sympathy and understanding must be lavishly dispensed, but the reward is to be found in that personal bond which forms the greatest satisfaction of the practice of medicine. One of the essential qualities of the clinician is interest in humanity, for the secret of the care of the patient is in caring for the patient.

Journal of the American Medical Association

Lawrence Joseph Henderson; 1936   **2409**

A physician and a patient taken together make up a social system. They do so because they are two and because they have relations of mutual dependence. Also they are heterogeneous, they manifest sentiments, they have economic interests, they talk, reason, pretend to reason, and rationalize.   *Transactions of the Association of American Physicians*

Ulysses Grant Dailey; 1943   **2410**

Don't expect your doctor to be able to diagnose all cases at the first examination.

Chicago Defender

Mary Elizabeth Bates; 1948   **2411**

One must understand a patient physically and psychologically; one must be sympathetic and firm in treating a patient; and you have to have quick reactions. You can't be pokey and slow when treating sick people.   *Minney D, Medical Women's Journal*

Richard Asher; 1948   **2412**

Mental cruelty is common and arises in three ways: 1) by saying too much; 2) by saying too little; and 3) by the patient being forgotten.   *The Seven Sins of Medicine*

Richard Asher; 1948   **2413**

Other forms of bad manners are: 1) impatience in taking a history from a slow-witted patient; 2) making jokes at the expense of the patient; and 3) reading the patient's newspaper which lies on his bed and displays headlines far more exciting than the story the patient is telling.   *The Seven Sins of Medicine*

Tinsley R. Harrison; 1950   **2414**

The patient is no mere collection of symptoms, signs, disordered functions, damaged organs, and disturbed emotions. He is human, fearful, and hopeful, seeking relief, help, and reassurance. To the physician, as to the anthropologist, nothing human is strange or repulsive.   *Principles of Internal Medicine*

William Carlos Williams; 1951   **2415**

For me the practice of medicine has become the pursuit of a rare element which may appear at any time, at any place, at a glance. It can be most embarrassing. Mutual recognition is likely to flare up at a moment's notice. The relationship between physician and patient, if it were literally followed, would give us a world of extraordinary fertility of the imagination which we can hardly afford. There's no use trying to multiply cases, it is there, it is magnificent, it fills my thoughts, it reaches to the farthest limits of our lives.

Autobiography

Roscoe L. Pullen; 1952   **2416**

The greatest single quality which the intern should develop is that of compassion for the sick, the afflicted and the suffering.... No single attribute of medical practice is more demanding, more difficult to acquire and more exacting to maintain than the bond which exists between the patient and the doctor.   *The Internship*

Michael Balint; 1957   **2417**

"Advice" is usually a well-intentioned shot in the dark, is nearly always futile, and that applies even more strongly to "reassurance." We have found that it is more profitable both for doctors and patients to diagnose the problem; more often than not, when that is done there will be no need either for advice or for reassurance.

The Doctor, His Patient, and the Illness

T.F. Main; 1957   **2418**

The sufferer who frustrates a keen therapist by failing to improve is always in danger of meeting primitive human behaviour disguised as treatment.

British Journal of Medical Psychology

[Anonymous]; 1959   **2419**

In medicine, as in stagecraft and propaganda, words are sometimes the most powerful drugs we can use.   *Sara Murray Jordan's obituary in The New York Times*

Carl Gustav Jung; 1963   **2420**

My patients brought me so close to the reality of human life that I could not help learning essential things from them. Encounters with people of so many different kinds and on so many different psychological levels have been for me incomparably more important than fragmentary conversations with celebrities. The finest and most significant conversations of my life were anonymous.   *Memories, Dreams, Reflections*

Robert Platt; 1963   **2421**

There is a side to human behavior in health and disease which is not a thing of the intellect, which is irrational and emotional but important. It is the mainspring of most of what we do and a great deal of what we think, but is in danger of being neglected by clinical science.... How often, indeed, do we physicians omit to enquire about the basic facts of happiness and unhappiness in our patients' lives. Yet all this is just as much the live fabric of medicine as biochemistry and applied physiology.   *Universities Quarterly*

John Berger; 1967   **2422**

An unhappy patient comes to a doctor to offer him an illness—in the hope that this part of him, at least (the illness) may be recognizable.... Clearly the task of the doctor—unless he merely accepts the illness on its face value... —is to recognize the man.   *A Fortunate Man*

John Ellard; 1968   **2423**

When the patient's condition is diagnosed he needs to be told three things, in words that he can understand. He needs to be told what is wrong with him, what it may possibly mean in the future, and what medical science has to offer him.   *Medical Journal of Australia*

H. Jonas; 1969   **2424**

In the course of treatment, the physician is obligated to the patient and to no one else. He is not the agent of society, nor of the interests of medical science, the patient's family, the patient's co-sufferers, or future sufferers from the same disease. The patient alone counts when he is under the physician's care.   *Daedalus*

Paul Ramsey; 1970   **2425**

Birth and death, illness and injury are not simply events the doctor attends. They are moments in every human life. The doctor makes decisions as an expert but also as a man among men; and his patient is a human being coming to his birth or to his death, or being rescued from illness or injury in between. Therefore, the doctor who attends the case has reason to be attentive to the patient as a person.   *The Patient as Person*

Philip A. Tumulty; 1970   **2426**

His thoughtful management of the total problems of the sick person makes mere treatment of a disease or a symptom seem woefully inadequate. He is inexhaustibly capable of infusing into his patients insight, self-discipline, optimism and courage. Those he cannot make well, he comforts. Versed in medical science, he also understands human nature and enjoys working with it.... The things he works with are intellectual capacity, unconfined clinical experience, and the perceptive use of his eyes, ears, hands and heart.

New England Journal of Medicine

L. Tushnet; 1971   **2427**

The milk of human kindness may not be as effective as the proper medicine for an illness, but it tastes better.   *The Medicine Men*

W. C. Watson; 1972   **2428**

The patient also has or ought to have some freedoms—to get appropriate medical attention where and when he needs it, to be kept informed up to the limits of his understanding, to die if he prefers death to a miserable living. The doctor is not his patient's keeper, but his counsellor. One is the convenient relationship of master and servant, the other the mature and more difficult relationship between free men.

Canadian Medical Association Journal

Philip A. Tumulty; 1978   **2429**

The principal function of a clinician is to give substance at all times to this universal reaching out for hope.... A wise clinician molds the truth so that it always contains some hope, for he realizes that a state of acute or chronic anxiety induces important physiological reactions, as well as destructive emotional and interpersonal ones.

Johns Hopkins Medical Journal

Philip A. Tumulty; 1978   **2430**

There must be time for the patient to communicate himself to you, and you to him. Without adequate time, you cannot possibly give suffently of yourself to your patients. Time is what they expect and what they need.   *Johns Hopkins Medical Journal*

Neil Kessel; 1979   **2431**

The deepest level of reassurance is reached when a patient is told that, whatever he may have to go through in this illness, he will be able to bear it, "with my help." That is a great deal, but that is the medical contract.   *The Lancet*

Franz J. Ingelfinger; 1980   **2432**

If you agree that the physician's primary function is to make the patient feel better, a certain amount of authoritarianism, paternalism, and domination are the essence of the physician's effectiveness.   *New England Journal of Medicine*

William H. Crosby; 1980   **2433**

As a physician I would rather be humane than encyclopedic. I can always look up the information, but where can I find humanity?   *Forum on Medicine*

Erma Bombeck; 1981   **2434**

Ever since I told a crowded room I had a Bavarian cyst and not only did no one laugh, but two others had the same thing, I've been convinced that doctor and patient do not speak the same language. They speak Latin. We speak Reader's Digest.   *Syndicated column*

Norman Cousins; 1981   **2435**

If a doctor cannot hear [a patient's] cry above the electronic clatter of his technological armamentarium, he is not meeting the main need being put before him.

Human Options

Norman Cousins; 1981   **2436**

Patients.... want to feel that the doctor who is examining them is thinking of nothing else. If his telephone rings, they feel a break in the circuit and are pained.   *Human Options*

Lewis Thomas; 1983   **2437**

There, I think, is the oldest and most effective act of doctors, the touching. Some people don't like being handled by others, but not, or almost never, sick people. They *need* being touched, and part of the dismay in being very sick is the lack of close human contact.

The Youngest Science

Robertson Davies; 1984   **2438**

What do you look like to your patients? You hope that you look like a trustworthy professional man, and so you do, in most cases, though not all. But you look like something else, to the wretch who sits in the chair on the other side of your desk. You look like a god. Oh, yes you do.... Your patient may not think so—not consciously. But about your head shines a divinity, and it is extremely likely that somewhere in your consulting room the identifying symbol of the god appears.   *The Merry Heart. Can a Doctor Be a Humanist?*

Robertson Davies; 1984   **2439**

Stupidity...seeps like a corrosive poison through every level of society, and lays its blighting hand on every aspect of social, professional, political and cultural life.... What can you—what, as humanist physicians, must you do—to fight stupidity? First, you must assure your own complete inoculation against this plague by massive daily applications of art, music, and literature. Then you must do the most difficult thing of all: you must be wholly honest with your patients.   *The Merry Heart. Can a Doctor Be a Humanist?*

Don DeLillo; 1985   **2440**

We...anticipated questions the doctor would ask and rehearsed our answers carefully. It seemed vital to agree on the answers even if we weren't sure they were correct. Doctors lose interest in people who contradict each other. This fear has long informed my relationship with doctors, that they would lose interest in me, instruct their receptionist to call other names before mine, take my dying for granted.   *White Noise*

Don DeLillo; 1985   **2441**

"I'm never in control of what I say to doctors, much less what they say to me. There is some kind of disturbance in the air."
"I know exactly what you mean."
"It's like having a conversation during a space walk, dangling in those heavy suits."
"Everything drifts and floats."
"I lie to doctors all the time."
"So do I."   *White Noise*

Philip G. Ney, P. Margot Ney; 1986   **2442**

Seven [unspoken] questions [of the patient] make up the basis for a good doctor-patient relationship.... Do you understand me? Is it serious? Can you help me? Will you stick with me? Will you always treat me? Will you take advantage of my dependency? Will you always promote my health?   *Canadian Medical Association Journal*

Steven Radlauer; 1986   **2443**

When you are exhausted from trying to beat the odds against recovery, when you want only to cash in your chips and let them fall where they may, you do not ask your doctor to gamble with your life but to *stop* gambling. The physician who overrules the request, insisting...on rolling the medical dice again and again to see how the inevitable can be postponed, is the one who is gambling.   *The New York Times*

Arnold S. Relman; 1987   **2444**

A physician cannot easily serve his patients as trusted counselor and agent when he has economic ties to profit-seeking businesses that regard those patients as customers.

New England Journal of Medicine

Warfield T. Longcope; 1987   **2445**

The relationship between doctor and patient partakes of a peculiar intimacy. It presupposes on the part of the physician not only knowledge of his fellow men but sympathy.... This aspect of the practice of medicine has been designated as the art; yet I wonder whether it should not, most properly, be called the essence.

Manning PR and DeBakey L, Medicine: Preserving the Passion

Norman Cousins; 1989   **2446**

Just the fact of medical care raises hope. The medical profession would cease to exist were it not for the hopes of patients. The wise physician hesitates to squelch hope. He knows that the emotional needs of patients can affect the course of the disease. Moreover, one of the prime advantages of developing the patient's emotional and intellectual resources is that it sets a stage for the physician to do his best. *Head First*

Anatole Broyard; 1992   **2447**

In learning to talk to his patients, the doctor may talk himself back into loving his work. He has little to lose and everything to gain by letting the sick man into his heart.

Intoxicated by My Illness. Intoxicated by My Illness

Anatole Broyard; 1992   **2448**

To the typical physician, my illness is a routine incident in his rounds, while for me it's the crisis of my life. I would feel better if I had a doctor who at least perceived this incongruity. *Intoxicated by My Illness. The Patient Examines the Doctor*

John Langone; 1995   **2449**

Medical practice requires men and women who are devoted to people as well as to their own egos. *Harvard Med*

John M. Thorp Jr., S.R. Wells, W.A. Bowes Jr., R.C. Cefalo; 1995   **2450**

The unique nature of the physician-patient relationship must never be used to coerce a patient into complying with her physician's morality. *Hastings Center Report*

Jerome Lowenstein; 1997   **2451**

The call for the "old-time physician" is not a call for a wise old man with a little black bag and a few harmless (and useless) nostrums, but a yearning for communication in a common language. *The Midnight Meal and Other Essays*

Lewis Mehl-Madrona; 1997   **2452**

From a modern doctor's perspective, a patient is a bundle of biological matter, a collection of tissues to be rolled in and out of treatment, x-ray, and operating rooms. A doctor needs to know nothing about the soul wrapped in those tissues. *Coyote Medicine*

Paul S. Bellet; 1997   **2453**

When physicians are at the bedside, patients want their physicians to talk to them, not about them in case presentations. *New England Journal of Medicine*

Dwight C. McGoon; Unknown   **2454**

How does one take that long walk from the operating room to look into the eyes of a pathetic, frightened, crushed mother to tell her her child is dead or dying of a deformed heart that we couldn't fix, and then squeeze the father's arm as he struggles to gulp back a wave of spiritual and physical nausea? Your compassion for your patients—trying to do the best for them—must be the major motivating force in your effort to remain competent. *Ecstasy, a Basis for Meaning in the World*

PATIENTS

Arnald of Villanova; [1240-1311]   **2455**

Don't take it [the pulse] when you first get there[since it may be abnormal], especially if the patient is conscious and has been eagerly expecting you. Of course, if he isn't conscious, then he won't react with joy or fear to the arrival of a physician and his pulse won't change at all. *McVaugh MR, Bulletin of the History of Medicine*

Peter Mere Latham; 1845   **2456**

There is hardly a man living, be his disease what it may, who will bear to believe himself beyond the possibility of restoration to health. *Aphorisms*

Claude Bernard; 1865   **2457**

A physician... is by no means physician... to the human race, but, rather, physician to a human individual, and still more physician to an individual in certain morbid conditions peculiar to himself and forming what is called his idiosyncrasy.

An Introduction to the Study of Experimental Medicine

Thomas Frazier Rumbold; 1880   **2458**

It is absurd to expect a patient can be successfully treated, while he continues to violate the laws of health. *Hygiene and Treatment of Catarrh*

Alonzo Clark; [1807-1887]   **2459**

Every man's disease is his personal property. *Savitz HA, A Jewish Physician's Harvest*

George Bernard Shaw; 1906   **2460**

You ask me to go into the question of whether my patients are of any use either to themselves or anyone else. Well, if you apply any scientific test known to me, you will achieve a *reductio ad absurdum*. You will be driven to the conclusion that the majority of them would be, as my friend Mr J. M. Barrie has tersely phrased it, better dead.

The Doctor's Dilemma, Act III

[Anonymous]; 1921   **2461**

Patients come to us with symptoms, not with diseases; they...often say, "Doctor, I've got a heavy cold on me," very rarely, "I'm afraid I am infected with the *Micrococcus catarrhalis*." *The Lancet*

Berkeley George Andrew Moynihan; [1865-1936]   **2462**

The most important person present at an operation is the patient.

Bevan PG, Journal of Medical Biography

Lawrence Joseph Henderson; 1936   **2463**

You may in theory analyze a person into aspects, in practice you may not do so with impunity. "Half a sheep is mutton." *Address to the Association of American Physicians*

Lawrence Joseph Henderson; 1936   **2464**

It is impossible to understand any man as a person without knowledge of [his] environment and especially of what he thinks and feels it is; which may be a very different thing.

Transactions of the Association of American Physicians

Marguerite Yourcenar; 1951   **2465**

It is difficult to remain an emperor in [the] presence of a physician, and difficult even to keep one's essential quality as [a] man. *Memoirs of Hadrian*

Joseph Fletcher; 1954   **2466**

The patient is not a problem; he is a person with a problem. *Morals and Medicine*

A.E. Clark-Kennedy; 1962   **2467**

Clearly no disease can exist without a person to suffer from it. A disease is an abstraction. The patient is the concrete reality. *Kelly M, Archives of Internal Medicine*

Alvan R. Feinstein; 1967   **2468**

The patient is neither a disease to be discussed, nor a showcase of pathologic interest, nor a dispassionate bystander. He is a sick person in the alien environment of the hospital, disturbed by his illness and involved in it at least as much as the doctors. He is anxious to know what is happening, entitled to find out, and generally able to make helpful contributions to all aspects of his clinical management. *Clinical Judgment*

Eric J. Cassell; 1986   **2469**
Sick people, then, are people who are forced to trust. *Daedalus*

Robertson Davies; 1994   **2470**
We were assured, with sincerity, that our task in life was to relieve suffering. But never once did I hear anyone explain that the word patient really means "a sufferer".... Often the suffering was simple fear. *The Cunning Man*

Wendell Berry; 2000   **2471**
The frequent imsultingness of modern... medicine is precisely its inclination to regard individual patients apart from their lives, as representatives or specimens of their age, sex, pathology, economic status, or some other category. *Life is a Miracle*

Abraham Verghese; 2001   **2472**
All patients we see, no matter how often we see them or how benign we consider their illnesses to be, are in the midst of a story. For patients, the story begins the moment they walk through the portals of the hospital or through the doors of out-clinics.... There is danger in the visit, even a "routine" one, for, say, a mammogram... They have the desire not to hear bad news, and therefore there is drama—and therefore there is a story. *Annals of Internal Medicine*

PEER REVIEW

Roger Egeberg; 1968   **2473**
Peer review is going to take a lot of sacrifice by the medical profession, but who the hell else is going to evaluate physicians? *Journal of the American Medical Association*

George V. Mann; 1977   **2474**
To be a dissenter was to be unfunded because the peer-review system rewards conformity and excludes criticism. *New England Journal of Medicine*

Barry Commoner; 1978   **2475**
The business of having a paper—or a grant proposal—rejected is something like venereal disease: it is a far more widespread phenomenon than one would guess from the frequency of personal accounts. Most victims are too ashamed of the event, or too worried about its effect on their careers, to talk about it. *Hospital Practice*

PELLAGRA

François Thiérry; 1755   **2476**
There is one [complication] which characterizes [this disease] and makes it very easy to distinguish. This is a horrible crust, dry, scabby, blackish, crossed with cracks, which causes much pain...and throws off a very foetid odor. This crust may be upon the elbows, the arms, the head, the abdomen.... [After the crusts dry up] there remain red and shiny marks, very smooth, and denuded of hair.... The patients are attacked by a perpetual shaking of the head and indeed of all the upper part of trunk. This trembling is so often marked that they can scarcely keep on their feet.... At night they feel a burning which often deprives them of slumber. *Journal de Medico-chirurgie et Pharmacologie*

Gaspar Casal y Julian; 1762   **2477**
The distinctive and inseparable symptoms of this disease are: ...constant trembling of the head,...the burning pain of the mouth, vesicles on the lips, and a coating on the tongue,...the distressing weakness of the entire body, especially of the legs,...the crusts of the metacarpals and metatarsals and a sort of collar on the upper part of the neck,...the scorching heat which torments them, especially in the chest[and] the heaviness, which...causes them to give way to a sad crying. *Historia Natural y Medica*

Francesco Frapolli; 1771   **2478**

I have retained the name *Pellagra* already employed to signify the entire disease....
Pellagra...is called by me a chronic malady of the entire body, in which the most common
symptoms are desquamation in the spring of the parts exposed to the sun, delirium, vertigo...pains in the spine and in the extremities, weakness of the lower parts.... Sig Odoardi
already recognizes, that Pellarina owed its origin to a deficiency of diet.

Animadversiones in Morbum

Joseph Goldberger; 1928   **2479**

One may ask, therefore, why, if the matter is so simple [a dietary deficiency] do so many
people continue to be stricken with the disease? The answer lies in the fact...that the
problem of pellagra is in the main a problem of poverty.

Address to the American Dietetic Association

PENICILLIN

Alexander Fleming; 1929   **2480**

A species of penicillium produces in culture a very powerful antibacterial substance which
affects different bacteria in different degrees.... The least sensitive bacteria are the Gram-
negative bacilli, and the most susceptible are the pyogenic cocci.... In addition to its possible use in the treatment of bacterial infections penicillin is certainly useful...for its
power of inhibiting unwanted microbes in bacterial cultures so that penicillin insensitive
bacteria can readily be isolated.... The name "penicillin" has been given to filtrates of both
cultures of the mould.   *British Journal of Experimental Pathology*

Ernest Boris Chain, H.W. Florey, A.D. Gardner, and others; 1940   **2481**

Penicillin is active in vivo against at least three of the organisms inhibited in vitro....
Penicillin does not appear to be related to any chemotherapeutic substance at present in
use and is particularly remarkable for its activity against the anaerobic organisms associated with gas gangrene.   *The Lancet*

Edward P. Abraham; Ernest Boris Chain, C.M. Fletcher, and others; 1941   **2482**

A description is given of the cultural and other conditions required for the effective production of penicillin by *Penicillium notatum*; and of methods of small-scale mass production and assay of material suitable for therapeutic use in man.... Penicillin was given intravenously to five patients with staphylococcal and streptococcal infections.... In all these
cases a favourable therapeutic response was obtained.   *The Lancet*

PENIS

Michel de Montaigne; 1580   **2483**

The indocile liberty of this member is very remarkable, so importunately unruly in its
tumidity and impatience, when we do not require it, and so unseasonably disobedient
when we stand most in need of it: so imperiously contesting in authority with the will,
and with so much haughty obstinacy denying all solicitation, both of hand and mind.

Essays. On the Force of Imagination

Nicholas Culpeper; 1660   **2484**

The Glans is the extreme part of the Yard, soft, and of an exquisite feeling, by reason of
thinness of the skin wherewith it is covered; it is covered with the Praeputiam, or fore skin,
which in some men cover the top of the Yard quite close, in others it doth not, which
moving up and down in the act of Copulation, brings pleasure both to the Man and
Women.   *A Directory for Midwives*

Robert Whytt; 1751   **2485**

We cannot, by an effort of the will, either command or restrain the erection of the penis;
and yet it is evidently owing to the mind; for sudden fear, or anything which fixes our

attention strongly and all at once, makes this member quickly subside, though it were ever so fully erected. *An Essay on the Vital and Other Involuntary Motions of Animals*

William H. Masters, Virginia E. Johnson; 1966   **2486**
The functioning role of the penis is as well established as that of any other organ in the body. Ironically, there is no organ about which more misinformation has been perpetrated. The penis constantly has been viewed but rarely seen. The organ has been venerated, reviled, and misrepresented with intent in art, literature, and legend through the centuries. *Human Sexual Response*

PEPTIC ULCER

Jean Cruveilier; 1829   **2487**
There is first an erosion of the mucosa.... The erosion or inflammation becomes an ulcer.... Simple ulcer...does not present other than a gross resemblance to cancerous ulcerÖ The best proof, however, that these ulcerations are not cancerous is their curability.... The [principal] symptoms are...loss of appetite or bizarre appetite, insurmountable distress, difficult digestion,...heavy pains in the epigastrium, and sometimes epigastric pain extremely sharp during the process of digestion or indeed when there is no food in the stomach.... The patient has the sensation of an enemy who is always present. *Anatomie Pathologique du Corps Humain*

Berkeley George Andrew Moynihan; 1910   **2488**
In the differentiation from gastric ulcer there is, as a rule, no great difficulty. If pain after food does not appear for two hours or more, it may be said with reasonable confidence that the ulcer is in the duodenum.... If pain appears early, within an hour or so, the ulcer is certainly in the stomach, probably on the lesser curvature.... The period of relief from pain conferred by the taking of a meal is then the first and a chief point to be considered in the differential diagnosis. *Duodenal Ulcer*

Bertram Welton Sippy; 1915   **2489**
The treatment consists essentially in accurately protecting the ulcer from gastric juice corrosion until healing of the ulcer takes place. *Journal of the American Medical Association*

William J. Mayo; 1915   **2490**
It is interesting to speculate as to what diagnoses were made in the cases of duodenal ulcers prior to our present knowledge. *Journal of the American Medical Association*

Albert E. Coates; 1946   **2491**
Patients [in prison camps] with peptic ulcer were regularly "milked" for acid which was used for patients suffering from hypochlorhydria. *Surgery*

Barry J. Marshall; 1983   **2492**
The...description of S-shaped spiral bacteria in the gastric antrum, by my colleague Dr. J. R. Warren, raises the following questions: ...are they pathogens...and are they campylobacters?... The pathogenicity of these bacteria remains unproven but their association with polymorphonuclear infiltration in the human antrum is highly suspicious. If these bacteria are truly associated with antral gastritis, as described by Warren, they may have a part to play in other poorly understood, gastritis associated diseases (i.e., peptic ulcer and gastric cancer). *The Lancet*

Barry J. Marshall, J. Robin Warren; 1984   **2493**
The bacteria [first called *Campylobacter*, but later corrected to *Helicobacter pylori*] were present in almost all patients with active chronic gastritis, duodenal ulcer, or gastric ulcer and thus may be an important factor in the aetiology of these diseases. *The Lancet*

Croatian proverb   **2494**
Troubles waste the stomach like rust wastes iron. *Proverb*

PERCUSSION

Leopold Auenbrugger (Elder von Auenbrugg); 1761   2495

The signs of scirrhus of the lungs—With the finding of the resonance impaired or totally suppressed in the affected parts of the thorax, the patients are more rarely afflicted with
a cough.   *On Percussion of the Chest*

Leopold Auenbrugger (Elder von Auenbrugg); 1761   2496

I here present the Reader with a new sign I have discovered for detecting diseases of the
chest. This consists in the Percussion of the human thorax, whereby, according to the
character of the particular sounds thence elicited, an opinion is formed of the internal
state of that cavity.   *On Percussion of the Chest*

PERIARTERITIS NODOSA

Adolf Kussmaul; 1866   2497

There is a certain affliction of the arteries...which we call periarteritis nodosa and...begins
in the intima, alters the contour of the arteries...and sometimes decreases the lumen and
hinders the flow of blood. Such a disease attacks...only the smaller arteries of selected
organs and systems, to be exact, the inner organs of the lower abdomen, of the heart and
voluntary muscles, and may develop acutely. Death may occur in a few weeks after the
first sign of serious illness.   *Deutsch Archiv der Klinische Medizin*

PERICARDIAL FLUID

Richard Lower; 1669   2498

When [the pericardial sac] is full in hydrops Cordis, and the walls of the organ are compressed...by the surrounding fluid to such an extent, that they are unable to dilate sufficiently to receive the blood, the heart beat diminishes greatly,...until at length it is completely suppressed...and syncope and death result. A similar process can be seen in
hydrops pectoris, where the lung is unable to distend sufficiently.   *A Treatise on the Heart*

PERICARDITIS

Guillaume de Baillou (Ballonius); 1735   2499

Water contained in the sac of the heart, likewise if the sac contain within either a fluid
putrid and smelling badly, or stones, it causes throbbing.... Adhesions of the pericardium
to the body of the heart itself...was observed in two dropsical patients.

Consiliorum Medicinalium

Albrecht von Haller; 1755   2500

The pericardium was everywhere attached to the heart...and all over the surface of the
pericardium there were white patches, some hard, others filled with a whitish material like
pus. Through these patches the heart was united to the pericardium.

Opuscula Pathologica

V. Collin; 1824   2501

We have only once observed the sound analogous to the creaking of new leather. It
occurred in a patient who died of chronic pericarditis. This sound continued for the first
six days of the disease, but disappeared as soon as the local symptoms indicated a slight
liquid effusion into the pericardium.... Perhaps this sound would be a constant symptom
of pericarditis before the occurance of liquid effusion fugacious in cases where the disease
runs its course in a short time, but of longer duration in chronic cases.

Sound Analogous to the Creaking of New Leather

Norman Chevers; 1842   2502

Complete and close adhesion of the pericardial surfaces, far from producing hypertrophy
dilatation, has a tendency to be followed by general diminution in the size of the heart

and its vessels and contraction of its cavities.... The principal cause of dangerous symptoms...of the above description appears to arise from the occurrence of gradual contraction in the layer of adhesive matter which has been deposited around the heart, compressing its muscular tissue and embarrassing its systolic and diastolic movement, but more particularly the latter. *Guy's Hospital Reports*

Walter Broadbent; 1895   2503

I am permitted to publish the notes of four cases...in each of which there is visible retraction, synchronous with the cardiac systole, of the left back in the region of the eleventh and twelfth ribs, and in three of which there is also systolic retraction of less degree in the same region of the right back. In all cases there is a definite history of pericarditis.

The Lancet

PERICARDIUM

Richard Lower; 1669   2504

Nature [has] placed various glands round the base of the heart. From these fluid trickles out [and] bathes the entire surface of the heart, and thereby renders its movement more ready and more easy of accomplishment.... This fluid is not entirely excretory...but rather part of the nutrient Serum oozing from the blood.... It sets into white jelly when heated only a very little. *A Treatise on the Heart*

PERITONITIS

William Gullen; 1792   2505

Among the inflammations of the abdominal region, I have given a place in our Nosology to the Peritonitis, comprehending under that title, not only the inflammations affecting the peritonaeum lining the cavity of the abdomen, but also those affecting the extensions of this membrane in the omentum and mesentery. *First Lines of the Practice of Physic*

PERNICIOUS ANEMIA

James Scarth Combe; 1824   2506

His face, lips and the whole extent of the surface, were of a deadly pale colour.... He complained...of weakness; his respiration...became hurried on the slightest exertion.... His bowels are very irregular, generally lax;...his stools are very dark and foetid;Ö[his] appetite impaired; of late his stomach has rejected almost every sort of food.... He is forty-seven years of age.... [Six months later] the oedema had extended over his face and upper extremities, and evident marks of effusion into the chest presented themselves. He died in a few weeks. *Transactions of the Medico-Chirurgical Society of Edinburgh*

Austin Flint; 1860   2507

The patients entered with intense anaemia.... Loss of appetite was a prominent symptom.... Diarrhoea was more or less prominent before death, but this was not due to intestinal lesions, as shown by examinations after death.... I suspect that in these cases there exists degenerative disease of the glandular tubuli of the stomach. *Lecture*

George Richards Minot, William Parry Murphy; 1926   2508

Forty-five patients with pernicious anemia...are continuing to take a special diet...for from about six weeks to two years...composed especially of foods rich in complete proteins and iron—particularly liver.... Following the diet, all the patients showed a prompt, rapid and distinct remission of their anemia, coincident with at least rather marked symptomatic improvement, except for pronounced disorders due to spinal cord degeneration.

Journal of the American Medical Association

William Bosworth Castle; 1929   2509

The foregoing experiments clearly demonstrate that the stomach contents of a normal man recovered during the digestion of a meal of beef muscle and subsequently incubated with additional hydrochloric acid contain a substance capable of causing remissions in certain cases of pernicious anemia comparable to those produced by moderate amounts of liver. *American Journal of Medical Science*

PERTUSSIS (WHOOPING COUGH)

Guillaume de Baillou (Ballonius); 1736   2510

Fevers attacked boys of four months, of ten months and a little older, countless numbers of whom died. Principally that common cough, which is usually called *Quinta* or *Quintana*.... Serious are the symptoms of this.... For they are without this troublesome coughing for...four or five hours...then this paroxysm of coughing returns, now so severe that blood is expelled with force through the nose and through the mouth.

Opera Omnia

PEUTZ-JEGHERS SYNDROME

Harold Jeghers, Victor A. McKusick, K.H. Katz; 1949   2511

This syndrome consists of two features: distinctive melanin spots of the buccal mucosa and lips... and polyposis... of the small intestine.... [It] appears to be inherited as a simple mendelian dominant. *New England Journal of Medicine*

PHARMACOLOGY

Richard Lower; 1669   2512

For many years at Oxford I saw others at work, and myself, for the sake of experiment, injected into the veins of living animals various and emetic solutions, and many medicinal fluids of that sort. *A Treatise on the Heart*

Johann Christian Reil; 1797   2513

Scientific pharmacology requires a complete knowledge of the nature of the drug in all its conditions, especially chemical.... We still do not know the specific and general constituents and especially not the quantitative condition of many medicines. As long as there are still gaps, a scientific treatment of pharmacology is not possible.... The only way to render pharmacology more complete is therefore to perform experiments, record the results accurately and subsume isolated experiences under higher laws.

Beitrag zu den Prinzipien für Jede Zukünstige Pharmakologie

John Jacob Abel; 1892   2514

This science tries to discover the physical and chemical changes that go in a living thing that has absorbed a substance capable of producing such changes, and it also attempts to discover the fate of the substance incorporated. It is not therefore an applied science, like therapeutics, but it is one of the biological sciences, using that word in its widest sense.

Pharmacology Era

PHARMACOPOEIA

Medical Society of the State of New York; 1818   2515

A uniform system of preparing, and compounding medicines, throughout the United States, would contribute much to the satisfaction of the practitioner.... The traveller finds different preparations, under the same name, in almost every village, town, or city...for so multifarious are the names of medicines, that a name which is common in one town may be unknown in another, or what is worse, be applied to a very different medicine. Therefore, Resolved, That it is expedient that a Pharmacopoeia should be formed for the use of the United States. *Anderson L and Higby GJ, The Spirit of Voluntarism*

PHILOSOPHY

Hugo Roesler; 1960   **2516**

A thesis which has never been written: "The Relations of the Theories of Philosophers to the Status of their Endocrine Organs."   *Temple University Medical Center Bulletin*

Earle P. Scarlett; 1972   **2517**

In these days we should be proclaiming the fact that uniformity and dull conformity are a crime against the intelligence and are indeed the sad abortion of creation. At a time when science both inside medicine and without is increasingly concerning itself with practical affairs and is ceasing to be related in any way to the fundamental problems of the meaning and purpose of life, it is imperative that a place be found for philosophy and its business of inquiring into the meaning of things.   *Roland CG, In Sickness and in Health*

PHRENOLOGY

Ambrose Bierce; 1906   **2518**

Phrenology, *n.* The science of picking the pocket through the scalp. It consists in locating and exploiting the organ that one is a dupe with.   *The Devil's Dictionary*

PHYSICAL EXAMINATION

Hippocrates; [460-375 BC]   **2519**

He should observe thus in acute diseases: first, the countenance of the patient, if it be like those of persons in health, and more so, if like itself, for this is the best of all; whereas the most opposite to it is the worst, such as the following: a sharp nose, hollow eyes, collapsed temples; the ears cold, contracted, and their lobes turned out; the skin about the forehead being rough, distended, and parched; the colour of the whole face being green, black, livid, or lead-coloured.   *The Book of Prognostics*

René-Théophile-Hyacinthe Laennec; 1819   **2520**

If auscultation by itself cannot, as Hippocrates supposed, detect the presence of a fluid in the chest, we obtain at least from the writings of this great man...a sign very characteristic of this affection, in one particular form of it. This method of exploration...consists in shaking the patient's trunk, and at the same time listening to the sounds thereby produced.   *Traité de l'Auscultation Médiate*

René-Théophile-Hyacinthe Laennec; 1819   **2521**

The natural sound of the chest, on percussion, fails over the whole space occupied by the fluid. From this result simply, we could not indeed be certain whether the disease is pleurisy or pneumonia.... But mediate auscultation...enables us to ascertain with precision, not merely the existence of the effusion, but its quantity. The signs by which the stethoscope effects this are, 1st, the total absence, or great diminution, of the respiratory sound; and, 2nd, the appearance, disappearance, and return of aegophony.   *Traité de l'Auscultation Médiate*

Josef Skoda; 1839   **2522**

That the lungs partially deprived of air, should yield a tympanitic, and when the quantity of air in them is increased, a non-tympanitic sound appears opposed to the laws of physics. The fact...is corroborated both by experiments on the dead body...and also by this constant phenomenon, viz.: that when the lower portion of a lung is entirely compressed by any pleuritic effusion, and its upper portion reduced in volume, the percussion-sound at the upper part of the thorax is distinctly tympanitic.   *Auscultation and Percussion*

William H. Byford; 1864   **2523**

I think we shall less frequently regret a thorough, although somewhat indelicate examination, when dictated by an honest and intelligent conviction of its necessity, than regret a neglect of such examination from too great a deference to the mere shame of our patients.   *Chronic Inflammation and Displacements of the Unimpregnated Uterus*

Robert Hall Babcock; 1891   **2524**

Physical signs that may exist in one individual without there being even a suspicion of tubercle, may afford in another indubitable evidence of their existence; hence, the term *normal*, so far as physical signs are concerned, is purely a relative one.

North American Practitioner

William Osler; *circa* 1900   **2525**

Failure to examine the throat is a glaring sin of omission, especially in children. One finger in the throat and one in the rectum makes a good diagnostician.   *Aphorisms*

William Osler; *circa* 1900   **2526**

The four points of a medical student's compass are: Inspection, Palpation, Percussion, and Auscultation.   *Aphorisms*

William Osler; *circa* 1900   **2527**

Make a thorough inspection. Never forget to look at the back of a patient. Always look at the feet. Looking at a woman's legs has often saved her life.   *Aphorisms*

William J. Mayo; 1938   **2528**

Sometimes I wonder whether today we take sufficient care to make a thorough physical examination before our patient starts off on the round of the laboratories, which have become so necessary that oftentimes we do not fully appreciate the value of our five senses in estimating the condition of the patient.

Collected Papers of the Mayo Clinic and Mayo Foundation

Maxwell M. Wintrobe; 1975   **2529**

Physical examination must be carried out with a watchful eye, a sensitive touch, discerning ears, and an alert sense of smell. Above all, what is needed is an alert mind, free of dogma and routine. Each clinical problem, no matter how routine it may appear to be on the surface, calls for an unprejudiced approach. Each possible clue must be pursued; nothing can be taken for granted.   *Medical Journal of St. Joseph Hospital*

PHYSICIAN-ASSISTED SUICIDE

Willard Gaylin, Leon R. Cass, Edmund D. Pelligrino, and others; 1988   **2530**

This issue touches medicine at its very moral center; if this...collapses, if physicians become killers or are even merely licensed to kill, the profession—and, therewith, each physician—will never again be worthy of trust and respect as healer and comforter and protector of life in all its frailty. For if medicine's power over life may be used equally to heal or to kill, the doctor is no more a moral professional but rather a morally neutered technician.   *Journal of the American Medical Association*

Jack Coulehan; 1997   **2531**

We should devote our attention to developing more compassionate medicine and a public policy that encourages more equitable care, rather than embarking precipitously on a policy of palliation-by-death. Dying patients do have a right to high-quality care and to a caring society that embraces its suffering members rather than discarding them.... The movement towards state-regulated physician-assisted suicide and euthanasia will surely move us somewhere, but not closer to each other.   *Annals of Internal Medicine*

PHYSICIAN HEALTH

Hippocrates; [460-375 BC]   **2532**

The dignity of a physician requires that he should look healthy, and as plump as nature intended him to be; for the common crowd consider those who are not of this excellent bodily condition to be unable to take care of others.   *The Physician*

Galen; [130-200]   **2533**
That physician will hardly be thought very careful of the health of his patients if he neglects his own.   *On Protecting the Health*

Marin Drzic; 1549   **2534**
Who was not sick cannot understand the ill.   *Tirena*

C. McKevitt, M. Morgan; 1997   **2535**
Doctors' ideas about their own illnesses are clearly bound up with questions about identity and role. Illness appears to compromise both.... Changing doctors' attitude to their own health, through the education of medical students,...will be insufficient if the organization of medical work does not facilitate taking sick leave and if prevailing generations of doctors, now employers and trainers, continue to transmit the notion that illness does not belong to doctors.   *Journal of the Royal Society of Medicine*

C. McKevitt, M. Morgan; 1997   **2536**
Illness doesn't belong to us. It belongs to them, the patients. Doctors need to be taught to be ill. We need permission to be ill and to acknowledge that we are not superhuman.
Journal of the Royal Society of Medicine

Herbert S. Waxman; 1997   **2537**
Unquestionably, my experiences as a patient changed my behavior as a physician. Although I had always thought of myself as a capable, caring internist and hematologist, my medical education had not prepared me to care for patients as well as did the added experience of having myself been a patient. How might it have been otherwise? It is hardly practical to require that every physician have a serious illness as part of the process of preparing to care for patients.... It may prove helpful, however, to listen carefully to physicians who have been patients.   *Annals of Internal Medicine*

PHYSICIANS

Homer; *circa* 700 BC   **2538**
For who ever himself seeks out and bids to the feast a stranger from afar, save only one of those that are craftsmen of the people, a prophet or a healer of ills, or a shipwright or even a godlike minstrel, who can delight all with his song? Nay, these are the men that are welcome over all the wide earth.   *The Odyssey*

Hippocrates; [460-375 BC]   **2539**
Many are physicians by repute, very few are such in reality.   *The Law*

Plato; [427-347 BC]   **2540**
Socrates, must we not have good physicians in our city? And they would be the most likely to be good who had treated the greatest number of healthy and diseased men.
The Republic

Plato; [427-347 BC]   **2541**
It is true enough of physicians that the ablest might prove to be men who, from childhood up, besides mastering their profession, had been in contact with the largest number of the worst cases, and moreover were not of a robust constitution and had themselves suffered from every malady.   *The Republic*

Ovid; [43 BC - 17 AD]   **2542**
A dire pestilence came upon my people.... So long as the scourge seemed of moral origin and the cause of the terrible plague was still unknown, we fought against it with the physician's art.... No one can control the pest, but it fiercely breaks out upon the very physicians, and their arts do but injure those who use them. The nearer one is to the sick and the more faithfully he serves them, the more quickly is he himself stricken to death.

Metamorphoses

Martial (Marcus Valerius Martialis); 40-104   **2543**
Jack supped - and drank - and went to bed.
Morn breaks - and finds him dead.
What caused this healthy man's perdition?
Alas! he dreamt of his Physician.   *Epigrams VI, 53*

[Anonymous]; *circa* 700   **2544**
He should keep his hair and nails clipped close and trim; he should be clean in his personal habits and should wear white garments. He should carry an umbrella, keep a walking stick and wear shoes. His dress should not be ostentatious and his mind should always be pleasantly disposed, his speech agreeable and his manners unpretentious. He should be a friend to all creatures and should see to it that he is given the proper assistance in his work.   *Ayurvedic medical text*

Desiderius Erasmus; 1518   **2545**
George. Diagnosis of the disease is a step toward sound health. Have you consulted no physician?
Livinus. Oh, yes, a great many.
George. What do they say?
Livinus. What Demipho's advisers say in the comedy: one says no, another yes, another decides he'll have to think it over.   *Colloquies. In Poor Health*

Paracelsus (Theophrastus Bombastus von Hohenheim); [1493-1541]   **2546**
You ought to know that at the time of Hippocrates, Rasis, Galen etc., it was a sheer pleasure to practice medicine. The reason: Purgatory was a small affair. But at present and henceforth, gradually less happiness may be found in medicine because evil is on the increase; for this reason there have never been so many bad physicians as there are now.
                                                    Volumen Medicinae Paramirum

Paracelsus (Theophrastus Bombastus von Hohenheim); [1493-1541]   **2547**
Ignorant physicians are satanic spirits sent by God to the patient.
                                                    Volumen Medicinae Paramirum

Martin Luther; *circa* 1566   **2548**
Able, cautious, and experienced physicians, are gifts of God. They are the ministers of nature, to whom human life is confided; but a moment's negligence may ruin everything. No physician should take a single step, but in humility and the fear of God; they who are without the fear of God are mere homicides.   *Of Sickness and of the Causes Thereof*

Francis Bacon; 1605   **2549**
The weakness of patients, and sweetness of life, and nature of hope, maketh men depend upon physicians with all their defects.   *The Advancement of Learning*

Francis Bacon; 1625   **2550**
Physicians are, some of them, so pleasing and conformable to the humor of the patient, as they press not the true cure of the disease; and some other are so regular, in proceeding according to art for the disease, as they respect not sufficiently the condition of the patient. Take one of a middle temper.   *Essays. Of Regimen of Health*

Thomas Fuller; 1642   **2551**
Physicians, like beer, are best when they are old.   *The Holy State and the Profane State*

Robert Boyle; *circa* 1660   **2552**
I look upon a good physician...as one, that is a counsellor and friendly assistant, who, in his patient's body, furthers those motions...conducive to the welfare and recovery of it.
                                        Kaplan BB, Divulging of Useful Truths in Physick

Molière (Jean-Baptiste Poquelin); 1665   **2553**
What will you do, sir, with four physicians? Is not one enough to kill any one body?
Love's the Best Doctor, Act II, Scene i

Molière (Jean-Baptiste Poquelin); 1665   **2554**
[Physicians] do nothing but receive the Glory of accidental success, and... may make profit of the Fortune of the Patient, and see all that may proceed from the Favours of Chance or the Force of Nature attributed... to Remedies.   *Don Juan*

Cotton Mather; 1724   **2555**
Of a *Distemper* we commonly say, *To know the Cause, is Half the Cure*. But, alas, how little Progress is there yett made in that *Knowledge*! *Physicians* talk about the *Causes of Diseases*. But their Talk is very *Conjectural*, very *Uncertain*, very *Ambiguous*; and often times a meer *Jargon*; and in it, they are full of *Contradiction* to One another.
The Angel of Bethesda

Benjamin Franklin; 1733   **2556**
He's the best physician that knows the worthlessness of most medicines.
Poor Richard's Almanac

Benjamin Franklin; 1736   **2557**
God heals, and the Doctor takes the Fees.   *Poor Richard's Almanac*

John Gregory; 1772   **2558**
I come now to mention the moral qualities peculiarly required in the character of a physician. The chief of these is humanity; that sensibility of heart which makes us feel for the distresses of our fellow creatures, and which of consequence incites in us in the most powerful manner to help them.   *Lectures on the Duties and Qualifications of a Physician*

Jean Jacques Rousseau; 1775   **2559**
Being subject...to so few causes of sickness, man, in the state of nature, can have no need of remedies, and still less of physicians.   *Origin of Inequality*

John Lettsom; 1780   **2560**
When people's ill, they comes to I,
I physics, bleeds, and sweat 'em;
Sometimes they live, sometimes they die,
What's that to I? I lets 'em.   *On Himself*

Edward Gibbon; 1781   **2561**
But the merit of the physician was received with universal favour and respect [by the Huns]: the Barbarians, who despised death, might be apprehensive of disease; and the haughty conqueror [Attila] trembled in the presence of a captive to whom he ascribed perhaps an imaginary power of prolonging or preserving his life.
The Decline and Fall of the Roman Empire

Samuel Johnson; 1781   **2562**
A physician in a great city seems to be the mere plaything of Fortune; his degree of reputation is, for the most part, totally casual; they that employ him, know not his excellence; they that reject him, know not his deficience.   *Lives of the Poets. Akenside*

Samuel Johnson; 1781   **2563**
Every man has found in physicians great liberality, and dignity of sentiment, very prompt effusion of beneficence, and willingness to exert a lucrative art, where there is no hope of lucre.   *Lives of the Poets. Garth*

William Patterson; 1795   **2564**
A physician, who is constantly busied, sees too much, and does not think enough.
Remarks on Some of the Opinions of Dr. Rush Respecting the Yellow Fever

William Heberden; 1802   **2565**

Plutarch says, that the life of a vestal virgin was divided into three portions; in the first of which she learned the duties of her profession, in the second she practiced them, and in the third she taught them to others. This is no bad model for the life of a physician.

Commentaries on the History and Cure of Diseases

Thomas Percival; 1803   **2566**

It is characteristic of a wise man to act on determinate principles; and of a good man to be assumed that they are conformable to rectitude and virture. The relations in which a Physician stands to his patients, to his brethren, and to the public, are complicated and multifarious; involving much knowledge of human nature and extensive moral duties.

Medical Ethics

Alexandre Dumas; 1845   **2567**

The physician has a sacred mission on earth; and to fulfil it he begins at the source of life, and goes down to the mysterious darkness of the tomb.   *The Count of Monte Cristo*

Claude Bernard; 1865   **2568**

Physicians, in their treatment, often have to take account of the so-called influence of the moral over the physical, and also of any number of family and social considerations which have nothing to do with science. Therefore, an accomplished practising physician should be not only learned in his science, but also upright and endowed with keenness, tact and good sense.   *An Introduction to the Study of Experimental Medicine*

Claude Bernard; 1865   **2569**

Medical personality is placed above science by physicians themselves; they seek their authority in tradition, in doctrines or in medical tact. This state of affairs is the clearest of proofs that the experimental method has by no means come into its own in medicine.

An Introduction to the Study of Experimental Medicine

Oliver Wendell Holmes; 1871   **2570**

The old age of a physician is one of the happiest periods of his life. He is loved and cherished for what he has been, and even in the decline of his faculties there are occasions when his experience is still appealed to, and his trembling hands are looked to with renewing hope and trust.... The young man feels uneasy if he is not continually doing something to stir up his patient's internal arrangements. The old man takes things more quietly, and is much more willing to let well enough alone.   *The Young Practitioner*

Christian Albert Theodor Billroth; 1876   **2571**

Culture is always an aristocratic thing. The physician, the school- teacher, the lawyer, the clergyman should be the best men of their village, of their city, of the circles in which they move. In order to be so they must have the super-power that comes with knowledge and skill, and this is acquired only through the hard work of study, and even more through the cultivation of the inner urge to study.   *The Medical Sciences in the German Universities*

Sarah Orne Jewett; 1884   **2572**

Nobody sees people as they are and finds the chance to help poor humanity as a doctor does. The decorations and deceptions of character must fall away before the great realities of pain and death. The secrets of many hearts and homes must be told to this confessor, and sadder ailments than the text-books name are brought to be healed by the beloved physicians.   *A Country Doctor*

Robert Louis Stevenson; 1887   **2573**

There are men and classes of men that stand above the common herd: the soldier, the sailor, and the shepherd not unfrequently; the artist rarely; rarelier still, the clergyman; the physician almost as a rule. He is the flower (such as it is) of our civilization; and when that stage of man is done with, and only to be marvelled at in history, he will be thought to have shared as little as any in the defects of the period, and most notably exhibited the virtues of the race.   *Underwoods, dedication*

Elizabeth Blackwell; 1889   **2574**

The true physician must possess the essential qualities of maternity. The sick are as help-less in his hands as the infant. They depend absolutely upon the insight and judgment, the honesty and hopefulness, of the doctor.

The Influence of Women in the Profession of Medicine

William Osler; 1897   **2575**

No class of men needs friction so much as physicians; no class gets less. The daily round of a busy practitioner tends to develop an egotism of a most intense kind.... The few set-backs are forgotten, the mistakes are often buried.... To this mental attitude the medical society is the best corrective, and a man misses a good part of his education who does not get knocked about a bit by his colleagues in discussions and criticisms.

The Functions of a State Faculty

Kerr Boyce Tupper; 1899   **2576**

Let a physician believe with all his heart that God meant him to be a physician, only a physician, wholly a physician, always a physician, then will he be a physician indeed, uncorrupted by the love of money, untainted by infection for fame, unintimidated by danger.... Have appetite for your life calling, and you will have aptitude for all its duties.

The Ideal Physician

Silas Weir Mitchell; 1900   **2577**

It is the power to reason from uncertain premises to conclusions as often unsure that makes the best physician. He practices an art not yet a science. It is based on many sci-ences. A man may know them all and be a less skilful healer than one who, knowing them less well, is master of the art to which they increasingly contribute.

Dr. North and His Friends

William Osler; *circa* 1900   **2578**

A physician who treats himself has a fool for a patient.   *Aphorisms*

Ambrose Bierce; 1906   **2579**

Physician, *n*. One upon whom we set our hopes when ill and our dogs when well.

The Devil's Dictionary

Alan Gregg; 1941   **2580**

The true physician cannot remain outside the manifold of the events he observes.

Bulletin of the New York Academy of Science

Thomas Addis; 1948   **2581**

A clinician is complex. He is part craftsman, part practical scientist, and part historian; so his several classifications involve, in varying degree, all these elements. It is only if we look at him when he is working with his patients that we find him pragmatic and utilitarian. His only design is to bring relief, and he is not at all scrupulous about how he does it.

Glomerular Nephritis

Tinsley R. Harrison; 1950   **2582**

No greater opportunity, responsibility, or obligation can fall to the lot of a human being than to become a physician. In the care of the suffering he needs technical skill, scientif-ic knowledge, and human understanding. He who uses these with courage, with humili-ty, and with wisdom will provide a unique service for his fellow man and will build an enduring edifice of character within himself. The physician should ask of his destiny no more than this; he should be content with no less.   *Principles of Internal Medicine*

John Parkinson; 1951   **2583**

The common duty required of a physician lies in the recognition and treatment of dis-ease. If he enlarges his study to cover life as affected by disease, and masters the psychol-ogy of the individual sick in body, he will widen his usefulness and reach a fuller life him-self as a physician.   *The Patient and the Physician*

Frank Lloyd Wright; 1953   **2584**

The physician can bury his mistakes, but the architect can only advise his client to plant vines.   *New York Times Magazine*

Thomas Mann; 1954   **2585**

The medical profession is not different from any other: its members are, for the most part, ordinary empty-headed dolts, ready to see what is not there and to deny the obvious.
                                        The Confessions of Felix Krull, Confidence Man

Henry E. Sigerist; 1960   **2586**

Hippocratic physicians were no demigods but just humble mortals, seeking the truth, erring, rejoicing, and suffering like ourselves.
                           Marti-Ibanez F, Henry E. Sigerist on the History of Medicine

Tinsley R. Harrison; 1962   **2587**

The true physician has a Shakespearean breadth of interest in the wise and the foolish, the proud and the humble, the stoic hero and the whining rogue. He cares for people.
                                                    Principles of Internal Medicine

René Jules Dubos; 1968   **2588**

The modern physician has at his command powerful remedies and has given up...props, but he cultivates nevertheless a...kind of bedside manner that contributes to his therapeutic effectiveness. He still believes...that "a miraculous moment comes when the doctor himself becomes the treatment."   *Man, Medicine, and Environment*

Earle P. Scarlett; 1972   **2589**

The essential loneliness of the conscientious physician, working in what is of necessity a highly individual role, burdened with the secrets of his patients, unable to share his thoughts and problems with anyone; above all finding little or no understanding of his particular role or his essential work among his circle of friends or even in his own family, except in some happy instances on the part of his wife.
                                                Roland CG, In Sickness and in Health

John Stone; 1978   **2590**

The old man asked, "Are you an Intern?" Hearing the young doctor's tired, "Yes," the old man followed with another question: "Do you know what it takes to be a good Intern? It takes the heart of a lion, the eye of an eagle, and the hand of a woman."
                                                           Abse D, My Medical School

Kenneth M. Ludmerer; 1985   **2591**

The thinking physician...is the one who in the practice of medicine asks not "What is there to do?" but "Should it be done?"   *Learning to Heal*

Matko Marusic; 1985   **2592**

A physician short in intelligence hides behind knowledge, one short in knowledge hides behind experience.   *Introduction to Medical Research*

Sherwin B. Nuland; 1994   **2593**

The very success of his esoteric therapeutics too often leads the physician to believe he can do what is beyond his doing and save those who, left to their own unhindered judgment, would choose not to be subjected to his saving.   *How We Die*

Sherwin B. Nuland; 1998   **2594**

Just as physicians must constantly admonish one another to seek the most subtle beginnings of disease, they must also forgive themselves when timing or circumstances frustrate their best intentions.   *American Scholar*

Douglas Arthur Kilgour Black; 2002   **2595**

A doctor who treats himself is dealing with two fools.   *Clinical Medicine*

Croatian proverb 2596
Seek old physician and young barber. *Proverb*

The Bible, The Apocrypha 2597
My son, when you are sick do not be negligent, but pray to the Lord, and he will heal you. Give up your faults and direct your hands aright, and cleanse your heart from all sin. Offer a sweet-smelling sacrifice, and a memorial portion of fine flour, and pour oil on your offering, as much as you can afford. And give the physician his place, the Lord created him; let him not leave you, for there is need of him. There is a time when success lies in the hands of physicians. *Ecclesiasticus 38:9-13*

Vladimir Jokanovic 2598
Some physicians went astray into medicine; unfortunately, nobody can show them the way out. *Loknar V, Croatian Medical Quotations*

PHYSICIANS AND THE PRESS

William Osler; 1897 2599
In the life of every successful physician there comes the temptation to toy with the Delilah of the press—daily and otherwise. There are times when she may be courted with satisfaction, but beware! sooner or later she is sure to play the harlot, and has left many a man shorn of his strength, viz., the confidence of his professional brethren. *Internal Medicine as a Vocation*

PHYSICIANS' WIVES

Ellen M. Firebaugh; 1894 2600
Physicians' wives have a motto. We have adopted it not from choice, but from necessity. It is "Watch and wait." The physician's wife, of all women, understands most fully what it means to watch and wait.... Let her find what consolation she can in the assurance of the old poet that they also serve who only stand and wait. *The Physician's Wife*

PHYSIOLOGY

John Morgan; 1765 2601
As every disease we labour under is a disorder of the vital, animal, or natural functions; a thorough acquaintance with these in their sound state is implied before we can pretend to understand their morbid affections, or how to remedy them. *A Discourse upon the Institution of Medical Schools in America*

Abraham Flexner; 1910 2602
Physiology is, in a sense, the central discipline of the medical school. It is the business of the physician to restore normal functioning: normal functioning is thus his starting-point in thought, his goal in action. *Medical Education in the United States and Canada*

Charles Horace Mayo; 1929 2603
Disease at times creates experiments that physiology completely fails to duplicate, and the wise physiologist can obtain clues to the resolution of many problems by studying the sick. *Address to the American College of Surgeons*

Matko Marusic; 1995 2604
The essence of physiology is its heroic attempt to explain life by laws of physics and chemistry. *Acta Facultatis Medicae Zagrabiensis*

PITUITARY TUMORS

Richard Lower; 1672 2605
A young student...suddenly [sleepy and lethargic] died in convulsions within two weeks.

In his brain the ventricles were found swollen with blood...which had gone down to the base of the skull.... The olfactory bulbs were not swollen at all. The pituitary gland...was completely blocked by a...viscous and gelatinous mass about the size of a small bean... Hence a dropsy of the brain ensued.   *De Catarrhis*

PITUITRIN

Alfred Fröhlich, L. von Frankl-Hochwart; 1910   **2606**
The uterus is stimulated by small doses...into strong, sometimes persistent contractions with pallor of the organ.... According to our studies pituitrin can be regarded as essentially non-toxic and should be considered by obstetricians and urologists in pertinent cases who might profit from the increased excitability which we have demonstrated in the animal experiments on the bladder and the uterus and use it therapeutically in such instances.   *Archives of Experimental Pathology*

PLACEBOS

Plato; [427-347 BC]   **2607**
[The cure for the headache] was a kind of leaf, which required to be accompanied by a charm, and if a person would repeat the charm at the same time that he sued the cure, he would be made whole; but that without the charm the leaf would be of no avail.
                                                          Dialogues. Charmides

Michel de Montaigne; 1580   **2608**
Why do the physicians possess, beforehand, their patients' credulity with so many false promises of cure, if not to the end, that the effect of imagination may supply the imposture of their decoctions? They know very well that a great master of their trade has given it under his hand, that he has known some with whom the very sight of physic would work.   *Essays. On the Force of Imagination*

Francis Bacon; 1625   **2609**
A king, when he presides in counsel, let him beware how he opens his own inclination too much, in that which he propoundeth; for else counsellors will but take the wind of him, and instead of giving free counsel, sing him a song of placebo.   *Essays. Of Counsel*

George Bernard Shaw; 1906   **2610**
You see, most people get well all right if they are careful and you give them a little sensible advice. And the medicine really did them good. Parrish's Chemical Food: phosphates, you know. One tablespoonful to a twelve-ounce bottle of water: nothing better, no matter what the case is.   *The Doctor's Dilemma, Act I*

John L. McClenahan; 1964   **2611**
It requires a great deal of faith for a man to be cured by his own placebos.   *Aphorism*

Howard Brody; 1982   **2612**
The lie that heals.   *Annals of Internal Medicine*

PLAGUE

Masanori Ogata; 1897   **2613**
Fleas on plague rats contain virulent plague bacilli, which, after the death of the rat, can convey the plague bacillus to man.   *Centralblat für Bakteriologie*

Ambrose Bierce; 1906   **2614**
Plague, *n.* In ancient times a general punishment of the innocent for admonition of their ruler, as in the familiar instance of Pharaoh the Immune. The plague as we of to-day have the happiness to know it is merely Nature's fortuitous manifestation of her purposeless objectionableness.   *The Devil's Dictionary*

Albert Camus; 1947   **2615**

The plague bacillus never dies or disappears for good; that it can lie dormant for years and years in furniture and linen-chests; that it bides its time in bedrooms, cellars, trunks, and bookshelves; and that perhaps the day would come when, for the bane and enlightening of men, it would rouse up its rats again and send them forth to die in a happy city.

The Plague

PLASMA CELLS

Paul Gerson Unna; 1910   **2616**

I suggested the name of plasma cell for this special cell. The rightness of this decision was recognized by Waldeyer in 1895. "The Unna plasma cells fit very well the definition which I gave in 1875 to the plasma cells; to distinguish the protoplasm poor cells in the connective tissue from other forms rich in protoplasm. I must accept the name given them by Unna." The plasma cell...is a frequent and important component of the infiltration of the skin in a number of diseases.   *Encyclopedia of Microscopic Technique*

PLATELETS (THROMBOCYTES)

Alfred Donné; 1842   **2617**

There exist in the blood three types of particles.... These globules are the product of chyle and show incessant diversity in the blood. They group into triplets and quartets, are enveloped by an albuminous coat while circulating in the blood, and in this manner constitute the white cells.   *Comptes Rendus de l'Académie des Sciences*

William Osler; 1874   **2618**

In many diseased conditions of the body, occasionally also in perfectly healthy individuals... careful investigation of the blood proves that, in addition to the usual elements, there exist pale granular masses, which on closer inspection present a corpuscular appearance.... In size, they vary greatly, from half or greater than that of a white blood-corpuscle, to enormous masses.   *Proceedings of the Royal Society of London*

PLEURISY

Aretaeus the Cappadocian; [81-138?]   **2619**

Under the ribs, the spine, and the internal part of the thorax as far as the clavicles, there is stretched a thin strong membrane, adhering to the bones.... When inflammation occurs in it, and there is heat with cough and parti-coloured sputa, the affection is named Pleurisy.... If it take a favourable turn...the resolution occurs on the fourteenth day. But if not so, it is converted into Empyema.   *On Pleurisy*

Ambroise Paré; 1575   **2620**

The Pleurisie is an inflammation of the membrane, investing the ribs, caused by subtile and cholerick blood.... If it tend to suppuration, it commonly infers a pricking pain, a Feaver and difficulty of breathing.... If nature being too weak...the disease is turned into an *Empyema*, wherefore the Chirurgeon must then be called, who...may make a vent between the third and fourth true and legitimate ribs.... The *pus* or matter must be evacuated by little and little at several times; and the capacity of the Chest cleansed from the purulent matter.   *Works*

Thomas Willis; 1674   **2621**

Both the sense of pain, as well as Anatomical Observations taken from the Patients dead of a Pleurisie do plainly attest, the seat of this Disease...consists in the Pleura or Membrane environing the inside of the ribs. And a true and singular Pleurisie is an inflammation of the Pleura it self...with a continual and acute Feaver, a pricking pain of the side, a Cough and difficulty of breathing.... If the Pleurisie be cured neither by it self, nor associating with a Peripneumonie...an Empyema or corruption between the Breast and Lungs succeeds.   *Pharmaceutice Rationalis*

PLEURITIS

Hippocrates; [460-375 BC]   2622

The lung is adherent and he has the feeling as though there were a heavy weight in the chest. Sometimes the pain is very severe. He has a friction like leather.

Peterson WF, Hippocratic Wisdom

PNEUMONIA

Hippocrates; [460-375 BC]   2623

Peripneumonia, and pleuritic affections, are to be thus observed: If the fever be acute, and if there be pains on either side, or in both, and if expiration be attended with pain, if cough be present, and the sputa expectorated be of a blond or livid colour, or likewise thin, frothy, and florid.... When pneumonia is at its height...it is bad if he had dyspnoea...and if sweat comes out about the neck and head, for such sweats are bad, as proceeding from the suffocation, rales, and the violence of the disease.

On Injuries of the Head

Aretaeus the Cappadocian; [81-138?]   2624

There is a sense of suffocation, loss of speech and of breathing, and a speedy death. This is what we call Peripneumonia, being an inflammation of the lungs, with acute fever, when they are attended with heaviness of the chest.... If any of the membranes, by which it is connected with the chest, be inflamed, pain also is present; respiration bad, and hot; they wish to get up into an erect posture, as being the easiest of all postures for the respiration.   *On Pneumonia*

PNEUMOTHORAX

James Carson; 1820   2625

The means we possess of reducing [a diseased lung] to a state of collapse, or of divesting it for a time of its peculiar functions, are equally simple and safe. In those cases in which the disease is placed in one of the lungs only, the remedy [i.e., induced pneumothorax] would appear to be simple, safe, and complete.   *Essays, Physiological and Practical*

POISONS

Thomas Love Peacock; 1831   2626

Next to him is Mr Henbane, the toxicologist, I think he calls himself. He has passed half his life in studying poisons and antidotes. The first thing he did on his arrival here, was to kill the cat; and while Miss Crotchet was crying over her, he brought her to life again.

Crotchet Castle

Ambrose Bierce; 1906   2627

Belladonna, *n.* In Italian a beautiful lady; in English a deadly poison. A striking example of the essential identity of the two tongues.   *The Devil's Dictionary*

POLIOMYELITIS

Michael Underwood; 1789   2628

The complaint...seems to arise from debility, and usually attacks children previously reduced by fever; seldom those under one, or more than four or five years old.... The first thing observed is a debility of the lower extremities...which after a few weeks are unable to support the body.   *Diseases of Children and Management of Infants from the Birth*

Walter Scott; 1808   2629

One night, I have been told, I showed great reluctance to be caught and put to bed, and after being chased about the room, was apprehended and consigned to my dormitory with some difficulty. It was the last time I was to show such personal agility. In the morning I was discovered to be affected with the fever which often accompanies the cutting of larger teeth. It held me three days. On the fourth, when they went to bathe me as usual, they discovered that I had lost the power of my right leg.

Lockhart JG, Memoirs of the Life of Sir Walter Scott

Giovanni Battista Monteggia; 1813   2630

[I should mention] a certain kind of paralysis limited to one or the other of the lower extremities.... It occurs in children who are nursing, or not much later; it begins with two or three days of fever, after which one of these extremities is found quite paralyzed, immobile, flabby, hanging down.... The fever ceases very soon, but the member remains immobile and regains with time only an imperfect degree of strength.

Instituzione Chirurgicale

John Badham; 1835   2631

A girl, aged 2 years...was found one morning to have lost the use...of the left arm.... The limb is now, after the lapse of nearly two months, hopelessly paralysed, and swings like a suspended object attached to the body.... The extraordinary youth of the patients is to be noticed.... Each case was either preceded by or ushered in by some apparent cerebral symptoms...in two by drowsiness. *London Medical Gazette*

Guillaume Benjamin Amand Duchenne; 1855   2632

The general or partial paralysis shows itself at the onset; it is accompanied, or not, by a few days of fever and sometimes it continues with a continuous or intermittent fever. The paralysed muscles lose, with variable degrees, their contractility and their sensitivity to electrical stimulation. *De l'Electrisation Localisée*

André-Victor Cornil; 1863   2633

Laurent... was placed with a wet nurse in the country at the time of the 1815 invasion in the Midi by the Allies. The wet nurse was obliged to take refuge in the woods where the little child suffered from the humidity and the cold. On the return to her parents, she was taken at the age of 2 years with paralysis of her lower limbs.

Comptes Rendus Societé de Biologie

Charles Fayette Taylor; 1867   2634

All those who have had experience in these cases have recommended the warm or hot local bath as of great value. My experience is that the value of local heat in these cases cannot be overestimated. *Infantile Paralysis and Its Attendant Deformities*

Jean-Martin Charcot; 1881   2635

The disease has an abrupt, sudden begining, generally ushered in by intense fever.... The paralytic symptoms show themselves with sudden completeness... and from the very outset, they have reached their summum in extent and intensity. *Lecture*

Jean-Martin Charcot; 1881   2636

In 1864, we had detected [in a case of infantile paralysis] the existence of an atrophy of the anterior cornua of the grey substance, and of the anterolateral white columns, in the region of the cord whence were given off the nerves going to supply the wasted muscles. *Lecture*

Philip Drinker, Charles F. McKhann; 1929   2637

A clinical test of a new apparatus for the administration of artificial respiration over prolonged periods indicates that it fulfils the desired clinical requirements. Artificial respiration was maintained almost continuously for 122 hours in a girl, aged 8 years, suffering from acute anterior poliomyelitis, without discomfort or apparent harm to the patient.... Death was believed due to cardiac failure. Examination of the lungs of the patient after death did not show any evidence of trauma due to overinflation.

Journal of the American Medical Association

Jonas Salk; 1953   **2638**

Antibody for all three immunologic types was induced by the inoculation of small quantities of...vaccines incorporated in a water-in-oil emulsion.... Levels of antibody induced by vaccination are compared with levels that develop after natural infection.... These studies...should not be interpreted to indicate that a practical vaccine is now at hand.

Journal of the American Medical Association

POLLUTION

Rachel Carson; 1962   **2639**

The most alarming of all man's assaults upon the environment is the contamination of air, earth, rivers, and sea with dangerous and even lethal materials. This pollution is for the most part irrecoverable; the chain of evil it initiates not only in the world that must support life but in living tissues is for the most part irreversible. In this now universal contamination of the environment, chemicals are the sinister and little-recognized partners of radiation in changing the very nature of the world—the very nature of its life.

Silent Spring

René Jules Dubos; 1965   **2640**

Almost daily and in every part of the world, new health hazards arise from modern technology. Some of these hazards make an immediate public impact.... Others attract less attention because they lack drama and are not obvious in their effects.... Such is the case for the dangers posed by certain pollutants of air, water, and food, which remain almost unnoticed despite their potential importance for public health.... Hardly anything is known of the *delayed* effects of pollutants on human life, even though they probably constitute the most important threats to health in the long run.   *Man Adapting*

POLONIUM

Pierre Curie, Marie Sklodowska Curie; 1898   **2641**

Very likely these minerals, with greater radioactivity than uranium or thorium, contain a new substance. We have attempted to isolate the substance from pitchblende to confirm our supposition.... We believe that the substance separated from pitchblende contains a metal unknown until today which is similar to bismuth in its analytical characteristics. If its existence is confirmed, we propose to call it polonium, according to the name of the country of origin of one of us.   *Comptes Rendus de l'Académie des Sciences*

POLYCYTHEMIA

Gabriel Andral; 1843   **2642**

The blood of plethoric persons...differs from ordinary blood in the greater quantity of globules and the much less quantity of water that it contains. Thus, before coagulation, the blood of plethoric people is remarkable for its high coloration, which is in relation with the large proportion of globules it contains.... Venesection will certainly modify it, by acting on the blood, whose globules it will infalliby diminish.

Essai d'Hématologie Pathologique

Louis Henri Vaquez; 1892   **2643**

Ten years ago...his extremities became progressively blue,...his veins were filled throughout his entire body, and then followed slowly shortness of breath and palpitations of the heart.... Attacks of vertigo commenced to appear.... The gums of the patient were tumefied, became fungoid, bleeding at the slightest contact.... [He had] an intense redness of the face.... Examination of the blood...showed the...figure of 8,900,000 red cells, that of the white cells remaining practically normal for this proportion.... We would be inclined to believe that there was a functional hyperactivity of the hematopoietic organs.

Comptes Rendus de la Société de Biologie

William Osler; 1903   **2644**

[The cyanosis] is most marked about the face and hands...but in both of my patients the skin of the entire body was of a dusky blue.... The viscidity [of the blood] is greatly increased. All observers have remarked not only upon the unusually dark, but upon the thick and sticky character of the blood drop. An extraordinary polycythaemia is a special feature of the affection.... In seven of the nine cases the spleen was enlarged. In four of these the enlargement may be termed great, reaching nearly to the navel.

American Journal of the Medical Sciences

POLYMERASE CHAIN REACTION (PCR)

K. Mullis, F. Faloona, S. Scharf, and others; 1986   **2645**

We have been exploring an alternative method for the synthesis of specific DNA sequences [consisting] of repetitive cyles of denaturation, hybridization, and polymerase extension.... This procedure [catalyzes] a doubling with each cycle in the amount of the fragment defined by the position of the 5' ends of the two primers on the template DNA.... The process can be continued for many cycles.... We have called this process *polymerase chain reaction*, or (inevitably) PCR.

Cold Spring Harbor Symposium on Quantitative Biology

POPULATION CONTROL

Thomas Robert Malthus; 1798   **2646**

Population, when unchecked, increases in a geometrical ratio. Subsistence increases only in an arithmetical ratio.   *An Essay on the Principle of Population*

Frank Laurence Lucas; 1961   **2647**

The first threat...is nuclear war; the second is world-wide overpopulation—a new Deluge, of a new kind, which *might* drown humanity in a Flood, not of water, but of themselves.... At times I have a vision of a crowd of villagers so anxiously intent on the heavings and rumblings of the mountain above them—will it erupt?—that they never notice how in smooth and sinister silence, from the far horizon behind them, there advances steadily and relentlessly the crest of a tidal wave.   *The Greatest Problem and Other Essays*

Frank Laurence Lucas; 1961   **2648**

Do we really want the earth turned into a human ant-heap, conurbanized or suburbanized from Calais to Vladivostok, with its wild nature disfigured and defiled, and the individual feeling himself more and more an impotent drop in a vast, but perhaps far from pacific, ocean of humanity?   *The Greatest Problem and Other Essays*

Julian Huxley; 1964   **2649**

We can and should devote ourselves with truly religious devotion to the cause of ensuring greater fulfillment for the human race in its future destiny. And this involves a furious and concerted attack on the problem of population; for the control of population is...a prerequisite for any radical improvement in the human lot.   *Essays of a Humanist*

Peter B. Medawar; 1984   **2650**

It is nonsense...to suppose that a human population could ever become so numerous as to be standing shoulder to shoulder upon the land surface of the earth. It is by no means nonsense, though, that unless the birth rate drops to a level commensurable with the death rate, the density-dependent factors that arrest the growth of the population will include the famine and pestilence expected of the Malthusian apocalypse.

The Limits of Science

Dennis V. Razis; 1994   **2651**

For Hippocratic medicine the reduction of the human death rate has always been an absolute goal, and concern about population growth has never been an accepted constraint on any public health measure. Yet medicine is largely responsible for the overpopulation, which could be one of the major causes of human extinction.... The application of Hippocratic medicine...has proven to be anti-biological; it...is largely responsible for the complete disorganization of the ecosystem of the Earth.

Journal of the Royal Society of Medicine

POST-PARTUM CARE

Grace Osler; 1903   2652
Take the advice of a strong woman and stay flat on your back as long as you can. You will never regret it and rarely have such a good excuse. Men—husbands & doctors—are always in such a hurry to get one up and it does make a difference later. And don't forget about the bandage if you want no stomach.   *Letter to Katherine Cushing*

POSTPARTUM PSYCHOSIS

Robert Gooch; 1820   2653
It is well known that some women, who are perfectly sane at all other times, become deranged after delivery, and that this form of the disease is called puerperal insanity.... The most common time for it to begin is a few days, or a few weeks, after delivery.... The nights are restless, and the temper is sharp; soon, however, there is an indescribable hurry, and peculiarity of manner, which a watchful and experienced observer and those accustomed to the patient will notice her conduct and language become wild and incoherent.

Medical Transactions

POVERTY

Elizabeth Blackwell; 1889   2654
It requires faith and courage to recognise the real human soul under the terrible mask of squalor and disease in these crowded masses of poverty, and then resist the temptation to regard them as "clinical material." The attitude of the student and doctor to the sick poor is a real test of the true physician.   *The Influence of Women in the Profession of Medicine*

Douglas Arthur Kilgour Black; 1999   2655
[Poverty] is basically a political problem, whose radical solution will require a return to distributive justice. Why write about it in a medical journal? Because doctors are also citizens; they have opportunities to observe and perhaps to mitigate the effects of poverty; and they should be, in Virchow's words, "the natural advocates of the poor."

Journal of the Royal College of Physicians

PREGNANCY

Hippocrates; [460-375 BC]   2656
All those who are pregnant have blemishes on the face and, at the beginning of pregnancy, lose their taste for wine, do not have a good appetite, are full of nausea and salivate.

On Sterile Women

Marsac; 1650   2657
[The fetus] jumps, turns, whirls, moves about freely, and is able to change its position frequently. The heart beats like a a millclapper and forges its spirit without blood or air.

Speert H, Obstetric and Gynecologic Milestones

Jacques Alexandre Lejumeau; 1822   2658
When I applied myself to following the movements of the fetus, I was suddenly struck by a sound the likes of which I had never noticed: it was as if a watch placed very near me produced a beating sound. [Double pulsations]   *Memoire sur l'Auscultation*

A.J.B. Parent-Duchatelet; 1837   **2659**

Examination of the genitals of prostitutes led M. [Ètienne Joseph] Jacquemin to the discovery of a new sign of pregnancy.... This sign consists of a violet coloration, sometimes like wine dregs, which the whole mucous membrane of the vagina acquires.... The sign is so obvious that M. Jacquemin is never misled by it. [He has been] able to determine the state of the mucous membranes in 4500 pregnant women. *Speert H, Obstetric and Gynecologic Milestones*

James Reed Chadwick; 1887   **2660**

[The] absence [of the bluish-violet color of the vaginal introitus] is not to be accepted as evidence that pregnancy does not exist, especially in the first three months, when satisfactory evidence is most needed.... From (and including) the second month, this color is generally present, and often of such a character as to be diagnostic. [Chadwick sign] *Transactions of the American Gynecological Society*

PREGNANCY TESTS

Selmar Aschheim, Bernhard Zondek; 1928   **2661**

Our test is carried out with morning urine.... The urine is injected subcutaneously into the infantile [mice].... Only the ovarian findings are of significance for the pregnancy reaction.... We have examined 78 cases of pregnancy. In 76 cases the reaction was definitely positive.... In [the] 198 control cases the reaction was positive twice.... The reaction thus has a precision that one cannot hope to surpass with a biologic method. [Aschheim-Zondek pregancy test] *Speert H, Obstetric and Gynecologic Milestones*

Maurice Harold Friedman, Maxwell Edward Lapham; 1931   **2662**

The urine is injected intravenously.... Forty-eight hours after the first injection the rabbit is killed. If the ovaries contain either fresh corpora lutea or large bulging corpora hemorrhagica, the reaction is positive and the patient who furnished the sample [of urine] is presumably pregnant. [Friedman pregnancy test] *Speert H, Obsetric and Gynecologic Milestones*

PREMENSTRUAL SYNDROME

Robert T. Frank; 1931   **2663**

The continued circulation of an excessive amount of female sex hormone in the blood may in labile persons produce serious symptoms, some cardiovascular, but the most striking definitely psychic and nervous (autonomic). These periodic attacks are incapacitating and lead occasionally to extreme unhappiness and family discord.... At present, in the severest cases of this nature, temporary or permanent amenorrhea, brought about by roentgen treatment, appears to be the proper procedure.
Archives of Neurology and Psychiatry

Raymond Greene, Katharina Dalton; 1953   **2664**

The term "premenstrual tension" is unsatisfactory, for tension is only one of the many components of the syndrome... We have preferred to use the term "premenstrual syndrome", but... this term is also unsatisfactory.... The first description of the syndrome is that of Frank (1931).... A large proportion of women... suffer a variety of distressing symptoms during the final week or so of the menstrual sycle.... They are probably produced by water-retention, and the evidence... suggests that this in its turn is due to abnormal elevation of the oestradiol/progesterone ratio. *British Medical Journal*

PRENATAL LIFE

Thomas Browne; 1643   **2665**

And surely we are all out of the computation of our age, and every man is some months elder then he bethinks him; for we live, move, have a being, and are subject to the actions

of the elements, and the malice of diseases, in that other World, the truest Microcosm, the Womb of our Mother.
Religio Medici

PRESCRIPTIONS

Benjamin Rush; 1811   **2666**
Sir Richard Nash was once asked by his physician if he had followed his prescription. "If I had," said Sir Richard, "I should certainly have broken my neck, for I threw it out of my window."
Brieger G, Medical America in the Nineteenth Century

Oliver Wendell Holmes; 1860   **2667**
Part of the blame of over-medication must, I fear, rest with the profession, for yielding to the tendency to self-delusion, which seems inseparable from the practice of the art of healing.
Currents and Counter-Currents in Medical Science

Oliver Wendell Holmes; 1860   **2668**
Pliny says, in so many words, that the cerates and cataplasms, plasters, collyria, and antidotes, so abundant in his time, as in more recent days, were mere tricks to make money.
Currents and Counter-Currents in Medical Science

Oliver Wendell Holmes; 1892   **2669**
Every man who does not take our prepared calomel, as prescribed by us in our Constitution and By-Laws, is and must be a mass of disease from head to foot; it being self-evident that he is simultaneously affected...with all possible...diseases...and he will certainly die, if he does not take freely of our prepared calomel, to be obtained only of one of our authorized agents.
The Professor at the Breakfast Table

Ambrose Bierce; 1906   **2670**
Prescription, *n*. A physician's guess at what will best prolong the situation with least harm to the patient.
The Devil's Dictionary

Arthur Hurst; [1879-1944]   **2671**
His writing was even more illegible than that of most busy doctors.... The wife of one of the Canons of Christ Church had invited Acland to dinner, but was quite unable to decipher his reply. The Canon suggested that she should take the letter to a chemist in the High, who would certainly be able to read the Regius Professor's writing.... He retired with it to the back of the shop. Five minutes later he reappeared. "That will be half-a-crown," he said, as he handed the lady a bottle of medicine.
Coope R, The Quiet Art

Barry Blackwell; 1973   **2672**
Too often a prescription signals the end to an interview rather than the start of an alliance.
New England Journal of Medicine

John F. Morrissey, Robert F. Barreras; 1974   **2673**
Before prescribing multiple doses of this size [physicians] should try several doses on themselves. The human stomach differs from a glass beaker...there is an intestine attached to the distal end of the stomach.
New England Journal of Medicine

PREVENTIVE MEDICINE

Huang Ti Nei Ching Su Wen; [2697-2597 BC]   **2674**
The superior physician helps before the early budding of the disease.... The inferior physician begins to help when [the disease] has already developed; he helps when destruction has already set in. And since his help comes when the disease has already developed it is said of him that he is ignorant.
The Yellow Emperor's Classic of Internal Medicine

Galen; [130-200]   **2675**
Since, both in importance and in time, health precedes disease, so we ought to consider first how health may be preserved, and then how one may best cure disease.
Hygiene

William Buchan; 1798   **2676**
Domestic medicine: an attempt to render medical art more generally useful by showing people what is in their own power, both with respect to the prevention and cure of diseases.   *Domestic Medicine*

Berkeley George Andrew Moynihan; 1910   **2677**
It is necessary for us now to devote our closest inquiry to the very earliest disturbances of health so that medical treatment of a condition whose authentic nature is known may be more purposeful, and surgical treatment, when necessary, adopted at an earlier, and in a safer, stage.   *The Pathology of the Living and Other Essays*

Henry Louis Mencken; 1922   **2678**
Hygiene is the corruption of medicine by morality. It is impossible to find a hygienist who does not debase his theory of the healthful with a theory of the virtuous. The whole hygienic art, indeed, resolves itself into an ethical exhortation. This brings it, at the end, into diametrical conflict with medicine proper. The aim of medicine is surely not to make men virtuous; it is to safeguard and rescue them from the consequences of their vices. The physician does not preach repentance; he offers absolution.   *Prejudices, 3rd series. The Physican*

Henry George Miller; 1968   **2679**
Preventive medicine all too often tells a person he's ill when he's feeling perfectly fit.   *World Neurology*

René Jules Dubos; 1968   **2680**
Whereas the prevention of disease can often be achieved at low cost, therapeutic medicine increasingly involves the use of expensive techniques, equipment, and supplies.   *Man, Medicine, and Environment*

René Jules Dubos; 1968   **2681**
Ideally the approach to disease control should be the same in all countries of the world.... Social and economic factors condition not only the incidence and manifestations of the various types of disease but also the extent to which medical knowledge can usefully be applied to their control. Each society must therefore have its own system of medicine and public health suited to its particular needs and to its resources.   *Man, Medicine, and Environment*

Ernst L. Wynder; 1975   **2682**
Clearly, if disease is man-made, then it can be man-prevented. It should be the function of medicine to help people die young as late in life as possible.   *Shenker I, The New York Times*

Petr Skrabanek; 1986   **2683**
Scaring people with disease and death is counterproductive and explains much of the failure of "health promotion" programmes: after a saturation dose from the moralists and cancer-mongers the populace find solace in fatalism. Anyway, what evidence have we that preventionists live more productive, happier, and longer lives than the targets of their exhortations?   *The Lancet*

Petr Skrabanek; 1986   **2684**
As religious faith declines, the dogmas of medicine grow. The shepherds of the soul have been replaced by the priests of prevention.   *The Lancet*

Paul Frame; 1996   **2685**
An ounce of prevention is a ton of work.   *Journal of the American Medical Association*

Croatian proverb   **2686**
More is spent to treat than to prevent.   *Proverb*

PRIAPISM

Aretaeus the Cappadocian; [81-138?]   2687
The Satyrs, sacred to Bacchus, in the paintings and statues, have the member erect, as the symbol of the divine performance. It is also a form of disease.... The appellation of Satyriasis being derived from its resemblance to the figure of the god. It is an unrestrainable impulse to connection; but neither are they at all relieved by these embraces, nor is the tentigo soothed by many and repeated acts of sexual intercourse.... Of the periods of life, it occurs principally in boys and striplings.... For the most part, the patients die on the seventh day.   *On Satyriasis*

PROFESSIONS

George Bernard Shaw; 1906   2688
It's always the way with the inartistic professions: when they're beaten in argument they fall back on intimidation. I never knew a lawyer yet who didn't threaten to put me in prison sooner or later. I never knew a parson who didn't threaten me with damnation. And now you threaten me with death. With all your talk you've only one real trump in your hand, and that's intimidation.   *The Doctor's Dilemma, Act III*

Louis D. Brandeis; 1925   2689
The peculiar characteristics of a profession as distinguished from other occupations, I take to be these: ... A profession is an occupation for which the necessary preliminary training is intellectual in character, involving knowledge and to some extent learning, as distinguished from mere skill.... It is an occupation which is pursued largely for others and not merely for one's self.... It is an occupation in which the amount of financial return is not the accepted measure of success.   *Business: A Profession*

PROGNOSIS

Hippocrates; [460-375 BC]   2690
Strong and continued headaches with fever, if any of the deadly symptoms be joined to them, are very fatal.   *The Book of Prognostics*

Hippocrates; [460-375 BC]   2691
The mildest class of fevers, and those originating with the most favorable symptoms, cease on the fourth day or earlier; and the most malignant, and those setting in with the most dangerous symptoms, prove fatal on the fourth day or earlier.   *The Book of Prognostics*

Hippocrates; [460-375 BC]   2692
In acute diseases, coldness of the extremities is bad.   *Aphorisms*

Hippocrates; [460-375 BC]   2693
He who would know correctly beforehand those that will recover, and those that will die, and in what cases the disease will be protracted for many days, and in what cases for a shorter time, must be able to form a judgment from having made himself acquainted with all the symptoms, and estimating their powers in comparison with one another.
                                                 The Book of Prognostics

Hippocrates; [460-375 BC]   2694
The physician who cannot inform his patient what would be the probable issue of his complaint, if allowed to follow its natural course, is not qualified to prescribe any rational treatment for its cure.   *Preliminary Discourse*

Théophile Bonet; 1684   2695
Let a Physician be doubtful in his Prognostick, unless there be most certain and infallible signs of death: Let him be moderate in his promises: Yet let him always give hopes rather of Health, than foretel certain Death.   *A Guide to the Practical Physician*

Jonathan Swift; 1726   2696
One great excellency in this tribe [physicians], is their skill at prognostics, wherein they seldom fail; their predictions in real diseases, when they rise to any degree of malignity, generally portending death, which is always in their power, when recovery is not: and therefore, upon any unexpected signs of amendment, after they have pronounced their sentence, rather than be accused as false prophets, they know how to approve their sagacity to the world, by a seasonable dose.   *Gulliver's Travels. Voyage to the Houyhnhnms*

Horace Walpole; 1785   2697
Prognostics do not always prove prophecies—at least the wisest prophets make sure of the event first.   *Letters. To Thomas Walpole*

Thomas Percival; 1803   2698
A physician should not be forward to make gloomy prognostications; because they savour of empiricism, by magnifying the importance of his services in the treatment or cure of the disease.   *Medical Ethics*

PROSTATISM

Edward Hyde, Earl of Clarendon; 1759   2699
He was very often, both in the Day and the Night, forced to make Water, seldom in any Quantity, because he could not retain it long enough.   *The Life of Edward, Earl of Clarendon*

PROSTITUTION

Denslow Lewis; 1895   2700
Few women become votaries of the vice from choice. In the great majority of cases the prostitute is what she is because man has in one way or another made her so.   *Medical Record*

PROTEIN

Francis Harry Compton Crick; 1958   2701
Protein synthesis is a central problem for the whole of biology, and... it is in all probability closely related to gene action.   *Symposia of the Society for Experimental Biology*

PROTEINURIA

Frederik Dekkers; 1673   2702
I cannot pass by that the urines in phthisics and those affected with consumption are limpid and clear, especially if not boiled.... If a drop or so of acetic acid be added and it is exposed to the cold air, soon a white coagulum falls to the bottom without doubt cheesy particles.   *Exercitationes Medicae Practicae circa Medendi Methodum*

Domenico Cotugno (Cotunnius); 1764   2703
I shall begin with urine, which everyone knows is not coagulable but which was seen to coagulate in those experiments of our[s] which I am about to describe.... A soldier...was suffering at this time with immense watery swellings of his whole body.... With two pints of this urine exposed to the fire, when scarcely half evaporated, the remainder made a white mass, already loosely coagulated like egg albumen. Thus it was shown for the first time that urine...can at some time contain a coagulable substance.

De Ischiade Nervosa Commentarius

William Charles Wells; 1812   **2704**

I have examined by means...of the tests which have been mentioned, the urine of one hundred and thirty persons, affected with dropsy from other causes than scarlet fever...and have found serum in that of seventy-eight.... In about a third of the cases in which serum was detected in the urine, its quantity was small.... On theother hand, the urine, after being exposed to the heat of boiling water, in five cases, became firmly solid.... [On opening the body of a dropsical soldier] the kidneys were much harder than they usually are.

Transactions of the Society for the Improvement of Medico-Chirurgical Knowledge

John Blackall; 1813   **2705**

The dropsy diffused through the cellular membrane, and in its progress usually involving the large cavities likewise, is a very common form of the disease. Its exciting causes are sometimes sufficiently remarkable.... One of these causes is scarlatina...another is courses of mercury imprudently conducted.... In the histories themselves the general character of the urine is given, and the extent of its coagulation by heat.

Observations on the Nature and Cure of Dropsies

PSEUDOHYPERTROPHIC MUSCULAR DYSTROPHY (DUCHENNE MUSCULAR DYSTROPHY)

Guillaume Benjamin Amand Duchenne; 1868   **2706**

The disease I am going to describe is characterized, first, by a weakening of movements, at the beginning, generally in the lower limbs, then extending progressively to the upper limbs... secondly, by increased volume, usually, of some of the paralyzed muscles... and thirdly by hyperplasia of the interstitial connective tissue of the paralyzed muscles with abundant production of fibrous tissue. *Archives Générales de Médecine*

PSEUDOHYPOPARATHYROIDISM

Fuller Albright, Charles Burnett, Patricia Smith, William Parson; 1942   **2707**

One should obtain essentially the same clinical picture from failure of an end-organ to respond to a hormone as from a decreased production or absence of said hormone. [We] report three cases with the clinical picture of hypoparathyroidism in each of which there is evidence that the cause of the disturbance is the failure of the organism to respond to the hormone. *Endocrinology*

PSORIASIS

John Updike; 1989   **2708**

[My mother], too, had psoriasis; I had inherited it from her. Siroil and sunshine and not eating chocolate were her only weapons in our war against the red spots, ripening into silvery scabs, that invaded our skins in the winter.... Only the sun... had real power over psoriasis; a few weeks of summer erased the spots from all of my responsive young skin that could be exposed.... You are forced to the mirror, again and again; psoriasis compels narcissism.

Self-consciousness. At War with My Skin

PSYCHIATRISTS

John Charles Bucknill; 1860   **2709**

The true mental physician transfers for the moment the mind of his patient into himself in order that, in return, he may give back some portions of his own healthful mode of thought to the sufferer. *Address*

David L. Bazelon; 1961   **2710**

The big terms of a psychiatrist's discourse under any rule are large ominous-sounding words which no one else in the courtroom really understands and which, as time goes by, clever lawyers are becoming adept at proving that the psychiatrist himself does not fully understand.   *Equal Justice for the Unequal*

Theodor Reik; 1966   **2711**
Some men not only suffer fools gladly but are interested in them and indefatigably study them: psychiatrists.   *The Many Faces of Sex*

Thomas Maeder; 1989   **2712**
A president of the American Academy of Psychotherapists once said, in an address to the members…"When I first visited a national psychiatric convention, in 1943, I was dismayed to find the greatest collection of oddballs, Christ beards, and psychoneurotics that I had ever seen outside a hospital." Yet this is to be expected; psychotherapists are those of us who are driven by our own emotional hunger.   *The Atlantic Monthly*

PSYCHIATRY

George Cheyne; 1733   **2713**
Of all the miseries that afflict human life and relate principally to the body, in this valley of tears I think nervous disorders in their extreme and last degrees are the most deplorable and beyond all comparison the worst.   *The English Malady*

Philippe Pinel; 1801   **2714**
It is…to be lamented, that regular physicians have indulged in a blind routine of inefficient treatment, and have allowed themselves to be confined within the fairy circle of antiphlogisticism, and by that means to be diverted from the more important management of the mind.   *Treatise on Insanity*

Philippe Pinel; 1801   **2715**
Few subjects in medicine are so intimately connected with the history and philosophy of the human mind as insanity. There are still fewer, where there are so many errors to rectify, and so many prejudices to remove. Derangement of the understanding is generally considered as an effect of an organic lesion of the brain, consequently as incurable; a supposition that is, in a great number of instances, contrary to anatomical fact.
                                                                                       Treatise on Insanity

Wilhelm Griesinger; 1868   **2716**
Psychiatry has undergone a transformation in its relationship to the rest of medicine…. This transformation rests principally on the realization that patients with so-called "mental illnesses" are really individuals with illnesses of the nerves and brain.
                                                                Archiv für Psychiatrie und Nervenkrankheiten

Theodor Meynert; 1890   **2717**
The more that psychiatry seeks, and finds, its scientific basis in a deep and finely grained understanding of the anatomical structure [of the brain], the more it elevates itself to the status of a science that deals with causes.   *Klinische Vorlesungen über Psychiatrie*

Daniel R. Brower; 1906   **2718**
I began thirty years ago the treatment of selected cases of acute insanity in general hospitals. Patients were admitted without any legal process, just as other sick people were, and from that time until the present I have never been without such cases, and believe that the results have been sufficiently satisfactory to urge this plan of treatment on the profession generally.   *Journal of the American Medical Association*

Elliott Emanuel; 1969   **2719**
Could it be that psychiatry has been made to seem so difficult and exotic a subject that a physician, a man who has had unique opportunities to study innumerable men and women and children, is afraid to stumble or make a fool of himself if he tries to unravel the predicament of another human being? If this is so, we psychiatrists have done a disservice.   *Canadian Medical Association Journal*

Henry George Miller; 1970   **2720**

As a clinical neurologist I have had the good fortune to work with and learn from a team of eclectic and realistic psychiatrists of outstanding calibre. They are the sort of psychiatrists who send the patient back to me with the polite suggestion that I have another look for the cerebral tumour—and they have an infuriating habit of being right. This is certainly one of his most important functions, and the psychiatrist whose knowledge and experience of the pleomorphism of organic disease is too insecurely based for its exercise is a danger to the patient.   *British Journal of Hospital Medicine*

Henry George Miller; 1970   **2721**

Psychiatry is neurology without physical signs, and calls for diagnostic virtuosity of the highest order.   *British Journal of Hospital Medicine*

Richard Hunter; 1972   **2722**

Psychiatrists do not diagnose their patients like other doctors do. They discard four of their senses and literally play it by ear. It is the no-touch technique adapted to new purpose.... Presenting symptoms are elevated to the status of a disease like varieties of fever were in the eighteenth century. The pharmaceutical industry provides corresponding antidotes and reinforces the illusion.   *Proceedings of the Royal Society of Medicine*

Robert L. Taylor; 1982   **2723**

Descriptive labeling does not provide causative understanding.   *Mind or Body*

[Anonymous]; 1991   **2724**

By use of such criteria the most prevalent psychiatric conditions, anxiety and depression, have been separated into adjustment disorders, generalized anxiety disorder, panic disorder, major depressive episode, and dysthymic disorder.... Thus, in the game of diagnostic "monopoly," players accumulate houses of operational criteria until they have sufficient to purchase diagnostic hotels, which remain on the same site till sold.   *The Lancet*

Edward Shorter; 1997   **2725**

Under the influence of Freud's teachings, American psychiatry accomplished the switch from psychosis to neurosis as the object of study, and from the asylum to Main Street as the venue for practice.   *A History of Psychiatry*

Edward Shorter; 1997   **2726**

What Nissl and Alzheimer could find under their microscopes they declared "neurology." What they couldn't find was psychiatry.   *A History of Psychiatry*

PSYCHOANALYSIS

Sigmund Freud; 1893   **2727**

The psychotherapeutic procedure...brings to an end the operative force of the idea which was not abreacted in the first instance, by allowing its strangulated affect to find a way out through speech; and it subjects it to associative correction by introducing it into normal consciousness (under light hypnosis) or by removing it through the physician's suggestion, as is done in somnambulism accompanied by amnesia.

On the Psychical Mechanism of Hysterical Phenomena

Sigmund Freud; 1893   **2728**

The ideas which have become pathological have persisted with such freshness and affective strength because they have been denied the normal wearing-away processes by means of abreaction and reproduction in states of uninhibited association.

On the Psychical Mechanism of Hysterical Phenomena

Sigmund Freud; 1893   **2729**

We found, to our great surprise at first, that each individual hysterical symptom immediately and permanently disappeared when we had succeeded in bringing clearly to light the memory of the event by which it was provoked and in arousing its accompanying affect, and when the patient had described that event in the greatest possible detail and had put the affect into words.   *On the Psychical Mechanism of Hysterical Phenomena*

W. Somerset Maugham; 1919   **2730**
The mystic sees the ineffable, and the psychopathologist the unspeakable.
The Moon and Sixpence

Carl Gustav Jung; 1963   **2731**
The brain is viewed as an appendage of the genital glands.   *Memories, Dreams, Reflections*

Karl Menninger, Martin Mayman, Paul Pruyser; 1963   **2732**
What psychoanalysis showed was that true love is more concerned about the welfare of the one loved than with its own immediate satisfactions, that it demands nothing, but is patient, kind, modest; that it is free from jealousy, boastfulness, arrogance, and rudeness; that it can bear all things, hope, and endure. So said Saint Paul. So said Freud.
The Vital Balance

Edward Shorter; 1997   **2733**
By helping to turn analysis into a temple devoted to the last remaining dinosaur ideology of the nineteenth century, the refugee analysts unwittingly guaranteed that the temple would soon come crashing down.   *A History of Psychiatry*

Edward Shorter; 1997   **2734**
Psychoanalysis was to therapy as expressionism was to art: Both represented exquisite versions of the search for insight.   *A History of Psychiatry*

PSYCHOSIS

Aretaeus the Cappadocian; [81-138?]   **2735**
The modes of mania are infinite in species, but one alone in genius. For it is altogether a chronic derangement of the mind, without fever.... Certain edibles, such as...hyoscyamus, induce madness: but these affections are never called mania; for, springing from a temporary cause, they quickly subside, but madness has something confirmed in it.... Dotage commencing with old age never intermits, but accompanies the patient until death; while mania intermits, and with care ceases altogether.   *On Madness*

François Boissier de Sauvages; 1772   **2736**
The distraction of our mind is the result of our blind surrender to our desires, our incapacity to control or to moderate our passions. Whence these amorous frenzies, these antipathies, these depraved tastes, this melancholy which is caused by grief, these transports wrought in us by denial, these excesses in eating, in drinking, these indispositions, these corporeal vices which cause madness, the worst of all maladies.
Nosologie methodique

Clifford Whittingham Beers; 1908   **2737**
No man can be born again, but I believe I came as near it as ever a man did. To leave behind what was in reality a Hell and, in less than one second, have this good green earth revealed in more glory than most men ever see in it, was a compensating privilege which makes me feel that my suffering was distinctly worth while.   *A Mind That Found Itself*

Angelo Mosso; 1915   **2738**
In politicians and men of business...overstrain is very common. In proof of this one need only think of the most terrible result of cerebral exhaustion, namely, madness.... American politicians in this respect far surpass the Jews of Europe. In the district of Columbia, which is the seat of government, there are 5.20 cases of insanity per thousand.   *Fatigue*

Manfred Joshua Sakel; 1934   **2739**
I have here indicated a method of treating schizophrenia, by the production of hypo-

glycemic states or severe hypoglycemic shocks by means of insulin.... The treatment is dangerous in unskilled hands, but I believe from what I have seen that it promises success. *Wiener Medizinische Wochenschrift*

John Frederick Joseph Cade; 1949   **2740**

There is no doubt that in mania patients improvement has closely paralleled treatment [with lithium].... The quietening effect on restless non-manic psychotics is additional evidence of the efficacy of lithium salts.... Lithium salts have no apparent hypnotic effect; the result is purely sedative. The effect on patients with pure psychotic excitement—that is, true manic attacks—is so specific that it inevitably leads to speculation as to the possible aetiological significance of a deficiency...in the genesis of this disorder.

Medical Journal of Australia

Thomas Szasz; 1973   **2741**

Doubt is to certainty as neurosis is to psychosis. The neurotic is in doubt and has fears about persons and things; the psychotic has convictions and makes claims about them. In short, the neurotic has problems, the psychotic has solutions. *The Second Sin*

PSYCHOSOCIAL MEDICINE

Irving J. Lewis, Cecil G. Sheps; 1983   **2742**

Unless our academic medical centers broaden the base of their activities and interests to give psychological elements as much continuing attention as is now given biological aspects, medicine's crisis and public disappointment and chagrin will continue and deepen. *The Sick Citadel*

PSYCHOSOMATIC MEDICINE

René-Théophile-Hyacinthe Laennec; 1826   **2743**

No pathological case presents with more obvious characteristics of an ailment due to a simple disturbance in nervous influence than does shortness of breath with puerile respiration. *Traité de l'Auscultation Médiate*

Peter Mere Latham; 1845   **2744**

Every day brought some fresh proof of how great was the influence of mental distress in augmenting bodily pain and sickness. Whatever circumstances were calculated to make a strong impression upon the spirits, threw them back at once from a state of convalescence, into absolute disease.... Passions and affections of the mind are wont to show their power over the body especially by the manner in which they influence the heart, even the healthy heart; rousing it to tumultuous and irregular action and engendering pain within it. *Aphorisms*

René Jules Dubos; 1968   **2745**

Clinical experience reveals that many, and perhaps all, disease states are the expressions of both organic and psychic factors. *Man, Medicine, and Environment*

Henry George Miller; 1970   **2746**

There are many circumstances when the patient with less serious psychiatric symptoms needs to be told very firmly that they are no more important than the low back pains that trouble so many of his contemporaries, or the piles or bunions that worry the rest.... If such self-denying stringency were more widely cultivated, abuse of the psychiatrist at every level of medicine and of society would be less conspicuous.

British Journal of Hospital Medicine

PSYCHOTHERAPY

William Shakespeare; 1606   **2747**
Canst thou not minister to a mind diseased,
Pluck from the memory a rooted sorrow,
Raze out the written troubles of the brain,
And with some sweet oblivious antidote
Cleanse the stuff'd bosom of that perilous stuff
Which weighs upon the heart?   *Macbeth, Act V, Scene iii*

Johann Wolfgang von Goethe; [1749-1832]   **2748**
When depression, hopelessness and lack of help do hurt
Healing that can last may still be achieved by a kindly word.
                                                            Nager F, Der Heilkundige Dichter

Edward Shorter; 1997   **2749**
The initial diffusion of psychotherapy had nothing to do with the discipline of psychiatry. The doctrine of "madness" had driven the patients from psychiatry, the panache of "nerves" luring them to the neurologist and the internist.   *A History of Psychiatry*

PSYCHOTROPIC DRUGS

Edward Shorter; 1997   **2750**
Following chlorpromazine, a veritable cornucopia of anti-psychotic, antimanic, and anti-depressant drugs poured forth, changing psychiatry from a branch of social work to a field that called for the most precise knowledge of pharmacology, the effect of drugs on the body.   *A History of Psychiatry*

PUBLIC HEALTH

Rudolf Ludwig Karl Virchow; [1821-1902]   **2751**
The improvement of medicine will eventually prolong human life, but the improvement of social conditions can achieve this result more rapidly and more successfully.
                                                    Eisenberg L, American Journal of Medicine

Abraham Flexner; 1910   **2752**
The overwhelming importance of preventive medicine, sanitation, and public health indicates that in modern life the medical profession is an organ differentiated by society for its own highest purposes, not a business to be exploited by individuals according to their own fancy.   *Medical Education in the United States and Canada*

Paul Ehrlich; 1910   **2753**
In syphilis, as in all infectious diseases, every improvement in the treatment of the individual is also of the greatest improvement to the community.
                                        Closing Notes on Experimental Chemotherapy of Spirilloses

Charles Horace Mayo; 1928   **2754**
When you want support for public health measures you have to educate the people. When you start to educate the people you should begin with the women because they will fight for the health of their children.   *Texas State Journal of Medicine*

George Rosen; 1958   **2755**
Throughout human history, the major problems of health that men have faced have been concerned with community life, for instance, the control of transmissible disease, the control and improvement of the physical environment (sanitation), the provision of water and food of good quality and in sufficient supply, the provision of medical care, and the relief of disability and destitution. The relative emphasis placed on each of these problems has varied from time to time, but they are all closely related, and from them has come public health as we know it today.   *A History of Public Health*

PUBLIC INFORMATION

George Bernard Shaw; 1911   **2756**
Keep the public carefully informed, by special statistics and announcements of individual cases, of all illnesses of doctors or in their families.   *The Doctor's Dilemma, Preface*

PUBLISHING

Thomas Dover; 1733   **2757**
I have spent the greatest Part of my Life without the least Thought of becoming an Author; and if it should be ask'd What makes me now appear in Print: I answer, That I have acquired in Physick, by my long Study and Practice, what I conceive may be for the common Benefit of Mankind; and therefore I publish my Observations.
The Ancient Physician's Legacy to his Country

Kurt Sprengel; 1786   **2758**
Our authors are not always what they should be. [They write out of] mere necessity, the need to make their names known through publication, or economic circumstance.
Kronick DA, A History of Scientific and Technical Periodicals

Johann Wolfgang von Goethe; [1749-1832]   **2759**
The artist may well be advised to keep his work to himself till it is completed, because no one can readily help or advise him with it…but the scientist is wise not to withhold a single finding or a single conjecture from publicity.   *Essay on Experimentation*

George Frederick Shrady; 1867   **2760**
The time is already past when any man can hope to rise to be an authority in any department of medical science through any royal road of social influence, political manipulations, or even personal charms. Those who are to be the leaders and guides of medical science for the coming generation must earn their position by persistent, original investigation, and by faithfully recording their experience in the permanent literature of the day.   *Medical Record*

William Osler; *circa* 1903   **2761**
In science the credit goes to the man who convinces the world, not to the man to whom the idea first occurs.   *Aphorisms*

William Osler; *circa* 1903   **2762**
Should your assistant make an important observation, let him publish it. Through your students and your disciples will come your greatest honor.   *Aphorisms*

Ulysses Grant Dailey; 1916   **2763**
[He excoriated the] publication of several articles on the same subject by the same author with a slightly different title, and with trifling alterations of the phraseology.
Journal of the National Medical Association

[Anonymous]; *circa* 1940   **2764**
Publish or perish.   *Commoner B, Hospital Practice*

Logan Wilson; 1942   **2765**
Results unpublished are little better than those never achieved…. One must write something and get it into print. Situational imperatives dictate a "publish or perish" credo within the ranks.   *The Academic Man*

Michael Faraday; 1950   **2766**
Work. Finish. Publish.   *Beveridge WIB, The Art of Scientific Investigation*

Warren O. Hagström; 1965   **2767**
Manuscripts submitted to scientific periodicals are often called "contributions," and they are, in fact, gifts. Authors do not usually receive royalties or other payments, and their

institutions may even be required to aid in the financial support of the periodical. On the other hand, manuscripts for which the scientific authors do receive financial payments, such as textbooks and popularizations, are, if not despised, certainly held in much lower esteem than articles containing original research results. *The Scientific Community*

Earle P. Scarlett; 1972 **2768**

It is bad enough to contemplate medicine being drowned in its own secretions as some fear. It is infinitely worse if those secretions are of a heavy, tawdry, and third-rate nature.
Roland CG, In Sickness and in Health

Michael A. Simpson; 1974 **2769**

We still consistently overvalue poor research and semi-literate publication; again, partly, because quantity, in number of publications, is easier to measure than quality.
The Lancet

Julius Comroe Jr.; 1976 **2770**

Almost every scientist working today can get his work published, somewhere, once he decides to "write it up"; maybe it will be in the Bulletin of the Podunk County Medical Society rather than in a journal with international prestige or readership, or maybe it will be published only as an abstract. The main determinant of what is or is not published therefore seems to be the scientist, for it is he who decides to become or not to become an author. *American Review of Respiratory Diseases*

Mack Lipkin; 1985 **2771**

Some bold souls are intimating that the prevailing pattern of having most clinical teaching and ward rounds done by teachers whose primary interest is really in research has led to a shortage of teacher models whose major interest and skill lies in the care of the sick.... Promotion committees know that the prestige of a department and of the medical school depends far more on the quality and quantity of publication than on the quality of teaching. *New England Journal of Medicine*

Edward Janavel Huth; 1986 **2772**

Why should the investigators confine themselves [they say] to one paper when they can slice up data and interpretations into two, three, five, or more papers that will better serve their needs when they face promotion or tenure committees? "Salami science" does not always equal baloney, but such divided publication is often an abuse of scientific publication. *Annals of Internal Medicine*

Arnold S. Relman; 1988 **2773**

The Journal undertakes review with the understanding that neither the substance of the article nor the figures or tables have been published or will be submitted for publication during the period of review. This restriction does not apply to abstracts published in connection with scientific meetings or to news reports based on public presentations at such meetings. *New England Journal of Medicine*

Matko Marusic; 1989 **2774**

Do not look for the titles of his publication, look for the journals where he has published his work! *Visible and Invisible Academia*

M. O'Donnell; 1995 **2775**

Scientific papers serve the needs of their authors above the needs of their readers.
Journal of the Royal College of Physicians

Donald Kennedy; 1997 **2776**

All the thinking, all the textual analysis, all the experiments and the data-gathering aren't anything until we write them up. In the world of scholarship we are what we write.

Academic Duty

PUERPERAL FEVER

Robert Gooch; 1826   2777

Lying-in women are subject to a disease called puerpural fever. In general it is of infrequent occurrence.... There are times, however, when this disease rages like an epidemic, and is very fatal. At these times circumstances occur which create a strong suspicion that the disorder may be communicated by a medical attendant or nurse from one lying-in woman to another.   *Quarterly Review*

Oliver Wendell Holmes; 1843   2778

In collecting, enforcing, and adding to the evidence accumulated upon this most serious subject, I would not be understood to imply that there exists a doubt in the mind of any well-informed member of the medical profession as to the fact that puerperal fever is sometimes communicated from one person to another, both directly and indirectly

.   *New England Quarterly Journal of Medicine*

Oliver Wendell Holmes; 1843   2779

The disease known as Puerperal Fever is so far contagious as to be frequently carried from patient to patient by physicians and nurses.   *New England Quarterly Journal of Medicine*

PULMONARY CIRCULATION

Michael Servetus (Villanovanus); 1553   2780

This communication [of the right ventricle of the heart to the left] however, does not take place through the septum, partition, or midwall of the heart, as commonly believed, but by another admirable contrivance, the blood being transmitted from the pulmonary artery to the pulmonary vein, by a lengthened passage through the lungs, in the course of which it is elaborated and becomes of a crimson colour.   *Christianismi Restitutio*

Matteo Realdo Colombo; 1559   2781

The blood is carried through the pulmonary artery to the lung and is there attentuated; then it is carried, along with air, through the pulmonary vein to the left ventricle of the heart.   *On Anatomy*

Richard Lower; 1669   2782

It occurred to me to make an experiment on a strangled dog, after sensations and life had completely deserted it, and to see if the still-fluid blood in the vena cava would all return equally bright in colour through the pulmonary vein, after being driven to the right ventricle and to the lungs. So I drove on the blood, and carried out a simultaneous insufflation to the perforated lungs. The result corresponded very well with my expectation, for the blood was discharged into the dish as bright-red in colour, as if it were being withdrawn from an artery in a living animal.   *A Treatise on the Heart*

Stephen Hales; 1733   2783

When we view in a strong Light the Blood circulating in the Lungs of a Frog, we see the Arteries as they pass on, sending Branches which spread like a fine Network over the Surface of each vesicle; and on some of these vesicles we may plainly see, the Blood when it has pass'd over little more than half their Surfaces, to enter corresponding capillary Veins.... I have... also seen the extream capillary Arteries, pour at right Angles their single Globules, into those much larger vessels.   *Statical Essays. Haemastaticks*

Paul H. Wood; 1954   2784

The behavior of the pulmonary vascular resistance is perhaps the most important physiological event in mitral stenosis, and to a large extent determines the course and pattern of the disease.... A high pulmonary vascular resistance saves the patient from drowning at the expense of a low cardiac output; a high venous pressure, hepatic distension, oedema, and fatigue replace haemoptysis, severe breathlessness, paroxysmal cardiac dyspnoea, and pulmonary oedema.   *British Medical Journal*

PULMONARY EMBOLISM

William Dock; 1984   2785

From my Stanford days... I had known that excessive bed rest gave rise to thromboembolic complications.... The death rate from thromboembolism was always much less at the County Hospital than it was at Stanford Hospital.... When [the County Hospital patients] got up to go to the bathroom[they] dislodged only tiny clots from their veins and these did not harm them when they got to the lungs and were dissolved, while the wealthier patients [at Stanford] who remained in bed and formed large clots in their legs and pelvises suffered the major consequences of large pulmonary emboli.

Weisse AB, Conversations in Medicine

PULMONARY EMPHYSEMA

Matthew Baillie; 1797   2786

The air-cells are seen much enlarged beyond their natural size, so as to resemble the air cells of the lungs in amphibious animals.   *Morbid Anatomy*

René-Théophile-Hyacinthe Laennec; 1819   2787

The pathognomic sign of this disease is furnished by a comparison of the indications derived from percussion and auscultation. The respiratory murmur is inaudible over the greater part of the chest, and is very feeble in the parts where it is audible; at the same time a very distinct sound is produced by percussion.... There is also heard, in the affected parts, an occasional slight sibilous rattle.   *Traité de l'Auscultation Médiate*

René-Théophile-Hyacinthe Laennec; 1819   2788

Both the local and general symptoms of pulmonary emphysema are rather equivocal.... The difficulty of breathing is constant.... The skin usually assumes a dull earthly hue, with a slight shade of blue here and there. The lips become violet, thick, and look swollen.... In every case...there existed an habitual cough.... The respiratory sound is inaudible over the greater part of the chest, and is very feeble in the points where it is audible.... The cylindrical form of the chest, and the slight lividity of the skin, will also help the diagnosis.

Traité de l'Auscultation Médiate

Oscar Auerbach, Edward Cuyler Hammond, David Kirman,
Lawrence Garfinkel; 1967   2789

Ten dogs smoked cigarettes daily in two sessions each day by voluntary inhalation through a tracheostomy tube.... Pulmonary fibrosis and emphysema, similar to those conditions in human beings, were found in all five of the smoking dogs killed. No such lung parenchymal changes were found in ten control dogs.   *Journal of the American Medical Association*

PULMONARY STENOSIS

James Hope; 1839   2790

It may be known that the murmur is not seated in the aorta, by its being inaudible, or comparatively feeble, two inches up that vessel; whereas, at a corresponding height up the pulmonary artery, it is distinct: also, by its being louder down the tract of the right ventricle than down that of the left.   *A Treatise on the Diseases of the Heart*

PULSUS ALTERNANS

Ludwig Traube; 1872   2791

The following case...shows us a variation of the Pulsus bigeminus; I designate it with the name of *Pulsus alternans*; ...it has to do with a succession of high and low pulses, in such a manner that a low pulse follows regularly a high pulse and this low pulse is separated from the following high pulse by a shorter pause than that between it and the preceding high pulse.   *Berliner Klinik Wochenschrift*

Thomas Lewis; 1913   **2792**

How grave is the condition of the patient whose heart produces this alternating pulse is often witnessed to by associated signs; angina, nocturnal dyspnoea, Cheyne-Stokes breathing or high blood pressure are often encountered in the same subject. But here lies its special significance: each and everyone of these signs may fail, and alternation may appear alone to foretell the future. Unexpected death is a common termination.

Clinical Disorders of the Heart Beat

Thomas Lewis; 1913   **2793**

It is the faint cry of an anguished and failing muscle, which, when it comes, all should strain to hear, for it is not repeated. A few months, a few years at most, and the end comes.

Clinical Disorders of the Heart Beat

PURPURA

Joao de Castello Branco Rodrigues (Amatus Lusitanus); 1556   **2794**

A boy referred to me without fever, completely covered with spots which were similar to flea bites and which moreover were quite black. So that it was quite astonishing that such a disease should be without fever.... Besides with two days of evacuations this boy passed much blood, black, fetid, foul smelling and escaped sound and free.

Curationum Medicinalium Centuriae Quator

Lazarus Riverius; 1668   **2795**

Purple-spots like Flea-bitings...are the proper and peculiar Signs of a Malignant Feaver.... Yet there do appear in other Diseases, spots very like unto those aforesaid, but springing from a far different Cause; viz. From the over thinness of the Blood.

The Practice of Physick

Paul Gottlieb Werlhof; 1735   **2796**

An adult girl, robust, without manifest cause, was attacked recently, towards the period of her menses with a sudden severe hemorrhage from the nose...together with a bloody vomiting of a very thick extremely black blood. Immediately there appeared about the neck and on the arms, spots partly black, partly violaceous or purple, such as are often seen in malignant smallpox.... The bleeding from the nose gradually stopped, the vomiting became less and the next day ceased; no lesions recurred.... The spots...disappeared the seventh day.   *Disquisito Medica et Philologica de Variolis et Anthracibus*

Eduard Heinrich Henoch; 1874   **2797**

If one compares these 4 cases, it is seen that they agree remarkably. Characteristic for all, is the combination of purpura and the striking intestinal symptoms, which are present in the form of colic, tenderness of the abdomen, vomiting (often a green mass), and in hemorrhages. Also the rheumatoid pains.... Characteristic, furthermore, is the appearance of these symptoms in attacks, with an interval of 8 days or more, so that in the usual cases 3 to 7 weeks passed before the process cleared up.... The rheumatoid pains in the joints...practically always preceded these attacks.   *Berliner Klinik Wochenschrift*

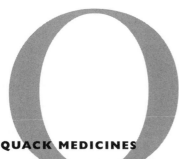

QUACK MEDICINES

Thomas Percival; 1803   **2798**

The use of quack medicines should be discouraged by the Faculty, as disgraceful to the profession, injurious to health, and often destructive even of life. Patients, however, under lingering disorders, are sometimes obstinately bent on having recourse to such as they see advertized, or hear recommended, with boldness and confidence, which no intelligent physician dares to adopt.... [The patient] may be apprized of the fallacy of his expectations, whilst assured... that diligent attention should be paid to the process of the experiment he is so unadvisedly making on himself, and the consequent mischiefs, if any, obviated as timely as possible.   *Medical Ethics*

QUACKERY

Aesop; *circa* 500 BC   **2799**

A frog once upon a time came forth from his home in the marsh and proclaimed to all the beasts that he was a learned physician, skilled in the use of drugs and able to heal all diseases. A Fox asked him, "How can you pretend to prescribe for others when you are unable to heal your own lame gait and wrinkled skin?"   *The Quack Frog*

Claude Deshais Gendron; 1700   **2800**

The cure of a disease labelled incurable by those who master the Art of Healing is not the privilege of those who excel in the practice of deception.   *Shimkin MB, Cancer*

Nathaniel Ames; 1733   **2801**

Where silly quacks are most respected, there honest doctors are neglected. Petty Attorneys and Quack Doctors are like Wolves and scabbed Sheep among the Flock. One devours and the other breeds the rot.   *Astronomical Diary*

Voltaire (François Marie Arouet); 1747   **2802**

The great doctor Hermes...visited the invalid and declared he would lose his eye. He even predicted the day and hour.... "Had it been the right eye," he said, "I could have cured it, but wounds on the left eye are incurable".... Two days later the abscess burst of its own accord and Zadig made a complete recovery. Hermes wrote a book in which he proved that he ought not to have recovered. Zadig did not read it.   *Zadig*

James Thacher; 1831   **2803**

Notwithstanding that in all the medical institutions in the United States, the most judicious energetic measures have been adopted to prevent the evils of quackery, there are ignorant and unprincipled imposters, who set at defiance all learning and theoretical knowledge, and practice the vilest acts and deceptions, sporting with the health and lives of their fellow-men without remorse. Such miscreants are too frequently encouraged by the heedless multitude, who, delighting in marvelous and magical airs, readily yield themselves dupes to the grossest absurdities.   *An Essay on Demonology, Ghosts, and Apparitions*

[Anonymous]; 1905   **2804**

Any physician who advertises a positive cure for any disease, who issues nostrum testimonials, who sells his services to a secret remedy, or who diagnoses and treats by mail patients he has never seen, is a quack.   *Adams SH, The Great American Fraud*

[Anonymous]; 1905   **2805**

Don't Dose Yourself with secret Patent Medicines, Almost all of which are Frauds and Humbugs. When sick Consult a Doctor and take his Prescriptions: it is the only Sensible Way and you'll find it Cheaper in the end.   *Adams SH, The Great American Fraud*

George Bernard Shaw; 1906   **2806**

Did I hear from the fireside armchair the bow-wow of the old school defending its drugs? Ah, believe me, Paddy, the world would be healthier if every chemist's shop in England were demolished. Look at the papers! full of scandalous advertisements of patent medicines! a huge commercial system of quackery and poison. Well, whose fault is it? Ours. I say, ours. We set the example. We spread the superstition. We taught the people to believe in bottles of doctor's stuff; and now they buy it at the stores instead of consulting a medical man.   *The Doctor's Dilemma, Act I*

George Frank Lydston; 1912   **2807**

The quack doesn't find out what the matter is but, to the patient's cost, he does find a lot of things that do not exist, and all because the reputable physician flouted as imaginary conditions which, to the patient's sensitive and morbid mind, are always terribly real.
          Medical Record

Joseph Garland; 1930   **2808**

After all is said and done, the cults, the quacks and the cranks are a boon to the medical profession for they give us something to keep our indignation in training on.
          The Doctor's Saddle-Bag

Wilfred Batten Lewis Trotter; 1932   **2809**

To adopt for a practical art a standard of attainment applicable to an applied science is not to improve its status, it is only to convert it into quackery.
          Art and Science in Medicine

Eugene A. Stead Jr.; 1997   **2810**

I've always been a quack. I've always been an excellent quack. The only difference between me and the quacks I don't like is that I don't try to get rich off my quackery, and I try to be honest about it.   *Hughes SG et al., The Pharos*

QUARANTINE

Alexander W. Kinglake; 1844   **2811**

If you dare to break the laws of the quarantine, you will be tried with military haste; the court will scream out your sentence to you from a tribunal some fifty yards off; the priest instead of whispering to you the sweet hopes of religion will console you at duelling distance, and after that you will find yourself carefully shot, and carelessly buried in the ground of the Lazaretto.   *Eothen*

QUECKENSTEDT TEST

Hans Heinrich Georg Queckenstedt; 1916   **2812**

The narrowed [spinal] channel impedes movement of fluid with an increase in pressure above the compression site.... The increment in pressure above the obstruction can be demonstrated by compression of the neck...which produces an increase in venous blood in the cranial cavity, with concomitant reduction in space for the cerebrospinal fluid.... The increased fluid pressure immediately transmitted throughout the system normally can be demonstrated with a...manometer attached to a lumbar puncture needle. In lesions of the cord the manometric change is greatly retarded.

Deutsche Zeitschrift für Nervenheilkunde

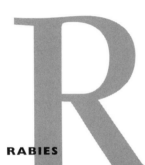

RABIES

William Shakespeare; 1592   **2813**

Take heed of yonder dog!
Look, when he fawns, he bites; and when he bites,
His venom tooth will rankle to the death:
Have not to do with him, beware of him;
Sin, death, and hell have set their marks on him.   *Richard III, Act I, Scene iii*

Louis Pasteur; 1885   **2814**

The death of this child appearing to be inevitable, I decided, not without lively and sore anxiety, as may well be believed, to try upon Joseph Meister the method which I had found constantly successful with dogs.... I thus made thirteen inoculations, and prolonged the treatment to ten days.... On the last days, therefore, I had inoculated Joseph Meister with the most virulent virus of rabies.... Three months and three weeks have elapsed since the accident, his state of health leaves nothing to be desired.

Comptes Rendus de l'Académie des Sciences

RADIOLOGY

Wilhelm Conrad Röntgen; 1895   **2815**

A discharge from a large induction coil is passed through a Hittdorf's vacuum tube, or through a well-exhausted Crookes' or Lenard's tube.... A piece of sheet aluminum, 15 mm. thick, still allowed the X-rays (as I will call the rays, for the sake of brevity) to pass.... The density of the bodies is the property whose variation mainly affects their permeability.... If the hand be held between the discharge-tube and the screen, the darker shadow of the bones is seen within the slightly dark shadow-image of the hand itself.   *Nature*

Robert Jones, Oliver Joseph Lodge; 1896   **2816**

Two preliminary short exposures to Roentgen rays indicated that the metal...was probably embedded among the bones of the wrist. The difficulty consisted in the opacity of those bones. I therefore took a tube with large electrodes.... Rather more than two hours' exposure was given.... The result was to bring out the wrist-bones clearly and to show the position of the pellet.   *The Lancet*

Godfrey Newbold Hounsfield; 1973   2817
In this procedure [MRI], absolute values of the absorption coefficient of the tissues are obtained. The increased sensitivity of computerized X-ray section scanning thus enables tissues of similar density to be separated and a picture of the soft tissue structure within the cranium to be built up.   *British Journal of Radiology*

Paul Christian Lauterbur; 1973   2818
The variations in water contents and proton relaxation times among biological tissues should permit the generation, with field gradients large compared to internal magnetic inhomogeneities, of useful zeugmatographic images from the rather sharp water resonances of organisms, selectively picturing the various soft structures and tissues. A possible application of considerable interest at this time would be to the *in vivo* study of malignant tumours.   *Nature*

Abraham Verghese; 1994   2819
What would it be like in a radiologist's shoes? To spend most of my day dealing with images of people: plain black-and-white x-ray images, or speckled images caused by sound waves bouncing off organs, or images caused by dyes outlining arteries and veins, or contrast medium filling loops of bowel, or images reconstructed by computers into cross sections of the body—all without speaking to a patient.   *My Own Country*

RADIOTHERAPY

Alexander Graham Bell; 1903   2820
The Crookes' tube, from which the Röntgen rays are emitted, is of course too bulky to be admitted into the middle of a mass of cancer, but there is no reason why a tiny fragment of radium sealed up in a fine glass tube should not be inserted into the very heart of the cancer, thus acting directly upon the diseased material.   *American Medicine*

Jean Alban Bergonié, Louis Mathieu Frédéric Adrien Tribondeau; 1906   2821
The effect of radiations on living cells is the more intense: (1) the greater their reproductive activity, (2) the longer their mitotic phase lasts, and (3) the less their morphology and function are differentiated.   *Comptes Rendus de l'Académie des Sciences*

RADIUM

Pierre Curie, Marie Sklodowska Curie, G. Bemont; 1898   2822
We have encountered a *second* strongly radioactive substance [that] seems to possess the chemical characteristics of barium.... We believe, however, that this substance, even though it contains a considerable proportion of barium, represents mainly the new element, emits radioactivity, and has chemical characteristics similar to barium.... Reasons, enumerated below, led us to believe that the new radioactive substance contained a new element which we propose to call radium.   *Comptes Rendus de l'Académie des Sciences*

RARE DISEASES

William Dock; *circa* 1970   2823
The most important thing to remember about rare diseases is that they are rare.
Medical Grand Rounds

RAYNAUD PHENOMENON

Maurice Raynaud; 1862   2824
It was the beginning of 1860 that one of the cases...attracted my attention. The case was one of spontaneous gangrene of the four extremities, which had occurred unexpectedly in a young woman aged 27 years.... It was necessary to admit the intervention of some influence up to that time ignored.... I consider syncope and local asphyxia as the first

delineation of a state much more grave, characterised by a cooling carried to the extreme by the formation of an eschar, and the fall of many parts of the phalanges of the hands and feet. *On Local Asphyxia and Symmetrical Gangrene of the Extremities*

Maurice Raynaud; 1862 **2825**

Under the influence of a very moderate cold, and even at the height of summer, she [case 1] sees her fingers become ex-sanguine, completely insensible, and of a whitish yellow colour.... One might indeed have suspected that the local asphyxia was connected with a spasmodic state of the vessels,...a functional trouble localized to the arterioles immediately contiguous to the capillaries.

On Local Asphyxia and Symmetrical Gangrene of the Extremities

READING

John of Arderne; *circa* 1400 **2826**

The use of books brings a doctor a good reputation because it is both noticed by others and he himself becomes wiser thereby. *On the Behaviour of a Leech*

[Anonymous]; 1773 **2827**

No one who wishes to practise medicine, either with safety to others, or credit to himself, will incline to remain ignorant of any discovery which time or attention has brought to light. But it is well known that the greatest part of those who are engaged in the actual prosecution of this art, have neither leisure nor opportunity for very extensive reading. Any expedient, therefore, which would serve to communicate new discoveries, without the necessity of examining a great variety of books, must have some influence in forwarding the improvement of the medical art. *Medical and Philosophical Commentaries*

Norman Moore; 1893 **2828**

The true use of reading in medicine is to make him think.... Perfect knowledge is that which has been thought over; imperfect knowledge that which has only been remembered. This is particularly noticeable in medicine, where a few observations well thought over will make a man far more useful than the mental retention of abstracts of hundreds of books. *The Principles and Practice of Medicine*

William Osler; 1901 **2829**

An old writer says that there are four sorts of readers: "Sponges which attract all without distinguishing; Howre-glasses which receive and powre out as fast; Bagges which only retain the dregges of the spices and let the wine escape, and Sives [Sieves] which retaine the best onely." A man wastes a great many years before he reaches the "sive" stage.

Books and Men

William Osler; 1901 **2830**

For the general practitioner a well-used library is one of the few correctives of the premature senility which is so apt to overtake him. Self-centred, self-taught, he leads a solitary life, and unless his everyday experience is controlled by careful reading or by the attrition of a medical society it soon ceases to be of the slightest value and becomes a mere accretion of isolated facts, without correlation. *Books and Men*

William Osler; 1903 **2831**

Start at once a bed-side library and spend the last half hour of the day in communion with the saints of humanity. *The Master-word in Medicine*

Joseph-François Malgaigne; 1905 **2832**

The physician who reads only medical books, will be a poor man and a very dull man.

Advice on the Choice of a Library

Joseph-François Malgaigne; 1905   **2833**

A well-balanced library should be divided into three parts. It should include, for the material needs, books on art or on vocation; for the heart, some books which improve or elevate; for the mind, books calculated to adorn or enlarge it.

Advice on the Choice of a Library

William Osler; 1909   **2834**

It is easier to buy books than to read them and easier to read them than to absorb them.

British Medical Journal

William Osler; 1909   **2835**

With half an hour's reading in bed every night as a steady practice, the busiest man can get a fair education before the plasma sets in the periganglionic spaces of his grey cortex.

British Medical Journal

RECONSTRUCTIVE SURGERY

Aulus Cornelius Celsus; 25 BC - AD 50   **2836**

Mutilations [of the ears, lips, and nostrils] can be treated if they are small; if they are large, either they are susceptible of treatment, or else may be so deformed by it as to be more unsightly than before.   *On Medicine*

Gaspare Tagliacozzi; 1597   **2837**

We bring back, refashion, and restore to wholeness the features which nature gave but chance destroyed, not that they may charm the eye but that they may be an advantage to the living soul, not as a mean artifice but as an alleviation of illness, not as becomes charlatans but as becomes good physicians and followers of the great Hippocrates. For although the original beauty of the face is indeed restored, yet this is only accidental, and the end for which the physician is working is that the features should fulfill their offices according to nature's decree.

Gnudi MT and Webster JT, The Life and Times of Gaspare Tagliacozzi

Joseph Pancoast; 1846   **2838**

Plastic surgery has for its object the restoration of parts that through accident or disease have been partially or altogether lost, by the transplantation of a portion of healthy integument [from a distant part of structures adjoint]. The birthplace of this branch of science appears to have been in India, where the reconstruction of the nose...has been practiced from time immemorial.   *A Treatise on Operative Surgery*

RECTAL EXAMINATION

Ulysses Grant Dailey, W.S. Grant; 1924   **2839**

We had almost come to the conclusion that the case [of vasovesiculitis] was one of acute appendicitis, but decided to make a rectal examination for the sake of completeness.

Medical Journal of Records

REFERRED PAIN

John Hilton; 1863   **2840**

Seeing that one branch of the obturator nerve goes to the hip-joint, a second to the interior of the knee, and a third to the inner side of that joint, I think we see how it occurs that disease in the interior of the hip-joint can produce "sympathetic" pain on the inner side of the knee, and in the interior of the knee joint.   *Rest and Pain*

REFLEX ACTION

Robert Whytt; 1751   2841

If a spark from the fire, or a drop of boiling water falls upon one's foot, the leg is instantly drawn in towards the body.... Therefore...the motion of the leg...be attributed to the pain...excited by the fire or boiling water, for avoiding of which the sentient principle is instantly determined...to remove the member from the offending cause.

Vital and Other Involuntary Motions of Animals

Marshall Hall; 1833   2842

Psychologists have hitherto enumerated only *three* sources or principles of muscular action—volition, the motive influence of respiration, and irritability. There is, however, a *fourth* source of muscular action distinct from any of these, though not hitherto distinguished, to which I have ventured to give the designation of the *reflex*.... The reflex function appears...to be the complement of the functions of the nervous system hitherto known.

Philosophical Transactions of the Royal Society

REFORM

Ernest Amory Codman; 1916   2843

[Richard C. Cabot] seems to want to reform the bottom of the profession, while I think the blame belongs at the top.   A *Study in Hospital Efficiency*

REFSUM'S DISEASE

Sigvald Bernhard Refsum; 1946   2844

In both families the parents [of the patients] were related to each other, being first cousins in family A and the children of cousins in family B.... The syndrome consists of hemeralopia... and atypical retinitis pigmentosa. [It] is also characterized by a condition suggestive of chronic polyneuritis, ataxia and other cerebellar phenomena. Three of the patients presented definitely pathological electrocardiograms... which in two cases resembled those of myocardial anoxia.   *Acta Psychiatrica et Neurologica Scandinavica, Supplementum*

REITER SYNDROME

Hans Conrad Reiter; 1916   2845

Characteristic of this disease, which I propose to call *spirochetosis arthritica*, is the course of fever...accompanied by regular night sweats. Outstanding clinical symptoms are the severe joint involvement, cystitis and conjunctivitis.   *Deutsche Medizinische Wochenschrift*

RELAPSING FEVER

John Rutty; 1770   2846

The latter part of July and the months of August, September, and October, were infested with a fever.... It was attended with an intense pain in the head. It terminated sometimes in four, for the most part in five or six days, sometimes in nine, and commonly in a critical sweat.... The crisis, however, was very imperfect, for they were subject to relapse, even sometimes to the third time, nor did their urine come to a complete separation.

A Chronological History of the Prevailing Diseases in Dublin

RELIGION

Santiago Ramón y Cajal; [1852-1934]   2847

When I consider the healthy color and the peace of mind of pious people, I think that religion possesses not only high moral value but also excellent nutritive worth. Faith strengthens and is conducive to flourishing longevity, while doubt sometimes condemns to sorrow and premature old age.   *Craigie EH and Gibson WC, The World of Ramón y Cajal*

REPRODUCTION

Aristotle; [384-322 BC]   2848

If the male is the active partner, the one which originates the movement, and the female qua female is the passive one, surely what the female contributes to the semen of the male will not be semen but material [for the semen to work upon]. And this in fact is what we find happening; for the natural substance of the menstrual fluid is to be classed as "prime matter."   *De Generatione Animalium*

Susan B. Anthony; 1857   2849

To be a Mother, to be a Father, is the last and highest wish of any human being—to reproduce himself or herself. The accomplishment of this purpose is only through the inciting of the sexes.... When we come into the presence of one of the opposite sex who embodies what to us seems the true and the noble, and the beautiful, our souls are stirred... It is a thrill of joy that such qualities are re-producible—and that we may be the agents, the artists in such reproduction.   *Letter to Elizabeth Cady Stanton*

RESEARCH

Hippocrates; [460-375 BC]   2850

Medicine... has discovered both a principle and a method, through which the discoveries made during a long period are many and excellent, while full discovery will be made, if the inquirer be competent, conduct his researches with knowledge of the discoveries already made, and make them his starting point.   *On Ancient Medicine*

Francis Bacon; 1620   2851

It is the peculiar and perpetual error of the human understanding to be more moved and excited by affirmatives than by negatives, whereas it ought duly and regularly to be impartial; nay, in establishing any true axiom, the negative instance is the most powerful.
                    Novum Organum. Aphorism 46

William Harvey; 1653   2852

Yet when we content ourselves with their discoveries [i.e., those of ancient Greece], and calmly believe (which is mere sleepiness) that there is now no more place for new inventions, the spritely edge of our own wit languisheth, and we extinguish the lamp which they lighted to our hands.   *Anatomical Exercitations*

Charles Darwin; 1859   2853

You would be surprised at the number of years it took me to see clearly what some of the problems were which had to be solved.... Looking back, I think it was more difficult to see what the problems were than to solve them.   *Letter to Charles Lyell*

Austin Flint; 1860   2854

I shall be ready to claim the merit of this idea when the difficult and laborious researches of someone have shown it be correct.   *American Medical Times*

Claude Bernard; 1865   2855

Devising an experiment...is putting a question; we never conceive a question without an idea which invites an answer. I consider it, therefore, an absolute principle that experiments must always be devised in view of a preconceived idea, no matter if the idea be not very clear nor well defined.   *An Introduction to the Study of Experimental Medicine*

Claude Bernard; 1865   2856

Where then...is the difference between observers and experimenters? It is here: we give the name observer to the man who applies methods of investigation...to the study of phenomena which he does not vary and which he therefore gathers as nature offers them. We give the name experimenter to the man who applies methods of investigation, whether simple or complex, so as to make natural phenomena vary, or so as to alter them with some purpose or other, and to make them present themselves in circumstances or conditions in which nature does not show them.

An Introduction to the Study of Experimental Medicine

Pierre-Charles-Alexandre Louis; [1787-1872]   **2857**

There is something rarer than the spirit of discernment; it is the need of truth; that state of the soul which does not allow us to stop in any scientific labors at what is only probable, but compels us to continue our researches until we have arrived at evidence.

Middleton WS, Annals of Medical History

Christian Albert Theodor Billroth; 1876   **2858**

The method of research, however, of positing the questions and solving the questions posited, is invariably the same, whether we have before us a blooming rose, a diseased grape-vine, a shining beetle, the spleen of a leopard, a bird's feather, the intestines of a pig, the brain of a poet or a philosopher, a sick poodle, or an hysterical princess.

The Medical Sciences in the German Universities

Hal C. Wyman; 1888   **2859**

Hunt up those oft tried, faithful and most efficient martyrs who give their lives to the cause of science—the dogs and rabbits.   *Abdominal Surgery*

Jean-Martin Charcot; 1889   **2860**

For the doctor, whether it is sad or not is not the issue. Let the patient live in illusions to the end...it is humane and the best way.... We are sometimes reproached for conducting incessant studies on the major neurologic diseases, which have, up to now, mostly been accurate. What use is it?.... Let us keep working, in spite of everything. Let us keep searching.   *Leçons du Mardi*

John Scott Haldane; 1922   **2861**

The growth of scientific medicine has been based on the study of the manner in which...the living body expresses itself in response to changes in environment, and reasserts itself in the face of disturbance and injury.   *Respiration*

Ronald Ross; 1923   **2862**

It is easy for persons to sit in arm-chairs and weave hypotheses; many imagined America before Columbus; but an ocean had to be traversed between the dream and the reality. Theorists who do not trouble to verify their own speculations deserve little credit.

Memoirs

Abraham Flexner; 1925   **2863**

Research, untrammeled by near reference to practical ends, will go on in every properly organized medical school; its critical method will dominate all teaching whatsoever.

Medical Education: A Comparative Study

Robert Bridges; 1929   **2864**

Wisdom will repudiate thee, if thou think to enquire WHY things are as they are or whence they came: thy task is first to learn WHAT IS, and in pursuant knowledge pure intellect will find pure pleasure and the only ground for a philosophy conformable to truth.   *The Testament of Beauty*

Harvey Cushing; 1935   **2865**

Among those who call themselves pure scientists, whatever their particular field, there are many who feel that they would demean themselves and lose caste among their fellows should they engage in researches which obviously point to some utilitarian purpose. This I have always regarded as an academic pose; for in the disinterested pursuit of knowledge, to stumble, as did Roentgen or the Curies or Banting, on something not only of great scientific importance but which at the same time was immediately applicable to human welfare, is certainly nothing to be ashamed of.   *Science*

Charles Scott Sherrington; 1946   **2866**
Essential to a great discoverer, in any field of Nature, would seem an intuitive flair for raising the right question. To ask something which the time is not ripe to answer is of small avail. There must be the means of reply and enough collateral knowledge to make the answer worthwhile.   *The Endeavour of Jean Fernel*

Robert A. McCance; 1950   **2867**
The medical profession has a responsibility not only for the cure of the sick and for the prevention of disease but for the advancement of knowledge upon which both depend. This third responsibility can only be met by investigation and experiment.
                    Proceedings of the Royal Society of Medicine

Harold G. Wolff; 1952   **2868**
Fixity of purpose requires flexibility of method.   *Stress and Disease*

Alphonse Raymond Dorchez; *circa* 1966   **2869**
You do one experiment in medicine to convince yourself, then 99 more to convince others.   *P&S Quarterly*

K-H Chen, G.F. Murray; 1976   **2870**
A rural Third World survey is the careful collection, tabulation, and analysis of wild guesses, half-truths, and outright lies meticulously recorded by gullible outsiders during interviews with suspicious, intimidated, but outwardly compliant villagers.
                    Marshall JF and Polgar S, Culture, Natality, and Family Planning

Peter B. Medawar; 1979   **2871**
Any scientist of any age who *wants to make important discoveries must study important problems*. Dull or piffling problems yield dull or piffling answers.... The problem must be such that it *matters* what the answer is.   *Advice to a Young Scientist*

G. Klein; 1981   **2872**
We must be wary of the ever-present occupational risk of the cancer researcher: generalization.   *Nature*

Walsh McDermott; 1982   **2873**
A physician's work has changed from seeing sick persons whose outcome is reasonably clear to seeing persons with [a] disease that has many far less recognizable subcategories, each with its own prognosis. We have lost our prognostic capability for most of the patients we see... Without [it] there can be no discriminating medicine.... What can we do?.... I have in mind... research and development aimed squarely at the actual process of medical practice, aimed at what the doctor does so that he may do it better.   *Annals of Internal Medicine*

Peter B. Medawar; 1984   **2874**
If the generative act in science is imaginative in character, only a failure of the imagination—a total inability to conceive what the solution of a problem *might* be—could bring scientific inquiry to a standstill. No such failure of the imagination—nor any failure of nerve that might be responsible for it—has yet occurred in science and there is not the slightest reason to suppose that it will ever do so.   *The Limits of Science*

Peter B. Medawar; 1984   **2875**
What is research but learning—and what scientist ever feels that, being complete, his research is now at last finished? The nature of science is such that a scientist goes on learning all his life—and must—and exults in the obligation upon him to do so.
                    The Limits of Science

Baruch S. Blumberg; 1987   **2876**
In research, and probably also in practice, maintaining and fostering curiosity—the ability to ask questions each time a new phenomenon occurs—is indispensable.
                    Manning PR and DeBakey L, Medicine: Preserving the Passion

Rita Levi-Montalcini; 1988   **2877**

I have become persuaded that, in scientific research, neither the degree of one's intelligence nor the ability to carry out one's tasks with thoroughness and precision are factors essential to personal success and fulfillment. More important... are total dedication and a tendency to underestimate difficulties, which cause one to tackle problems that other, more critical and acute persons instead to opt to avoid.   *In Praise of Imperfection*

Robert A. McCance, Elsie M. Widdowson; 1993   **2878**

If your results don't make physiological sense, think! You may have made a mistake or you may have made a discovery.   *Ashwell M, A Scientific Partnership of 60 Years*

Joshua Lederberg; 1995   **2879**

The promulgation of fraud is an outrage, striking at the roots of the scientific enterprise.... A much larger toll is exacted from inadequate experimental design and sloppy execution. The lost effort that is expended in straightening out muddy claims, or merely plowing through their presentation in the literature, greatly exceeds what can be attributed to intentional fraud.   *The Scientist*

Curtis L. Meinert; 1996   **2880**

In research, data speak.   *Clinical Trials Dictionary*

RESPIRATION

[Anonymous]; *circa* 1500 BC   **2881**

As for "the breath which enters the nose," it enters into the heart and the lungs. It is they which give to the entire body.   *Ebers Papyrus*

Aretaeus the Cappadocian; [81-138?]   **2882**

Animals live by two principal things, food and breath (spirit, pneuma); ...of these by far the most important is the respiration, for if it be stopped, the man will not endure long, but immediately dies.   *On Pneumonia*

Galen; [130-200]   **2883**

What is the use of breathing? That it is not a trifling use is clear from our inability to survive for even the shortest time after it has stopped.... It remains, then, that we breathe for regulation of heat. This, then, is the principal use of breathing, and the second is to nourish the psychic pneuma.   *On Respiration and the Arteries*

Robert Boyle; *circa* 1660   **2884**

The inspired and exspired air may be sometimes very useful, by condensing and cooling the blood...through the lungs; I hold that...not only one of the ordinary, but one of the principal uses of respiration.   *Kaplan BB, Divulging of Useful Truths in Physick*

Robert Hooke; 1666   **2885**

As the bare Motion of the Lungs *without fresh air* contributes nothing to the life of the Animal, he being found to survive as when they were not mov'd as when they were; so it was not the subsiding or movelessness of the Lungs, that was the immediate cause of Death, or the stopping of the Circulation of the Blood through the Lungs, but the *want* of a sufficient *supply* of fresh air.   *Philosophical Transactions of the Royal Society*

Richard Lower; 1669   **2886**

On this account [i.e., observation of a "cake of blood" *in vitro*] it is extremely probable that blood takes in air in its course through the lungs, and owes its bright color entirely to the admixture of air. Moreover, after the air has in large measure left the blood again within the body and the parenchyma of the viscera, and has transpired through the pores of the body, it is equally consistent with reason that the venous blood, which has lost its air, should forthwith appear darker and blacker.   *A Treatise on the Heart*

John Mayow; 1674   **2887**

It is quite certain that animals in breathing draw from the air certain vital particles which are also elastic. So that there should be no doubt at all now that an aërial something absolutely necessary to life enters the blood of animals by means of respiration.

Tractatus Quinque Medico-physici

Robert Boyle; 1682   **2888**

That portion of Air which hath once served the respiration of Animals as much as it could, is no longer useful for the respiration of another Animal, at least of the same kind.

The Spring and Weight of the Air

Antoine-Laurent Lavoisier; 1777   **2889**

Respiration acts only on the portion of pure or dephogisticated air [oxygen], contained in the atmosphere;... the residuum or mephitic part [nitrogen] is a merely passive medium which enters into the lungs, and departs from them nearly in the same state, without change or alteration.

Experiments on Animal Respiration

John Hutchinson; 1844   **2890**

The subject of this paper resolves itself under the following heads: First—the quantity of air expelled from the lungs... Second—the absolute capacity of the thorax... Third—the respiratory movements and mobility of the chest. Fourth—the inspiratory and expiratory muscular power. Fifth—the elasticity of the ribs, and estimate of the voluntary respiratory power.... Seventh—General and practical deductions, to detect disease by the spirometer, with the method of its application.

Medico-Chirurgical Transactions

John Scott Haldane, J.G. Priestly; 1914   **2891**

The experiments...indicate clearly that under normal conditions the regulation of the lung-ventilation depends on the pressure of CO_2 in the alveolar air. Even a very slight rise or fall in the alveolar CO_2 pressure causes a great increase or diminution in the lung-ventilation.... For each individual the normal alveolar CO_2 pressure appears to be an extraordinarily sharply defined physiological constant.

Journal of Physiology

Susan Ott; 1981   **2892**

Roses are red,
Violets are blue,
Without your lungs,
Your blood would be too.

New England Journal of Medicine

RESPIRATORY GASES

Per Frederik Scholander; 1947   **2893**

A volumetric gas analyzer is described which will determine carbon dioxide, oxygen, and nitrogen in 0.5 cc samples or less, with an accuracy of ± 0.015 volume per cent. It handles samples containing from zero to over 99 per cent absorable gases. The analysis requires from 6 to 8 minutes.

Journal of Biological Chemistry

RESPONSIBILITY

Charles Warrington Earle; 1880   **2894**

It is becoming altogether too customary in these days to speak of a vice as a disease, and to excuse men and women for the performance and indulgence of certain acts which not only ruin themselves and families, but bring burden on the community, simply because they are not responsible for the act[and] excuse them because they have a disease.

Chicago Medical Review

Harold M. Schoolman; 1977   **2895**

Clinical decision making...in teaching hospitals evolves through a series of subspecialists.... The diffusion of responsibility for decision making is tolerated, if not promoted.... The physician [can] deal with his discomfort by...allowing decisions to be made by others.... The result is that no one is responsible for the patient. Decisions are now made not by a patient advocate, but rather by a therapeutic advocate.

New England Journal of Medicine

REST

John Hunter; 1794   **2896**

The first and great requisite for the restoration of injured parts, is rest, as it allows that action, which is necessary for repairing injured parts, to go on without interruption, and as injuries often excite more action than is required, rest becomes still more necessary.

A Treatise on the Blood, Inflammation, and Gun-Shot Wounds

John Hilton; 1863   **2897**

By Therapeutics, however, I do not mean to imply the action of drugs, which more especially belongs to the department of the physician; but rather the influence of what I may venture to call "Natural Therapeutics" in the cure of surgical diseases. The chief of these is one so apparently simple as to make me almost apologize to you for selecting it. It is Rest—Physiological as well as Mechanical Rest.   *Rest and Pain*

RESTLESS LEG SYNDROME

Thomas Willis; [1621-1675]   **2898**

Wherefore to some, when being a Bed they betake themselves to sleep, Presently in the Arms and Leggs, Leapings and Contractions of the Tendons, And so great a Restlessness and Tossing of their Members ensue, that the diseased are no more able to sleep, Than if They were in a place of the greatest Torture.   *The Practice of Physick*

F. Gerard Allison; 1943   **2899**

This... ailment.... occurs most often when the legs get warm in bed, and prevents going to sleep.... A curious unlocalized restlessness is felt in one or both legs. It is not quite a pain, but is distinctly unpleasant. A combination of voluntary movement and involuntary jerks of the affected limb fails to find rest. In ten minutes to an hour the "jitters" depart and sleep comes.... The disagreeable sensation stops at once on chewing one-onehundredth grain of nitroglycerine, suggesting that the cause is vascular.

Canadian Medical Association Journal

Karl-Axel Ekbom; 1944   **2900**

When the syndrome is complete, it consists of the following symptoms: peculiar and characteristic paresthesia in the lower legs mostly during the night, weakness or clumsiness of the legs while walking, and a sensation of cold in the legs or feet. The paresthesia was called "anxietas tibiarum" in the middle of the previous century.   *Acta Medica Scandinavica*

Karl-Axel Ekbom; 1945   **2901**

Asthenia crurum paraesthetica is a disease (or syndrome) mainly characterized by peculiar, deep-lying paresthesia ("crawling") in the extremities, particularly the legs, which sets in only when the patient is resting and forces him to keep moving the affected limbs.... There is decided reason to believe in the existence of definite hereditary factors.

Acta Medica Scandinavica, Supplementum

RESUSCITATION

W.U. McClenahan; 1974   2902

When giving mouth-to-mouth resuscitation, the important thing to remember is to remove your denture first.   *G.P.*

RETINITIS PIGMENTOSA

Charles H. Usher; 1935   2903

I shall refer to but a single pedigree of retinitis pigmentosa in which some of the members have been known to me since 1897.... Of particular importance is the limitation of the disease to one sex.... Only males are affected... and transmission of the disease takes place through unaffected females.

Transactions of the Ophthalmological Society of the United Kingdom

RHEUMATIC FEVER

John Haygarth; 1805   2904

The Rheumatick Fever...begins with chilly fits; succeeded by increased heat; frequent pulse; thirst; loss of appetite; and prostration of strength. The symptom peculiar to this disease is an inflammation of the joints, which often increases to great violence, with swelling, soreness to the touch, and sometimes redness of the skin.... This is a very formidable and extremely painful disease[and] generally continues for many weeks.... The consequences of this disorder are often painfully felt for many years.

A Clinical History of Diseases

RHEUMATIC HEART DISEASE

William Charles Wells; 1810   2905

Dr. David Pitcairn, about the year 1788, began to remark, that persons subject to rheumatism were attacked more frequently than others, with symptoms of an organic disease of the heart. Subsequent experience having confirmed the truth of this observation, he concluded, that these two diseases often depend upon a common cause, and...called the latter disease rheumatism of the heart.

Transactions of the Society for the Improvement of Medical and Chirurgical Knowledge

Jean-Baptiste Bouillaud; 1835   2906

The newest and the most curious point of view of these researches is, without doubt, the coincidence of inflammation of the sero-fibrinous internal and external tissues of the heart (rheumatismal endocarditis and pericarditis) with acute articular rheumatism.... In auscultating the sounds of the heart in some individuals still labouring under, or convalescing from, acute articular rheumatism, I was not a little surprised to hear a strong file, saw, or bellows sound; such as I had often met with in chronic or organic induration of the valves, with contraction of the orifices of the heart.   *Cliniques des Maladies du Coeur*

RHEUMATISM

Guillaume de Baillou (Ballonius); 1736   2907

The whole body becomes painful, the face in some becomes red, the pain rages especially about the joints, so that indeed neither the foot nor the hand, nor the finger can be moved...without pain and outcry.... Although the arthritis is in a certain part, this rheumatism itself is in the entire body.   *Opera Medica Omnia*

William Heberden; 1802   2908

The rheumatism is a common name for many aches and pains, which have yet got no peculiar appellation, though owing to very different causes.

Commentaries on the History and Cure of Diseases

RHEUMATOID ARTHRITIS

Guillaume de Baillou; 1642   **2909**
Now what articular gout [arthritis] is in any limb, exactly so is rheumatism in the whole body, as regards pain, tension and the "feeling" of burning heat—as I call it—others say sensation. Both complaints are somewhat painful, but the gouty pain in the joint is repeated at definite times and periods. Not so this rheumatism.... The rheumatic disease may finally... bring about a state of generalized gout or "arthritic diathesis".   *On Rheumatism*

Jean-Baptiste Emile Vidal; 1855   **2910**
The articulation of the wrist and of the hand is very painful, reacting to the slightest touch.... The right forearm is in a position of forced pronation, while supination is impossible. The patient holds his hand towards the ulnar side with the dorsal surface presenting.... All joints may be affected, even the spine and the jaw.... These findings accompany the atrophic type of primary chronic articular rheumatism. The mechanism of its development is different from the other types.

Considerations on Chronic Primary Articular Rheumatism

George Frederick Still; 1897   **2911**
There is a disease, occurring in children, and beginning before the second dentition, which is characterized clinically by elastic fusiform enlargement of joints without bony change, and also by enlargement of glands and spleen. This disease has...been called rheumatoid arthritis, but it differs from that disease in adults, clinically in the absence of bony change...and pathologically in the absence, even in an advanced case, of the cartilage changes which are found quite early in that disease, and also in the absence of osteophytic change.   *Medico-Chirurgical Transactions*

Philip Showalter Hench, Edward Calvin Kendall, Charles H. Slocomb, Howard F. Polley; 1949   **2912**
Certain clinical and biochemical features of rheumatoid arthritis have been markedly improved by the daily intramuscular injection of either the adrenal cortical hormone, 17-hydroxy-11-dehydrocorticosterone (compound E), or the pituitary adrenocorticotropic hormone, ACTH.   *Proceedings of Staff Meetings of the Mayo Clinic*

RHEUMATOID SPONDYLITIS

Ernst Adolph Gustav Gottfried von Strümpell; 1887   **2913**
[Some] cases...are confined mainly to the vertebral column.... It leads very gradually and painlessly to a complete anchylosis of the entire spinal column and the hip-joints, so that the head, trunk, and thighs are firmly united and completely stiffened, while all the other joints retain their normal mobility.   *A Textbook of Medicine for Students and Practitioners*

RICKETS

Daniel Whistler; 1645   **2914**
The epiphyses at the joints are massive and large out of proportion to the age.... Knotty swellings also grow out on the sides [of the chest] where the cartilaginous parts join the bony.... The whole bony system is in truth flexible like wax.... The tibiae...become bent.... These children have enlargement of the head.... The teeth are cut late and with excessive trouble.... Other accompaniments are narrowness of the chest, prominence of the sternum, and asymmetry.   *Disputatio Medica Inauguralis*

Francis Glisson; 1650   **2915**
There appeareth the unusual bigness of the Head.... Certain swellings and knotty excrescences, about some of the joynts are observed.... These are chiefly conspicuous in the Wrists.... The like Tumors also are in the tops of the Ribs where they are conjoyned with gristles in the Breast.... Some Bones wax crooked, especially the Bones called the Shank-

bone.... The Breast...becomes narrow on the sides, and sticking up foreright, so that it may not be unaptly compared to the Keel of a Ship inverted.

De Rachitide sive Morbo Puerili

Cotton Mather; 1724   **2916**

In our Countrey, it is now a Very Common Malady.... Tis a Melancholy Spectacle, which the *Rickety Children* afford unto us, when we see their *Heads* growing into an unporportionable Magnitude; with diverse uncomely Protuberances: Their *Breasts* troublesomely straitened and mishapen; the *Sternum* Sticking out; Their *Bellies* enormously Swelled; Their *Backs* and *Bones* Crooked; Their *Joints* tumified; Their *Breath* short.

The Angel of Bethesda

RICKETTSIALPOX

Robert Joseph Huebner, W.L. Jellison, C. Pomerantz; 1946   **2917**

An organism having the morphologic and cultural characteristics of a rickettsia has been isolated from a patient during the course of an unusual outbreak of disease [with a vesicular-papular eruption] occurring in New York.   *Public Health Reports*

RIGHTS OF CHILDREN

Billy F. Andrews; 1968   **2918**

That when and if correction is deemed necessary it will be applied with the greatest of respect and care and without mental or physical abuse.   *The Children's Bill of Rights*

RINGWORM (TINEA CAPITIS)

Raymond Jacques Adrien Sabouraud; 1905   **2919**

The apparatus...has allowed me to form regulations for the use of the X-rays in the treatment of ringworm.... This yellow paper [with platino-cyanide of barium] becomes brown under the influence of the X-rays and acts as a control apparatus.... The sitting is then terminated and the scalp of the patient has received the quantity of X-rays necessary to cause total alopecia of the region exposed, without provoking erythema or radiodermatitis and without preventing restoration later. A patch of ringworm is thus cured at a single sitting.   *Elementary Manual of Regional Topographical Dermatology*

RURAL MEDICINE

Abraham Flexner; 1910   **2920**

The small town needs the best and not the worst doctor procurable. For the country doctor has only himself to rely on: he cannot in every pinch hail specialist, expert, and nurse. On his own skill, knowledge, resourcefulness, the welfare of his patient altogether depends. The rural district is therefore entitled to the best trained physician that can be induced to go there.   *Medical Education in the United States and Canada*

Abraham Flexner; 1910   **2921**

It might conceivedly become the duty of the several states to salary district physicians in thinly settled or remote regions—surely a sounder policy than the demoralization of the entire profession for the purpose of enticing ill trained men where they will not go.

Medical Education in the United States and Canada

David Lloyd George; 1912   **2922**

Anyone who lived in these mountain regions knows what sickness means there. There are miles of track, broken and rutted by the winter rains, before you even reach the high road. The people there never sent for medical aid for petty ailments. Doctors not even summoned for important family events are called in when life is in jeopardy.   *Speech*

SAINT JOHN'S WORT

Samuel Stearns; 1801   **2923**

Hypericum perforatum. It is called a mild detergent, corroborant, and vulnerary. It was formerly used to strengthen the system, kill worms, promote urine, heal wounds, cure
ulcers[and] hypocondrical, hysterical, and maniacal disorders; but it is not employed in
the present practice.   *The American Herbal*

SALICYLATES

Pedanius Dioscorides (Anazarbeus); [40?-90?]   **2924**

Salix is a tree known to all, whose fruit and leaves and bark and juice have astringent qualities.... The juice out of the leaves and bark, being warmed with Rosaceum in a cup of
Malum Punicum, doth help the griefs of the ears, and the decoction of them is an excellent fomentation for the Gout.   *De Materia Medica*

Thomas John MacLagan; 1876   **2925**

A remedy would most hopefully be looked for among those plants and trees whose
favourite habitat presented conditions...under which the rheumatic miasm seemed most
to prevail.... The plants whose haunts best corresponded...were the various forms of willow.... The bark contains salicin.... The idea of treating acute rheumatism by salicin
occurred to me in November, 1874.... We have in salicin a valuable remedy.... The relief
of pain is always one of the earliest effects produced. In acute cases, relief of pain and a
fall of temperature generally occur simultaneously.   *The Lancet*

SALIVARY DUCTS (STENSEN DUCT)

Niels Stensen; 1661   **2926**

[Three weeks after arriving at the anatomy laboratory of Gerhard Blasius in Amsterdam]
fortune so favored me that in the first sheep's head, which I...was dissecting alone in my
room, I found a duct which, so far as I knew, had been described by no one before.
                                                                         Letter to Thomas Bartholin

SANITATION

Jacob Riis; 1901   **2927**
You can kill a man with a tenement as easily as you can kill a man with an ax.
How the Other Half Lives

SARCOCELE

Samuel Johnson; 1783   **2928**
My case, which you guessed at not amiss, is a Sarcocele; a dreadful disorder which however, I hope, God will not suffer to destroy me. Let me have your prayers. I have consulted Mr. Mudge of Plymouth who strongly presses an immediate operation. I expect Dr. Heberden's advice tomorrow.
Letter to Bennet Langton

SARCOIDOSIS

Ernest Besnier; 1889   **2929**
Finally, three years later, the nose has doubled in size, and shows an extreme lividity; the varicosities are larger; the involved area that covers almost all of the deformed portion is livid with the color of wine, and has enlarged sebaceous pores and small necrotic erosions at the nares. [Lupus pernio]
Annales de Dermatologie et de Syphiligraphie

Caesar Peter Moeller Boeck; 1899   **2930**
We find in a middle-aged... man groups of lymph nodes much swollen [and] a widespread, somewhat symmetrical, eruption, firm nodules of varying sizes on head and extensor surfaces of trunk and extremities... [involving] the whole skin.... The color of the early nodules is bright red, becoming darker and finally yellowish or brown.... The nodules disappear.... leaving... a loss of substance in the skin.... The disease seems benign.... The... new growth might be described as perivascular sarcomatoid tissue built up by excessively rapid proliferation of epithelioid connective-tissue cells.... The term "multiple benign sarcoid" perhaps will not be found unsuitable.
Journal of Cutaneous and Genitourinary Diseases

SCARLET FEVER

Daniel Sennert; 1633   **2931**
The entire body appears red and as if on fire, and also as if it suffered from a universal erysipelas. In declination the redness itself diminishes and wide red spots again appear as in the beginning, which however disappear the seventh or ninth day with the skin falling off like scales. This disease indeed is grave and dangerous and often lethal. *De Febribus*

Thomas Sydenham; 1676   **2932**
This attacks infants most, and that towards the end of summer. Shivers and chills at the commencement; but no great depression. The whole skin is marked with small, red spots, more frequent, more diffused, and more red than in measles. These last two or three days. Then they disappear; leaving the skin covered with branny *squamulae*, as if powdered with meal.
Febris scarlatina

William Heberden; 1802   **2933**
The scarlet fever begins with the common symptoms of other fevers. On the first or second day an unusual redness appears on the skin, and there is a slight pain of the throat. At the same time in some patients there are swellings under each ear, or in other glands, which are not always dispersed without coming to suppuration.
Commentaries on the History and Cure of Diseases

SCHIZOPHRENIA

John Haslam; 1809   2934

Connected with the loss of memory, there is a form of insanity which occurs in young persons.... The attack is almost imperceptible.... The sensibility appears to be considerably blunted... They do not bear the same affection towards their parents and relations... As their apathy increases they are negligent of their dress, and inattentive to personal cleanliness. Thus in the interval between puberty and manhood, I have painfully witnessed this hopeless and degrading change, which in a short time has transformed the most promising and vigorous intellect into a slavering and bloated ideot.

Observations on Madness and Melancholy

Clifford Whittingham Beers; 1908   2935

In telling the story of my life, I must relate the history of another self—a self which was dominant from my twenty-fourth to my twenty-sixth year. During that period I was unlike what I had been, or what I have been since. The biographical part of my autobiography might be called the history of a mental civil war.   *A Mind That Found Itself*

Eugen Bleuler; 1911   2936

By the term... "schizophrenia" we designate a group of psychoses whose course is at times chronic, at times marked by intermittent attacks, and which can stop or retrograde at any stage.... The disease is characterized by a specific type of alterations of thinking, feeling, and relation to the external world which appears nowhere else in this particular fashion.

Dementia Praecox

Eugen Bleuler; 1911   2937

We are left with no alternative but to give the disease a new name.... I am well aware of the disadvantages of the proposed name but I know of no better one.... I call dementia praecox "schizophrenia" because... the "splitting" of the different functions is one of its most important characteristics. For the sake of convenience, I use the word in the singular although it is apparent that the group includes several diseases.   *Dementia Praecox*

SCIENCE

St. Bernard; [1091-1153]   2938

We see more and farther than our predecessors, not because we have keener vision or greater height, but because we are lifted up and borne aloft on their gigantic stature.

John of Salisbury, The Metalogica of John of Salisbury

Robert Boyle; 1663   2939

The Requisites of a good Hypothesis are:
That it be Intelligible.
That it neither Assume nor Suppose
anything Impossible, unintelligible,
or demonstrably False.
That it be consistent with itself.
That it be fit and sufficient to Explicate
the *Phaenomena*, especially the chief.
That it be, at least, consistent with the
rest of the *Phaenomena* it particularly
relates to, and do not contradict any other
known *Phaenomena* of nature, or manifest
Physical Truth.   *Kaplan BB, Divulging of Useful Truths in Physick*

Abraham Cowley; [1618-1669]   2940
Thus Harvey sought for Truth in Truth's own Book
The Creatures, which by God himself was writ;
And wisely thought 'twas fit,
Not to read Comments only upon it,
But on th' Original itself to look.   *Ode upon Doctor Harvey*

Isaac Newton; [1642-1727]   2941
No great discovery is ever made without a bold guess.   *Beveridge WIB, The Art of Scientific*
Investigation

Alexander Pope; 1733   2942
Trace Science then, with Modesty thy guide;
First strip off all her equipage of Pride.   *An Essay on Man. Epistle II*

John Hunter; 1775   2943
Why do you ask me a question, by the way of solving it? I think your solution is just; but
why think, why not trie the Expt?   *Letters to Edward Jenner*

Lazzaro Spallanzani; [1729-1799]   2944
If I set out to prove something, I am no real scientist—I have to learn to follow where the
facts lead me—I have to learn to whip my prejudices.   *Coope R, The Quiet Art*

René-Théophile-Hyacinthe Laennec; *circa* 1821   2945
[Broussais] defies me, he waits for me...he addresses me by private name and collective
name and in choosing me somehow [makes me] champion of doctors, who with me profess Hippocratic empiricism, enlightened by the observation of the living and the dead,
by the relationship of facts, and by the very reserved use of the inductive method.... Only
an invalid could refuse to defend such a beautiful cause.   *Manuscript in Musée Laennec*

Johannes Müller; 1824   2946
Observation is simple, indefatigable, industrious, upright, without any preconceived
opinion. Experiment is artificial, impatient, busy, digressive, passionate, unreliable.
                        Inaugural lecture as docent of physiology at University of Bonn

Pierre-Charles-Alexandre Louis; 1829   2947
It behooves those who devote themselves to observation to be impressed by this truth
[i.e., that many "facts" grow old] and to realize that the best work is only good in relation
to its time and that it awaits another, more exact and more complete.   *Recherches*
Anatomiques, Pathologiques et Therapeutiques

Johann Wolfgang von Goethe; [1749-1832]   2948
You are engrossed in botany? in optic? What are you doing?
Is it not much nicer to move a tender heart?
Ah well, those tender hearts! A bungler can easily move them;
Let my only happiness be to stay in touch with you, Oh Nature!
                        Otto R, Romische Elegien und Venezianische Epigramme

Johann Wolfgang von Goethe; [1749-1832]   2949
We see only what we know.   *Beveridge WIB, The Art of Scientific Investigation*

William Beaumont; 1833   2950
Truth, like beauty, is "when unadorned, adorned the most," and, in prosecuting these
experiments and inquiries, I believe I have been guided by its light.
                        Experiments and Observations on the Gastric Juice

Constantine Hering; 1843   2951
Among men of deliberate and acute reflection, no difference of opinion can exist relative
to the truth of a discovery which rests upon the basis of actual experiment.
                        Hahnemann S, Organon of Homeopathic Medicine

Jan Evangelista Purkyně; *circa* 1850   **2952**
For the one science is the noble gift of Heaven, yet for the other only the cow to milk, so that there is butter enough.   *Poems and Translations*

Claude Bernard; 1852   **2953**
Art is myself, science is ourselves.
Illustrated Manual of Operative Surgery and Surgical Anatomy

Karl Friedrich Gauss; [1777-1855]   **2954**
I have the result but I do not yet know how to get it.
Beveridge WIB, The Art of Scientific Investigation

Oliver Wendell Holmes; 1858   **2955**
Scientific knowledge, even in the most modest persons, has mingled with it a something which partakes of insolence. Absolute, peremptory facts are bullies.
The Autocrat of the Breakfast Table

Oliver Wendell Holmes; 1860   **2956**
A Pseudo-science does not necessarily consist wholly of lies.... When we have one fact found us, we are very apt to supply the next out of our own imagination.
The Professor at the Breakfast Table

Claude Bernard; 1865   **2957**
The application of mathematics to natural phenomena is the aim of all science.
An Introduction to the Study of Experimental Medicine

Claude Bernard; 1865   **2958**
There never are any unsuccessful experiments: they are all successful in their own definite conditions, so that negatives cannot nullify positive results.
An Introduction to the Study of Experimental Medicine

Claude Bernard; 1865   **2959**
No man's opinion, formulated in a theory or otherwise, may be deemed to represent the whole truth in the sciences. It is a guide, a light, but not an absolute authority. The revolution which the experimental method has effected in the sciences is this: it has put a scientific criterion in the place of personal authority. The experimental method is characterized by being dependent only on itself, because it includes within itself its criterion—experience.   *An Introduction to the Study of Experimental Medicine*

Claude Bernard; 1865   **2960**
True science teaches us to doubt and, in ignorance, to refrain.
An Introduction to the Study of Experimental Medicine

Ralph Waldo Emerson; 1870   **2961**
Men love to wonder, and that is the seed of science.   *Society and Solitude*

Samuel Wilks; 1877   **2962**
Discoveries are made by the age and not by the individual.   *Guy's Hospital Reports*

Charles Darwin; 1888   **2963**
I am not very skeptical—a frame of mind which I believe to be injurious to the progress of science. A good deal of skepticism in a scientific man is advisable to avoid much loss of time, but I have met with not a few men, who, I feel sure, have often thus been deterred from experiment or observations, which would have proved directly or indirectly serviceable.   *Darwin F, The Life and Letters of Charles Darwin*

William Osler; 1894   **2964**
To the physician particularly, a scientific discipline is an incalculable gift, which leavens his whole life, giving exactness to habits of thought and tempering the mind with that judicious faculty of distrust which can alone, amid the uncertainties of practice, make

him wise unto salvation. For perdition inevitably awaits the mind of the practitioner who has never had the full inoculation with the leaven, who has never grasped clearly the relations of science to his art, and who knows nothing and perhaps cares less, for the limitations of either. *The Leaven of Science*

William Thomson, Lord Kelvin; 1894   **2965**
When you can measure what you are speaking about, and express it in numbers, you know something about it; but when you cannot measure it, when you cannot express it in numbers, your knowledge is of a meager and unsatisfactory kind: it may be the beginning of knowledge, but you have scarcely, in your thoughts, advanced to the stage of science.
Popular Lectures and Addresses

Louis Pasteur; [1822-1895]   **2966**
My only strength is my tenacity. *Beveridge WIB, The Art of Scientific Investigation*

Frances Dickinson; 1900   **2967**
I know no facts, when listed for scientific purposes, to be "indelicate, indecent, obscene, or nasty." These adjectives express relative conditions in social life. The varied conditions of human beings from physical and psychological standpoints should be handled without sentiment and prejudice if scientific conclusions are to be reached and present conditions bettered. *The Gynecologic Consideration of the Sexual Act*

Abraham Flexner; 1910   **2968**
Scientific medicine...brushes aside all historic dogma. It gets down to details immediately. No man is asked in whose name he comes—whether that of Hahnemann, Rush, or of some more recent prophet. But all are required to undergo rigorous cross-examination. Whatsoever makes good is accepted, becomes in so far part, and organic part, of the permanent structure. *Medical Education in the United States and Canada*

Karl Pearson; 1911   **2969**
Every great advance of science opens our eyes to facts which we failed before to observe, and makes new demands on our powers of interpretation. This extension of the material of science into regions where our great-grandfathers could see nothing at all...is one of the most remarkable features of modern progress.... Where they discovered the circulation of the blood, we see the physical conflict of living poisons within the blood, whose battles would have been absurdities for them. *Coope R, The Quiet Art*

Jules-Henri Poincaré; [1854-1912]   **2970**
Science is built of facts the way a house is built of bricks; but an accumulation of facts is no more science than a pile of bricks is a house. *Toronto Globe and Mail*

Miguel de Unamuno; 1913   **2971**
Science is a cemetery of dead ideas, even though life may issue from them.
The Tragic Sense of Life

Miguel de Unamuno; 1913   **2972**
True science teaches, above all, to doubt and to be ignorant. *The Tragic Sense of Life*

Charles Horace Mayo; 1926   **2973**
The scientist is not content to stop at the obvious.
Collected Papers of the Mayo Clinic and Mayo Foundation

Wilfred Batten Lewis Trotter; 1930   **2974**
The truly scientific mind is altogether unafraid of the new, and while having no mercy for ideas which have served their turn or shown their uselessness, it will not grudge to any unfamiliar conception its moment of full and friendly attention, hoping to expand rather than to minimize what small core of usefulness it may happen to contain.
British Medical Journal

Ludwik Fleck; 1935   **2975**

Once a structurally complete and closed system of opinions consisting of many details and relations has been formed, it offers constant resistance to anything that contradicts it.

Genesis and Development of a Scientific Fact

Walter Bradford Cannon; 1945   **2976**

This time element is essential. The investigator may be made to dwell in a garret, he may be forced to live on crusts and wear dilapidated clothes, he may be deprived of social recognition, but if he has time, he can steadfastly devote himself to research. Take away his free time and he is utterly destroyed as a contributor to knowledge.

Beveridge WIB, The Art of Scientific Investigation

Alfred North Whitehead; [1861-1947]   **2977**

The aim of science is to seek the simplest explanation of complex facts. We are apt to fall into the error of thinking that the facts are simple because simplicity is the goal of our quest. The guiding motto in the life of every natural philosopher should be "Seek simplicity and distrust it." *Journal of Electrocardiology*

Albert Einstein; [1879-1955]   **2978**

The most beautiful thing we can experience is the mysterious. It is the source of all art and science. *Maslow AH, Motivation and Personality*

Jacob Bronowski; 1965   **2979**

I once told an audience of school children that the world would never change if they did not contradict their elders. I was chagrined to find next morning that this axiom outraged their parents. Yet it is the basis of the scientific method. A man must see, do and think things for himself, in the face of those who are sure that they have already been over all that ground. In science, there is no substitute for independence. *Science and Human Values*

Peter B. Medawar; 1967   **2980**

The scientific method is not deductive in character: it is a well-known fallacy to regard it as such. *The Art of the Soluble*

Peter B. Medawar; 1967   **2981**

Nowadays we all give too much thought to the material blessings or evils that science has brought with it, and too little to its power to liberate us from the confinements of ignorance and superstition. The greatest liberation of thought achieved by the scientific revolution was to have given human beings a sense of future in this world.

The Art of the Soluble

Barry Commoner; 1971   **2982**

There is, indeed, a specific fault in our system of science, and in the resultant understanding of the natural world.... This fault is reductionism, the view that effective understanding of a complex system can be achieved by investigating the properties of its isolated parts. The reductionist methodology, which is so characteristic of much of modern research, is not an effective means of analyzing the vast natural systems that are threatened by degradation.

The Closing Circle

Edward de Bono; 1971   **2983**

Pouncing on an idea as soon as it appears kills the idea. Too early and too enthusiastic logical attention either freezes the idea or forces it into the old moulds. Concentration on an idea isolates it from its surroundings and arrests its growth. The glare of attention inhibits the fertile semi-conscious processes that go to develop an idea. *New Think*

Edward de Bono; 1971   **2984**

When you have got somewhere interesting, that is the time to look back and pick out the surest way of getting there again. Sometimes it is very much easier to see the surest route to a place only after you have arrived. You may have to be at the top of a mountain to find the easiest way up. *New Think*

John R. Henderson; 1971   **2985**

Almost anybody can have an idea. Ideas are the small change of science: it is conviction—zany, indestructible belief—that is the real pot of gold.   *Guy's Hospital Gazette*

C.R. Lowe; 1974   **2986**

It is impossible to prove that an hypothesis is true, one can only accumulate evidence, in an infinite series, to support it. On the other hand, one observation can refute it.... A "good" scientific hypothesis is one that can be disproved. An hypothesis that can be adjusted, like an expanding suitcase, to accommodate an increasing variety of observed facts is scientifically worthless.   *Proceedings of the Royal Society of Medicine*

James Bryant Conant; [1893-1978]   **2987**

The stumbling way in which even the ablest of the scientists in every generation have had to fight through thickets of erroneous observations, misleading generalizations, inadequate formulations, and unconscious prejudice is rarely appreciated by those who obtain their scientific knowledge from textbooks.   *Science and Common Sense*

Howard E. Gruber; 1979   **2988**

The power and the beauty of science do not rest upon infallibility, which it has not, but on corrigibility, without which it is nothing.   *New York Times Book Review*

Eric J. Cassell; 1984   **2989**

The changes in medicine that are occurring today are part of a larger social upheaval.... This social movement...is marked by a turning away from science and technology—even, on occasion, from reason itself.... With time it will become apparent again that science and technology are not the enemies; and..."reason" is not *inherently* atomistic or reductionist, nor science the enemy of persons. Then the search for the solutions to the problems faced by medicine...will inevitably involve the development of new and exciting intellectual tools.   *The Place of the Humanities in Medicine*

Peter B. Medawar; 1984   **2990**

The most heinous offense a scientist as a scientist can commit is to declare to be true that which is not so; if a scientist cannot interpret the phenomenon he is studying, it is a binding obligation upon him to make it possible for another to do so.   *The Limits of Science*

Peter B. Medawar; 1984   **2991**

It is a layman's illusion that in science we caper from pinnacle to pinnacle of achievement and that we exercise a Method which preserves us from error. Indeed we do not; our way of going about things takes it for granted that we guess less often right than wrong, but at the same time ensures that we need not persist in error if we earnestly and honestly endeavor not to do so.   *The Limits of Science*

Peter B. Medawar; 1984   **2992**

Philosophers and logicians since the days of Bacon have been entirely clear on this point: deduction merely makes explicit information that is already there. It is not a procedure by which new information can be brought into being.   *The Limits of Science*

Peter B. Medawar; 1984   **2993**

Science can only proceed on a basis of confidence, so that scientists do not suspect each other of dishonesty or sharp practice, and believe each other unless there is very good reason to do otherwise.   *The Limits of Science*

Peter B. Medawar; 1984   **2994**

Science is a great and glorious enterprise—the most successful, I argue, that human beings have ever engaged in. To reproach it for its inability to answer all the questions we should like to put to it is no more sensible than to reproach a railway locomotive for not flying or, in general, not performing any other operation for which it was not designed.

The Limits of Science

Peter B. Medawar; 1984   **2995**

Science will persevere just as long as we retain a faculty we show no signs of losing: the ability to conceive—in no matter how imperfect or rudimentary a form—what the truth *might* be and retain also the inclination to ascertain whether our imaginings correspond to real life or not.   *The Limits of Science*

Robertson Davies; 1984   **2996**

Science, during the past 150 years, has gained formidable new authority, and it is to Science that we owe the increased longevity of the race, and the control of many of the terrible ills that afflict mankind. Science may cure disease, but can it confer health? Like all powerful gods, Science seeks to be the One True God, and as it writhes about the staff of Hermes it seeks to diminish and perhaps drive out the other god, the god of Humanism.   *The Merry Heart. Can a Doctor Be a Humanist?*

Matko Marusic; 1988   **2997**

Nature is really fascinating! It is packed with my scientific views!   *Personal communication*

Neil Cossons; *circa* 1990   **2998**

Science's function is to describe how things work, not what they mean. That is a role for philosophers, artists, and writers.   *Dean M, The Lancet*

Colin Tudge; 1993   **2999**

The true role of science is not to change the universe but more fully to appreciate it.   *The Engineer in the Garden*

Londa Schiebinger; 1993   **3000**

Only recently have we begun to appreciate that who does science affects the kind of science that gets done. How, then, has our knowledge of nature been influenced by struggles determining who is included in science and who is excluded, which projects are pursued and which ignored, whose experiences are validated and whose are not, and who stands to gain in terms of wealth or well-being and who does not?   *Nature's Body*

Londa Schiebinger; 1993   **3001**

Objectivity in science cannot be proclaimed, it must be built.   *Nature's Body*

David Kerr; 1996   **3002**

It is...willingness to accept that your ideas may prove wrong, and require revision, that characterizes science.   *Journal of the Royal College of Physicians*

Marcia Angell; 1996   **3003**

Litigation, fear, bias, and greed can interfere with scientific efforts to answer an important public health question. Perhaps most troubling of all,...in deciding about health risks, our courts and a substantial segment of the American public seem comfortable with methods that can only be described as antiscientific and irrational. Yet, like it or not, science and the rules of evidence and reason are the only reliable tools we have to investigate risks to human health.   *New England Journal of Medicine*

Leon Eisenberg; 2002   **3004**

Medical science is only a series of approximations.   *The New York Times*

SCIENTISTS

Wilhelm Conrad Röntgen; 1894   **3005**

Every genuine scientist, whatever his line, who takes his task seriously, fundamentally follows purely ideal goals and is an idealist in the best sense of the word.   *Glasser O, Wilhelm Conrad Röntgen and the Early History of the Roentgen Rays*

Henry Louis Mencken; 1922   **3006**

What actually moves him is his unquenchable curiosity—his boundless, almost pathological thirst to penetrate the unknown, to uncover the secret, to find out what has not been found out before. His prototype is not the liberator releasing slaves, the good Samaritan lifting up the fallen, but a dog sniffing tremendously at an infinite series of rat-holes. *Prejudices, 3rd series. The Scientist*

Peter Frank; 1949 **3007**
I have little patience with scientists who take a board of wood, look for the thinnest part, and drill a great number of holes where the drilling is easy. *Reveiw of Modern Physics*

Heinz Hartmann; 1960 **3008**
Every avenue which could lead to an increase of our knowledge deserves to be followed, regardless of the consequences. This is the professional code, or rather one of the professional codes, we find in men of science. *Psychoanalysis and Moral Values*

[Anonymous]; 1981 **3009**
Scientists are human. If you prick them, do they not bleed? If you approve their results, shall they not receive grants? If you publish their papers, shall their careers not prosper? *The Lancet*

SCLERODERMA

Ferdinand von Hebra, Moriz Kaposi; 1874 **3010**
By the term *Scleroderma adultorum*, we understand an idiopathic, morbid change in the skin which is chiefly known by a diffuse and remarkable induration, rigidity, and comparative shortening of the affected part.... The morbid change appears on various parts of the body, mostly on the upper extremities.... If the skin of the face be affected the features are rigid, quite immovable, as if "petrified," like those of a marble bust. Neither pain nor joy causes the "stony" countenance to alter. *On Diseases of the Skin*

William Osler; 1898 **3011**
In its more aggravated forms diffuse scleroderma is one of the most terrible of all human ills. Like Tithonus to "wither slowly" and like him to be "beaten down and marred and wasted" until one is literally a mummy, encased in an evershrinking, slowly contracting skin of steel, is a fate not pictured in any tragedy, ancient or modern. *Journal of Cutaneous Genitourinary Diseases*

SCREENING

William Keith C. Morgan; 1969 **3012**
While it is conceded that the routine physical examination may detect a few diseases while the patient is still asymptomatic and also pick up a few biochemical abnormalities, with one or two doubtful exceptions it has not been shown that the prognosis of the disease diagnosed under such circumstances has been improved one jot or tittle. *Medical Journal of Australia*

SCURVY

Jacques Cartier; [1491-1557] **3013**
Some did lose all their strength, and could not stand on their feete, then did their legges swel.... Others also had all their skins spotted with spots of blood of a purple color.... Their mouth became stincking, their gummes so rotten, that all the flesh did fall off, even to the rootes of the teeth, which did also almost all fall out.... Domagaia...had been very sicke with that disease.... Our Captaine seeing him whole and sound...asked...how he had done to heale himselfe: he answered, that he had taken the juice and sappe of the leaves of a certain Tree. *Hakluyt R, The Principall Navigations*

Cotton Mather; 1724 **3014**
Spirit of *Sal Armoniac*, now and then taken in a glass of Wine, is an excellent Thing for

the *Scurvy*. And so is *Whey*, with the Juice of Orange or Lemon in it. *Limons* do Wonders for the Relief of the *Scurvy*.
The Angel of Bethesda

James Lind; 1753 **3015**
I come...to an additional, and extremely powerful cause, observed at sea to occasion this disease, and in which...progress of time, seldom fails to breed it. And this is, the want of fresh vegetables and greens.... The difficulty of obtaining them at sea, together with a long continuance in the moist sea-air, are the true causes of its so general and fatal malignity upon that element.
A Treatise on the Scurvy

James Lind; 1753 **3016**
I selected twelve patients in the scurvy, on board the *Salisbury* at sea.... They all in general had putrid gums, the spots and lassitude, with weakness of their knees.... The most sudden and visible good effects were perceived from the use of oranges and lemons; one of those who had taken them, being at the end of six days fit for duty.
A Treatise on the Scurvy

John Huxham; 1757 **3017**
The Fleet returns to its Port; fresh Air, wholesome Liquor, fresh Provisions, especially proper Fruits and Herbage, soon purify the Blood and...restore their Health.... Apples, Oranges, and Lemons, alone, have been often known to do surprising Things in the Cure of very deplorable scorbutic Cases, that arose...in Long Voyages. But what will cure will prevent.
A Method for Preserving the Health of Seamen

Gilbert Blane; 1785 **3018**
The principal source of scurvy is a vitiated or scanty diet, and that it is very much promoted by cold, moisture, filth, sloth, and dejection of mind. Fresh vegetables are the most effectual antiscorbutics.... There is something in a particular class of fruit of the lemon and orange kind, which far surpasses every other remedy.
Observations on the Diseases Incident to Seamen

SEBORRHEIC DERMATITIS

Paul Gerson Unna; 1887 **3019**
Seborrhoeal eczema is quite a different matter; here the skin was not previously very healthy, and a few weeks after birth, there has existed...an extensive seborrhea of the scalp. This often spreads over the ears, forehead and cheeks after it has taken on a moist character.... It spreads upon the shoulders and upper arm in the form of dry, scaly or fatty plaques.... The differential diagnosis is to be made from other forms of chronic eczema, and from psoriasis.
Mittheilungen der Praktische Dermatologie

SELF

Alexander Pope; 1733 **3020**
Know then thyself, presume not God to scan;
The proper study of Mankind is Man.
An Essay on Man. Epistle II

Vaclav Havel; 1994 **3021**
The more thoroughly all our organs and their functions, their internal structure and the biochemical reactions that take place within them are described, the more we seem to fail to grasp the spirit, purpose and meaning of the system that they create together and that we experience as our unique "self."
Speech

SERUM THERAPY

Arthur L. Bloomfield; 1958 **3022**
The 1890's were the beginning of the golden age of serum therapy. Doctors, "like stout

Cortez when with eagle eyes he stared at the Pacific," saw a vast ocean of opportunity and dreamed of curing all infections by appropriate sera.

A Bibliography of Internal Medicine: Communicable Diseases

SERVICE

Thomas Sydenham; [1624-1689]   3023
I have weighed in a nice and scrupulous balance whether it be better to serve men or be praised by them, and I prefer the former. *Coope R, The Quiet Art*

SEX

Hippocrates; [460-375 BC]   3024
Sexual intercourse reduces, moistens, and warms. It warms owing to the fatigue and the excretion of moisture; it reduces owing to the evacuation; it moistens because of the remnant in the body of the matters melted by the fatigue. *Regimen*

Aristotle; [384-322 BC]   3025
At the same time of life that semen begins to appear in males and is emitted, the menstrual discharge begins to flow in females, their voice changes and their breasts begin to become conspicuous. *De Generatione Animalium*

Moses Maimonides; *circa* 1190   3026
The indulgence of sexual intercourse is one of the requirements for the maintenance of health, providing that there should be adequate abstinence between periods of indulgence, so that no noticeable enfeeblement or weakness ensue; rather one's body should feel [better] than before the act.

Rosner F and Munter S, The Medical Aphorisms of Moses Maimonides

Thomas Browne; 1643   3027
I could be content that we might procreate like trees, without conjunction, or that there were any way to perpetuate the World without this trivial and vulgar way of union: it is the foolishest act a wise man commits in all his life; nor is there any thing that will more deject his cool'd imagination, when he shall consider what an odd and unworthy piece of folly he hath committed. *Religio Medici*

Nicholas Culpeper; 1660   3028
Lust is the cause of begetting more children than the desire of the blessings of God.

A Directory for Midwives

John Hill; 1771   3029
As for a moderate commerce with the other sex, far from enfeebling nature, it preserves her in a right state: it was intended in our construction; and is required by our constitution. *The Management of Gout in Diet, Exercise, and Temper*

Benjamin Rush; 1812   3030
When indulged in an undue or a promiscuous intercourse with the female sex, or in onanism, it produces seminal weakness, impotence, dysury, tabes dorsalis, pulmonary consumption, dyspepsia, dimness of site, vertigo, epilepsy, hypochondriasis, loss of memory, manalgia, fatuity, and death. *Diseases of the Mind*

Mary Putnam Jacobi; 1877   3031
Physiologists and physicians again, while demonstrating the slavery that results from abuse of the sexual functions, have hinted of no danger consequent upon their normal exercise. On the contrary, their stimulating effects upon the rest of the economy have been portrayed in brilliant colors by even sober pens.

The Question of Rest for Women During Menstruation

Denslow Lewis; 1899   **3032**

She [the bride] should be informed that it is a consecration of the marriage vows and a bond of union between her husband and herself. She should be told that it is right and proper for her to experience pleasure in its performance...it is only fair for the girl to understand that there is no immodesty in her active participation, but on the contrary that such action on her part will increase the interest of the event for both her husband and herself.

Transactions of the Section of Obstetric Diseases in Women of the American Medical Association

Elizabeth Blackwell; 1902   **3033**

Although physical sexual pleasure is not attached exclusively, or in woman chiefly, to the act of coition, it is a well-established fact that in healthy loving women...increasing physical satisfaction attaches to the ultimate physical expression of love. A repose and general well-being results from this natural occasional intercourse, whilst the total deprivation of it produces irritability.   *The Human Element in Sex*

Denslow Lewis; 1903   **3034**

If we note the existence of the sexual instinct in the adolescent it is said to be nasty and obscene. If we attempt, even in this association, to consider anything pertaining to sex relationship, some one will remark that the discussion of the subject is attended with filth and besmirch ourselves by discussing it in public.   *Medico-Legal Journal*

Miguel de Unamuno; 1913   **3035**

Sexual love is the generative type of every other love.   *The Tragic Sense of Life*

Henry Louis Mencken; 1919   **3036**

The mystery of sex presents itself to the young, not as a scientific problem to be solved, but as a romantic emotion to be accounted for. The only result of the current endeavor to explain its phenomena by seeking parallels in botany is to make botany obscene.

Prejudices, 1st series. The Blushful Mystery

Margaret Sanger; 1920   **3037**

There is nothing in the church code of morals to protect the woman, either from unwilling submission to the wishes of her husband, from undesired pregnancy, nor from any other of the outrages only too familiar to many married women. Nothing is said about the crime of bringing an unwanted child into the world.... [The code] is man-made; [its] vital factor, as [applied] to woman, is submission to the man.... Closely associated with... the principle of submission, has been the doctrine that the sex life is in itself unclean.

Woman and the New Race

Evelyn Waugh; 1930   **3038**

All this fuss about sleeping together. For physical pleasure I'd sooner go to my dentist any day.   *Vile Bodies*

Theodor Reik; 1945   **3039**

The third thousandth year of the Christian era will bring at least a clarification, if not a solution, of many problems of sex and love. The year three thousand nine hundred will...see decided progress in subduing the tension between the sexes, the removal of a great deal of envy and possessiveness, and will usher in a new education of both sexes for companionship.   *Psychology of Sex Relations*

Evelyn Millis Duvall; 1967   **3040**

Sex is a part of life. It can be fine and full and very beautiful. It can be painful, restricting and shameful. Like every other source of power, it must be harnessed or it runs wild and becomes destructive. Electricity wired into your home will light your house, cook your meals, warm your feet, and perform all kinds of miracles. Left unleashed, as lightning, it can destroy everything your care about in one burning holocaust. So it is with sex.

Love and the Facts of Life

Edward Shorter; 1975   3041

No subject is more forbidding to study in *la vie intime* than marital sexuality. Next to nothing is known about it, because among all the things the popular classes didn't discuss in the Bad Old Days, what they did in bed was foremost (second only to where they hid their money).   *The Making of the Modern Family*

Edward O. Wilson; 1978   3042

If insemination were the sole biological function of sex, it could be achieved far more economically in a few seconds of mounting and insertion. Indeed, the least social of mammals mate with scarcely more ceremony. The species that have evolved long-term bonds are also, by and large, the ones that rely on elaborate courtship rituals.... Love and sex do indeed go together.   *On Human Nature*

Richard Gordon; 1993   3043

All the world loves loving, but it entails the bothersome inconveniences of pregnancy and disease.   *The Alarming History of Medicine*

Roy Porter; 1997   3044

Until the Victorian era, "unnatural acts" were regarded mainly as vices which might be indulged by various immature, profligate, impressionable, foreign, or over-sexed individuals, succumbing to lust, intoxication, libertinism, opportunity, or necessity.... Medical sexual science invented and popularized all the sexual-ists and -isms.... The groups identified have wavered between rejecting such names (...stigmatizing) and embracing them (...exonerating and empowering). The medicalization of sexuality may thus be either a threat or a blessing.   *The Greatest Benefit to Mankind*

William Ian Miller; 1998   3045

Sex has to be procreative to be, finally, enjoyable. All the embarrassing activities that constitute sex, the tristesse, the loss of dignity, are on occasion rewarded after a time by the pleasures of baby flesh.   *American Scholar*

SEX EDUCATION

Denslow Lewis; 1899   3046

Sexual matters should be taught to the young at an early age. Girls expecially should know the usual consequence of sexual intercourse. Their modesty may be shocked but their virtue will be saved.   *Transactions of the Section of Obstetric Diseases in Women of the AMA*

C. Everett Koop; 1986   3047

You can't talk of the danger of snake poisoning and not mention snakes.   *Time*

SEX HORMONES

Arnold Adolph Berthold; 1849   3048

So far as voice, sexual urge, belligerence, and growth of combs and wattles are concerned[the] birds remain true cockerels [after testicular transplantation]. The results...are determined by the productive function of the testes...by their action on the blood stream, and then by corresponding reaction of the blood upon the entire organism.
                                          Archiv für Anatomie, Physiologie und Wissenschaftliche Medicin

SEXISM

Cotton Mather; 1724   3049

Poor Daughters of *Eve*, Languishing under your *Special Maladies*, Look back on your *Mother*, the *Woman*, who being *Deceived*, was first *in the Transgression*, that has brought upon us, *all our Maladies*.   *The Angel of Bethesda*

Mary Wortley Montagu; 1758   **3050**

I am charmed with [Sydenham's] taking off the reproach which you men so saucily throw on our sex, as if we alone were subject to vapours. He clearly proves that your wise honourable spleen is the same disorder and arises from the same cause; but you vile usurpers do not only engross learning, power, and authority to yourselves, but will be our superiors even in constitution of mind, and fancy you are incapable of the woman's weakness of fear and tenderness. Ignorance!   *Letter to Sir James Steuart*

Alfred Stillé; 1871   **3051**

Another disease has become epidemic. "The woman in question" in relation to medicine is only one of the forms in which the *pestis muliebris* vexes the world. In other shapes it attacks the bar, wriggles into the jury box, and clearly means to mount upon the bench; it strives, thus far in vain, to serve at the altar and thunder from the pulpit; it raves at political meetings, harangues in the lecture-room, infects the masses with its poison, and even pierces the triple brass that surrounds the politician's heart.   *Address*

Mary Putnam Jacobi; 1877   **3052**

The sex that is supposed to be limiting in its nature, is nearly always different from that of the person conducting the inquiry.   *The Question of Rest for Women During Menstruation*

Anatole France (Jacques Anatole François Thibault); 1912   **3053**

We have medicines to make women speak; we have none to make them keep silence.
                                              The Man Who Married a Dumb Wife, Act II, Scene iv

SEXUALLY TRANSMITTED DISEASES

Jacques de Bethencourt; 1527   **3054**

The venereal disease is a condition of the body proceeding from sexual intercourse and contagion: at the onset causing ulcers on the genitalia or point of contagion: then corrupting the humors especially the phlegm, the organs of generation: by which pustules, tumors, ulcers and pains are produced.   *Nova Peonitentialis Quadragesima*

Cotton Mather; 1724   **3055**

Among other *Judgments* which even in This World overtake the Vicious, who *being past all Feeling, have given themselves over unto Lasciviousness, to Work all Uncleanness with Greediness*; there is of Later time, inflicted a *Foul Disease*; the Description whereof, and of the Symptoms that attend it, would be such a *Nasty Discourse*, that Civility to the Readers will Supercede it; and the Sheets of the Treatise now before him, Shall not be stained with so much Conspurcation.   *The Angel of Bethesda*

Johann Wolfgang von Goethe; [1749-1832]   **3056**

The solitude at night in bed is so depressing.
Yet how revolting is the fear of the snakes that threaten the road of love,
And the fear of the poison among the roses of lust,
When in the moment sublime of the complete surrender,
Whispers of worry to follow are beginning to approach your mind about to relax.
                                              Unseemly Matters

Abraham Colles; 1837   **3057**

A child born of a mother who is without any obvious venereal symptoms, and which, without being exposed to any infection subsequent to its birth, shows this disease when a few weeks old...will infect the most healthy nurse, whether she suckle it, or merely handle and dress it; and yet this child is never known to infect its own mother, even though she suckle it while it has venereal ulcers of the lips and tongue.
                                              Practical Observations on the Venereal Diseases

Samuel Solly; 1868   **3058**

Dr. Samuel Solly, President of the Royal Medical and Chirurgical Society giving evidence to a government committee, said of syphilis that it was self-inflicted, it is avoidable by refraining from sexual activity and was intended as a punishment for our sins and that we should not interfere in the matter.   *Abse D, Doctors and Patients*

John Hinchman Stokes, Herman Beerman, Norman R. Ingraham; 1945   **3059**

The purveying of sexual pleasure used to be a professional specialty. The hip flask, the automobile, and the sexification of young and old...have made it an amateur sport.... The zipper, the simplification of clothing, the car, the tourist camp, the invariable presence of alcohol—the ounce too much—has spread the transmission of the venereal diseases all over the place.   *Modern Clinical Syphilology*

Theresa Crenshaw; 1987   **3060**

You're not sleeping with just one person, you're sleeping with everyone they ever slept with.   *NBC-TV Interview: Men, Women, Sex, and AIDS*

SHOCK

Walter Bradford Cannon, J. Fraser, A.N. Hooper; 1918   **3061**

The first noteworthy characteristic of the blood in shock is a high capillary red count.... When hemorrhage as a complicating factor tending to reduce the blood count is considered, these high counts are striking. They indicate that in shock a concentration of the blood occurs, at least in the superficial capillaries.   *Journal of the American Medical Association*

Alfred Blalock; 1930   **3062**

The experiments... presented in this paper offer no evidence that trauma to an extremity produces a toxin that causes a general dilatation of capillaries with an increase in capillary permeability and a general loss of fluid from the blood stream.... There was sufficient loss of blood volume into the traumatized area in all of these experiments on dogs anesthetized by barbital to account for the reduction in blood pressure.   *Archives of Surgery*

SICKLE CELL DISEASE

James Bryan Herrick; 1910   **3063**

The patient was an intelligent negro of 20.... Most of the ulcers had been on the legs.... For about a year he had noticed some palpitation and shortness of breath which he had attributed to excessive smoking. There had been times when he thought he was bilious and when the whites of the eyes had been tinged with yellow.... The red corpuscles varied much in size, many microcytes being seen and some macrocytes.... The shape of the reds was very irregular, but what especially attracted attention was the large number of thin, sickle-shaped and crescent-shaped forms.   *Archives of Internal Medicine*

James V. Neel; 1949   **3064**

In a genetic situation such as appears to obtain here, where the heterozygote, who may be termed the genetic carrier of the disease, may be readily distinguished from normal and from the homozygote, it is possible to predict with a high degree of accuracy which marriages should result in homozygous individuals—in this case, children with sickle cell anemia.   *Science*

Linus C. Pauling, H.A. Itano, S.J. Singer, I.C. Wells; 1949   **3065**

A significant difference exists between the electrophoretic mobilities of hemoglobin derived from erythrocytes of normal individuals and from those of sickle cell anemic individuals.... The hemoglobin derived from erythrocytes of individuals with sicklemia, however, appears to be a mixture of the normal hemoglobin and sickle cell anemia hemoglobin in roughly equal proportions.   *Science*

Vernon Martin Ingram; 1957   **3066**

I have... found that out of nearly 300 amino-acids in [the globin of normal and sickle cell anaemia], only one is different; one of the glutamic acid residues of normal haemoglobin is replaced by a valine residue in sickle cell anaemia haemoglobin.... It is now possible to show, for the first time, the effect of a single gene mutation as a change in one amino-acid of the haemoglobin polypeptide chain for the manufacture of which that gene is responsible.   *Nature*

SIGMOIDOSCOPY

Henry George Miller; 1968   **3067**

Annual sigmoidoscopy for all, after their fortieth birthday: something to look forward to.
                                                                 World Neurology

SINOATRIAL NODE

Arthur Keith, M.W. Flack; 1907   **3068**

There is a remarkable remnant of primitive fibers persisting at the sino-auricular junction in all the mammalian hearts examined. These fibres are in close connection with the vagus and sympathetic nerves and have a special arterial supply; in them the dominating rhythm of the heart is believed to normally arise.   *Journal of Anatomy and Physiology*

SJÖGREN SYNDROME

Henrik Sjögren; 1933   **3069**

In keratoconjunctivitis sicca there are besides the ocular change and the diminished, on occasions absent, lachrymal secretion, several other symptoms. This permits us to regard the disease as a general disease which attacks chiefly the eyes as well as the lachrynal and salivary glands. Histological investigations have supported this.

                                                         Acta Ophthalmologica Scandinavica

SKULL FRACTURE

Hippocrates; [460-375 BC]   **3070**

Of these modes of fracture, the following require trepanning: the contusion, whether the bone be laid bare or not; and the fissure, whether apparent or not. And if, when an indentation (*hedra*) by a weapon takes place in a bone it be attended with fracture and contusion, and even if contusion alone, without fracture, be combined with the indentation, it requires trepanning.   *On Injuries of the Head*

SLEEP

Hippocrates; [460-375 BC]   **3071**

Sleep or sleeplessness, in undue measure, these are both bad symptoms.   *Aphorisms*

Thomas Browne; 1643   **3072**

We term sleep a death; and yet it is waking that kills us, and destroys those spirits that are the house of life. 'Tis indeed a part of life that best expresseth death; for every man truely lives, so long as he acts his nature, or some way makes good the faculties of himself.

                                                                 Religio Medici

Johann Wolfgang von Goethe; [1749-1832]   **3073**

Heavenly Morpheus, in vain do you wave the poppies;
My eye will remain awake, if Amor will not close it.

                          Otto R, Romische Elegien und Venezianische Epigramme

Eugene Aserinsky, Nathaniel Kleitman; 1953   **3074**

The fact that these [rapid, jerky] eye movements, EEG pattern, and autnomic nervous system activity are significantly related and do not occur randomly suggests that these physiological phenomena, and probably dreaming, are very likely all manifestations of a particular level of cortical activity which is encountered normally during sleep. [REM sleep]

Science

Aldous Huxley; [1894-1963]   **3075**

That we are not much sicker and much madder than we are is due exclusively to that most blessed and blessing of all natural graces, sleep.   *Coren S, Sleep Thieves*

SLEEP DEPRIVATION

Stanley Coren; 1996   **3076**

It may...come to pass that someday the person who drives or goes to work while sleepy will be viewed as being as reprehensible, dangerous, or even criminally negligent as the person who drives or goes to work while drunk. If so, perhaps the rest of us can all sleep a little bit more soundly.   *Sleep Thieves*

SLEEPING SICKNESS (TRYPANOSOMIASIS)

Thomas Masterman Winterbottom; 1803   **3077**

The Africans are very subject to a species of lethargy, which they are much afraid of.... It is called by the Soosoos, kee kóllee kondee, or sleepy sickness.... The appetite declines, and the patient gradually wastes away.... The disposition to sleep is so strong, as scarcely to leave a sufficient respite for the taking of food; even the repeated application of a whip...is hardly sufficient to keep the poor wretch awake.... The disease...usually proves fatal with three or four months.   *An Account of the Native Africans in the Neighborhood of Sierra Leone*

Aldo Castellani; 1903   **3078**

On November 12th, 1902, when examining a specimen of cerebro-spinal fluid...from a well-marked case of sleeping sickness, I was surprised to observe a living trypanosoma.... I would suggest as a working hypothesis...that sleeping sickness is due to the species of trypanosoma I have found in the cerebro-spinal fluid.   *British Medical Journal*

Ambrose Bierce; 1906   **3079**

Tzetze (or Tsetse) Fly, n. An African insect (*Glossina morsitans*) whose bite is commonly regarded as nature's most efficacious remedy for insomnia, though some patients prefer that of the American novelist (*Mendax interminabilis*).   *The Devil's Dictionary*

SMALLPOX

Rhazes (Abu Bakr Muhammad Ibn Zakariya al-Razi); [864-930]   **3080**

The bodies most disposed to the Small-Pox are in general such as are moist, pale, and fleshy; the well-coloured also, and ruddy, as likewise the swarthy when they are loaded with flesh; those who are frequently attacked by acute and continued fevers, bleeding at the nose, inflammation of the eyes, and white and red pustules, and vesicles.

A Treatise on the Small-Pox and Measles

Thomas Babington Macaulay; 1848   **3081**

The havoc of the plague had been far more rapid: but the plague had visited our shores only once or twice within living memory; and the small pox was always present, filling the church-yards with corpses, tormenting with constant fears all whom it had not yet stricken, leaving on those whose lives it spared the hideous traces of its power, turning the babe into a changeling at which the mother shuddered, and making the eyes and cheeks of the betrothed maiden objects of horror to the lover.   *History of England*

SMALLPOX IMMUNIZATION

Mary Wortley Montagu; 1717   3082
The small pox, so fatal and so general amongst us, is here rendered entirely harmless by
the invention of ingrafting, which is the term they give it. There is a set of old women
who make it their business to perform the operation every autumn....The old woman
comes with a nutshell full of the matter of the best sort of smallpox, and asks what veins
you please to have opened. She immediately rips open that you offer to her with a large
needle...and puts into the vein as much venom as can lie upon the head of her needle,
and after binds up the little wound with a hollow bit of shell.   *Letter to Sara Chiswell*

Edward Jenner; 1798   3083
This disease has obtained the name of the cow-pox.... The disease makes its progress from
the horse to the nipple of the cow, and from the cow to the human subject.... What renders the cow-pox virus so extremely singular is that the person who has been thus affected is forever after secure from the infection of the small-pox; neither exposure to the var-
iolous effluvia, nor the insertion of the matter into the skin, producing this distemper.
An Inquiry into the Causes and Effects of the Variolae Vaccinae

Benjamin Waterhouse; 1800   3084
I have procured some of the vaccine matter, and therewith inoculated seven of my family. The inoculation has proceeded in six of them exactly as described by Woodville and
Jenner; but my desire is to confirm the doctrine by having some of them inoculated [with
smallpox] by you.... If you accede to my proposal, I shall consider it as an experiment in
which we have co-operated for the good of our fellow citizens, and relate it as such in the
pamphlet I mean to publish on the subject.   *A Prospect of Exterminating the Smallpox*

Edward Jenner; 1801   3085
A hundred thousand persons, upon the smallest computation have been inoculated in
these realms. The number who have partaken of its benefits throughout Europe and other
parts of the globe are incalculable; and it now becomes too manifest to admit of controversy, that the annihilation of the Small Pox, the most dreadful scourge of the human
species, must be the final result of this practice.   *The Origin of the Vaccine Inoculation*

Thomas Jefferson; 1806   3086
Medicine has never before produced any single improvement of such utility. You have
erased from the calendar of human afflictions one of its greatest.
Letter to Dr. Edward Jenner

SMELL

Richard Axel, Linda Buck; 1991   3087
To address the problem of olfactory perception at a molecular level, we have cloned and
characterized 18 different members of an extremely large multigene family that encodes
seven transmembrane domain proteins whose expression is restricted to the olfactory
epithelium. The members of this novel gene family are likely to encode a diverse family
of odorant receptors.   *Cell*

SMOKING

James I; 1604   3088
A custom loathsome to the eye, hateful to the nose, harmful to the brain, dangerous to
the lungs, and in the black stinking fume thereof, nearest resembling the horrible Stygian
smoke of the pit that is bottomless.   *A Counter Blaste to Tobacco*

James I; 1604   3089
And for the vanities committed in this filthy custom, is it not both great vanity and
uncleaness, that at the table, a place of respect, of cleanliness, of modesty, men should

not be ashamed to sit tossing tobacco pipes, and puffing of the smoke of tobacco one to another, making the filthy smoke and stink thereof, to exhale athwart the dishes and infect the air, when very often, men that abhor it are at their repast?

A Counter Blaste to Tobacco

Cotton Mather; 1724   **3090**
There is a Caustic Salt communicated unto the Mass of Blood, by the too frequent Smoking of Tobacco: From which there cannot but follow many Infellicities. And I pray what will the Flech be the better for being so Baconized? *The Angel of Bethesda*

Cotton Mather; 1724   **3091**
I must and will insist upon it; That a *Slavery* to the *Custome* of *Smoking Tobacco*, is a Thing, by no means Consistent with the Dignity of a *Rational Creature*; and much less of a *Vertuous Christian*. The *Nature of Man* is debased and is disgraced by such a *Slavery*.

The Angel of Bethesda

Samuel Thomas von Soemmerring; 1795   **3092**
Carcinoma of the lips occurs most frequently where men indulge in pipe smoking; the lower lip is particularly affected by cancer when it is compressed between the tobacco pipe and the teeth. *De Morbis Vasorum Absorbentium Corporis Humani*

Benjamin Waterhouse; 1822   **3093**
I am entirely convinced that smoking and chewing injures ultimately the hearing, smell, taste, and teeth.... The practice of smoking is productive of indolence; and tends to confirm the lazy in their laziness. Instead of exercising in the open air, as formerly, you sit down before large fires and smoke tobacco. *Cautions to Young Persons Concerning Health*

Johann Wolfgang von Goethe; [1749-1832]   **3094**
Smoking is...markedly impolite, an impertinent unsociability. Smokers poison the air near and far and suffocate every honest person who cannot defend himself by smoking in his turn. Who on earth can enter the room of a smoker without getting nauseated? And who could stay there and not perish? *Nager F, Der Heilkundige Dichter*

Ernest Ludwig Wynder, Evarts Ambrose Graham; 1950   **3095**
Among 605 men with bronchiogenic carcinoma... 96.5 per cent were moderately heavy to chain smokers for many years, compared with 73.7 per cent among the general male hospital population without cancer.... The occurrences of carcinoma of the lung in a male nonsmoker or minimal smoker is a rare phenomenon (2.0 per cent).

Journal of the American Medical Association

William Richard Shaboe Doll, Austin Bradford Hill; 1950   **3096**
The risk of developing carcinoma of the lung increases steadily as the amount smoked increases.... The relative risks become 6, 19, 26, 49, and 65 when the number of cigarettes smoked a day are 3, 10, 20, 35, and, say, 60.... The risk seems to vary in approximately simple proportion with the amount smoked. *British Medical Journal*

Edward Janavel Huth; 1964   **3097**
The physician who has smoked and stopped can present himself in that most convincing of social roles—the man who is both *superior* and *human*—betrayed as human by his eloquent account of the acute though temporary agonies of abstention, stamped as superior because he did win.... If enough of us who were smokers take this stand, we may succeed with snobbery where reason and fear would fail. *Annals of Internal Medicine*

Surgeon General's Advisory Committee on Smoking and Health; 1964   **3098**
Cigarette smoking is causally related to lung cancer in men; the magnitude of the effect of cigarette smoking far outweighs all other factors.... The risk of developing lung cancer increases with duration of smoking and the number of cigarettes smoked per day, and is diminished by discontinuing smoking. *Smoking and Health*

Surgeon General's Advisory Committee on Smoking and Health; 1964   **3099**
The overwhelming evidence points to the conclusion that smoking—its beginning, habituation, and occasional discontinuation—is to a large extent psychologically and socially determined. *Smoking and Health*

Oscar Auerbach, Edward Cuyler Hammond, David Kirman,
Lawrence Garfinkel; 1970   **3100**
86 dogs [were] trained to smoke through a tracheostoma.... Early invasive squamous cell carcinoma was found in bronchi of two of 12 group H [filter tip cigarettes] dogs which were killed. *Archives of Environmental Health*

SOCIAL WELFARE

Harvey Cushing; 1935   **3101**
Let us hope that when some...student of this confused and disconcerting period in our history, comes to tell of it, he will be able to say; that at the very time when such progress in their subjects was being made as never before,...the scientists and the engineers of the country temporarily abandoned the investigations dear to their hearts...to concentrate on problems the most difficult of all to solve—those that have to do with the social well-being of the community at large. *Science*

SPECIALIZATION

Herodotus; [484-424 BC]   **3102**
[Egyptians split up] the practice of medicine...into separate parts, each doctor being responsible for the treatment of only one disease. There are, in consequence, innumerable doctors, some specializing in diseases of the eyes, others of the head, others of the teeth, others of the stomach, and so on; while others, again, deal with the sort of troubles which cannot be exactly localized. *The Histories*

Andreas Vesalius; 1543   **3103**
Great harm is caused by too wide a separation of the disciplines which work toward the perfection of each individual art, and much more by the meticulous distribution of the practices of this art to different workers. *The Fabric of the Human Body*

John Morgan; 1765   **3104**
If Physic, Surgery, and Pharmacy were in different hands, practitioners would then enjoy much more satisfaction in practice. *A Discourse upon the Institution of Medical Schools in America*

James V.Z. Blaney; 1854   **3105**
Should you aim at more than mediocrity in the profession, let me recommend to you to select as early as possible some one department of Medical Science, to which your tastes or your locality may direct you, and devote yourself to its study and advancement. *Valedictory address*

George Frederick Shrady; 1885   **3106**
Specialism is an established feature of modern medicine. It...cannot be cried down, for already, in the face of opposition and distrust, it has steadily increased, and will surely continue to do so. It is not an artificial addition to medicine, but a natural and inevitable development. It has its dangers, against which we can utter warnings; it has its defects and insufficiencies, which should be pointed out. But to attempt to check its growth would not only be useless, but would work an injury to the profession. *Medical Record*

Oliver Wendell Holmes; 1891   **3107**
The specialist is much like other people engaged in lucrative business. He is apt to magnify his calling, to make much of any symptom which will bring a patient within range of his battery of remedies. *Over the Teacups*

William Osler; 1892   **3108**
No more dangerous members of our profession exist than those born into it, so to speak, as specialists. Without any broad foundation in physiology or pathology, and ignorant of the great processes of disease, no amount of technical skill can hide from the keen eyes of colleagues defects which too often require the arts of the charlatan to screen from the public.   *Remarks on Specialism*

Prince Albert Morrow; 1893   **3109**
The genius of modern medical literature is clearly in the direction of division of labor and associated effort.   A *System of Genito-Urinary Diseases, Syphilology, and Dermatology*

Richard Austin Freeman; 1926   **3110**
Take the case of an aurist. You think that he lives by dealing with obscure and difficult middle and internal ear cases. Nothing of the kind. He lives on wax. Wax is the foundation of his practice. Patient comes to him deaf as a post. He does all the proper jugglery—tuning fork, otoscope, speculum, and so on, for the moral effect. Then he hikes out a good old plug of cerumen, and the patient hears perfectly. Of course he is delighted. Thinks a miracle has been performed.   *The D'Arblay Mystery*

Henry George Miller; 1947   **3111**
The worst mistakes...must be laid at the door of the specialist rather than the general practitioner, who, from his intimate contact with sick people in their natural surroundings, often has a lively understanding of the nervous patient, and is able to see him and his problems as a whole.   *The Practitioner*

John Berger; 1967   **3112**
Increasing specialization encourages an increasingly scientific view of illness.
     A Fortunate Man

Macfarlane Burnet; 1968   **3113**
We may well find that the men who staff the hospitals of next century will include many who are much more mathematicians and biochemists than physicians as we know them today, but there will still be wide range of surgical and other specialists.... I fancy that those men will still need to be able to apply common sense, courage, and compassion in dealing with all the human difficulties that escape the machines.   *Changing Patterns*

Rosemary Stevens; 1971   **3114**
In the whole process of reassessment...of the medical profession...has come the recognition of medicine as an interdependent, not independent, profession and as one consisting of a complex of specialties rather than one general discipline.
     American Medicine and the Public Interest

SPHINCTER ANI

Walter C. Bornemeier; 1960   **3115**
The sphincter ani can do it. The sphincter apparently can differentiate between solid, fluid and gas. It apparently can tell whether its owner is alone or with someone, whether standing up or sitting down, whether its owner has his pants on or off. No other muscle in the body is such a protector of the dignity of man, yet so ready to come to his relief.
     American Journal of Proctology

SPHYGMOGRAPH

James Mackenzie; 1902   **3116**
However eloquent may be the words of a writer, he cannot in a page convey as clear an idea of the rhythm of a heart as a simple pulse-tracing; and if writers had given us more pulse-tracings, their works would have been greatly enhanced in value.
     The Study of the Pulse

SPINAL CORD

[Anonymous]; *circa* 2500 BC   **3117**

If thou examinest a man having a dislocation in a vertebra of his neck, shouldst thou find him unconscious of his two arms (and) his two legs on account of it, while his phallus is erected on account of it, (and) urine drops from his member without his knowing it; his flesh has received wind; his two eyes are bloodshot; it is a dislocation of a vertebra of his neck extending to his backbone which causes him to be unconscious of his two arms (and) his two legs.   *The Edwin Smith Surgical Papyrus*

Hippocrates; [460-375 BC]   **3118**

The spinal cord... would suffer, if the luxation due to jerking out of a vertebra had made so sharp a curve [forward[; the vertebra in springing out would press on the cord, even if it did not break it. The cord, then, being compressed and intercepted, would produce complete narcosis of many large and important parts.   *On Joints*

Galen; [130-200]   **3119**

Probably then, provident nature made the nerves grow out from the spinal medulla right at the point where the lateral parts of the vertebrae come to an end, so that the nerves may not suffer in any way.   *On the Usefulness of the Parts of the Body*

Galen; [130-200]   **3120**

All limbs but not the face are deprived of motion and sensation, when a condition has arisen at the level of the spinal cord where the first nerves leave, since this prevents a flow of the faculties from the brain to the limbs. Likewise, when only half [of the spinal cord] where these nerves originate is affected, the paralysis does not involve all the parts further down but only those, of course, at the right or left side.   *On the Affected Parts*

SPIROMETRY

John Hutchinson; 1846   **3121**

If a man breathes into the Spirometer 200 cubic inches, it is neither 199 or 201 cubic inches; it requires no delicate training of the judgment, nor sense of sight, to come to such a conclusion; therefore, for the purpose of determining a *fact*, the Spirometer is ready and definite, without a long system of education, but by education, I am inclined to think it becomes an important means of diagnosis.   *Medico-Chirurgical Transactions*

SPLEEN

Richard Blackmore; 1725   **3122**

On attentive Enquiry into the Office of that Organ [the spleen], it evidently appears to me, that it was not formed for the Benefit and Preservation of the Animal, of which it is a Part; and therefore it is of no use at all in respect of the Individual.... I myself have opened the Side of a Dog, and torn off with my Fingers the Spleen from the Parts to which it grew; yet without so much as tying up the Vessels, the Wound in the Side being sowed up, the Creature soon recovered, and shewed no sign of any Damage.

A Treatise of the Spleen and Vapours

SPLENOMEGALY

Guido Banti; 1894   **3123**

Splenic anemia is a progressive idiopathic anemia, accompanied by idiopathic hypertrophy of the spleen and often of the liver, without leukemia.... The disease sets in with splenic hypertrophy, which progresses in an insidious manner, so that when it is noticed by the patient or his physician, the spleen has attained a considerable size.... Anaemic symptoms follow upon tumefaction of the spleen and consist, as a rule, in increasing debility, with pallor of the skin...dyspnoea and palpitation consequent upon the slightest effort.

Sperimentale

SPRUE

Vincent Ketelaer; 1669   3124
The Blisters are whitish on the top and inside of the mouth, and especially occur in the vicinity of the organs of respiration and of swallowing.... If finally it attacks precipitately the abdomen, it brings on a phalanx of symptoms, and among these a most pernicious diarrhoea, which leaves behind scarcely any juice for his body and fuel for his strength.
Commentarius Medicus

William Hillary; 1759   3125
The Patient who labours under this Disease, usually first complains of an uneasy Sensation, or slight burning Heat about the Cardia, or upper Mouth of the Stomach.... Little small Pustulae, or Pimples, filled with a clear acrid Lymph...begin to rise; generally first on the End and Sides of the Tongue.... When the Humour falls upon the Intestines, it produces a Diarrhoea with a Sense of Heat, and sometimes a Griping...and sometimes with hot Stools...so that most of the nutricious Juices run off that Way, which greatly wastes and sinks the Patient.
Observations on the Changes of the Air

STATE MEDICINE

Katherine Ott; 1996   3126
Bureaucratic management of tuberculosis was the first permanent attempt by the state to control disease.
Fevered Lives

STATISTICS

Galen; [130-200]   3127
For [the empiricists] say that a thing seen but once cannot be accepted nor regarded as true, neither what was seen a few times only. They believe something can only be accepted and considered true, if it has been seen very many times, and in the same manner every time.
On Medical Experience

Leonardo da Vinci; [1452-1519]   3128
There is no certainty where one can neither apply any of the mathematical sciences nor any of those which are based upon the mathematical sciences.
Treatise on Painting

Gottfried Leibniz; 1704   3129
When we cannot decide a question absolutely, we might still determine the degree of likelihood from the data, and can consequently judge reasonably which side is the most likely.
New Essays on Human Understanding

Joseph Butler; 1736   3130
Probability is the very guide of life.
The Analogy of Religion

Thomas Bayes; 1763   3131
The probability of any event is the ratio between the value at which an expectation depending on the happening of the event ought to be computed and the value of the thing expected upon its happening.
Philosophical Transactions of the Royal Society

John Gregory; 1772   3132
The advancement of the sciences... requires only an attention to probabilities... a quick discernment where the greatest probability lies, and habits, of acting in consequence of this with facility and vigor.
Lectures on the Duties and Qualifications of a Physician

Gilbert Blane; 1785   3133
There is... a great difficulty attending all practical inquiries in medicine; for in order to ascertain truth, in a manner that is satisfactory to a mind habituated to chaste investigation, there must be a series of patient and attentive observations upon a great number of

cases, and the different trials must be varied, weighed, and compared in order to form a proper estimate of the real efficacy of different remedies and modes of treatment.

Observations on the Diseases Incident to Seamen

Pierre-Simon Laplace; 1825   3134

Studies on illnesses may... shed a great light on psychology when physicians join to the knowledge of their art and accessory sciences the spirit of precision and of criticism that is provided by the study of mathematics and in particular by the knowledge of probabilities.

Philosophical Essay on Probabilities

Francis Bisset Hawkins; 1829   3135

Statistics has become the key to several sciences... and there is reason to believe, that a careful cultivation of it, would materially assist the completion of a philosophy of medicine.... Medical statistics affords the most convincing proofs of the efficacy of medicine.

Elements of Medical Statistics

Pierre-Charles-Alexandre Louis; 1834   3136

As to different methods of treatment, it is possible for us to assure ourselves of the superiority of one or other...by enquiring if the greater number of individuals have been cured by one means than another. Here it is necessary to count. And it is, in great part at least, because hitherto this method has not at all, or rarely been employed, that the science of therapeutics is so uncertain.

Essay on Clinical Instruction

Carl Emil Fenger; 1839   3137

The use of the numerical method in medicine is not essentially new. From the time of Hippocrates to our day any doctor would say that this symptom is rare in a particular disease, but that one common; that this cause is more common than that one; that this treatment cures more patients than that one.

Ugeskrift für Léger

George Cheyne Shattuck Jr.; 1839   3138

Some seem to have been misled by the term numerical system, which has been said to be that of M. Louis. They seem to have thought that his peculiarity consists in this merely, that he counts.... We call some experienced, scientific. Is it not by comparing individual cases, by adding what they have observed in one to what they have observed in another, by *counting*, that they have become so?

Researches on the Yellow Fever

Thomas Carlyle; 1839   3139

A judicious man...looks at Statistics, not to get knowledge, but to save himself from having ignorance foisted on him.

Chartism

Elisha Bartlett; 1844   3140

[An] average result is not to be taken as the positive and absolute expression of the law before us. The result is still subject to a certain degree of variableness...the amount of which can be ascertained...by the *calculation of probabilities*.

An Essay on the Philosophy of Medical Science

Claude Bernard; 1865   3141

The first requirement in using statistics is that the facts treated shall be reduced to comparable units.

An Introduction to the Study of Experimental Medicine

Claude Bernard; 1865   3142

The goal of scientific physicians...is to reduce the indeterminate. Statistics therefore apply only to cases in which the cause of the facts observed is still indeterminate.

An Introduction to the Study of Experimental Medicine

Claude Bernard; 1865   3143

Only when a phenomenon includes conditions as yet undefined, can we compile; we must learn, therefore, that we compile statistics only when we cannot possibly help it.

An Introduction to the Study of Experimental Medicine

Claude Bernard; 1865   **3144**

When a physician is called to a patient, he should decide on the diagnosis, then the prognosis, and then the treatment.... Physicians must know the evolution of the disease, its duration and gravity in order to predict its course and outcome. Here statistics intervene to guide physicians, by teaching them the proportion of mortal cases; and if observation has also shown that the successful and unsuccessful cases can be recognized by certain signs, then the prognosis is more certain.   *An Introduction to the Study of Experimental Medicine*

[Anonymous]; 19th century   **3145**

There are three kinds of lies: lies, damn lies, and statistics.

Mencken HL, A New Dictionary of Quotations

Francis Galton; 1883   **3146**

The object of statistical science is to discover methods of condensing information concerning large groups of allied facts into brief and compendious expressions suitable for discussion. The possibility of doing this is based on the constancy and continuity with which objects of the same species are found to vary.   *Statistical Methods*

John Shaw Billings; 1889   **3147**

Statistics are somewhat like old medical journals, or like revolvers in newly opened mining districts. Most men rarely use them, and find it troublesome to preserve them so as to have them easy of access; but when they do want them, they want them badly.

Medical Record

William Osler; 1897   **3148**

Louis introduced what is known as the Numerical Method, a plan which we use every day, though the phrase is not now very often on our lips.... To get an accurate knowledge of any disease it is necessary to study a large series of cases and to go into all the particulars—the conditions under which it is met, the subjects specially liable, the various symptoms, the pathological changes, the effects of drugs. This method, so simple, so self-evident, we owe largely to Louis.   *The Influence of Louis on American Medicine*

Student (William Sealy Gosset); 1908   **3149**

An experiment may be regarded as forming an individual of a "population" of experiments which might be performed under the same conditions. A series of experiments is a sample drawn from this population. Now any series of experiments is only of value in so far as it enables us to form a judgment as to the statistical constants of the population to which the experiments belong. In a great number of cases the question finally turns on the value of a mean, either directly, or as the mean difference between the two quantities.   *Biometrika*

Student (William Sealy Gosset); 1908   **3150**

A curve has been found representing the frequency distribution of standard deviations of samples drawn from a normal population. A curve has been found representing the frequency distribution of values of the means of such samples, when these values are measured from the mean of the population in terms of the standard deviation of the sample.... Tables are given by which it can be judged whether a series of experiments, however short, have given a result which conforms to any required standard of accuracy or whether it is necessary to continue the investigation.   *Biometrika*

Andrew Lang; [1844-1912]   **3151**

He uses statistics as a drunken man uses lampposts—for support rather than for illumination.   *Strauss MB, Familiar Medical Quotations*

[Anonymous]; 1921   **3152**

Is the application of the numerical method to the subject-matter of medicine a trivial and time-wasting ingenuity as some hold, or is it an important stage in the development of our art, as others proclaim?   *The Lancet*

Ronald Aylmer Fisher; 1925   **3153**

It is...fortunate that the distribution of *t*, first established by "Student" in 1908, in his study of the probable error of the mean, should be applicable, not only to the case thus treated, but to the more complex, but even more frequently needed problem of the comparison of two mean values.   *Statistical Methods for Research Workers*

Student (William Sealy Gosset); 1925   **3154**

The present tables have...been constructed with argument $t = zn$, where *n* is now one less than the number in the sample, which we may call *n?*.... Table I extends from $t = 0$ to $t = 6$, at intervals of 0.1, from $n = 1$ to $n = 20$, inclusive.... Table II gives values beyond $t = 6$.... Table III gives...values of *p*.   *Metron*

Thomas Lewis; 1934   **3155**

The statistical method of testing treatment is never more than a temporary expedient.... Little progress can come of it directly; for in investigating cases collectively, it does not discriminate between cases that benefit and those that do not, and so fails to determine criteria by which we know beforehand in any given case that treatment will succeed.

Clinical Science, Illustrated by Personal Experiences

[Anonymous]; 1937   **3156**

Statistics are curious things. They afford one of the few examples in which the use, or abuse, of mathematical methods tends to induce a strong emotional reaction in non-mathematical minds. This is because statisticians apply, to problems in which we are interested, a technique we do not understand.... It requires more equanimity than most of possess to acknowledge that the fault is in ourselves.   *The Lancet*

M.J. Moroney; 1951   **3157**

A statistical analysis, properly conducted, is a delicate dissection of uncertainties, a surgery of suppositions.   *Facts from Figures*

John Punnett Peters; 1953   **3158**

The statistical correlation of two variables does not *ipso facto* signify that either one is the cause or effect of the other.   *Yale Journal of Biology and Medicine*

Amos Tversky, Daniel Kahneman; 1971   **3159**

The believer in the law of small numbers practices science as follows.... He gambles his research hypothesis on small samples without realizing that the odds against him are unreasonably high. He overestimates power.... He has undue confidence in early trends...and in the stability of observed patterns. He overestimates significance.... He rarely attributes a deviation of results from expectations to sampling variability, because he finds a causal "explanation" for any discrepancy.   *Psychological Bulletin*

Austin Bradford Hill; 1971   **3160**

The essence of an experiment in the treatment of a disease lies in comparison.... Though...human beings are not unique in their responses to some given treatment, there is no doubt that they are likely to be variable, and sometimes extremely variable. Two or three observations may, therefore, give, merely through the customary play of chance, a favourable picture in the hands of one doctor, an unfavourable picture in the hands of another.   *Principles of Medical Statistics*

Alvan R. Feinstein; 1977   **3161**

The widespread acceptance of [the] rigid categories of "statistical significance" [based on the *p* value] is a lamentable demonstration of the credulity with which modern scientists will abandon biology in favor of any quantitative ideology that offers the specious allure of a mathematical replacement for sensible thought   *Clinical Biostatistics*

Lewis Thomas; 1977   **3162**

Hunches and intuitive impressions are essential for getting the work [of building a solid underpinning of biostatistical and epidemiological knowledge] started, but it is only through the quality of the numbers at the end that the truth can be told.   *Science*

Thomas Sherwood; 1978   **3163**

It is a nice idea, of course, that numbers must prove something true: after all, one patient is a case-report, two are a series. But all that numbers can do is tell us what is probable, and probability can lead us into terrible mistakes—like Bertrand Russell's chicken. Day in, day out, throughout its life, the chicken got breakfast as the farmer arrived in the morning. Thus it had clearly discovered a highly probable natural law: farmer = food—until, that is, the morning when the farmer very naturally arrived to wring its neck instead.

The Lancet

Kenneth J. Rothman; 1986   **3164**

Confidence intervals convey information about both magnitude of effect and precision and therefore are preferable to p values.... Confidence intervals should be viewed... as a quantitative lens, focusing on the measure of effect. Rather than putting emphasis on exactly where the boundaries of a confidence interval lie, the limits should be thought of as gray zones, with the interval merely defining a region of probable measurement.

Annals of Internal Medicine

Lawrence L. Weed; 1996   **3165**

You use probabilities in direct proportion to your ignorance of the uniqueness of the individual.   *Address to the New York Academy of Family Physicians*

Sherwin B. Nuland; 1998   **3166**

For any specific person suffering from a specific disease in a specific setting being treated in a specific environment by a specific doctor, a statistic is nothing more than a statement of relative probability.   *American Scholar*

STETHOSCOPE

René-Théophile-Hyacinthe Laennec; 1819   **3167**

I had not imagined it would be necessary to give a name to such a simple device, but others thought differently. If one wants to give it a name, the most suitable would be "stethoscope."   *Traité de l'Auscultation Médiate*

René-Théophile-Hyacinthe Laennec; 1819   **3168**

I happened to recollect a...well-known fact in acoustics...the augmented impression of sound when conveyed through...solid bodies.... I rolled a quire of paper into a...cylinder and applied one end of it to the region of the heart and the other to my ear... I could perceive the action of the heart in a manner much more clear and distinct than I had ever been able to do by the immediate application of the ear.... This instrument I commonly designate simply the Cylinder, sometimes the Stethoscope.

Traité de l'Auscultation Médiate

William Stokes; 1825   **3169**

The stethoscope is an instrument, not, as some represent it, the bagatelle of a day, the brain-born fancy of some speculative enthusiast, the use of which, like the universal medicine of animal magnetism, will be soon forgotten, or remembered only to be ridiculed. It is one of those rich and splendid gifts which Science now and then bestows upon her most favoured votaries, which, while they extended our views and open to us wide and fruitful fields of inquiry, confer in the meantime the richest benefits and blessings on mankind.   *An Introduction to the Use of the Stethoscope*

[Anonymous]; 1834   **3170**

That [the stethoscope] will ever come into general use, notwithstanding its value [is] extremely doubtful; because its beneficial application requires much time and gives a good bit of trouble both to the patient and the practitioner; because its hue and character are foreign and opposed to all our habits and associations.... There is something even ludicrous in the picture of the grave physician proudly listening to a long tube applied to the patient's thorax.   *The Times [London]*

William H. Byford; 1858   **3171**

The flexible stethoscope is a very handy instrument to relieve us from a fatiguing and not very delicate posture.   *Chicago Medical Journal*

Matko Marusic; 1994   **3172**

Physicians wear their stethoscopes primarily in cafeterias.   *Lijecnicki Vjesnik*

STIFF-PERSON SYNDROME (STIFF-MAN SYNDROME)

H.W. Woltman, F.P. Moersh; 1956   **3173**

In the summer of 1924, an Iowa farmer, aged 49 years, came to the [Mayo] Clinic because of "muscle stiffness and difficulty in walking". His disability had begun insidiously 4 years earlier and had become so serious he could not do his work.... The rigidity has been punctuated by intermittent and moderately painful spasms.... We could not make a diagnosis but we nicknamed it the "stiff-man syndrome".... A metabolic basis for the malady should be considered.   *Mayo Clinic Proceedings*

M. Solimena, F. Folli, S. Denis-Donini, and others; 1988   **3174**

The serum and the cerebrospinal fluid [of this 49-year old woman] produced an identical, intense staining of all gray-matter regions when used to stain brain sections [with an immunofluorescence method].... The staining patterns were identical to those produced by antibodies to glutamic acid decarboxylase. A band comigrating with glutamic decarboxylase in sodium dodecyl sulfate polyacrylamide gels appeared to be the only nervous tissue antigen recognized by cerebrospinal fluid.... These findings... raise the possibility of an autoimmune pathogenesis.   *New England Journal of Medicine*

F. Gorin, B. Baldwin, R. Tait, and others; 1990   **3175**

Our data support the hypothesis that patients with stiff-man syndrome have an autoimmune disorder directed against suprasegmental or spinal inhibitory GABA[gamma-aminobutyric acid]ergic neurons.... These two patients have type I diabetes and stiff-man syndrome, and both... have islet cell, gastric parietal cell, and thyroid microsomal autoantibodies in addition to antibodies directed against GABAergic neurons.

Annals of Neurology

STREPTOMYCIN

Albert Schatz, Elizabeth Bugie, Selman A. Waksman; 1944   **3176**

A new antibacterial substance, designated as streptomycin, was isolated from two strains of an actinomyces related to an organism described as *Actinomyces griseus*. This substance resembles streptothricin in...its selective activity against gram-negative bacteria, and its limited toxicity to animals. However, the two substances differ in the nature of their respective bacteriostatic spectra.   *Procedures of the Society of Experimental Biological Medicine*

STRESS

Hans Selye; 1956   **3177**

Stress is not necessarily bad for you: it is also the spice of life, for any emotion, any activity, causes stress.   *The Stress of Life*

STROKES

Samuel Johnson; 1783   3178

[I] waked and sat up...when I felt a confusion and indistinctness in my head which lasted, I suppose about half a minute; I was alarmed and prayed God, that however he might afflict my body he would spare my understanding.... Soon after I perceived that I had suffered a paralytick stroke, and that my Speech was taken from me.   *Letter to Mrs. Thrale*

SUBARACHNOID HEMORRHAGE

Johann Jakob Wepfer; 1658   3179

The Abbot by chance wished to decide with him the fate of the servants, found [him] prostrate upon the ground, insensible to shouts, to shaking and pinching of the body...senseless.... I saw him livid from pallor, deprived of all sensation and animate motion.... The first hour after midday of the same day he ceased to live.... By the indulgence of the Most Reverend Lord Abbot... I opened the head.... Much blood flowed from the space.... The [blood] covered [the brain] all over.... The ventricles laid open, I found them all filled up with blood.   *Observationes Anatomicae*

SUFFERING

François, Duc de la Rochefoucauld; 1678   3180

Consolation for unhappiness can often be found in a certain satisfaction we get in looking unhappy.   *Moral Reflections, Sentences, and Maxims*

Wilhelm Nero Pilatus Barbellion (Bruce Frederick Cummings); 1920   3181

Suffering does not only insulate. It drops its victim on an island in an ocean desert where he sees men as distant ships passing. I not only feel alone, but very far away from you all.   *A Last Diary*

SUICIDE

Seneca; [8 BC - 65 AD]   3182

I will not relinquish old age if it leaves my better part intact. But if it begins to shake my mind, if it destroys its faculties one by one, if it leaves me not life but breath, I will depart from the putrid or tottering edifice.... If I must suffer without hope of relief, I will depart.   *Nuland SB, How We Die*

William Shakespeare; 1600   3183

To be, or not to be—that is the question.   *Hamlet, Act III, Scene i*

Ludwig von Beethoven; 1810   3184

Had I not read somewhere that a man ought not of his own free will take away his life so long as he could still can perform a good action, I should long ago have been dead—and, indeed, by my own hand.   *Letter to Dr. F.G. Wegeler*

John Keats; 1820   3185

I have been half in love with easeful Death.   *Ode to a Nightingale*

John Chalmers Da Costa; 1910   3186

When civilization reaches some higher level in some dim future century, we will recognize that some suicides are reasonable, natural and justifiable. We will then have a suicide tribunal, as Sir Thomas More devised for his Utopia. In Utopia the priests and magistrates are to permit or actually direct those afflicted with incurable disease to commit suicide.   *Address to the American Philosophical Society*

John Chalmers Da Costa; 1910   3187
It seems a law of nature that the race must pay a penalty for development, and while some develop others must degenerate, hence insanity and suicide must increase as civilization and material progress advance.   *Address to the American Philosophical Society*

Thomas Merton; 1966   3188
We fear the thought of suicide, and yet we need to think rationally about it, if we can, because one of the characteristics of our time is precisely that it is a suicidal age.... For the well-to-do—and they are the ones most suicidal—there is comfort, security, no end of distraction, life should be livable and even happy.   *Conjectures of a Guilty Bystander*

Robert P. Hudson; 1983   3189
In 1967 the head of the National Institute of Mental Health officially pronounced suicide a disease.... Centers to prevent suicide sprang up, some with the assistance of taxpayers' money. A medical journal, *The Bulletin of Suicidology*, was founded. Conferences were held at which learned men pondered the causes, treatment, and prevention of the new disease. It is reasonable to inquire what brought all of this about. The phenomenon of self destruction had not changed.... Yet what had been a sin in the eighteenth century and a crime in the nineteenth was now a disease in the twentieth.   *Disease and Its Control*

SULFONAMIDES

Lionel Ernest Howard Whitby; 1938   3190
2-(*p*-aminobenzene sulphonamide) pyridine is chemotherapeutically active in experimental infections in mice against pneumococci of Types I, II, III, V, VII, VIII and especially against Types I, VII, and VIII.... It is as active as sulphanilamide against haemolytic streptococcus and meningococcus.   *The Lancet*

Maxwell Finland, Elias Strauss, Osler L. Peterson; 1941   3191
Sulfadiazine was used in the treatment of 446 patients with various infections. It appeared to be highly effective in the treatment of...pneumococcic, staphylococcic and...pneumonias; meningococcic infections; acute infections of the upper respiratory tract including sinusitis; erysipelas; acute infections of the urinary tract, particularly those associated with Escherichia coli bacilluria, and acute gonorrheal arthritis.... Toxic effects...were relatively mild and infrequent.   *Journal of the American Medical Association*

SURGEONS

Aulus Cornelius Celsus; 25 BC - AD 50   3192
A surgeon should be youthful or at any rate nearer youth than age; with a strong and steady hand which never trembles, and ready to use the left hand as well as the right; with vision sharp and clear, and spirit undaunted; filled with pity, so that he wishes to cure his patient, yet is not moved by his cries to go too fast or cut less than is necessary, but does everything just as if the cries of pain cause him no emotion.   *On Medicine*

Martial (Marcus Valerius Martialis); [40-104]   3193
Both as surgeon and sexton it must be confessed
Old Sawyer's helped many a man to his rest.   *Epigrams I, 30*

Lanfrancho of Milan; 1296   3194
Each practitioner is a theoretician: each surgeon is a practitioner: therefore each surgeon is a theoretician.   *Garrison FH, An Introduction to the History of Medicine*

Theodoric, Bishop of Cervia; 1297   3195
There is no need...to be rash or daring, but let them be foresighted, gentle, and circumspect, in order that with the greatest deliberateness and gentleness under all circumstances they may operate with what gentleness they can, and especially around cerebral membranes, sensitive parts, and other ticklish places.... They must needs be well-read,

and even if they be aided sometimes by experience, yet frequently will they fall into error and into confusion. I scarcely think that anyone can understand surgery without schooling.

The Surgery of Theodoric

Henri de Mondeville; [1260-1320]   **3196**

The surgeon should be fairly audacious [yet] he should operate with prudence and sagacity; he should never commence perilous operations unless he has provided everything in order to avoid danger; ...he should not sing his own praises; he should not cover his colleagues with blame; he should not cause envy among them; he should work always with the idea of acquiring a reputation of probity; he should be reassuring to his patients by kind words and acquiesce to their requests when nothing harmful will result from them as to their cure.

Cumston CG, Buffalo Medical Journal

Guy de Chauliac; 1363   **3197**

The conditions necessary for the surgeon are four: first, he should be learned; second, he should be expert; third, he must be ingenious, and fourth, he should be able to adapt himself.... Let the surgeon be bold in all sure things, and fearful in dangerous things.

Brennan WA, On Wounds and Fractures

Paracelsus (Theophrastus Bombastus von Hohenheim); *circa* 1550   **3198**

In judicando ye are a physician, in curando a surgeon. The patient asks for cure—surgery—and not for theory—medicine—it is the doctor who needs the latter. That is: there can be no surgeon who is not also a physician; the latter begets the surgeon and the surgeon tests the physician by the result of his work.

Spitalbuch

John Halle; 1565   **3199**

A chirurgien should have three dyvers properties in his person. That is to say, a harte as the harte of a lyin, his eyes like the eyes of a hawke, and his handes the handes of a woman.

Daniels AM, Times Literary Supplement

John Jones; 1775   **3200**

A judicious surgeon will always find his powers and abilities of assisting the wretched, proportionable to the time he has spent, and the pains he has bestowed in acquiring the proper knowledge of his profession.... [The surgeon] ought to have firm steady hands, and be able to use both alike, and above all, a mind calm and intrepid, yet humane and compassionate, avoiding every appearance of terror and cruelty to his patients, amidst the most severe operations.

Plain, Concise, Practical Remarks on Treatment of Wounds and Fractures

Joseph Lister; 1854   **3201**

I must not expect to be a Liston or a Syme, still I shall get on. Certain it is, I love Surgery more and more, and this is one great point; and I believe my judgement is pretty sound, which is another important point. Also I trust I am honest, and a lover of truth, which is perhaps as important as anything. As to brilliant talent, I know I do not possess it; but I must try to make up as far as I can by perseverance.

Coope R, The Quiet Art

Samuel David Gross; 1887   **3202**

It is impossible for any man to be a great surgeon if he is destitute...of the finer feelings of our nature.... I do not think that it is possible for a criminal to feel much worse the night before his execution than a surgeon when he knows that upon his skill and attention must depend the fate of a valuable citizen, husband, father, mother or child. Surgery under such circumstances is a terrible task master, feeding like a vulture upon a man's vitals.

Autobiography

Lois Wright (Lucy Waite); 1901   **3203**

Objection is often made to the vaginal route, that it is a blind method of operating. Yes—surely to the surgeon who has not eyes in the ends of his fingers; but as the musician fingers the strings of his instrument until he can play with his eyes closed, so must the skilled pelvic surgeon be able to distinguish by the touch the line of cleavage between normal and pathological tissue.

American Journal of Surgery and Gynecology

John Chalmers Da Costa; 1915   **3204**

A fashionable surgeon, like a pelican, can be recognized by the size of his bill.

New York Medical Journal

Wilfred Batten Lewis Trotter; 1932   **3205**

It is sometimes asserted that a surgical operation is or should be a work of art...fit to rank with those of the painter or sculptor.... That proposition does not admit of discussion. It is a product of the intellectual innocence which I think we surgeons may fairly claim to possess, and which is happily not inconsistent with a quite adequate worldly wisdom.

Address

Thomas Findley; 1944   **3206**

The surgeon...is a man of action. He lives in an exhilarating world of knives, blood, and groans. His tempo is of necessity rapid. He is inclined to look at his less kinetic colleague with an air of puzzled condescension but may, in a relaxed moment, admit that the medical man is occasionally able to assist uncomfortable dowagers in the selection of a cathartic.

Surgery

Oliver St. John Gogarty; 1951   **3207**

Let Surgeon MacCardle confirm you in Hope.
A jockey fell off and his neck it was broke.
He lifted him up like a fine, honest man;
And he said "He is dead; but I'll do all I can."

The Three

Richard Selzer; 1991   **3208**

In the operating room the patient must be anaesthetized in order that he or she feel no pain. The surgeon too must be anaesthetized, insulated against the emotional heat of the event so that he can perform this act of laying open the body of a fellow human being, which, take away the purpose for which it is being done, is no more than an act of assault and battery. A barbaric act. So the surgeon dons a carapace which keeps him from feeling. It is what gives many surgeons the appearance of insensitivity.   *The Surgeon as Writer*

SURGERY

Hippocrates; [460-375 BC]   **3209**

The things relating to surgery, are—the patient; the operator; the assistants; the instruments; the light, where and how; how many things, and how; where the body, and the instruments; the time; the manner; the place.   *On Surgery*

Hippocrates; [460-375 BC]   **3210**

Let those who look after the patient present the part for operation as you want it, and hold fast the rest of the body so as to be all steady, keeping silence and obeying their superior.   *On Surgery*

Hippocrates; [460-375 BC]   **3211**

Those diseases that medicines do not cure are cured by the knife. Those that the knife does not cure are cured by fire. Those that fire do not cure must be considered incurable.

Aphorisms

Hippocrates; [460-375 BC]   **3212**

In surgical operations that consist in incising or cautery, speed or slowness are commended alike, for each has its value.... Where the surgery is performed by a single incision, you must make it a quick one; for since the person being cut usually suffers pain, this suffering should last for the least time possible.... When many incisions are necessary, you must employ a slow surgery, for a surgeon that was fast would make the pain sustained and great, whereas intervals provide a break for the patients.   *On Physicians*

Aretaeus the Cappadocian; [81-138?]   **3213**

But if the stone is not very large, there is frequent suppression of urine; for by falling readily into the neck of the bladder, it prevents the escape of the urine. Although it be safer to cut in these cases than for the large stones, still the bladder is cut; and although one should escape the risk of death, still there is a constant drain of water; and although this may not be dangerous, to a freeman the incessant flow of urine is intolerable, whether he walk or whether he sleep; but is particularly disagreeable when he walks.

On Those in the Bladder

John Evelyn; 1650   **3214**

The sick creature was strip'd to his shirt, and bounde arms and thighs to an high Chaire, 2 men holding his shoulders fast down: then the Chirurgion with a crooked Instrument prob'd til he hit on the stone, then...he made Incision thro the Scrotum about an Inch in length, then he put in his forefingers to get the stone as neere the orifice of the wound as he could, then with another Instrument like a Cranes neck he pull'd it out with incredible torture to the Patient.   *Diary*

John Evelyn; 1672   **3215**

That morning my Chirurgeon cut off a poore creaturs Leg, a little under the knee, first cutting the living and untainted flesh above the Gangreene with a sharp knife, and then sawing off the bone in an instant; then with searing and stoopes stanching the blood, which issued abundantly; the stout and gallant man, enduring it with incredible patience, and that without being bound to his chaire, as is usual in such painefull operations, or hardly making a face or crying oh.   *Diary*

R. Yeo; 1732   **3216**

The work was in a moment done.
If possible, without a groan:
So swift thy hand, I could not feel
The progress of the cutting steel....
For quicker e'en than sense, or thought,
The latent ill view was brought;
And I beheld with ravish'd eyes,
The cause of all my agonies.
And above all the race of men,
I'll bless my GOD for Cheselden.   *The Grateful Patient*

John Jones; 1775   **3217**

It might... be of singular advantage to young surgeons, particularly before they begin an operation to go through every part of it attentively in their own minds, to consider every possible accident which may happen, and to have the proper remedies at hand in case they should; and in all operations of delicacy and difficulty to act with deliberation.

Plain, Concise, Practical Remarks on Treatment of Wounds and Fractures

John Jones; 1776   **3218**

The exterior of this science, has nothing pleasing or attractive in it, but is rather disgusting to nice, timid, and delicate persons:—Its objects too, except in time of war, lying chiefly among the poor and lower classes of mankind, do not excite the industry of the ambitious or avaritious, who find their best account among the rich and great.

Plain, Concise, Practical Remarks on Treatment of Wounds and Fractures

John Syng Dorsey; 1813   **3219**

An American, although he must labour under many disadvantages in the production of an elementary treatise, is in one respect better qualified for it than an European surgeon. He is—at least he ought to be—strictly impartial, and therefore adopts from all nations their respective improvements.   *Elements of Surgery*

Ephraim McDowell; 1817   **3220**

Having never seen so large a substance extracted, nor heard of an attempt, or success attending any operation such as this required, I gave to the unhappy woman...information of her dangerous situation.... The tumor...appeared full in view, but was so large we could not take it away entire.... We took out fifteen pounds of a dirty, gelatinous looking substance. After which we cut through the fallopian tube, and extracted the sac, which weighed seven pounds and one half.... In five days I visited her, and much to my astonishment found her making up her bed.   *Eclectic Repertory and Analytical Review*

John Murray Carnochan; 1857   **3221**

While respect for life will dictate to the surgeon the greatest prudence—will counsel him to attempt no operation which he would not be willing to perform on his own child, it will also teach him, that if the extremes of boldness are to be shunned, pusillanimity is not the necessary alternative.   *Contributions to Operative Surgery*

Emily Dickinson; 1859   **3222**

Surgeons must be very careful
When they take the knife!
Underneath their fine incisions
Stirs the Culprit - Life!   *Surgeons Must Be Very Careful*

Valentine Mott; 1863   **3223**

This discovery [of anesthesia] has not only taken from surgery its greatest horrors, but has also very much increased the facility and safety of operations; and in this way, "The domain of surgery is extended."   *Pain and Anaesthetics*

Christian Fenger; 1882   **3224**

We must naturally ask ourselves: Does suffering humanity gain anything by this operation? or, in other words, Does the operation enable us to save, or only to prolong, life, and is it worth while for patients having uterine cancer to undergo this severe operation?
                                                       The Total Extirpation of the Uterus

John Homans; 1887   **3225**

Deaths for which I am inclined to think I am at fault, have occurred generally towards the end of many daily ovariotomies, when I may have been tired or possibly unclean.
                                               Three Hundred and Eighty-Four Laparotomies

Oliver Wendell Holmes; 1887   **3226**

Which would give the most satisfaction to a thoroughly humane and unselfish being, of cultivated intelligence and lively sensibilities: to have written all the plays Shakespeare has left as an inheritance for mankind, or to have snatched from the jaws of death more than a hundred fellow-creatures...and restored them to sound and comfortable existence?
                                                              Our Hundred Days in Europe

Lois Wright (Lucy Waite); 1896   **3227**

Modern gynecological surgery stands for much more than the mere saving of life. The day is gone by when the successful surgeon is the one who can report the greatest number of cases discharged from the hospital cured at the end of three or four weeks, to drag out as many years or it may be the remainder of their days in hopeless invalidism.
                                                                    Chicago Medical Record

Lois Wright (Lucy Waite); 1908   **3228**

We are rapidly becoming a nation of scars.   *Medical Record*

George Bernard Shaw; 1911   **3229**

It is not the fault of our doctors that the medical service of the community, as at present provided for, is a murderous absurdity. That any sane nation, having observed that you could provide for the supply of bread by giving bakers a pecuniary interest in baking for you, should go on to give a surgeon a pecuniary interest in cutting off your leg, is enough to make one despair of political humanity. But that is precisely what we have done. And the more appalling the mutilation, the more the mutilator is paid.

The Doctor's Dilemma, Preface

George Bernard Shaw; 1911   **3230**

We do not go to the operating table as we go to the theatre, to the picture gallery, to the concert room, to be entertained and delighted; we go to be tormented and maimed, lest a worse thing should befall us.... The experts on whose assurance we face this horror and suffer this mutilation should have no interests but our own to think of; should judge our cases scientifically; and should feel about them kindly.   *The Doctor's Dilemma, Preface*

Harvey Cushing; 1911   **3231**

Why not put the surgical age of retirement for the attending surgeon at sixty and the physician at sixty-three or sixty-five, as you think best? I have an idea that the surgeon's fingers are apt to get a little stiff and this makes him less competent before the physician's cerebral vessels do. However, as I told you, I would like to see the days when somebody would be appointed surgeon somewhere who had no hands, for the operative part is the least part of the work.   *Letter to Dr. Henry Christian*

William Williams Keen; 1912   **3232**

As my colleague in the Chair of Pathology was a sceptic as to the role of these "bugs" as he disdainfully called the bacteria, I felt it to be of the utmost importance that this subject should be the foundation of a new Text-Book of Surgery, which I at once planned.

Autobiography (unpublished)

Roscoe C. Giles; 1922   **3233**

It cannot be too often emphasized, however, that the post-operative treatment is as essential as the operation, and the surgeon is as much responsible for the post-operative treatment as for the operation.   *Journal of the National Medical Association*

Thomas Clifford Allbutt; 1922   **3234**

From the time of Hippocrates surgery has ever been the salvation of inner medicine. In inner medicine physicians have dwelt too much in dogmas, opinions and speculations; and too often their errors passed undiscovered to the grave. The surgeon, for his good, has had a sharper training on facts; his errors hit him promptly in the face.   *The Lancet*

Charles Horace Mayo; 1935   **3235**

Carry out the two fundamental surgical requirements: see what you are doing and leave a dry field.   *Collected Papers of the Mayo Clinic and Mayo Foundation*

Edward W. Archibald; 1935   **3236**

Fingers replace brains, and handicraft outruns science.   *Annals of Surgery*

Berkeley George Andrew Moynihan; [1865-1936]   **3237**

Every operation in surgery is an experiment in bacteriology.   *Journal of Medical Biography*

Berkeley George Andrew Moynihan; [1865-1936]   **3238**

Surgery should be a merciful art; the cleaner and gentler the act of operating, the less the patient suffers.   *Journal of Medical Biography*

William J. Mayo; 1938   **3239**

I think all of us who have worked years in the profession understand that many very skillful operators are not good surgeons.   *Surgery, Gynecology, and Obstetrics*

Allen O. Whipple; 1949   **3240**

Actual operative skill cannot be gained by observation, any more than skill in playing the violin can be had by hearing and seeing a virtuoso performing on that instrument.

Surgery

Edward Johnson Wayne; 1960   **3241**

I made up my mind to become a physician rather than a member of the cutting trades when I was a house surgeon. My boss at that time described me as "The best ambisinistrous surgeon in the business" and remarked, after I had performed a circumcision, "I can only hope the functional result will be better than the cosmetic!"   *Speech*

John Heysham Gibbon Jr.; 1960   **3242**

Many are the trysts I've had
With the mortals here,
Their bodies offered to my trust,
To cut and sew and maybe cure.   A *Dream of the Heart*

John Kirklin; 1963   **3243**

Surgery is always second best. If you can do something else, it's better.   *Time*

Rosemary Stevens; 1971   **3244**

The tangled past has produced an oddly structured medical profession in America. The decline of general practice is one phenomenon. A second notable characteristic is the predominance of surgeons.... Nearly one out of every three physicians...is in a field that involves surgery.... The question must arise: Is this balance appropriate? But the next question must be: Appropriate to what? And the next still: Who is to make the estimations?   *American Medicine and the Public Interest*

Michael E. DeBakey; 1991   **3245**

It became popular in recent years to divide medicine into cognitive and noncognitive disciplines—a throwback to the schism between medicine and surgery in the Dark Ages, when use of the hands was demeaned and the status of surgery, and indeed of all medicine, declined significantly. But the labeling of surgery as a noncognitive discipline is fallacious and totally unsupported by its history and achievements.   *Annals of Surgery*

Joseph Epstein; 1999   **3246**

I looked upon this surgery as tantamount to having a vicious bully, who was going to beat the hell out of me, but it was the price of getting back into school, and since I wanted back in, there was nothing for it but to take my beating.   *The New Yorker*

Sherwin B. Nuland; 2001   **3247**

The surgeon attempts to replicate a perfection that can be reached only by removing himself from the emotion of the moment.   *The American Scholar*

SYMPTOMS

William S. Haubrich; 1955   **3248**

The world's population can be divided into two groups: some people feel well; some people do not. The presence or absence of disease has relatively little to do with which group you might be included.   *Personal communication*

Arthur Barsky, Jonathan Borus; 1995   **3249**

Not every symptom denotes disease.   *Journal of the American Medical Association*

SYNAPSE

Charles Scott Sherrington; 1897   **3250**

We are led to think that the tip of a twig of the aborescence [of the axon of a neuron] is not continuous with but merely in contact with the substance of the dendrite or cell-body on which it impinges. Such a special connection of one nerve-cell with another might be called a "synapsis." ["synapsis" eventually became "synapse"]
                          A *Text-book of Physiology. The Central Nervous System*

SYNDROME

Samuel Daniel; 1606   3251
Welcome, faire nimph, come let me try your pulse.
I cannot blame you t'hold you selfe not well.
Some thing amisse, quoth you; here's all amisse.
Th'whole Fabrick of your distempred is;
The Systole and Dynastole of your pulse,
Do shew your passions most hystericall.
It seems you have not very carefull bene,
T'observe the prophilactick regiment
Of your owne body, so that we must now
Descend unto the Therapeuticall;
That so we may prevent the syndrome
Of symptomes, and may afterwards apply
Some analepticall Elexipharmacum,
That may be proper for your maladie.   *The Queenes Arcadia, Act III, Scene ii*

SYNOVIAL MEMBRANE

John Hilton; 1863   3252
Synovial membrane is merely a modification of serous membrane, and as such is endowed
with secreting and absorbing powers.   *Rest and Pain*

SYPHILIS

Niccolo Leoniceno; 1497   3253
A disease of an unusual nature has invaded Italy and many other regions. In the begin-
ning pustules are on the private parts, soon on the whole body and frequently located on
the face itself besides causing great hideousness as well as a great deal of pain. Moreover
to this disease the physicians of our time do not yet give a name, but is called by the common name of French disease, as if this contagion were imported from France into Italy or
because Italy was invaded at the same time both by the disease itself and and the armies
of the French.   *Libellus de Morbo Gallico*

Juan Almenor; 1502   3254
It is concluded...that this disease which amongst the Italians is called *Gallicus*, that is to
say, the French disease, should now be named *Patursa*,...a disease filthie and Saturnall. It
is a filthie disease, because it maketh women to be esteemed unchast and irreligious....
There is a twofold kinde of causes.... The first is the only influence or corruption of the
aire, from whence we must charitably thinke, that it infected those which were religious.
The second is conversation, as by kissing and sucking, as appeareth in children, or by car-
nall copulation.   *De Morbo Gallico*

Johannis (Giovanni) de Vigo; 1514   3255
In the year 1494...there appeared...throughout almost all Italy, a malady of a nature
unknown to that time.... The contagion which gives rise to it comes particularly from
coitus; that is, sexual commerce of a healthy man with a sick woman or the contrary....
The first symptoms of this malady appear almost invariably upon the genital organs, that
is, upon the penis or the vulva.... These pimples are circumscribed by a ridge of callous-
like hardness.   *Practica in Arte Chirurgia Copiosa*

Ulrich von Hutten; 1519   **3256**

In the Year of Christ 1493, or thereabouts, this Evil began amongst the People.... It is thought that this Disease in our days ariseth not, unless by infection from carnal Contact, as in copulating with a diseased Person, since it appears now that young Children, old Men and others, not given to fornication or bodily lust, are very rarely diseased: Also the more a Man is addicted to these Pleasures, the sooner he catcheth it.... In Women the Disease resteth in their secret Places, wherein are little pretty Sores, full of venomous Poison, being very dangerous such as unknowingly meddle with them.   *De Morbo Gallico*

Fracastorius (Girolamo Fracastoro); 1530   **3257**

A shepherd once (distrust not ancient fame)
Possest these Downs, and Syphilus his Name....
Some destin'd Head t'attone the Crimes of all,
On Syphilus the dreadful Lot did fall....
Through what adventures this unknown Disease
So lately did astonisht *Europe* seize,
Through *Asian* coasts and *Libyan* Cities ran,
And from what Seeds the Malady began,
Our Song shall tell: to *Naples* first it came
From France, and justly took from *France* his Name,
Companion of the War—   *Syphilis sive Morbus Gallicus*

Ambroise Paré; [1510-1590]   **3258**

A certain very good Citizen of this City of Paris granted to his wife [that] she should have a nurse in the house to ease her of some part of the labour: by ill hap, the nurse they took was troubled with this disease; wherefore she presently infected the child, the child the mother, the mother her husband, and he two of his children, who frequently accompanied him to bed and board.   *Collected Works*

Giovanni Maria Lancisi; 1728   **3259**

The lymph that abounds in Gallic salts...moves...within the outermost substance of the coat of the artery, begins to eat it away, and next distends it into an aneurysm.... A Gallic aneurysm is known not only by the...signs of venereal disease that has already spread to other parts...but above all it is identified by the manner in which a definite place is attacked by aneurysm.   *De Motu Cordis et Aneurysmatibus*

Phillippe Ricord; 1838   **3260**

My clinical observations have led me to the following classification of the symptoms of syphilis.... Primary symptom (accident primitif), chancre from the direct action of the virus which it produces, and by means of which it propagates itself.... Secondary symptoms, or symptoms of general infection.... Tertiary symptoms (accidents tertiares) occurring at indefinite periods, but generally long after the cessation of the primary affection.   *A Practical Treatise on Venereal Diseases*

Phillippe Ricord; 1838   **3261**

Alexander Benedictus, a Veronese physician, was the first to admit, as a contagious principle, a venereal taint produced in the sexual organs of women by the alteration of humors which they exhale; this was admitted by Fernel, and received the name of lues venerea, poison, venereal virus, &c., and since that time most writers on syphilis have acknowledged the existence of a specific cause, of a peculiar deleterious principle.   *A Practical Treatise on Venereal Diseases*

Elisha Bartlett; 1844   **3262**

Syphilis.... the offspring of excessive and irregular animal indulgence and its terrible scourge and avenger; its poison, when received into the system, and not counteracted by appropriate treatment, extends and multiplies itself, till the entire economy becomes its prey, till every fibre and every fluid of the body is involved in its foul contamination, and this fair and goodly fabric, "the cunning'st pattern of excelling nature," is changed to a reeking mass of loathsomeness and abomination.

Essay on the Philosophy of Medical Science

Jonathan Hutchinson; 1861   **3263**

It is the permanent set [of teeth] only which show any peculiarities. The milk teeth of syphilitic infants...show no peculiarities of form.... The central upper incisors are the test-teeth.... The teeth are short and narrow. Instead of becoming wider as they descend from the gum, they are narrower at their free edge than at their crowns.... In the centre of their free edge is a deep verticle notch.

British Medical Journal

Fritz Schaudinn, Erich Hoffman; 1905   **3264**

In the group of medical cases this spirochetal form, visible as a "pale figure", is seen only in cases with evidence of syphilis.... I coin for the zoological nomenclature the name *Sp. pallida* for this pale form, which is consistent with the name for the preceding dark form, *Sp. refringens.* [subsequently named *Treponema pallidum*]

Arbeiten aus dem Kaiserlichen Gesundheitsamte

August von Wassermann, A. Neisser, C Bruck; 1906   **3265**

On one hand we can determine in vitro whether a human serum or animal immune serum contains antibodies specific for substances of the syphilitic agent and we will be able to quantitate these antibodies. On the other hand, in using the described reaction, it is possible to demonstrate whether a particular organ contains syphilitic substances.

Deutsche Medizinische Wochenschrift

Paul Ehrlich; 1910   **3266**

It has been shown to be possible, by deliberately planned and chemotherapeutic approach, to discover curative agents which act specifically and aetiologically against diseases due to protozoal infections, and especially against the spirilloses, and amongst these against syphilis in the first place. Further evidence for the specificity of the action of dihydroxydiaminoarsenobenzene [Salvarsan, "606"] is the disappearance of the Wasserman reaction, which reaction must...be regarded as indicative of a reaction of the organism to the constituents of the spirochaetes.

Closing Notes on Experimental Chemotherapy of Spirilloses

John Friend Mahoney, R.C. Arnold, A. Harris; 1943   **3267**

Four male patients have been treated [with penicillin] and observed for a period sufficiently long to permit comparison with results produced by more conventional forms of treatment.... The results of the blood studies indicate that the therapy was responsible for a more or less rapid and complete disappearance from the blood stream of the reacting substance...which is usually associated with activity in early syphilis.

Venereal Disease Informatics

TEACHERS

William Osler; 1892   **3268**

The function of the teacher is to teach and to propagate the best that is known and taught in the world. To teach the current knowledge of the subject he professes—sifting, analyzing, assorting, laying down principles. To propagate, i.e., to multiply, facts on which to base principles—experimenting, searching, testing.   *Teacher and Student*

William Osler; 1895   **3269**

The very best instructor for students may have no conception of the higher lines of work in his branch, and contrariwise, how many brilliant investigators have been wretched teachers?   *Teaching and Thinking*

William Osler; 1905   **3270**

The teacher's life should have three periods—study until 25, investigation until 40, profession until 60, at which age I would have him retired on a double allowance.

Valedictory address

TELEOLOGY

Ernst Wilhelm von Bruecke; [1819-1892]   **3271**

Teleology is a lady without whom no biologist can live. Yet he is ashamed to show himself with her in public.   *Johns Hopkins Hospital Bulletin*

Lawrence Joseph Henderson; 1917   **3272**

According to the theory of probabilities[the] connection between the properties of matter and the process of evolution cannot be due to mere contingency. Therefore, since the physicochemical functional relationship is not in question, there must be admitted a functional relationship of another kind, somewhat like that known to physiology. This functional relationship can only be described as teleological.   *The Order of Nature*

TEMPORAL ARTERITIS

Jonathan Hutchinson; 1890   **3273**

The "red streaks" proved, on examination, to be his temporal arteries, which on both sides were found to be inflamed and swollen. The streaks extended from the temporal region almost to the middle of the scalp, and several branches of each artery could be distinctly traced. *Archives of Surgery*

TESTES

Nicholas Culpeper; 1660   3274

The Stones are called in Latin, *Testes*, that is Witness because they witness one to be a man, ask the Pope else, he will tell you I say true.... I need not tell you where they are placed, for Every Boy that knows his right hand from his left, knows that.... The use of the stones is, 1. To convert blood spirit into seed for the procreation of man...2. They add heat, strength, and courage to the Body. *A Directory for Midwives*

TESTS

Robert Hall Babcock; 1911   3275

In my experience as consultant I have become deeply impressed with the general reliance on laboratory methods shown by practitioners recently out of college, and at the same time with their inability accurately to observe or appreciate the significance and value of symptoms as compared with the findings of the microscope or test-tube.... Is there not danger of the science of medicine so overshadowing as to obscure the art of healing? *Lancet Clinic*

William J. Mayo; 1923   3276

I have been surprised to note the readiness with which high-grade young men, graduates from medical institutions which are models of our time, yield to the temptation of machine-made diagnoses. *Surgery, Gynecology, and Obstetrics*

John W. Todd; 1968   3277

A useful exercise before ordering any investigation is to ask: "Whatever the result, will my opinion be changed?" If the answer, as it so often is, is No, there is no point in performing it.... This is a sensitive area, since clinicians mostly take it for granted that if they want an investigation, that settles the matter. *The Lancet*

Archibald Leman Cochrane; 1972   3278

I was brought up in an older tradition. I was told, "Before ordering a test decide what you will do if it is (a) positive or (b) negative, and if both answers are the same don't do the test." *Effectiveness and Efficiency*

Joseph E. Hardison; 1979   3279

The "As long as he is in the hospital, we might as well" excuse. When I ask, "If the patient had not been admitted to the hospital, would you have ordered this test?", the answer often is, "No." There apparently is a law: the more available and accessible a test or procedure, the greater the indication to do it. *New England Journal of Medicine*

Joseph E. Hardison; 1979   3280

The less the indication there is for a test, the more likely a positive result is falsely positive. *New England Journal of Medicine*

Norman Cousins; 1979   3281

There were other tests, some of which seemed to me to be more an assertion of the clinical capability of the hospital than of concern for the well-being of the patient. *Anatomy of an Illness*

Marcia C. Schmidt; 1984   3282

Overreliance on laboratory tests is...part of what is known as the quantitative fallacy. That widespread misapprehension—which is by no means limited to physicians or even to scientists generally—centers on the assumption that if some variable can be expressed in numbers, it must mean something. On occasion, it also involves the converse assumption: that anything that *cannot* be quantified is meaningless or unimportant. *Hospital Practice*

Horton A. Johnson; 1991   **3283**

In the quest for diagnostic certainty, one can be led into a false sense of accomplishment by the results of sensitive, specific, and well-executed diagnostic tests that provide little or no diagnostic information. This is a consequence of the fact that as one approaches diagnostic certainty the useful information returned by diagnostic tests and observations approaches zero.   *Journal of the American Medical Association*

TETANUS

[Anonymous]; *circa* 1500 BC   **3284**

It is painful for him to open his mouth. His heart beats too slowly (or weakly) for speech. You observe his saliva falling from his lips, but not falling completely.... He suffers stiffness in his neck. He does not find he can look at his two shoulders and his breast.

Ebers Papyrus

Hippocrates; [460-375 BC]   **3285**

The master of a large ship mashed the index finger of his right hand with the anchor. Seven days later a somewhat foul discharge appeared; then trouble with his tongue—he complained he could not speak properly. The presence of tetanus was diagnosed, his jaws became pressed together, his teeth were locked, then symptoms appeared in his neck: on the third day opisthotonos appeared with sweating. Six days after the diagnosis was made he died.   *Beck T, Hippokrates Erkenntnisse*

Aretaeus the Cappadocian; [81-138?]   **3286**

Tetanus...is a spasm of an exceedingly painful nature, very swift to prove fatal.... They are affections of the muscles and tendons about the jaws; but the illness is communicated to the whole frame.... "Spasm from a wound is fatal." And women also suffer from this spasm after abortion; and, in this case, they seldom recover.   *On Tetanus*

William Heberden; 1802   **3287**

On the sixth day after the extirpation of a scirrhous testicle, the patient began to complain of a difficulty of swallowing, or rather of a sudden sense of suffocation; and in two days the jaw became immoveably locked, and the patient soon died.

Commentaries on the History and Cure of Diseases

TEXTBOOKS

Michael Foster; [1836-1907]   **3288**

Never write a textbook; if it is a failure it is time thrown away and worse than wasted; if it is a success, it is a millstone around your neck for the rest of your life.

Rolleston HD, The Cambridge Medical School

Wilburt C. Davison; [1892-1972]   **3289**

In contrast to many pediatric books which too often resemble the old-fashioned hoop skirt in covering the subject without touching it, this book is like a G-string in touching the subject without any pretense of covering it.   *Barnes RH, The Pharos*

Eric J. Cassell; 1997   **3290**

I went to the bookstore and looked at many textbooks of medicine. They reminded me of the Irish elk of evolutionary fame whose antlers, it is said, became even larger in the course of its evolution until it could no longer get through the forests and perished from the earth.   *Annals of Internal Medicine*

THERMOMETRY

Thomas Clifford Allbutt; 1870   **3291**

I have found that the mercurial thermometer is the best for common use.... I...set to work with Messrs. Harvey and Reynolds to manufacture...an accurate thermometer of a new form.... It is a matter of much regret that these instruments are all made by the Fahrenheit scale.... It has the...disadvantage of making English and foreign observers mutually unintelligible.... I nearly always make use of the mouth in observing myself.... For patients I always use the axilla.... If patients allow of single rectal observation...they will certainly rebel against their frequent repetition.

British and Foreign Medico-Chirurgical Review

THINKING

Charles Bell; 1811   3292

All ideas originate in the brain: the operation producing them is the remote effect of an agitation or impression on the extremities of the nerves of sense; directly they are consequences of a change or operation in the proper organ of the sense which constitutes a part of the brain, and over these organs, once brought into action by external impulse, the mind has influence.

The Idea of a New Anatomy of the Brain

Charles Darwin; 1887   3293

If I had to live my life again I would have made a rule to read some poetry and listen to some music at least once a week; for perhaps the parts of my brain now atrophied could thus have been kept active through use.

Autobiography

John Maynard Keynes; 1933   3294

Anyone who has ever attempted a pure scientific or philosophical thought knows how one can hold a problem momentarily in one's mind and apply all one's power of concentration to piercing through it, and how it will dissolve and escape and you find that what you are surveying is a blank.

Essays in Biography

THIOURACIL DRUGS

William Dock; 1984   3295

[Alan Chesney] was studying something that had to do with rabbits but, along the way, noted that his rabbits got goiters during certain times of the year when they were eating nothing but cabbage for greens. He looked into this and found that it was a thiocompound in the greens that gave them the goiter. And this is where all those antithyroid drugs—thiouracil, and so on—come from. He was the one that opened up that field.... This was serendipity, but when he stumbled over something he knew that he had "bumped his shins."

Weisse AB, Conversations in Medicine

THOMAS HIP-SPLINT

Hugh Owens Thomas; 1875   3296

I assert that a fractured thigh, if treated by extension only, would be accompanied with vastly more muscular irritability than if the same case was placed in a modern appliance, in which the limb was immoveably in the strict meaning of the term fixation.

Diseases of the Hip, Knee, and Ankle Joints

THROMBOANGIITIS OBLITERANS (BUERGER DISEASE)

Leo Buerger; 1908   3297

The disease [occurs] in young adults between the ages of twenty and thirty-five or forty years.... Upon examination we see that one or both feet are markedly blanched, almost cadaveric in appearance, cold to the touch, and that neither the dorsalis pedis nor the posterior tibial artery pulsates.... After months...trophic disturbances make their appearance.... Even before the gangrene, at the ulcerative stage, amputation may become imperative because of the intensity of the pain.

American Journal of the Medical Sciences

THROMBOCYTES (BLOOD PLATELETS)

William Osler; 1874   **3298**

Careful investigation of the blood proves that, in addition to the usual elements, there exist pale granular masses, which on closer inspection present a corpuscular appearance. In size they vary greatly from half or quarter that of a white blood-corpuscle, to enormous masses.... They have a compact solid look...while in specimens examined without any reagents the filaments of fibrin adhere to them.   *Proceedings of the Royal Society*

THROMBOPHLEBITIS

Rudolf Ludwig Karl Virchow; 1860   **3299**

That therefore, which according to the ordinary nomenclature is called suppurative phlebitis, is neither suppurative, nor yet phlebitis, but a process which begins with a coagulation, with the formation of a thrombus in the blood, and afterwards presents a stage in which the thrombi soften, so that the whole history of the process is contained in the history of the thrombus.   *Cellular Pathology*

Alistair Cooke; 1986   **3300**

Perhaps the secret of avoiding blood clots lay in the humble admonition of the London bobby: "Keep moving!"   *The Patient Has the Floor*

THYROID GLAND

Thomas Wilkinson King; 1836   **3301**

[The thyroid gland] has no very evident mechanical or local office to fulfill.... Yet we may one day be able to show, that a particular material principle is slowly formed, and partially kept in reserve; and that this principle [serves] important subsequent functions in the course of the circulation.... Something analogous to a reservoir function obtains in this part.   *Guy's Hospital Report*

Victor Alexander Haden Horsley; 1885   **3302**

The practical surgical question as to whether the cretinous symptoms following thyroidectomy are due to— (1.) Chronic asphyxia, as believed by Kocher; (2.) Injury of the sympathetic and other nerve trunks; (3.) Arrest of function of the thyroid gland; is almost settled in favor of the third view, and with it also the pathology of Myxoedema.

Proceedings of the Royal Society

Robert Hutchison; 1896   **3303**

The thyroid contains two proteids—a nucleo-albumin and the colloid matter.... The colloid is present in large amount and is contained in the acini. It contains a small amount of phosphorus and a considerable proportion of iodine.... The colloid matter is the only active constituent of the gland.   *Journal of Physiology*

David Marine, C.H. Lenhart; 1909   **3304**

Iodin is necessary for normal thyroid activity.... Iodin is taken up rapidly by the thyroid, the rapidity depending on the degree of active hyperplasia.... In endemic cretinism the fibrous overgrowth with atrophy of the gland is consequent on active hyperplasia and is associated with a very low iodin content. In myxedema the anatomical and iodin changes are similar to those of cretinism.   *Archives of Internal Medicine*

Jack Gross, Rosalind Venetia Pitt-Rivers; 1953   **3305**

3:5:3'-Triiodothyronine has been isolated from ox thyroid gland and has been identified in tryptic hydrolysates of thyroids from rats previously injected with sodium [^{131}I] iodide.

Biochemical Journal

THYROID-STIMULATING HORMONE

Leo Loeb, R.B. Bassett; 1929   3306
We prepared, from dried and powdered anterior pituitary of cattle, acid as well as alkaline extracts...which we injected daily 1 cc. intraperitoneally in each of a series of 19 guinea pigs.... There resulted in every case hypertrophy of the thyroid gland.... [The findings suggest] very strongly...that administration of the extracts caused an increased elimination of thyroid hormones...and thus caused an increase in metabolism.
Proceedings of the Society for Experimental Biology and Medicine

THYROXINE

Edward Calvin Kendall; 1915   3307
The iodin-containing compound has been isolated in pure crystalline form.... Its...chemical properties are best expressed by di-iodo-di-hydroxy-indol.... The amount of the A iodin-containing compound necessary to produce symptoms is extremely small. One-half milligram (1/120 of a grain) per day produced marked effects in a cretin weighing 15 kilos.
Transactions of the Association of American Physicians

TIME

Benjamin Franklin; 1738   3308
Time is an herb that cures all Diseases.   *Poor Richard's Almanac*

TOBACCO

James I; 1604   3309
It is alleged to be found true by proof, that by the taking of tobacco...very many do find themselves cured of diverse diseases.... In this argument there is...a great mistaking.... When a sick man hath had his disease at the height, he hath at that instant taken tobacco, and afterward his disease taking the natural course of declining, and consequently the patient of recovering his health, O then the tobacco forsooth, was the worker of that miracle.
A Counter Blaste to Tobacco

John Hill; 1761   3310
Whether or not polypusses, which attend Snuff-takers, are absolutely caused by that custom; or whether the principles of the disorder were there before, and Snuff only irritated the parts, and hastened the mischief, I shall not pretend to determine: but even supposing the latter only to be the case, the damage is certainly more than the indulgence is worth.... No man should venture upon Snuff, who is not sure that he is not so far liable to a cancer: and no man can be sure of that.   *Cautions Against the Immoderate Use of Snuff*

Samuel Auguste David Tissot; 1769   3311
The use of tobacco is another abuse in which one would not have thought that Learned People would indulge.... Tobacco...is a kind of henbane which troubles the brain like opium. It causes the same effects on our senses as inebriating beverages, and those who start to smoke are in the same state as those who have drunk too much; if this does no longer occur later, it is because one gets used to smoking as one gets used to drinking.
About the Health of Learned People

Samuel Auguste David Tissot; 1769   3312
I am not afraid to say that whilst tobacco does not cause harm to all, at least it causes much harm to the majority of people, albeit less to some than to others, and it is necessary to none. Smokers will not listen to this any more than drunkards listen to a discourse on the dangers of wine, but I shall be content if I can prevent young people, who have not yet become enslaved, to take up the habit and if I can open the eyes of those who take care of the education on that subject, which, upon examination, will perhaps appear more worthy of their attention than they have hitherto thought.   *About the Health of Learned People*

V.R. Khanolkhar, L.D. Sanghvi, K.C.M. Rao; 1955   3313

The habit of chewing was associated with cancer of the oral cavity; ...the combined habit of smoking and chewing was associated with cancer of the hypopharynx and base of the tongue; and...only smoking was associated with cancer of the oropharynx and oesophagus.

British Medical Journal

TOURETTE SYNDROME

Jean-Marc-Gaspard Itard; 1825   3314

Madame de Dampierre, now 26 years old, was taken, at the age of 7, with convulsive contractions of the hands and arms which manifested themselves mainly when she practised writing.... [Now] in the midst of a conversation... suddenly, without being able to prevent it, she interrupted what she was saying or listening to with bizarre cries and extraordinary words that contrasted deplorably with her distinguished manner. These words were, for the most part, gross curses, obscene terms.   *Archives Générales de Médecine*

George Miller Beard; 1880   3315

The [Maine jumpers] could not help repeating the word or sound that came from the person that ordered them any more than they could help striking, dropping, throwing or jumping, or starting; all of these phenomena were indeed but part of the general condition known as jumping..... The jumper's liability to jump was a life-long condition.... Jumping was hereditary and ran in families... Once a jumper, always a jumper.

Journal of Nervous and Mental Disease

H. A. O'Brien; 1883   3316

Those subjects who appear to be affected [start] unduly at the sound of an unexpected and loud noise, or at the sight of an unexpected... incident.... Their irresistible impulse seems to be to strike out at the nearest object, animate or inanimate, and... their involuntary exclamation is always characterized by what I must call obscenity.... This element is never absent from the cry of a startled latah, who may, on ordinary occasions, appear the essence of propriety.   *Journal of the Straits Branch of the Royal Asiatic Society in Singapore*

Georges Gilles de la Tourette; 1884   3317

This illness is hereditary; it is characterized by motor incoordination in the form of abrupt muscular jerks that are often severe enough to make the patient jump;... the incoordination may be accompanied by articulated or inarticulated sounds. When articulated, the words are often repetitions of words which the patient may have just heard.... Among the expressions which the patient may repeatedly utter... some may have the special character of being obscene (coprolalia);... the physical and mental health of these patients is otherwise basically normal. The condition seems incurable and life long, with onset in childhood.   *Archives de Neurologie*

William A. Hammond; 1884   3318

The captain... , running up to [the steward], suddenly clapping his hands at the same time, accidently slipped and fell hard on the deck; without having been touched by the captain, the steward instantly clapped his hands and shouted, and then, in powerless imitation, he too fell as hard and almost precisely in the same manner and position.... [The disorder] is known to Russians by the name of "Miryachit".... It will at once... be perceived that there are striking analogies between "Miryachit" and [the] disorder of the "Jumping Frenchmen" of Maine.   *New York Medical Journal*

TOXINS

Croatian proverb   3319

All mushrooms are edible, but some only once.   *Proverb*

TRAVEL

William Osler; 1897   **3320**
The all-important matter is to get breadth of view as early as possible, and this is difficult without travel.   *Internal Medicine as a Vocation*

Sherwood L. Gorbach; 1982   **3321**
Travel expands the mind and loosens the bowels.   *New England Journal of Medicine*

TREATMENT

[Anonymous]; *circa* 2500 BC   **3322**
Now when thou findest that the skull of that man is split, thou shouldst not bind him, (but) moor (him) at his mooring stakes until the period of his injury passes by. His treatment is sitting. Make for him two supports of brick, until thou knowest he has reached a decisive point.... As for: "Moor (him) at his mooring stakes," it means putting him on his customary diet, without administering to him a prescription. As for: "until thou knowest he has reached a decisive point," it means (until) thou knowest whether he will die or he will live.   *The Edwin Smith Surgical Papyrus*

[Anonymous]; *circa* 1550 BC   **3323**
When thou examinest the obstruction in his abdomen and thou findest that he is not in a condition to leap the Nile, his stomach is swollen and the chest asthmatic, then say thou to him: "It is the Blood that has got itself fixed and does not circulate." Do thou cause an emptying by means of a medicinal remedy.   *Ebers Papyrus*

Confucius; [551-478 BC]   **3324**
Because the newer methods of treatment are good, it does not follow that the old ones were bad: for if our honorable and worshipful ancestors had not recovered from their ailments, you and I would not be here today.   *Brallier JM, Medical Wits and Wisdom*

Hippocrates; [460-375 BC]   **3325**
Whenever the illness is too strong for the available remedies, the physician surely must not expect that it can be overcome by medicine. To attempt futile treatment is to display an ignorance that is allied to madness.   *Basta LL, A Graceful Exit*

Hippocrates; [460-375 BC]   **3326**
The prime object of the physician in the whole art of medicine should be to cure that which is diseased; and if this can be accomplished in various ways, the least troublesome should be selected; for this is more becoming a good man, and one well skilled in the art, who does not covet popular coin of base alloy.   *On the Articulations*

Hippocrates; [460-375 BC]   **3327**
For extreme diseases, extreme methods of cure...are most suitable.   *Aphorisms*

Hippocrates; [460-375 BC]   **3328**
Diseases caused by over-eating are cured by fasting; those caused by starvation are cured by feeding up. Diseases caused by exertion are cured by rest; those caused by indolence are cured by exertion. To put it briefly: the physician should treat disease by the principle of opposition to the cause of the disease according to its form.   *Hippocratic Writings*

Aulus Cornelius Celsus; 25 BC - AD 50   **3329**
Treatment is to be always directed to the part which is mostly in trouble.   *On Medicine*

Seneca; [8 BC - 65 AD]   **3330**
Nothing hinders a cure so much as frequent change of medicine.   *Epistles*

Thomas Aquinas; [1225?-1274]   **3331**
The physician strengthens nature, and employs food and medicine, of which nature makes use for the intended end.   *Summa Theologica*

Baltasar Gracián y Morales; 1637   **3332**

Remedies often worsen evil.... The wise physician knows when to prescribe and when not to, and sometimes it takes skill not to apply remedies.... There is no better remedy for disorder than to leave it alone to correct itself.   *The Art of Worldly Wisdom*

Robert Boyle; *circa* 1660   **3333**

Honored with the title of *Generous Remedies*...are Bleeding, Vomiting, Purging, Sweating, and Spitting, of which I briefly observe in General, that they are sure to weaken or discompose when they are imployed, but do not certainly cure afterwards.

Kaplan BB, Divulging of Useful Truths in Physick

Thomas Sydenham; [1624-1689]   **3334**

It is a great mistake to suppose that Nature always stands in need of the assistance of Art...nor do I think it below me to acknowledge that, when no manifest indication pointed out to me what was to be done, I have consulted the safety of my patient and my own reputation effectually by doing nothing at all.   *Coope R, The Quiet Art*

Edward Baynard; 1719   **3335**

For in ten words the whole Art is comprised;
For some of the ten are always advised.
Piss, Spew, and Spit,
Perspiration and Sweat;
Purge, Bleed, and Blister,
Issues and Clyster....
Most other specifics
Have no visible effects,
But the getting of fees,
For a promise of ease;
(Much like the South Seas).   *Shorter E, Doctors and Their Patients*

Jean Jacques Rousseau; 1775   **3336**

However useful medicine, properly administered, may be among us, it is certain that, if the savage, when he is sick and left to himself, has nothing to...fear but from his disease; which renders his situation often preferable to our own.   *Origin of Inequality*

Thomas Reid; 1785   **3337**

The art of medicine is to follow Nature, to imitate and assist her in the cure of diseases.

Inquiry into the Human Mind on the Principles of Common Sense

William Withering; 1785   **3338**

It is much easier to write upon a disease than upon a remedy. The former is in the hands of nature and a faithful observer, with an eye of tolerable judgment, cannot fail to delineate a likeness. The latter will ever be subject to the whims, the inaccuracies and the blunders of mankind.   *An Account of the Foxglove and Some of Its Medical Uses*

William Heberden; 1802   **3339**

New medicines, and new methods of cure, always work miracles for a while.

Commentaries on the History and Cure of Diseases

Thomas Jefferson; 1807   **3340**

Where...we have seen a disease, characterized by specific signs or phenomena, and relieved by a certain natural evacuation or process, whenever that disease recurs under the same appearances, we may reasonably count on producing a solution of it, by the use of such substances as we have found produce the same evacuation or movement. Thus, fulness of the stomach we can relieve by emetics; disease of the bowels, by purgatives; inflammatory cases, by bleeding; intermittents, by the Peruvian bark; syphilis by mercury; watchfulness, by opium.   *Chuinard EG, Only One Man Died*

Thomas Jefferson; 1807   **3341**
I would wish the young practitioner especially, to have deeply impressed on his mind, the real limits of his art, & that when the state of his patient gets beyond these, his office is to be a watchful, but quiet spectator of the operations of nature, giving them fair play by a well-regulated regimen, & by all the aid they can derive from the excitement of good spirits and hope in the patient.   *Letter to Dr. Casper Wistar*

James Gregory; [1753-1821]   **3342**
Young men kill their patients; old men let them die.   *Horae Subsecivae*

Jacques André Rochoux; 1836   **3343**
In any case, every method has reverses; every method successes; from which it follows that the problem to pose should not be the old problem: given a certain malady, find the treatment; but rather the following: given this particular case, deduce from it the treatment.
Bulletin de l'Academie Nationale de Medicine

Jacob Bigelow; 1854   **3344**
[Physicians] should not allow [the patient] to be tormented with useless and annoying applications, in a disease of settled destiny. It should be remembered that all cases are susceptible of errors of commission as well as omission, and that by an excessive application of means of art, we may frustrate the intentions of nature, when they are salutary, or embitter the approach of death when it is inevitable.   *Nature in Disease*

Pierre Marie; 1883   **3345**
There is, we believe, both in pathogenesis and in therapeutics: much remedy, little cure; much theory, little truth.   *Archives de Neurologie*

Alfred Stillé; 1884   **3346**
When [no therapy] avails to ward off the fatal ending, it is still no small portion of [the physician's] art to rid his patient's path of thorns if he cannot make it bloom with roses. *Address*

Charles Warrington Earle; 1891   **3347**
Do not waste time and annoy the patient by doctoring a symptom; attack the disease.
Archives of Pediatrics

William Osler; *circa* 1900   **3348**
The physician without physiology and chemistry practices a sort of popgun pharmacy, hitting now the malady and again the patient, he himself not knowing which.   *Aphorisms*

George Bernard Shaw; 1911   **3349**
There is at bottom only one genuinely scientific treatment for all diseases, and that is to stimulate the phagocytes. Stimulate the phagocytes. Drugs are a delusion.
The Doctor's Dilemma, Preface

Stephen Leacock; 1911   **3350**
Consider the advance of the science on its practical side. A hundred years ago it used to be supposed that fever could be cured by the letting of blood; now we know positively that it cannot. Even seventy years ago it was thought that fever was curable by the administration of sedative drugs; now we know that it isn't. For the matter of that, as recently as thirty years ago, doctors thought that they could heal a fever by means of low diet and the application of ice; now they are absolutely certain that they cannot. This instance shows the steady progress made in the treatment of fever.   *How To Be a Doctor*

Santiago Ramón y Cajal; [1852-1934]   **3351**
The sun, the open air, silence, and art are great physicians. The first two are tonics for the body, the last two still the vibrations of sorrow, free us from all our own ideas, which are sometimes more virulent than the worst of microbes, and guide our sensibilities towards the world about us, the font of the purest and most refreshing pleasures.
Craigie EH and Gibson WC, The World of Ramón y Cajal

Harvey Cushing; 1935   **3352**

In a certain sense every drug a doctor administers and every operation a surgeon performs is experimental in that the result can never be mathematically calculated, the doctor's judgment and the patient's response being variables indeterminable by any law of averages.

Science

Fuller Albright; 1951   **3353**

One cannot possibly practice good medicine and not understand the fundamentals underlying therapy. Few if any rules for therapy are more than 90 per cent correct. If one does not understand the fundamentals, one does more harm in the 10 per cent of instances to which the rules do not apply than one does good in the 90 per cent to which they do apply.   *Diseases of the Ductless Glands*

Wystan Hugh Auden; 1969   **3354**

Healing...is not a science, but an intuitive wooing of Nature.   *The Art of Healing*

Archibald Leman Cochrane; 1972   **3355**

The most important type of inefficiency [in treatment] is really a combination of two separate groups, the use of ineffective therapies and the use of effective therapies at the wrong time.   *Effectiveness and Efficiency*

Tinsley R. Harrison; 1973   **3356**

Hope, like sleep, food, and smiles, is among the most potent of all therapeutic measures.

Journal of the American Medical Association

Richard Gordon; 1993   **3357**

Among the greatest discoveries of medicine are the generally belated ones that some treatments are utterly useless.   *The Alarming History of Medicine*

TREMOR

Melvin D. Yahr; 1981   **3358**

The common practice of referring to tremor as the hallmark of Parkinson's disease is unfortunate; like all reductionist thinking, it does not simplify but only complicates the work of diagnosis. Since tremor is symptomatic of a wide variety of disorders, using this as the sole identifier of a given disease is like calling any red fruit a tomato simply because it is red. Parkinson's disease is a multifaceted disorder; as such, it cannot be defined by tremor or any other single finding.   *Hospital Practice*

TRENDELENBURG POSITION

Friedrich Trendelenburg; 1890   **3359**

If one places the body of a patient on the operating table in such a way that the sym-physis pubis forms the highest point of the trunk and the long axis of the trunk forms an angle of at least 45 degrees with the horizontal, then the various organs, especially the liver, spleen and mesentery fall into the concavity of the diaphragm by virtue of their weight.

Medical Classics

TRICHINOSIS

Ambrose Bierce; 1906   **3360**

Trichinosis, *n*. The pig's reply to proponents of porcophagy.   *The Devil's Dictionary*

TRIGEMINAL NEURALGIA

William Heberden; 1802 3361

When such a topical intermittent infests the head or face, as it often does, there is as exquisite an anguish suffered as from any distemper to which the body is subject, if we may judge by the expressions of it, which are wrung from the most patient tempers.

Commentaries on the History and Cure of Diseases

TROUSSEAU SIGN

Armand Trousseau; 1868 3362

In the upper limbs, the thumb is forcibly and violently adducted; the fingers are pressed closely together, and semi-flexed over the thumb...the hand assumes a conical shape, or better the shape which the accoucheur gives to it when introducing it into the vagina.... I discovered this influence of pressure by chance... I saw a paroxysm return in the hand on the same side when the bandage was applied round the arm.

Lectures on Clinical Medicine

TRUTH

Benjamin Rush; 1789 3363

Preserve upon all occasions a composed or cheerful countenance in the room of your patients, and inspire as much hope of a recovery as you can, consistent with truth, especially in acute diseases. *Duties of a Physician*

William Osler; 1889 3364

In seeking absolute truth we aim at the unattainable, and must be content with finding broken portions. *Aequanimitas. Aequanimitas*

William Osler; 1905 3365

No human being is constituted to know the truth, the whole truth, and nothing but the truth; and even the best of men must be content with fragments, with partial glimpses, never the full fruition. *The Student Life*

W.P. Lucas; 1927 3366

In meeting most of the mental and spiritual problems of childhood, the force of example is the strongest weapon. Physicians must not lie to their small patients, or allow others to do so. If we must hurt them, tell them so. If you tell him that he is not going to be hurt, and then do so, you have lost his confidence, and given him a lesson in untruthfulness which he will try out for himself. *The Modern Practice of Pediatrics*

Lewis Thomas; 1979 3367

It is not so bad being ignorant if you are totally ignorant; the hard thing is knowing in detail the reality of ignorance. *The Medusa and the Snail*

TUBERCULOSIS

Hippocrates; [460-375 BC] 3368

Phthisis most commonly occurs between the ages of eighteen and thirty-five years.

Aphorisms

Bernard de Gordon; 1495 3369

Phthisis is an ulcer of the lung that consumes the whole body. *Pratiqum*

Johannis (Giovanni) de Vigo; 1514 3370

Phthisis, in greke signifieth wasting...a consumption as we call it.

Practica in Arte Chirurgica Copiosa

Fracastorius (Girolamo Fracastoro); 1546   3371

Similar to the contagious are the hereditary forms of phthisis [i.e., tuberculosis]. About this it is wonderful to know that some families have died from this disease for six generations running, and many of their members at the same age.

De Contagione et Contagiosis Morbis

François de le Boe (Sylvius); 1679   3372

Among the Conditions Causing *Ulcerations* of the *Lungs*, and which is commonly followed by a condition causing *Feebleness of the entire body*.... Not infrequently Pus collected in the Cavity of the Chest forms an *Empyema*, from whose acrid humor the Lungs are frequently attacked and *Phthisis* is produced.... We do not understand by the name of Phthisis every Consumption but only that which *follows Ulcer of the Lung*.   *De Phthisis*

Samuel Garth; 1699   3373

Whilst meagre Phthisis gives a silent bow,
Her strokes are sure, but her advances slow.
No loud alarms, nor fierce assaults are shown:
She starves the fortress first, then takes the town.   *The Dispensary*

Cotton Mather; 1724   3374

A DREADFUL Disease! But so incident unto *Us*, that Foreigners call it, *The English Disease*. What is the *Spectacle* that we have before us, when we see a Friend, with a *Consumption* upon him.... We see the Body Wasting with a Lingering *Fever*; and for the most Part a tedious *Cough*, proceeding from ill-figured Particles in the *Blood*, with which the Lungs are grievously corroded.   *The Angel of Bethesda*

William Stark; 1788   3375

In the cellular substance of the lungs are found roundish firm bodies (named tubercles) of different sizes, from the smallest granule, to about half an inch in diameter, the latter often in clusters.... The cavities of less than half an inch diameter are always shut up; those... a little larger have... a round opening made by a branch of the trachea. At this period... there being a communication between the cavity of it and the open air, it is proper to change the name of tubercle to that of vomica.   *Works*

William Heberden; 1802   3376

I have observed several die of consumptions, in whom infection seemed to be the most probable origin of their illness, from their having been the constant companions, or bedfellows, of consumptive persons.   *Commentaries on the History and Cure of Diseases*

William Heberden; 1802   3377

Consumptive women readily conceive, and during their pregnancy the progress of the consumption seems to be suspended; but as soon as they are delivered, it begins to attack them with redoubled strength; the usual symptoms come on, or increase with great rapidity, and they very soon sink under their distemper.

Commentaries on the History and Cure of Diseases

William Heberden; 1802   3378

Dissections of those who have died of pulmonary consumptions, have acquainted me, that their lungs are full of little glandular swellings, many of which are in a state of suppuration.   *Commentaries on the History and Cure of Diseases*

René-Théophile-Hyacinthe Laennec; 1818   3379

I must conclude that Pectoriloquy is a true pathognomonic sign of pulmonary phthisis and that it detects the disease with certainty long before any other [sign] can raise suspicions. I ought to add that it is the only sign that can be regarded as certain.

Académie des Sciences

René-Théophile-Hyacinthe Laennec; 1819   3380

When miliary tubercles are accumulated in great numbers in the upper portions of the lungs, the sound resulting from percussion of the clavicles becomes less, and is usually unequal.... When the tubercles begin to soften...the cough gives rise to a kind of guggling.... The cough, transformed to *cavernous*, indicates the formation of a pulmonary excavation. In proportion as this empties itself, the respiration also assumes the cavernous character [and] points out the increasing extent of the cavity.

Traité de l'Auscultation Médiate

John Keats; 1820   3381

That is blood from my mouth.... I know the colour of that blood—it is artificial blood—I cannot be deceived in that colour—that drop of blood is my death warrant—I must die.

Letter written on the occasion of his first haemoptysis

René-Théophile-Hyacinthe Laennec; 1826   3382

Whatever the form in which the tuberculous matter develops, it begins as a grey, semi-transparent matter that little by little becomes yellow, opaque, and dense. Then it softens, and slowly acquires a liquidity like pus, and, when it is expelled through the airways, it leaves cavities, commonly called ulcers of the lung, that we will designate as tuberculous excavations.

Traité de l'Auscultation Médiate

Gaspard Laurent Bayle; 1838   3383

One should call pulmonary phthisis *every lesion of the lung, which left to itself, produces a progressive disintegration of this organ, as the result of which ulceration appears and finally death*. One recognizes ordinarily phthisis with the aid of the following artificial characteristics: ...*cough, difficulty in breathing, emaciation, hectic fever, and sometimes purulent expectoration*.

Encyclopedie des Sciences Médicales

William Budd; 1867   3384

The idea that phthisis is a self-propagating zymotic disease and that the leading phenomena of its distribution may be explained by supposing that it is disseminated through society by specific germs in the tuberculous matter cast off by persons already suffering from the disease first came into my mind, unbidden, so to speak, while I was walking on the Observatory Hill at Clifton in that second week of August 1856

The Lancet

Jean-Antoine Villemin; 1868   3385

Tuberculosis...pursues the course of a general affection, resulting from a morbid agent which infects the entire organism, that it developes and is propagated under conditions common to zymotic diseases, that it has the greatest analogy with syphilis, but especially with glanders...and we have been led to suppose that it ought to be inoculable like the diseases it resembles. The experiments which form the subject of this study have fully confirmed our hypothesis, as one can readily see.

Etudes sur la Tuberculose

Joseph Marie-Jules Parrot; 1876   3386

In this period of life [1 to 7 years] there is no pulmonary condition that is not clearly reflected in the bronchial lymph nodes; they are like the mirror of the lungs, and, reciprocally, there is no bronchial adenopathy that does not have a pulmonary origin. [Primary tuberculous complex of childhood]

Comptes Rendus Societé de Biologie

Carlo Forlanini; 1882   3387

I see the proposition of artificial pneumothorax in phthisis suggested, moreover as a necessary, logical, obvious offspring of clinical facts, the worth of which cannot be doubted.... When by experimentation on animals it will have been demonstrated that the physician can qualify with precision artificial pneumothorax and always control its volume...then this operative procedure should seem logical and legitimate.

Gazetta degli Ospedali e delle Cliniche di Milano

Paul Ehrlich; 1882   3388

The differentiation of the tubercle bacilli proceeds only very slowly with vesuvin, so that it is necessary to use acid.... Within a few seconds one can see the preparation fade under the acid treatment.... One would see that everything had been decolorized except the bacteria, and they had remained intensely colored.... All of these cases which I examined were frank cases of Phthisis pulmonum. I examined in all 26 cases and in all of them the bacillus could be demonstrated.   *Deutsche Medizinische Wochenschrift*

Robert Koch; 1882   3389

On the basis of my numerous observations I state it to be proved that the bacteria designated by me as the tubercle bacilli are present in all cases of tuberculosis disease of man and animals, and that they may be differentiated from all other microorganisms by their characteristic properties.... If the conviction that tuberculosis is an exquisite infectious disease makes its way among the doctors, then the question of a purposeful attack on tuberculosis certainly will come under discussion and it will develop of itself.

Berliner Klinische Wochenschrift

Robert Koch; 1882   3390

In order to gain some idea as to the presence of tubercle bacilli in the sputum of phthisical patients, I have examined repeatedly the sputa from a large series of patients with pulmonary tuberculosis and have found that in many of them none is present, but in about half the cases, they are extraordinarily numerous, some...containing spores.... It was noted that, in a number of tests of patients not having phthisis, the tubercle bacilli were never found. Animals injected with this fresh sputum containing bacilli became tuberculous just as surely as after inoculation with miliary tubercles.

Berliner Klinische Wochenschrift

Gustav Riehl, R. Paltauf; 1886   3391

In the most highly developed lesion the horny layer over the wart-like papilla was unusually thick.... The principal alterations were seen in the upper layers of the cutis.... The papillae were increased in all dimensions.... Several papilli contained caseous foci.... The infiltrates showed all of the properties of giant cell tubercles. The process is easily recognized as a particular form of skin tuberculosis.

Vierteljahr-Schrift für Dermatologie und Syphilologie

Eliza H. Root; 1904   3392

Climate will not cure tuberculosis any more than cod liver oil will.

Woman's Medical Journal

Ambrose Bierce; 1906   3393

King's Evil, *n.* A malady that was formerly cured by the touch of the sovereign, but has now to be treated by the physicians.   *The Devil's Dictionary*

Clemens Peter Freiherr von Pirquet; 1907   3394

If one arranged the hundred cases according to age, more than one third of all of them and more than one half of the cases free of tuberculosis fall into the first year; of 33 cases that were older than three years one could find only 6 free of tuberculous changes. [Pirquet test for the diagnosis of tuberculosis]   *Wiener Klinische Wochenschrift*

Ernst Ferdinand Sauerbruch; 1913   3395

Five phrenicotomies in humans have shown that his operation is simple to perform and not severe on the patient.... The first patient suffered from advanced tuberculosis on the right side of the lung.... The interruption of the phrenic nerve relieved the annoying compulsive cough, which ceased at once.... In the fourth and fifth cases, both with tuberculosis, the coughing stopped and the sputum decreased after the phrenicotomy.

Munchen Medizinische Wochenschrift

Edward Livingston Trudeau; 1916   **3396**
The tubercule bacillus bore cheerfully a degree of medication which proved fatal to its
host!   *An Autobiography*

Eugene Lindsay Opie; 1917   **3397**
Tuberculosis infection is practically universal. Dissemination of the disease among adults
is so widespread that readily recognizable tuberculous lesions have been found in all of
fifty individuals above the age of 18.... Tuberculosis of children does not select the apices
of the lungs, is accompanied by massive tuberculosis of regional lymphatic nodes, and
exhibits the characters of tuberculosis in a freshly infected animal, whereas tuberculosis
which occurs in the pulmonary apices of adults has the characters of a second infection.
Almost all human beings are spontaneously "vaccinated" with tuberculosis before they
reach adult life.   *Journal of Experimental Medicine*

Milton Rosenau; 1927   **3398**
In man the balance between immunity and susceptibility to tuberculosis is delicately
adjusted: there is a small factor of safety.   *Preventive Medicine and Hygiene*

William Hugh Feldman, Horton Corwin Hinshaw; 1944   **3399**
Streptomycin is an antibiotic substance well tolerated by guinea pigs, which is capable
under the conditions imposed of exerting a striking suppressive effect on the pathogenic
proclivities in guinea pigs of the human variety of *Mycobacterium tuberculosis.* The results
with streptomycin are comparable to those observed previously with certain drugs of the
sulfone series.   *Proceedings of the Staff Meetings of the Mayo Clinic*

Horton Corwin Hinshaw, William Hugh Feldman; 1945   **3400**
From preliminary impressions obtained from the study of thirty-four patients who had
tuberculosis and were treated with streptomycin during the past nine months it appears
that streptomycin has exerted a limited suppressive effect.... While the reproduction of
Mycobacterium tuberculosis may have been temporarily inhibited by the treatment...we
obtained no convincing evidence of rapidly effective antibacterial action.
                                                                         Proceedings of Staff Meetings of the Mayo Clinic

Horton Corwin Hinshaw, William Hugh Feldman; 1945   **3401**
From preliminary impressions obtained from the study of thirty-four patients who had
tuberculosis and were treated with streptomycin during the past nine months it appears
probable that streptomycin has exerted a limited suppressive effect, especially on some of
the more unusual types of pulmonary and extrapulmonary tuberculosis in this small series
of patients.   *Proceedings of the Staff Meetings of the Mayo Clinic*

Jörgen Lehmann; 1946   **3402**
I have investigated more than 50 derivatives of benzoic acid with the purpose of finding
a substance possessing bacteriostatic properties against the tubercle bacillus.... The most
active substance found was 4-aminosalicylic acid (*p*-aminosalicylic acid).... The treatment
of tuberculosis in man started parallel with the animal experiments.... In many cases... a
prompt fall in temperature... was accompanied by improvement in the patient's general
condition as indicated by a gain in appetite and weight... and a decrease in the erythro-
cyte sedimentation rate.   *The Lancet*

Edward Heinrich Robitzek, Irving J. Selikoff; 1952   **3403**
Forty-four cases of acute febrile, progressive caseous-pneumonic tuberculosis have been
treated with two hydrazine derivatives of isonicotinic acid.... All patients experienced
rapid and marked reversal of their original toxic states, as evidenced by gain in weight,
return of appetite, defervesence, and a sharp return in sense of well-being. Cough and
expectoration have been eliminated or markedly reduced. Sputum bacillary contents have
been reduced in 38 cases and, in 8 cases...smears have been repeatedly negative.
                                                                         American Review of Tuberculosis

René Jules Dubos; 1952   3404

Obviously, the equilibrium between man and the tubercle bacillus is very precarious. If war can so rapidly upset it, other unforeseen events might also cause recurrences of the tuberculosis epidemic in the Western world.... In the final analysis, the fight against tuberculosis can be carried along two independent approaches, by preventing the spread of the bacilli through procedures of public health, and by increasing the resistance of man through a proper way of life.   *The White Plague*

TYPHOID FEVER AND TYPHUS

Girolamo Cardano (Jerome Cardan); 1536   3405

The thirty-sixth fatal error is, in that disease, which produces in the body, marks like the bites of fleas. For they seek to call this by the name of measles, we shall call it from its resemblance pulicaris.... Measles are elevated above the skin.... Morbus pulicaris is wholly without elevations, and only spots on the skin are present, in its nature deadly.

De malo recentiorum medicorum medendi usu libellus

Fracastorius (Girolamo Fracastoro); 1584   3406

There are other fevers...usually called malignant rather than pestilent: such were those which in the years 1505 & 1528 first appeared in Italy...it was called "lenticulae" or "puncticulae," it produced lenticular spots or spots like the bites of fleas.... This fever...is contagious, but not rapidly, nor by fomites & from the distance, but only by the handling of the sick.   *Complete Works*

William Wood Gerhard; 1837   3407

The typhus fever, which is so common throughout the British dominions, is not attended with ulceration or other lesions of the glands of Peyer.... It would seem that there is no constant anatomical lesion, but that the lungs present traces of the disease more frequently than any other organ.... The lesion of the glands of Peyer is now well known to the British physicians, but an error frequently committed by them is that they regard this affection (dothinenteritis) [typhoid fever] as a mere complication of their ordinary typhus, or a modified form of it.   *On the Typhus Fever*

William Budd; 1856   3408

This species of fever has two characteristics: the first is that it is an essentially contagious disorder; the second that by far the most virulent part of the specific poison by which the contagion takes effect is contained in the diarrhoeal discharges which issue from the diseased and exanthematous bowel.   *The Lancet*

Charles Jules Henri Nicolle; 1909   3409

Many observations have led us to limit our hypothesis to the louse. At the hospital of Tunis, the patients on admission are washed and re-dressed with clean clothing; no case of inside contagion has been observed, notably during the epidemics of 1902 and 1906, in spite of the absence of any isolation and the presence of numerous bedbugs in the wards.... These experiments show that it is possible to transmit the typhus of the infected bonnet-macaque to a new monkey by means of the body louse.... Measures to combat typhus should have as their aim, a destruction of the parasites; they live principally on the body, linen, clothes, and bed-clothes of the patients.

Comptes Rendus de l'Académie des Sciences

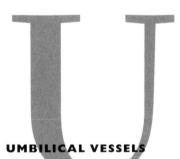

UMBILICAL VESSELS

Hieronymus Fabricius; 1649   **3410**

Why do they meet this most unfortunate and lamentable fate? Have these vessels committed some great crime, that you, O Nature, a just and provident mother to all other parts of the body, have become a stepmother to these alone, so that they deserve to be visited with an affliction so dire, a punishment so severe as wasting and death? Did not the vein continuously supply blood to the fetus? Did not the arteries give life to it? Were they not the means of bestowing increase and nutrition upon the fetus?   *Surgical Works*

UNIVERSITIES

Wilhelm Conrad Röntgen; 1894   **3411**

The university is a nursery of scientific research and mental education, a place for the cultivation of ideals for students as well as for teachers. Her significance as such is much greater than her practical usefulness.

Glasser O, Wilhelm Conrad Röntgen and the Early History of the Roentgen Rays

Wilder Penfield; 1963   **3412**

Universities, at best, can do little more than lead men to the threshold of their understanding, teach them how to educate themselves.   *The Second Career*

URINALYSIS

Thomas Addis; 1948   **3413**

When the patient dies the kidneys may go to the pathologist, but while he lives the urine is ours. It can provide us day by day, month by month, and year by year, with a serial story of the major events going on within the kidney.   *Glomerular Nephritis*

URINARY TRACT CALCULUS

Hippocrates; [460-375 BC]   **3414**

In those cases where there is a sandy sediment in the urine, there is calculus in the bladder (or kidneys).   *Aphorisms*

Cotton Mather; 1724   **3415**

The Times whereat you often in a day have the *Urinary Excretion* performed with *Ease*, are times which invite you very frequently to lift up your Hearts unto God with such an Acknowledgment as This; O, *My most merciful God, I bless thee, that the grinding Torments of the Stone, are not now grinding of me.*   *The Angel of Bethesda*

UROSCOPY

John Harington; 1596   **3416**

He called for his urinall and having made water in it, he cast it, & viewed it (as Physicians do) a prettie while; at last he sware soberly, he saw nothing in that mans water, but that he might live.   *The Metamorphosis of Aiax*

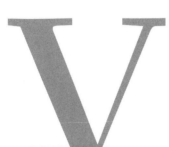

VACCINATION

Pierre-Simon Laplace; 1825   **3417**

By one of those mysteries that nature so often offers us, the vaccine is as sure a preventive of smallpox as the variola virus, and there is no risk attached to it. It does not expose one to any disease, and it calls for only very little care. Thus its use has quickly spread, and to make it universal one has only to overcome the natural inertia of people, against which it is necessary to struggle constantly, even when their dearest interests are concerned.   *Philosophical Essay on Probabilities*

VAGINISMUS

James Marion Sims; 1862   **3418**

I attempted to make a vaginal examination, but failed completely. The slightest touch at the mouth of the vagina [caused] most intense suffering.... She shrieked aloud, her eyes glaring wildly, while tears rolled down her cheeks.... This lady's husband threatened to obtain a divorce.... By the term *Vaginismus* I propose to designate involuntary spasmodic closure of the mouth of the vagina [forming] a complete barrier to coition.   *Transactions of the Obstetrical Society of London*

VAGOTOMY

Benjamin Collins Brodie; 1814   **3419**

In an inquiry which I had formerly instituted, respecting the functions of the stomach, I divided these nerves [the vagi] in the neck of a dog, for the purpose of ascertaining the influence which they possess on the secretion of the gastric juice.... We may conclude that the suppression of the secretions...sufficiently demonstrate, that the secretions of the stomach and intestines are very much under the control of the nervous system.   *Transactions of the Royal Society*

VALSALVA MANEUVER

Antonio Maria Valsalva; 1704   3420

Thus (in order to offer one of many proofs) if someone would instill a medicinal fluid into the tympanic cavity...or in the outer portion of the auditory meatus and if now, with mouth and nose closed, an attempt is made to compress the air, fluid would flow copiously from the auditory meatus. I recommend this for a prompt evacuation of a suppurative lesion since this may be remedial for the illness which might not occur by itself.... However, many more benefits may be derived from the physician's knowledge of these functions.

The Human Ear

VALVULAR HEART DISEASE

William Cowper; 1706   3421

The Symptoms in his Illness plainly shewed what must follow, from the disorders of these Valves, as they are rendered more or less useless: For as their Offise is to prevent the return of the Blood into the Heart, in its Diastole, by exactly shutting up the passage of the Aorta (as the Flaps in Water Engines) so if by any accident they are hinder'd from doing their duty, as they were by the Petrifactions mentioned, the consequences must be, not only a regurgitation of Blood into the Heart, but they baulk its impulsive force.

Philosophical Transactions of the Royal Society

VASCULAR SURGERY

John Benjamin Murphy; 1897   3422

A row of sutures was placed around the edge of the overlapping distal end [of the femoral artery], the sutures penetrating only the media of the proximal portion; the adventitia was then drawn over the line of union and sutured. The clamps were removed. Not a drop of blood escaped at the line of suture. Pulsation was immediately restored in the artery below the line of approximation.... A pulsation could be felt in the dorsalis pedis on October 11th, four days after the operation. There were no oedema of the leg and no pain.

Medical Record

VEINS

Hieronymus Fabricius; 1603   3423

Doorlets of veins is the name I give to some extremely delicate little membranes in the lumen of veins. They occur at intervals, singly or in pairs, especially in the limb veins. They open upwards in the direction of the main venous trunk, and are closed below, while, viewed from the outside.... Two evils are avoided... , undernutrition of the upper parts of the limbs , and a permanently swollen condition of the hands and feet.

De Venarum Ostiolis

VELPEAU BANDAGE

Alfred Armand Louis Marie Velpeau; 1832   3424

I have designed a bandage from a long strip of fabric which is suitable in sternoclavicular luxations...also in acromioclavicular luxations.   *New Elements of Operative Surgery*

VENIPUNCTURE

Richard Lower; 1672   3425

The lancet should be made in such a fashion and driven into the vein [so that] mishaps are easily avoided.... In its lower part, where it has to be applied to the skin, it should be blunt and a little rounded.... The rest of the bottom edge of the lancet is rounded (but not thick) so that the underlying skin will not be lacerated while the blade itself is driven into the vein.... Constrict the limb and let the vein swell.... Then...cut the vein gradually in a slanting way.   *De Catarrhis*

VENTRICULAR DEFIBRILLATION

Peter Christian Abildgaard; 1775   3426

With a shock to the head, the animal was rendered lifeless, and arose with a second shock to the chest; however, after the experiment was repeated rather often, the hen was completely stunned, walked with some difficulty, and did not eat for a day and night; then later it was very well and even laid an egg.   *Societatis Medicae Havniensis*

Claude Schaeffer Beck, E.C. Weckesser, F.M. Barry; 1956   3427

Now it appears that the resuscitation procedure has application beyond the operating room. Perhaps even beyond the hospital, and, if so, this is a new medical project for development.... The death factor in coronary artery disease is often small and reversible. It is comparable to turning the ignition switch in an automobile or to stopping and starting the pendulum of a clock. The heart wants to beat, and often it needs only a second chance.   *Journal of the American Medical Association*

VENTRICULAR FIBRILLATION

John Alexander MacWilliam; 1889   3428

A sudden, unexpected, and irretrievable cardiac failure may, even in the absence of any prominent exciting cause, present itself in the form of an abrupt onset of fibrillar contraction (ventricular delirium). The cardiac pump is thrown out of gear, and the last of its vital energy is dissipated in a violent and prolonged turmoil of fruitless activity in the ventricular walls.   *British Medical Journal*

VINBLASTINE

M.E. Hodes, R.J. Rohn, W. Bond; 1959   3429

Extracts of Vinca rosea produce bone marrow depression in animals. Several alkaloids have been isolated from the plant. One, vincaleukoblastine... not only causes marrow depression but has produced 50-150% prolongation of life in DBA/2 mice grafted with leukemia P-1534. This study concerns the effect of this agent in human beings.... Complete hematologic remission has been achieved in acute lymphocytic and monocytic leukemia. In those situations where hematologic remission was not achieved, tumor cell infiltrates have decreased in size.   *Journal of Laboratory and Clinical Medicine*

VISION

Oliver Wendell Holmes; 1858   3430

Spectacles. I don't use them. All I ask is a large, fair type, a strong daylight or gas-light, and one yard of focal distance, and my eyes are as good as ever.

    The Autocrat of the Breakfast Table

VISITORS

Samuel Johnson; 1783   3431

Visitors are no proper companions in the chamber of sickness. They come when I could sleep, or read, they stay till I am weary, they force me to attend, when my mind calls for relaxation, and to speak when my powers will hardly actuate my tongue.

    Letter to Mrs. Thrale

VITALISM

Claude Bernard; 1865   3432

When an obscure or inexplicable phenomenon presents itself, instead of saying "I do not know," as every scientific man should, physicians are in the habit of saying, "This is life"; apparently without the least idea that they are explaining darkness by still greater darkness.... Life is nothing but a word which means ignorance, and when we characterize a phenomenon as vital, it amounts to saying that we do not know its immediate cause or its conditions.   *An Introduction to the Study of Experimental Medicine*

VITAMIN A

Elmer Vernier McCollum, Marguerite Davis; 1913   3433

We have found that the failure of rats to make further growth, after being brought to this "critical" point on mixtures of isolated food substances, is due to a lack of certain ether-soluble substances in the diet. These can be supplied by the ether-extract of egg or butter.\   *Journal of Biological Chemistry*

Sidney Q. Cohlan; 1953   3434

The administration of excessive amounts of vitamin A to pregnant rats produces a diminished litter rate and characteristic malformations [such as extrusion of the brain, macroglossia, harelip, cleft palate, gross defects in eye development] among the surviving group.   *Science*

VITAMIN B_1 (THIAMINE)

Casimir Funk; 1911   3435

Polyneuritis in birds...is due to the lack of an essential substance in the diet. The substance is only present in minute amount, probably not more than 1 grm. per kilo of rice. The substance which is absent in polished rice and is contained in rice-polishings is an organic base.... The curative dose of the active substance is small; a quantity of substance which contains 4 mgr. of nitrogen cured pigeons.   *Journal of Physiology*

VITAMIN B_3 (NICOTINAMIDE)

Joseph Goldberger, G.A. Wheeler, R.D. Lillie, L.M. Rogers; 1926   3436

We feel justified in adopting...the working hypothesis that black tongue of dogs is the analogue of pellagra in man. Accordingly, it may tentatively be assumed that factor P-P is the dietary essential primarily concerned in the prevention and causation of both black tongue and pellagra.   *U.S. Public Health Reports*

Conrad A. Elvehjem, Robert J. Madden, F.M. Strong, D.W. Woolley; 1938   3437

Nicotinic acid and nicotinic acid amide are active in the cure and prevention of canine black tongue.... It is impossible to conclude...that [nicotinic acid] will prove useful in the treatment of human pellagra. However, Spies has used nicotinic acid in four cases...and reports...that the fiery red color associated with pellagrous dermatitis, stomatitis, and vaginitis improved promptly.   *Journal of Biological Chemistry*

VITAMIN B_5 (PANTOTHENIC ACID)

Roger J. Williams, Carl M. Lyman, George H. Goodyear, and others; 1933   3438

We conclude that the ability of [extracts of very diverse tissues] to stimulate yeast growth is due to the presence of a single acid substance which appears to be of universal biological occurrence. We have tentatively designated it as "pantothenic" acid, the name being derived from the Greek, meaning *from everywhere*.... Several similarities suggest its close relationship to vitamin G (B_2).   *Journal of the American Chemical Society*

VITAMIN B₁₂ (CYANOCOBALAMIN)

Edward Lawrence Rickes, N.G. Brink, F.R. Koniusky, and others; 1948   **3439**

Further purification of clinically active liver fractions has led to the isolation, in minute amounts, of a crystalline compound which is highly active for the growth of *L. lactis*. This compound is being called vitamin B_{12}.... We may in the future wish to designate a name based upon chemical structure.   *Science*

Mary Shaw Shorb; 1948   **3440**

Vitamin B_{12} is either wholly or partially responsible for the LLD growth activity observed for liver extracts.   *Science*

Randolph West; 1948   **3441**

Vitamin B_{12} has produced a positive hematological response in three patients following single intramuscular injections of 3, 6, and 150 mcg, respectively.   *Science*

VITAMIN C (ASCORBIC ACID)

Jack Cecil Drummond; 1919   **3442**

The dietary requirements of the higher animals include in addition to a satisfactorily balanced ration of protein, fats, carbohydrate and mineral salts, an adequate supply of three accessory food factors: 1. Fat-soluble A. 2. Water-soluble B, or antineuritic factor. 3. Water-soluble C, or antiscorbutic factor.   *Biochemical Journal*

Albert Szent-Györgyi; 1928   **3443**

The hexuronic acid from oranges and cabbages...forms an essential part of the reducing factor, the chemistry of which is discussed.   *Biochemical Journal*

VITAMIN D

Elmer V. McCollum, Nina Simmonds, J. Ernestine Becker, P.G. Shipley; 1922   **3444**

Cod liver oil oxidized for 12 to 20 hours does not cure xerophthalmia in rats. It does, however, cause the deposition of calcium in the bones of young rats which are suffering from rickets.... The evidence...demonstrates that the power of certain fats to initiate the healing of rickets depends on the presence in them of a substance which is distinct from fat-soluble [vitamin] A.   *Journal of Biological Chemistry*

VITAMIN E

Herbert McLean Evans, Katherine Scott Bishop; 1922   **3445**

Rats may be reared on a dietary regime consisting of "purified" protein, fat, and carbohydrate to which an appropriate salt mixture and adequate doses of the growth vitamins Fat Soluble A and Water Soluble B have been added.... Such animals are sterile.... We have...been able to witness a comparatively sudden restoration of fertility...by the administration of fresh green leaves of lettuce.   *Science*

VITAMIN K

Hugh Butt, Albert Snell; 1938   **3446**

The administration of vitamin K together with bile or bile salts [to those] who have jaundice has reduced elevated prothrombin times to within normal limits and in certain cases probably has prevented hemorrhage.... The prevention and control of the hemorrhagic diathesis of the jaundiced patient may be attained in the not too distant future.   *Proceedings of the Staff Meetings of the Mayo Clinic*

VITAMINS

Casimir Funk; 1912   **3447**

It is now known that all these diseases, with the exception of pellagra, can be prevented
and cured by the addition of preventive substances; the deficient substances, which are
of the nature of organic bases, we will call "vitamines." *Journal of State Medicine*

Jack Cecil Drummond; 1920   **3448**

The suggestion is now advanced that the final "-e" [of Funk's "vitamine"] be dropped, so
that the resulting word Vitamin is acceptable under the standard scheme of nomenclature adopted by the Chemical Society.... It is recommended that the somewhat cumbrous
nomenclature introduced by McCollum (Fat-soluble A, Water-soluble B), be dropped,
and that the substances be spoken of as Vitamin A, B, C, etc. *Biochemical Journal*

Richard Gordon; 1993   **3449**

Vitamins are chemicals in food clinically conspicuous by their absence.

The Alarming History of Medicine

VIVISECTION

Samuel Johnson; 1758   **3450**

Among the inferiour professors of medical knowledge, is a race of wretches whose lives are
only varied by varieties of cruelty, whose favourite amusement is to nail dogs to tables and
open them alive. *The Idler*

Samuel David Gross; 1887   **3451**

I am naturally fond of dogs, and my sympathies were often wrought to the highest pitch,
especially when I happened to get hold of an unusually clever specimen. Anesthetics had
not yet been discovered, and I was therefore obliged to inflict severe pain.

Autobiography

Walter Bradford Cannon; 1908   **3452**

And just as the future growth in the physical world must wait further discoveries and new
applications of knowledge, so in the realm of biology and medicine, the hope of progress
must rest on a continuation of the method which has brought us thus far out of the darkness of the unknown—it must rest on the study of normal and pathologic processes that
go on in living animals. *Journal of the American Medical Association*

VOLKMANN ISCHEMIC CONTRACTURES

Richard von Volkmann; 1881   **3453**

For years I have called attention to the fact that the pareses and contractures of limbs following application of tight bandages are caused not by pressure paralysis of nerves, as formerly assumed, but by the rapid and massive deterioration of contractile substance and
by...reactive and regenerative processes. *Zentralblatt für Chirurgerie*

VULNERABILITY

Austin Flint; 1881   **3454**

The term *vulnerability* has been, of late, applied to a condition of the system favorable for
the morbific operation of any causes, either ordinary or specific. The sense of this term
differs from that of *predisposition*, the latter denoting a tendency to a particular form of
disease, whereas *vulnerability* denotes a susceptibility to all morbific agents. Vulnerability,
thus, in contradistinction to predisposition, does not determine the nature of the diseases
produced by different causes. The term *vulnerability*, in fact, means neither more nor less
than a general susceptibility to the causes of disease.

A Treatise on the Principles and Practice of Medicine

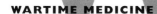

WARTIME MEDICINE

B. Markowski; 1945   **3455**

To take blood from other prisoners, overworked and exhausted, was not practicable. Many times my colleagues and I had to give our own blood immediately after an operation to save a man's life. We did not get any stored blood whatsoever from the Germans.

British Medical Journal

Albert E. Coates; 1946   **3456**

The local manufacture of catgut from ox peritoneum, the distillation of alcohol, our main antiseptic, from rice, and the spinal use of cocaine as an anaesthetic helped to make surgery less barbaric than it might have been.   *Medical Journal of Australia*

E.E. Dunlop; 1946   **3457**

Some of the special problems in the treatment of dysentery have been.... The ever-embarrassing shortage, and in many cases the complete absence, of specific amoebicidal drugs. For example, in working camps providing the most wretched conditions of life, at times not even magnesium sulphate could be obtained, and recourse was had to such pathetic devices as the administration of charcoal manufactured locally. Emetine, when available, was often obtained only sporadically, in clandestine ways, and had to be used with the utmost economy, with a view not to cure but to prolong life.   *British Medical Journal*

Jacob Markowitz; 1946   **3458**

Those who developed debilitating diseases died in droves. We, therefore, worked on the principle that blood is all things to all tissues, being meat to the hungry, blood to the malarious, and life-giving fluid to the collapsed and to those losing protein by the discharge of albuminous exudates.   *Journal of the Royal Army Medical Corps*

Jacob Markowitz; 1946   **3459**

By the application of simple Listerian principles we found that the mortality from [amputation of the thigh] per se was negligible. Although conditions in the wards approximated to those described by Florence Nightingale in the Crimean War, it was possible to perform even a bilateral amputation of the thigh safely with smooth recovery.

Journal of the Royal Army Medical Corps

WARTS

May Kennedy McCord; 1964   **3460**

Another "sleight" for getting rid of a wart is merely to prick it with a thorn until it bleeds, then throw the thorn over the left shoulder and walk away without looking back.

Randolf V, Ozark Superstitions

WELCH BACILLUS

William Henry Welch, George Henry Falkiner Nuttall; 1892   **3461**

In endeavoring to select a name suitable for the bacillus described in this article we have thought of several designations.... Upon the whole we prefer the first name, bacillus aerogenes capsulatus. The presence of a capsule does not appear to be constant, but it is common and forms a characteristic feature of the morphology of the bacillus.

Johns Hopkins Hospital Bulletin

WISDOM

William Osler; *circa* 1900   **3462**

Common-sense nerve fibers are seldom medullated before forty—they are never seen even with a microscope before twenty.

Aphorisms

Robertson Davies; 1984   **3463**

Knowledge may enable you to memorize the whole of Gray's *Anatomy* and Osler's *Principles and Practice of Medicine*, but only wisdom can teach you what to do with what you have learned.

The Merry Heart. Can a Doctor Be a Humanist?

Robertson Davies; 1994   **3464**

Knowledge and Wisdom and they are not the same, because Knowledge is what you are taught, but Wisdom is what you bring to it.

The Cunning Man

WOMEN

Cotton Mather; 1724   **3465**

The sex that is called, *The Weaker Vessel*, has not only a share with us, in the most of our Distempers, but is liable to many that may be called, Its *Peculiar Weaknesses*.... I have readd...that Physicians have *Two Women-Patients to One Man*.... But inasmuch as both Sexes Dy in a more Equal Proportion, This is very much for the Honour of the Physicians, who cure them.

The Angel of Bethesda

Mary Putnam Jacobi; 1883   **3466**

To the extent to which women continue to isolate themselves, or to submit to enforced isolation from [the] vast current of intellectual life, it is inevitable that their own must become apathetic.

Commencement address

Alfred Jarry; 1899   **3467**

O the despair of Pygmalion, who might have created a statue and only made a woman!

L'Amour Absolu

Denslow Lewis; 1903   **3468**

Times have changed during the past ten years and our young American women are becoming truly independent in thought and action. They are advancing because they are acquiring knowledge.

Medico-Legal Journal

Margaret Sanger; 1920   **3469**

American womanhood is blasting its way through the debris of crumbling moral and religious systems toward freedom.

Woman and the New Race

Simone de Beauvoir; 1952 **3470**

People have tirelessly sought to prove that woman is superior, inferior, or equal to man. Some say that, having been created after Adam, she is evidently a secondary being; others say on the contrary that Adam was only a rough draft and that God succeeded in producing the human being in perfection when he created Eve.... If we are to gain understanding, we must get out of these ruts; we must discard the vague notions of superiority, inferiority, equality which have hitherto corrupted every discussion of the subject and start afresh. *The Second Sex*

Sophie Tucker; [1884-1966] **3471**

From birth to 18 a girl needs good parents. From 18 to 35, she needs good looks. From 35 to 55, good personality. From 55 on, she needs good cash. I'm saving my money
. *Freedland M, Sophie*

WOMEN IN MEDICINE

Medical school student body vote; 1847 **3472**

Resolved, That one of the radical principles of a Republican Government is the universal education of both sexes; that to every branch of scientific education the door should be open equally to all; that the application of Elizabeth Blackwell to become a member of our class meets our unanimous approbation. *Talbott JH, A Biographical History of Medicine*

William H. Byford; 1884 **3473**

The question is not whether women, as a class, are as strong as men, but whether they possess the strength necessary to become efficient practitioners. In view of the facts of the past and the present, I can have no doubt they are. *Chicago Medical Examiner*

Elizabeth Blackwell; 1889 **3474**

What are the spiritual principles...which constitute the distinctive...domain of women? They are the subordination of self to the welfare of others; the recognition of the claim which helplessness and ignorance make upon the stronger and more intelligent; the joy of creation and bestowal of life; the pity and sympathy which tend to make every woman the born foe of cruelty and injustice; and hope...the realization of the unseen—which foresees the adult in the infant, the future in the present.
The Influence of Women in the Profession of Medicine

Elizabeth Blackwell; 1889 **3475**

We must understand what the special contribution is, that women may make to medicine, what the aspect of morality which they are called upon to emphasize. It is not blind imitation of men, nor thoughtless acceptance of whatever may be taught by them that is required, for this would be to endorse the widespread error that the race is men. Our duty is loyalty to right and opposition to wrong, in accordance with the essential principles of our own nature. *The Influence of Women in the Profession of Medicine*

Lois Wright (Lucy Waite); 1891 **3476**

To see two real live women physicians, not mid-wives nor nurses, but bona fide doctors, was to be an era in his existence. He had heard that there were such abnormal specimens of womanhood abroad in the land, but had never had any curiosity to see them, avoiding them as he would any monstrosities shocking to the sensibilities. *Doctor Helen Rand*

Mary Putnam Jacobi; 1891 **3477**

Have you ever had an opportunity of watching a woman originally "charming" deteriorate under the influence of medicine? If not, how do you know that those whom you have met, medical and charmless, were not always so, even before they had taken the fatal plunge? And have you compared the influence of millinery, dress making, traveling, journalism, authorship, business, etc., etc. with that of medicine in this respect?
Letter to Silas Weir Mitchell

William Osler; 1894   3478

I come here today, with...sorrow at my heart, to tell you that coeducation has proved an absolute failure, from our standpoint. When I tell you that 33.3 per cent of the ladies, students, admitted to Johns Hopkins Hospital at the end of our short session are to be married, then I tell you that coeducation is a failure. If 33.3 per cent fall victims at the end of one session, what will happen at the end of the fourth?   *Boston Medical and Surgical Journal*

Abraham Flexner; 1910   3479

Now that women are freely admitted to the medical profession, it is clear that they show a decreasing inclination to enter it. More schools in all sections are open to them; fewer attend and fewer graduate. True enough, medical schools generally have shrunk; but as the opportunities of women have increased, not decreased, and within the period during which entrance requirements, so far as they are concerned, not materially altered, their enrolment should have augmented, if there is any strong demand for women physicians or any strong ungratified desire on the part of women to enter the profession. One or the other of these conditions is lacking—perhaps both.

Medical Education in the United States and Canada

Perrin H. Long; 1964   3480

We have never understood just why there are not more women in surgery. We once heard Dr. Edward D. Churchill jokingly say, speaking of the difference between a surgeon and an internist, that the surgeon was the captain of the team, while an internist never had a team. Does this mean that women don't make good captains?   *Resident Physician*

Carol L. Joseph; 1994   3481

This was not the first time a female physician had told me she had sent her child away to a distant relative in order to complete some portion of training. The first time I had heard of this, I thought it was just an aberration. How could she do it, I wondered. She must not feel the way I do. Perhaps she lacks some maternal instinct. Maybe she just didn't bond. But confronted with this second instance, I raged inwardly against a system that pretends to teach humanism while destroying humanity. "Can our medical schools make no concession to the next generation?" I asked.   *Annals of Internal Medicine*

WORK

William Osler; 1899   3482

As to your method of work, I have a single bit of advice, which I give with the earnest conviction of its paramount influence in any success which may have attended my efforts in life—*Take no thought for the morrow*. Live neither in the past nor in the future, but let each day's work absorb your entire energies, and satisfy your widest ambition.

After Twenty-five Years

William Osler; 1903   3483

The master-word looms large in meaning. It is the open sesame to every portal, the great equalizer in the world, the true philosopher's stone, which transmutes all the base metal of humanity into gold.... It is directly responsible for all advances in medicine during the past twenty-five centuries.... Not only has it been the touchstone of progress, but it is the measure of success in every-day life.... And the master-word is Work.

The Master-word in Medicine

William Osler; 1905   3484

Men will not take time to get to the heart of a matter. After all, concentration is the price the modern student pays for success. Thoroughness is the most difficult habit to acquire, but it is the pearl of great price, worth all the worry and trouble of the search. The dilettante lives an easy, butterfly life, knowing nothing of the toil and labor with which the treasures of knowledge are dug out of the past, or wrung by patient research in the laboratories.

The Student Life

Bertrand Russell; 1930 **3485**

One of the symptoms of approaching nervous breakdown is the belief that one's work is terribly important, and that to take a holiday would bring all kinds of disaster. If I were a medical man, I should prescribe a holiday to any patient who considered his work important. *The Conquest of Happiness*

Richard A. Kern; 1951 **3486**

Work is a prime means to preserve vigor. The wheel that doesn't turn, rusts.... Faculties and skills, as well as muscles that are not used, weaken and atrophy. *The Care of the Aged*

WOUNDS

[Anonymous]; *circa* 2500 BC **3487**

One having a wound in his eyebrow. An ailment which I will treat. Treatment [of a wound in the eyebrow]: Now after thou hast stitched it[thou shouldst bind] fresh meat upon [it] the first day. If thou findest that the stitching of this wound is loose, thou shouldst draw it together for him with two strips (of plaster), and thou shouldst treat it with grease and honey every day until he recovers. *The Edwin Smith Surgical Papyrus*

WRITING

John Maynow; 1668 **3488**

Disease, as it stalks the land, cannot keep pace with the incurable vice of scribbling about it. *De Rachitide*

[Anonymous]; 1865 **3489**

We have frequent occasion to observe [the] tendency to neologism, and the avidity with which second and third rate writers especially cover a certain crudity of reasoning and obscurity of thought, or endeavour to give weight to a shallow theory, by the selection of the very longest and most technical words which the medical vocabulary will supply. This is an error to be deplored and reprobated. *The Lancet*

Ferdinand von Hebra; [1816-1880] **3490**

I confess freely my ignorance upon [causes of acne rosacea] rather than, with other writers, to repeat over and over again names and phrases which are either meaningless or unsupported by proof.

Stillians AW, Quarterly Bulletin of the Northwestern University Medical School

John Shaw Billings; 1881 **3491**

First have something to say, say it as briefly as possible, and stop when you have said it. *British Medical Journal*

Samuel David Gross; 1887 **3492**

It was written when I was a young man, without any one to advise or guide me, in my leisure hours, often snatched from sleep, and under the exhaustion of fatigue, when one is ill-qualified for healthful mental exertion. *Autobiography*

Samuel David Gross; 1887 **3493**

What compensation does the reader think I obtained for this hard work, this excessive toil of my brain, including original composition, the correction and improvement of new editions, and the proof-reading, in itself a horrible task, death to brain and eyes.... Eighty-five cents a copy, all told, and no extra dividends! *Autobiography*

Samuel David Gross; 1887 **3494**

I generally spent from five to eight hours a day upon my manuscript, subject of course to frequent and sometimes annoying interruptions by patients. *Autobiography*

Denslow Lewis; 1896   **3495**

The hot weather has been too much for me and I have not been able to get my brain in
working order so that I could complete the article in time for your next issue.

Letter to George Henry Cleveland

Rudolf Ludwig Karl Virchow; [1821-1902]   **3496**

Brevity in writing is the best insurance for its perusal.

Garrison FH, Bulletin of the New York Academy of Medicine

Thomas Clifford Allbutt; 1904   **3497**

All writers, however, even the least skillful, are, in the degree of their skill, at some care
how to begin. An unpractised writer, for sheer helplessness at the outset, may never begin;
he may abandon his work in despair.... Of ends I will only say, "Do not end anyhow;" let
your leave-taking be easy, gracious, and impressive in proportion to the theme; not ponderous, pompous, epigrammatic, or austere.   *Notes on the Composition of Scientific Papers*

Thomas Mann; 1939   **3498**

Medicine and writing go well together, they shed light on each other and both do better
by going hand in hand. A doctor possessed of the writer's art will be the better consoler
to anyone rolling in agony; conversely, a writer who understands the life of the body, its
powers and its pains, its fluids and functions, its blessings and banes, has a great advantage over him who knows nothing of such things.   *Joseph the Provider*

Alan Gregg; 1941   **3499**

Good writing in our professional journals is pitifully rare. Discriminating use of adverbs
and adjectives is no mere literary embellishment. It is essential to the accurate and unambiguous wording of precise or complicated relationships.

Bulletin of the New York Academy of Science

[Anonymous]; 1954   **3500**

A medical paper should be like a lady's dress—short enough to be interesting but long
enough to cover the subject.   *DeBakey S, Journal of the American Medical Association*

Heinz Edgar Lehmann, Gordon E. Hanrahan; 1954   **3501**

Between May and July 1953[Lehmann] gave the patients the [chlorpromazine] and
recorded the results, writing up his findings as a "unique" new therapeutic agent. The
director of the asylum told him, "You never use the word 'unique' in anything that you
publish, because you always regret it later on—there is no such thing as unique."

AMA Archives of Neurology and Psychiatry

Richard M. Hewitt; 1957   **3502**

Authorship cannot be conferred; it may be undertaken by one who will shoulder the
responsibility that goes with it.... Thou shalt not allow thy name to appear as a co-author
unless thou hast some authoritative knowledge of the subject concerned, hast participat-
ed in the underlying investigation, and hast labored on the report to the extent of weighing every word and quantity therein.   *The Physician-Writer's Book*

George White Pickering; 1961   **3503**

If we are to advance knowledge and not destroy it—for knowledge is a unity, and the sum
total of its parts—we must set our faces against loose or obscure or unnecessary jargon.
We must pay attention to the meaning of words we use, ensuring that we use only words
whose meaning we understand, and, so far as possible, words whose meaning others
understand.   *The Lancet*

Joseph Garland; 1964   **3504**

The principle of good writing consists of trying to make oneself understood by the greatest possible number of readers.... I suspect that the physical act of writing has become easy, and...easy writing makes hard reading.... Let me state my own addiction to a soft lead pencil that needs to be sharpened at short intervals and bears an eraser at its proximal end.   *New England Journal of Medicine*

Austin Bradford Hill; 1965   **3505**

Why did you start, what did you do, what answer did you get, and what does it mean anyway? This [seems to me to be] a logical order for a scientific paper.   *British Medical Journal*

Charles Percy Snow; 1966   **3506**

I do not think doctors suffer from the other great weaknesses of engineers, that is, their complete lack of verbalism. Engineers can often be extremely clever but they cannot spell and they cannot speak. The doctors I have known are extremely articulate. I suspect the descriptive processes they have to go through, both themselves and presumably with their patients, are extremely good verbal training, and I do not think it is an accident that the one thing the medical profession has done, apart from producing doctors, is to produce writers.   *Lecture*

Walker Percy; 1971   **3507**

The prayer of the scientist if he prayed, which is not likely: Lord, grant that my discovery may increase knowledge and help other men. Failing that, Lord, grant that it will not lead to man's destruction. Failing that, Lord, grant that my article in *Brain* be published before the destruction takes place.   *Love in the Ruins*

Archibald Leman Cochrane; 1972   **3508**

In publishing...papers I have inevitably adopted that standard MRC [Medical Research Council] style of writing which passes for scientific English. There is a lot to be said for it. It is accurate, meticulous, and almost bias-proof. Personal prejudice is concealed. The only drawback...is that I find it almost unreadable.   *Effectiveness and Efficiency*

Earle P. Scarlett; 1972   **3509**

While it is perhaps inevitable that a certain verbal greyness should characterize our scientific and medical language, it is still essential that precision and discipline should prevail.   *Roland CG, In Sickness and in Health*

Franz J. Ingelfinger; 1976   **3510**

Many medical writers appear seriously addicted to "significant" in its nonstatistical sense. The word is convenient, for it implies so much and means so little. One may even find five wearisome "significants" on one typed double-spaced page!

New England Journal of Medicine

Earle P. Scarlett; 1978   **3511**

The pencil is greater than the stethoscope.   *Interview*

J.R.A. Mitchell; 1982   **3512**

These examples illustrate the time problems which must beset the editors of huge multiauthor texts and they make me question their very existence. Dinosaurs died out because they were too big, could not adapt to change, and because their brains were too far from their genitalia.   *The Lancet*

Curtis L. Meinert; 1996   **3513**

A scientific paper should be short on claims and long on data and facts.

Clinical Trials Dictionary

X

XANTHOMA DIABETICORUM

Thomas Addison; 1848   **3514**

On the 18th August, 1848, a patient was admitted into the hospital...for diabetes.... On the 25th January of the following year,...an eruption somewhat suddenly appeared on the arms.... It consisted of scattered tubercles of various sizes, some being as large as a small pea.... When incised with a lancet they were found to consist of firm tissue.... They were of a yellowish colour, mottled with a deepish rose-tint.... [At the beginning of March] many of the tubercles began to subside.   *A Collection of the Published Writings*

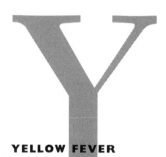

YELLOW FEVER

Mathew Carey; 1793   **3515**

The malignant fever, which has committed such ravages in Philadelphia, made its appearance here, about the end of July.... On the origin of the disorder, there prevails a very great diversity of opinion.... "The general opinion was, that the disorder originated from some damaged coffee, or other putrefied and animal matters".... Thousands were swept off in three or four weeks.
A Short Account of the Malignant Fever

Benjamin Rush; 1794   **3516**

I did not hesitate to name [the fever] the *bilious remitting yellow fever*. I had seen it epidemic in Philadelphia, in the year 1762.... "The patients were generally seized with rigours, which were succeeded with violent fever, and pains in the head and back. The pulse was full, and sometimes irregular. The eyes were inflamed, and had a yellowish cast, and a vomiting almost always attended.... An excessive heat and burning about the region of the liver, with cold extremities, portended death to be at hand."
An Account of the Bilious Remitting Yellow Fever

Pierre-Charles-Alexandre Louis; 1839   **3517**

But the most remarkable lesion of the liver was the alteration of its color.... This alteration consisted in a discoloration, the liver being sometimes the color of fresh butter, sometimes of a straw color, sometimes of the color of coffee and milk.
Anatomical, Pathological, and Therapeutic Researches on the Yellow Fever

Carlos Juan Finlay; 1881   **3518**

Should it be finally proven that the mosquito-inoculation not only reproduces the yellow fever, but that it constitutes the regular process through which the disease is propagated, the conditions of existence and of development for the dipterous insect would account for the anomalies hitherto observed in the propagation of yellow fever, and while we might, on one hand, have the means preventing the disease from spreading, non-immunes might at the same time be protected by a mild inoculation.
Anales de Academia de Ceincias Medicas de Habana

Carlos Juan Finlay; 1881   **3519**

From the evidence adduced in the preceding pages, I conclude that while yellow fever is incapable of propagation by its own unaided efforts, it may be artificially communicated by inoculation, and only becomes epidemic when such inoculations can be verified by some external natural agent, such as the mosquito.... This disease appears incapable of propagation wherever tropical mosquitoes do not or are not likely to exist.

Anales de Academia de Ceincias Medicas de Habana

Walter Reed; 1901   **3520**

1. The mosquito—*C. fasciatus*—serves as intermediate host for the parasite of yellow fever.

2. Yellow Fever is transmitted to the non-immune individual by means of the bite of the mosquito that has previously fed on the blood of those sick with this disease....

10. The spread of yellow fever can be most effectually controlled by measures directed to the destruction of mosquitoes and the protection of the sick against the bites of these insects.   *Journal of the American Medical Association*

Walter Reed; 1901   **3521**

Thus within the period of one week—December 9 to December 15—we had succeeded in producing an attack of yellow fever in each of the four individuals whom we had caused contaminated insect to bite, and in all save one of the five non-immunes whom we had originally selected for experimentation.   *Medical Record*

ZOLLINGER-ELLISON SYNDROME

Robert M. Zollinger, Edwin H. Ellison; 1955   **3522**

Fortunate indeed is the surgical service that does not have one or more problem cases of recurrent marginal ulceration despite the adequacy of the surgical attack.... We have observed two such problem cases of benign ulceration of the upper jejunum associated with extremely high gastric acid production over a 12-hour period.... Of particular interest is the fact that a non-Beta cell adenoma, with no clinical or laboratory evidence of insulin production, was found at the time of autopsy in one patient, and at the time of total gastrectomy in the surviving patient.   *Annals of Surgery*

Author–Citation Index

Order

Citations are arranged alphabetically by the last name of the quotation's author. When more than one citation is given for a particular author, they are listed alphabetically by the title of the work (see section on Author Quoted from More Than One Source below).

Content

Aside from full bibliographic information for each source, each citation includes the topic name (in SMALL CAPS) under which the corresponding quotation appears and its quotation number (in **bold face**).

> **Balint, Michael.** *The Doctor, His Patient, and the Illness.* New York: International Universities Press; 1957, p. 292. PATIENT-PHYSICIAN RELATIONS **2417**

Here a quotation from Michael Balint's book, *The Doctor, His Patient, and the Illness*, appears under the heading PATIENT-PHYSICIAN RELATIONS and is quotation number **2417**. Note that because there is only one quotation listed, the page number of the original work is given, appropriately, after the date. However, if a particular source is quoted more than once, the appropriate page numbers of the original source are given in square brackets after the bold quotation number.

> **Cassell, Eric J.** *The Healer's Art: A New Approach to the Doctor-Patient Relationship.* New York: J.B. Lippincott; 1976. DECISION MAKING **692** [16], ILLNESS **1406** [48], MEDICAL EDUCATION **1793** [44], SCIENCE **2989** [6]

Here four quotations are cited from Eric J. Cassell's *The Healer's Art*. The topics and quotation numbers are given as in the first example; the individual pages on which each quotation appears in Cassell's book are listed in brackets.

Brackets are also used to specify other pertinent information, primarily to indicate a secondary source if the original was missing data (e.g., page numbers) or was difficult to obtain because of scarcity or age. In these instances, bracketed page numbers correspond to the secondary source. If we did not have a secondary source, [Limited data] is used.

> **Adams, Samuel Hopkins.** *The Great American Fraud*, 1906 [In: Accardo P. *The Medical Almanac*. Totowa, NJ: Humana Press; 1992, p. 198]. MEDICAL PROFESSION **1995**

> **Albucasis.** *Cyrurgia Albucasis cum Cauteriis & Aliis Instrumentis.* Venice: 1500 [In: Shimkin MB, *Contrary to Nature: Cancer*, p. 39 (q.v.)]. CANCER **374**

> **Brownlee, John.** *Germinal Vitality: A Study of the Growth of Nations as an Instance of a Hitherto Undescribed Factor in Evolution.* Glasgow: Carter & Pratt; 1908 [Limited data]. EPIDEMICS **967**

NOTE: *q.v.* used after a frequently cited secondary source indicates that its full citation exists elsewhere in the index. Occasionally, the date of the edition cited is much later than the date of the quotation. The text gives the original date of the quotation.

Although these examples illustrate the main characteristics of the citations listed on the following pages, they merely depict the basic format for an author quoted from his or her own book. Below you will find examples of the other specific citation formats.

Author Quoted in Another Author's Book

The author or editor of the work from which the quotation is taken is given after the quoted author.

> **Alvarez, Walter C.** In Scott DH (ed). *American Man of Medicine.* New York: Van Nostrand Reinhold; 1976, p. 8. MEDICAL HISTORIES **1886**

Author Quoted from His or Her Own Medical Journal Article

We adopted the style employed by the *Annals of Internal Medicine* to cite medical journals. When there was only one author, we opted to give the full name when known.

> **Hollister JH, Cook EP, Hamilton JL.** Report on drugs and medicines. *Trans Ill State Med Soc.* 1873;23:118-29. CONTINUING EDUCATION **591**

> **Houston, Charles S.** Acute pulmonary edema of high altitude. *N Engl J Med.* 1960;263:478-9. HIGH-ALTITUDE MEDICINE **1285**

Author Quoted in Another Author's Medical Journal Article

Fisher, Martin H. In Fred HL. *South Med J*. 1986;79:351. NOMENCLATURE 2259

Author Quoted from His or Her Own Newspaper or Magazine Article

Porter, Roy. Offering resistance: the checkered history and contemporary travails of cancer immunotherapy [Review of Hall SS. *A Commotion in the Blood*]. *The New York Times*. 29 June 1997, p. 9. MEDICINE 2138

Author Quoted in Another Author's Newspaper or Magazine Article

Banting, Frederick Grant. In Hemingway E. "An absolute lie," says Dr. Banting of serum report. *The Toronto Star*. 11 Oct 1923 [Limited data]. INSULIN 1459

Author Quoted from More than One Source

The author's name is set above the citations and his or her works listed in alphabetical order. The works of other authors or editors who quote that author follow; these secondary sources begin with the word "In."

Latham, Peter Mere.
   A Word or Two on Medical Education, 1864 [In: Martin R (ed). *The Collected Works of Dr. P.M. Latham*, vol II. London: The New Sydenham Society; 1878, p. 560]. MEDICAL EDUCATION 1746
   General Remarks on the Practice of Medicine, 1836. [In: Martin R (ed). *The Collected Works of Dr. P.M. Latham*, vol. II. London: The New Sydenham Society; 1878, p. 466]. DRUGS 884 [376], EXPERIENCE 1027 [466]
   In Bean WB (ed). *Aphorisms from Latham*. Iowa City: Prairie Press; 1962. CLINICAL OBSERVATION 509 [90], DIAGNOSIS 759 [101], MEDICAL PRACTICE 1922 [26], 1924 [22]; MEDICAL PROFESSION 1982 [19], PATIENT-PHYSICIAN RELATIONS 2386 [101], PATIENTS 2456 [101], PSYCHOSOMATIC MEDICINE 2744 [56]
   In Martin R (ed). *The Collected Works of Dr. P.M. Latham*. London: The New Sydenham Society; 1878. DIAGNOSIS 740 [vol. I; lecture XIV: p. 173], MEDICAL PRACTICE 1923 [II;II:23], MURMURS 2207 [I;II:17], 2208 [I;II:3]

Abel JJ, Crawford AC. On the blood-pressure raising constituent of the suprarenal capsule. *Bull Johns Hopkins Hosp.* 1897;8:151-7. EPINEPHRINE (ADRENALINE) **982**

Abel JJ, Rowntree LG, Turner BB. On the removal of diffusible substances from the circulating blood of living animals by dialysis. *J Pharmacol Exp Ther.* 1914;5:275-316. HEMODIALYSIS **1264**

Abel, John Jacob.
> The methods of pharmacology, with experimental illustration. *Pharm Era.* 1892;7:105. PHARMACOLOGY **2514**
>
> Ueber den blutdruckerregenden bestandtheil der nebenniere, das epinephrin. *Hoppe-Seyl Z Physiol Chem.* 1899;28:318-62. EPINEPHRINE (ADRENALINE) **983**

Abildgaard, Peter Christian. Tentamina electrica in animalibus instituta. *Societatis Medicae Havniensis.* 1775;2:157-61. VENTRICULAR DEFIBRILLATION **3426**

Abraham EP, Chain EB, Fletcher CM, and others. Further observations on penicillin. *Lancet.* 1941;2:177-88. PENICILLIN **2482**

Acosta, José de. *Historia Natural y Moral de las Indias.* Seville: 1590. [In: Major RH., *Classic Descriptions of Disease*, p. 603 (q.v.).] HIGH-ALTITUDE MEDICINE **1284**

Adams, John. *The Anatomy and Diseases of the Prostate Gland.* London: 1851. CANCER OF THE PROSTATE GLAND **408**

Adams, Robert. Cases of diseases of the heart, accompanied by pathological observations. *Dublin Hosp Rep.* 1827;4:353-453. BRADYCARDIA **335**, CORONARY ARTERY DISEASE **616**, HEART BLOCK **1237**

Adams, Samuel Hopkins. *The Great American Fraud*, 1906. [In: Accardo P. *The Medical Almanac*. Totowa, New Jersey: Humana Press; 1992, p. 198.] MEDICAL PROFESSION **1995**

Addis, Thomas. *Glomerular Nephritis: Diagnosis and Treatment.* New York: Macmillan; 1948. CLASSIFICATION **500** [125], PHYSICIANS **2581** [120], DIAGNOSIS **748** [126], DISEASE **789** [4], URINALYSIS **3413** [2]

Addison, Thomas.
> *Elements of the Practice of Medicine*, 1839. APPENDICITIS **223**
>
> *On the Constitutional and Local Effects of Disease of the Supra-renal Capsules.* London: 1855. ADRENAL GLANDS **42**, ADRENOCORTICAL INSUFFICIENCY (ADDISON DISEASE) **45**, ADRENOCORTICAL INSUFFICIENCY (ADDISON DISEASE) **46**, PATHOPHYSIOLOGY **2358**
>
> In Wilks, Daldy (eds). *A Collection of the Published Writings of the Late Thomas Addison, MD, Physician to Guy's Hospital.* London: The New Sydenham Society; 1868:160. XANTHOMA DIABETICORUM **3514**

Adrian, Edgar Douglas. *The Mechanism of Nervous Action: Electrical Studies of the Neurone.* Philadelphia: University of Pennsylvania Press; 1935:12. NERVOUS SYSTEM **2243**

Aesop.
> *The Old Man and Death.* Fables. DYING **901**
>
> *The Quack Frog.* Fables. QUACKERY **2799**

Aetius of Amida. *Liborum Medicinalium Tomus Primusi.* Venice: 1534. CANCER OF THE BREAST **391**, CANCER OF THE UTERUS **416**

Ahlquist RP. A study of the adrenotropic receptors. *Am J Physiol.* 1948;153:586-600. ADRENERGIC RECEPTORS **44**

Albright F, Bauer W, Ropes M, Aub JC. Studies of calcium and phosphorus metabolism. Part IV: The effect of the parathyroid hormone. *J Clin Invest.* 1929;7:139-81. [In: *Ann Intern Med.* 1970;72:326.] PARATHYROID GLANDS **2338**

Albright F, Bloomberg E, Smith PH. Postmenopausal osteoporosis. *Trans Assoc Am Phys.* 1940;55:298-305. OSTEOPOROSIS **2303**

Albright F, Burnett CH, Smith PH, Parson W. Pseudo-hypoparathyroidism: an example of "Seabright-Bantam Syndrome": report of three cases. *Endocrinology.* 1942;30;922-32. PSEUDOHYPOPARATHYROIDISM **2707**

Albright, Fuller.
> Diseases of the ductless glands. In Cecil RL, Loeb RF (eds). *A Textbook of Medicine*, 8th ed. Philadelphia: WB Saunders; 1951. DOCTORS **850** [1217], HYPOGONADISM **1380** [1216], TREATMENT **3353** [1217]
>
> Hair. *Ann Intern Med.* 1970;72:4;546. HIRSUTISM **1291**
>
> Osteoporosis. *Ann Intern Med.* 1947;27(6):861-82. OSTEOPOROSIS **2304**
>
> Polyostotic fibrous dysplasia: a defence of the entity. *J Clin Endocrinol.* 1946;7:307-24. EPONYMS **986**
>
> What endocrinology is and is not. *Ann Intern Med.* 1970;72:4;504. HOMOSEXUALITY **1312**

Albucasis. *Cyrurgia Albucasis cum Cauteriis & Aliis Instrumentis.* Venice: 1500. [In: Shimkin MB, *Contrary to Nature: Cancer*, p. 39 (q.v.).] CANCER **374**

Alcott, John V. *World Medical News.* Aug 1986 [Limited data]. DERMATOLOGY **722**

Aldrich, Thomas Bell. A preliminary report on the active principle of the suprarenal gland. *Am J Physiol.* 1901;5:457-61. EPINEPHRINE (ADRENALINE) **984**

Allbutt, Thomas Clifford.

Lancet, 1922. SURGERY **3234**

Notes on the Composition of Scientific Papers. London: 1904. WRITING **3497**

On Professional Education, with Special Reference to Medicine. London: Macmillan; 1906:50. MEDICAL EDUCATION **1761**

Visceral Neuroses, Being the Gulstonian Lectures on Neuralgia of the Stomach and Allied Disorders. London: 1884. [In: Keynes M, Butterfield J. Sir Clifford Allbutt: physician and refius professor, 1892-1925. *J Med Biography* 1993;1:67-75.] HYPOCHONDRIA **1371**

In Asher R. *A Sense of Asher: A New Miscellany.* The Keynes Press, British Medical Association, 1983 [Limited data from contriubtor]. MEDICAL RESEARCH **2028**

In Coope R (ed). *The Quiet Art,* p. 124 (q.v.). PATIENT-PHYSICIAN RELATIONS **2407**

Medical thermometry. *Br Foreign Med-Chir Rev.* 1870;45:429-41. MEDICAL EDUCATION **1748**, THERMOMETRY **3291**

Senile plethora or high arterial pressure in elderly persons: Hunterian Society Lecture, February 27th, 1895. *Trans Hunterian Soc.* 1896:38-57. HYPERTENSION **1348**

Sir William Osler. *Br Med J.* 1920;1:64. AGING **79**

Allen, Edgar. The menstrual cycle of the monkey, *Macacus rhesus:* observations on normal animals, the effects of removal of the ovaries and the effects of injection of ovarian and placental extracts into the spayed animals. *Contrib Embryol Carneg Inst.* 1927;98:1-44. MENSTRUATION **2153**

Allison, F. Gerard. Obscure pains in chest, back or limbs. *Can Med Assoc J.* 1943;48:36-8. RESTLESS LEG SYNDROME **2899**

Almenor J. *De Morbo Gallico.* Venice: 1502. [In: Major RH. *Classic Descriptions of Disease,* pp. 22-4.] SYPHILIS **3254**

Alsop, Stewart. *Stay of Execution: A Sort of Memoir.* Philadelphia: J.B. Lippincott; 1973. DEATH **677** [32], DYING **923** [299]

Altschule, Mark D. The making of a physician according to John Stuart Mill. *Med Counterpoint.* 1970;2:5. MEDICAL EDUCATION **1786**

Alvarez, Walter C. In Scott DH (ed). *American Man of Medicine.* New York: Van Nostrand Reinhold; 1976, p. 8. MEDICAL HISTORIES **1886**

Alving AS, Miller BF. A practical method for the measurement of glomerular filtration rate (inulin clearance) with an evaluation of the clinical significance of this determination. *Arch Intern Med.* 1940;66:306-18. KIDNEY FUNCTION **1499**

Alzheimer, Alois. Über eigenartige Erkrankung der Hirnrinde. *Allg Zeitschr Psychiatrie.* 1907;64:146-8. [In: Wilkins RH, Brody IA. Alzheimer's disease. *Arch Neurol.* 1969;21:109-10.] ALZHEIMER'S DISEASE **132**

Amberson JB Jr, McMahon BT, Pinner M. A clinical trial of sanocrysin in pulmonary tuberculosis. *Am Rev Tuberc.* 1931;24:401-35. CLINICAL TRIALS **543**

American Dental Association. [Advertisement]. *Time.* 11 February 1985, p. 21. DENTAL HEALTH **699**

American Medical Association, Bureau of Medical Economics. *Economics and the Ethics of Medicine.* Chicago: American Medical Association; 1935, pp. 49-50. [In: Starr P. *The Social Transformation of American Medicine.* New York: Basic Books; 1982, p. 217.] MEDICAL ECONOMICS **1710**

American Medical Association, House of Delegates. AMAgrams. *JAMA.* 1970;213:359. ABORTION **11**

American Public Health Association. Recommended standards for abortion services. Adopted by the Executive Board of the APHA at the 98th Annual Meeting in Houston, Texas. *Am J Public Health.* 1971:;61(2):396-8. ABORTION **13**

Ames, Nathaniel. *Astronomical Diary for the Year 1734.* Boston: Booksellers; 1733. [In: McCarter D. Dr. Ames defines his profession. *Trans Studies Coll Phys Phila.* 1995;17:115-31.] QUACKERY **2801**

Amis, Kingsley. *One Fat Englishman,* London: 1963. CHILDREN **463**

Anderson, Charles M. *Richard Selzer and the Rhetoric of Surgery.* Carbondale: Southern Illinois University Press; 1989, p. 1. HEALERS **1162**

Andes, George M. Mark Twain's cat. *Ann Intern Med.* 1998;128:1043-4. CARETAKERS **429**

Andral G, Gavarret LDJ. Recherches sur la quantité d'acide carbonic exhalé par le poumon humaine. *Annal Chimie Physique.* 1853; serie 3, 8:129-50. METABOLISM **2160**

Andral, Gabriel.

Essai d'Hématologie Pathologique. Paris: 1843. ANEMIA **156**, LEAD POISONING **1521**, POLYCYTHEMIA **2642**

Lecture on the grippe, or epidemic influenza. In Dunglison R (ed). *Medical and Surgical Monographs.* Philadelphia: A. Waldie; 1838:143-8. INFLUENZA **1442**

Andrews, Billy F.

The Children's Bill of Rights. 19 May 1968. CHILDREN **464-466**, INFORMED CONSENT **1447**, RIGHTS OF CHILDREN **2918**

Medicine is more than a profession [Poem]. *South Med J.* 1991;84:1018. MEDICAL PROFESSION **2015**

Andrews, Edmund.

Complete record of the surgery of the battles fought near Vicksburg, December 27-30, 1862. *Chicago Med Examiner.* 1863;4:12-58. [In: Beatty WK. Edmund Andrews: surgeon, inventor, and record-keeper. *Proc Inst Med Chicago.* 1985;38:59-69.] MILITARY SURGERY **2181, 2182**

Two extraordinary forms of rectal fistula. *Chicago Med Examiner* . 1868;9:577-80. [In: Beatty WK, Edmund Andrews: surgeon, inventor, and record-keeper. *Proc Inst Med Chicago.* 1985;38:59-69.] NOMENCLATURE **2256**

Andric, Ivo. *The Chronicle of Travnik.* 1945 [Limited data]. DISEASE **788**

Andry de Bois-Regard, Nicolas.

An Account of the Breeding of Worms in the Human Body, 1700. PARASITOLOGY **2334**

Book 4, Means of preventing and correcting the deformities of the hand. In: *Orthopaedia,* 1741. ANEMIA **155**

Preface to *Orthopaedia,* 1741. ORTHOPAEDICS **2295**

Angell, Marcia.

Evaluating the health risks of breast implants: the interplay of medical science, the law, and public opinion. *N Engl J Med.* 1996;334:1513-8. SCIENCE **3003**

Fixing medicare. *N Engl J Med.* 1997;337:192-4. MEDICARE **2072**

Angier, Robert Crane. The structure and synthesis of the liver *L. casei* factor. *Science.* 1946;103:667-9. FOLIC ACID **1065**

Annas, George A. In Otten AL. Parents and newborns win new legal rights to sue for negligence. *The Wall Street Journal.* 7 June 1985, p. 1. MALPRACTICE **1616**

Anonymous.

[Letter]. *Med Trans R Coll Phys London.* 1785;3:1. ANGINA PECTORIS **179**

The Times [London]. STETHOSCOPE **3170**

Greek Anthology, II, Book 7. Paton, WR; translator. Sepulchral Epigrams. Cambridge, MA; Loeb Classical Library, Harvard University Press; 1960:77-9. HIPPOCRATES **1286**

Medical and Philosophical Commentaries, 2nd ed. Volume I, Part I. London: John Murray; 1774:6; first edition, 1773. READING **2827**

Russian Proverbs. Mount Vernon, NY: Peter Pauper Press; 1960. DRUGS **898**

The School of Salernum: Regimen Sanitatis Salerni. Translated by Harington J. Salerno: Ente Provinciale per Il Turismo; 1966. DIET **759** [24], HEALTH **1170** [22], LIVING **1566** [28]

Washington Post Magazine. Oct 1990 [Limited data]. HEALTH **1206**

A new clinical entity? *Lancet.* 1956;1:789-90. BENIGN MYALGIC ENCEPHALOMYELITIS **296**

Ancient Egyptian medical papyrus. In: *The Edwin Smith Surgical Papyrus,* vol. 1. Translated by Breasted JH. Chicago: University of Chicago Press; 1930. CIRCULATION **484** [430], CRANIAL TRAUMA **638** [438], DISLOCATIONS **805** [449], HEMIPLEGIA **1263** [437-8], SPINAL CORD **3117** [452-3], TREATMENT **3322** [432-3], WOUNDS **3487** [440]

Bedside medicine: the Oslerian reliquary. *Med J Aust.* 1971;1:1251-2. MEDICAL EDUCATION **1787**

Benign intracranial hypertension [Editorial]. *Lancet.* 1976;2:1007. OPHTHALMOSCOPY **2294**

Dishonest toil [Editorial]. *Lancet.* 1981;1:1403. SCIENTISTS **3009**

Dr. Sara M. Jordan, co-founder of the Lahey Clinic, is dead at 75 [Obituary]. *The New York Times,* 23 Nov 1959, p. 86. PATIENT-PHYSICIAN RELATIONS **2419**

Group practice: a menace or a blessing? [Editorial]. *JAMA.* 1921;76:452-3. MEDICAL ECONOMICS **1709**

Hospitals and general practitioners [Editorial]. *Natl Hosp Rec.* 1907;41:187. HOSPITAL STAFFS **1316**

How to read a journal [Editorial]. *S Afr Med J.* 1971;45:514. MEDICAL JOURNALS **1903**

In *Ebers papyrus.* [In: Carmichael AG, Ratzan RM (eds). *Medicine: A Treasury of Art and Literature.* New York: Hugh Lauter Levin Associates; 1991:29.] TREATMENT **3323**

In *Ebers papyrus.* [In: Nunn JF. *Ancient Egyptian Medicine.* Norman: University of Oklahoma Press; 1996.] ABSCESS **16** [76], BRAIN **337** [50], CORONARY ARTERY DISEASE **607** [87], LAXATIVES **1514** [159], RESPIRATION **2881** [55], TETANUS **3284** [181]

In Adams SH. *The Great American Fraud*. New York: Collier & Sons; 1905. QUACKERY **2804** [39], **2805** [84]

In an Ayurvedic medical text, *c*. 700. [In: On beginning practice. *Ann Intern Med*. 1972;76:442.] PHYSICIANS **2544**

In Byams-pa 'Phrin Las, Wang Lei. *Tibetan Medical Thangas of the Four Medical Tantras*. Lhasa: People's Publishing House of Tibet; 1990. [In: Clarke CRA. Three journeys to high altitude: medicine, Tibetan thangkas, and Sepu Kangri. *J R Coll Phys Lond*. 1999;33:78-84.] PATIENT-PHYSICIAN RELATIONS **2374**

In Clendening L. *Source Book of Medical History*, ch. 30. New York: Paul B. Hoeber/Harper & Bros.; 1942:333. NURSES **2267**

In Commoner B. Peering at peer review. *Hosp Practice*. 1978;13:25-29. PUBLISHING **2764**

In Coope R (ed). *The Quiet Art*, p. 165 (q.v.). PATHOLOGY **2357**

In Dana CL. Evil spoken of physicians. *Proc Charaka Club*. 1902;1:77-90. MEDICINES **2141**

In DeBakey S. Suggestions on preparation of medical papers. *JAMA*. 1954;155:1573-77. WRITING **3500**

In England now. *Lancet*. 1991;337:727. HYPOCHONDRIA **1378**

In Kekez J. *Svaki je Kamen da se Kuca Gradi*. Osijek: Publishing Center of the Open University; 1990 [Limited data]. EATING **936**

In Kendall PL. *The Relationship Between Medical Educators and Medical Practitioners*. Evanston, IL: Association of American Medical Colleges; 1965:82. MEDICAL EDUCATION **1783**

In Kinnier WJV. Diseases of Babylon: an examination of selected texts. *J Royal Soc Med*. 1996;89:135-40. BRUXISM **353**

In O'Donnell M. The toxic effect of language on medicine. *J R Coll Phys Lond*. 1995;29:525-9. CASES **438**

In Sprague JS (ed). *Medical Ethics and Cognate Subjects*. Toronto: Sparling; 1902, p. 39. PATIENT-PHYSICIAN RELATIONS **2399**

In Starr P. *The Social Transformation of American Medicine*. New York: Basic Books; 1982:166. HOSPITAL STAFFS **1317**

In Stille A. Latin fanatic: a profile of Father Reginald Foster. *American Scholar*. 1994;63:497-526. DOCTORS **866**

In Talbott JH. At the bedside. *N Eng J Med*. 1967;277:109. MEDICAL JOURNALS **1902**

In Wilson JVK. Diseases of Babylon: an examination of selected texts. *J R Soc Med*. 1996;89:135-40. GANGRENE **1076**

Mathematics and medicine [Editorial]. *Lancet*. 1937;1:31. STATISTICS **3156**

Medical statistics. *Lancet*. 1921;1:985-8. CLINICAL RESEARCH **528**, PATIENTS **2461**, STATISTICS **3152**

Plain English. *Lancet*. 1865;2:378-9. WRITING **3489**

Recurrent brief depression and anxiety [Editorial]. *Lancet*. 1991;337:586-7. PSYCHIATRY **2724**

Round the world: uniformity of style in journals. *Lancet*. 1981;1:1414. MEDICAL JOURNALS **1905**

Sprague JS (ed). *Medical Ethics and Cognate Subjects*. Toronto: Sparling; 1902, p. 39. MEDICAL PRACTICE **1934**

The psalm of the addict. *Congressional Record*. 31 Jul 1971, vol. 31, no. 117, p. 28511. HEROIN **1281**

Anthony, Susan B. Letter to Elizabeth Cady Stanton, 29 September 1857. In: Gordon AD, editor. *The Selected Papers of Elizabeth Cady Stanton and Susan B. Anthony. Volume 1, In the School of Anti-Slavery, 1840 to 1866*. New Brunswick, NJ: Rutgers University Press; 1997:352-7. REPRODUCTION **2849**

Aquinas, Thomas. *Summa Theologica*, vol 1. TREATMENT **3331**

Archibald EW. Higher degrees in the profession of surgery. *Ann Surg*. 1935;102:481-95. [481]. SURGERY **3236**

Archimathaeus. *The Coming of a Physician to His Patient*. Translated by Walsh JJ. [In: Strauss MB, *Familiar Medical Quotations*, p. 163 (q.v.).] EXAMINATION **1015**

Aretaeus the Cappadocian.

On Arthritis and Schiatica. In Adams F (ed). *The Extant Works of Aretaeus the Cappadocian*, book II, chap. XII. Birmingham, AL: Classics of Medicine Library; 1990, pp. 362-3. ARTHRITIS **234**

On Asthma. In Adams F (ed). *The Extant Works of Aretaeus the Cappadocian*, book I, ch. XI. Birmingham, AL: Classics of Medicine Library; 1990. ASTHMA **249** [316-7], ORTHOPNEA **2296** [316]

On Cephalaea.. In Adams F (ed). *The Extant Works of Aretaeus the Cappadocian*, book I, ch. V. Birmingham, AL: Classics of Medicine Library; 1990, pp. 294-5. MIGRAINE **2163**

On Cholera. In Adams F (ed). *The Extant Works of Aretaeus theCappadocian*, book II, ch. V. Birmingham, AL: Classics of Medicine Library; 1990, pp. 273-4. CHOLERA **469**

The Seven Sins of Medicine [Lecture given to the University College Hospital Medical Society, March 17, 1948]. [In: *Lancet*. 1949;2:358-60.] MEDICAL SINS **2057**

Malingering. *Trans Med Soc London*, vol. LXXV. 1959. [In: *Richard Asher Talking Sense*. London: Pitman Medical; 1972, p. 153.] MUNCHAUSEN SYNDROME **2205**

Munchausen's syndrome. *Lancet*. 1951;1:339-41. MUNCHAUSEN SYNDROME **2204**

The dangers of going to bed. *Br Med J*. 13 Dec 1947, p. 967-8. EARLY AMBULATION **934**

The seven sins of medicine. *Lancet*. 1949;2:358-60. PATIENT-PHYSICIAN RELATIONS **2412, 2413**

Asimov, Isaac A. In Basta LL. *A Graceful Exit: Life and Death on Your Own Terms*. New York: Insight Books, Plenum Press; 1996, p. 90. PAIN **2329**

Askey, Vincent. *The Land of Hypochondriacs* [Speech given at Bakersfield, California, October 20, 1960]. [In: Simpson JB, *Contemporary Quotations*, p. 177 (q.v.).] HEALTH **1195**, HYPOCHONDRIA **1375**

Astwood, Edwin Bennett. Treatment of hyperthyroidism with thiourea and thiouracil. *JAMA*. 1943;122:78-81. HYPERTHYROIDISM **1365**

Atlee, Washington Lemuel. *General and Differential Diagnosis of Ovarian Tumors, with Specific References to the Operation of Ovariotomy and Occasional Pathological and Therapeutical Considerations*, preface. Philadelphia: J.B. Lippincott; 1873. [In: Rutkow M, *The History of Surgery in the United States*, p. 304 (q.v.).] MEDICAL ERROR **1809**

Auden, Wystan Hugh. The Art of Healing. In: *Collected Poems*. Edited by Mendelson E. London: Faber & Faber; 1976:626. TREATMENT **3354**

Auenbrugger, Leopold. *On Percussion of the Chest*. Vienna: 1761 [Translated by Forbes J. Baltimore: Johns Hopkins University Press; 1936]. PERCUSSION **2495, 2496**

Auerbach O, Hammond EC, Garfinkel L. Smoking in relation to atherosclerosis of the coronary arteries. *N Engl J Med*. 1965;273:775-9. CORONARY ARTERY DISEASE **629**

Auerbach O, Hammond EC, Kirman D, Garfinkel L.

Effects of cigarette smoking on dogs. Part II: Pulmonary neoplasms. *Arch Environ Health*. 1970;21:754-68. SMOKING **3100**

Emphysema produced in dogs by cigarette smoking. *JAMA*. 1967;199:241-6. PULMONARY EMPHYSEMA **2789**

Auerbach O, Stout AP, Hammond EC, Garfinkel L. The role of smoking in the development of lung cancer. *Proc Natl Cancer Conf*. 1964;5:497-501. CANCER OF THE LUNG **406**

Augustine, Saint.

Confessions IV, 401. PATIENT-PHYSICIAN RELATIONS **2368**

In Pope Pius XI. Casti connubi: encyclical of Pope Pius XI on Christian marriage, December 31, 1930. In Carlen C. *The Papal Encyclicals, 1903-1939*, sec. 55. Raleigh, NC: McGrath Publishing; 1981, p. 399. CONTRACEPTION **599**

Avery OT, MacLeod CM, McCarty M. Studies on the chemical nature of the substance inducing transformation of pneumococcal types: induction of transformation by a deoxyribonucleic acid fraction isolated from pneumococcus type III. *J Exp Med*. 1944;79:137-58. DEOXYRIBONUCLEIC ACID (DNA) **705**

Avicenna.

Liber canonis. Mediolani: P. de Lavagna; 1473. CANCER **373**

In Gruner OC. *A Treatise on the Canon of Medicine of Avicenna: Incorporating a Translation of the First Book*. London: Luzac; 1930, p. 25. MEDICINE **2081**

Axel R, Buck L. A multigene family may encode odorant receptors: a molecular basis for odor recognition. *Cell*. 1991;65(1):175-87. SMELL **3087**

Ayr, Washington. *The Semi-Centennial of Anaesthesia* [an account of an eyewitness to the first public demonstration of ether anesthesia at the Massachusetts General Hospital, October 16, 1846]; 1897. ANESTHESIA **167**

Babcock, Robert Hall.

Cardiac hypochondriacs. *N Y Med J*. 1914;100:7-10. HYPOCHONDRIA **1374**

Certain normal physical signs and their liability to lead to false diagnosis. *North Am Pract*. 1891;3:375-81. [In: Beatty WK. Robert Hall Babcock: acute diagnostician and physicians' physician. *Proc Inst Med Chicago*. 1984;37:130-44.] PHYSICAL EXAMINATION **2524**

Medical tendencies. *Lancet Clinic*. 1911;106:414-48. TESTS **3275**

President's address: the limitations of drug therapy. *Trans Am Clin Climatol Assoc*. 1901;17:1-13. NUTRITION **2277**

Babington, Benjamin Guy. Proceedings of societies: Hunterian Society, March 18, 1829. *Lond Med Gazette*. 1829;3:555. LARYNGOSCOPE **1512**

Babinski, Joseph-François-Félix. Sur le reflexe cutane plantaire dans certaines affections organiques du systeme nerveau central. *C R Seances Soc Biol.* 1896;48:207-8. BABINSKI REFLEX 275

Back, James de. A Discourse of the Heart. In: Harvey, William. *Anatomical Exercises.* London: 1653. HEMATOLOGY 1260

Bacon, Francis.
Essays. Of Counsel, 1625. PLACEBOS 2609
Essays. Of Deformity, 1625. DEFORMITY 695
Essays. Of Regimen of Health, 1625. HEALTH 1173, PHYSICIANS 2550
Maxims of the Law. Preface, 1630. MEDICAL ETHICS 1816
Novum Organum. Aphorism 46, 1620. RESEARCH 2851
The Advancement of Learning, 1605. MEDICINE 2085, PHYSICIANS 2549

Bacot, John. *A Treatise of Syphilis, in Which the History, Symptoms, and Methods of Treating Every Form of That Disease Are Fully Considered.* London: Longman, et al.; 1829, p. 49. [In: Bloomfield AL, *Communicable Diseases,* p. 303.] CLINICAL RESEARCH 526

Baden, Michael. In Johnston L. Artist's death: a last statement in a thesis on "self-termination." *New York Times.* 17 Jun 1979, p. 1,10. CANCER 385

Badham, John. Paralysis in childhood: four remarkable cases of suddenly induced paralysis in the extremities, occurring in children, without any apparent cerebral or cerebro-spinal lesion. *Lond Med Gazette.* 1835;17:215-8. POLIOMYELITIS 2631

Baer, Karl Ernst von. *On the Genesis of the Ovum of Mammals and of Men* [Latin]. Leipzig: L. Voss; 1827. [In: O'Malley CD (tr). *Isis.* 1956;47:121-53.] OVARIES 2309

Bagliavi, Duro Armeno. *Dubrovnik Archives.* 1668-1707 [Limited data]. MEDICINE 2090

Bailey, Charles P. In Weisse AB. *Conversations in Medicine: The Story of Twentieth-Century American Medicine in the Words of Those Who Created It.* New York: New York University Press; 1984, p. 136. MITRAL-VALVE SURGERY 2195

Baillie, Matthew.
The Morbid Anatomy of Some of the Most Important Parts of the Human Body, 2nd ed. London: 1797. [In: Major RH. *Classic Descriptions of Disease* (q.v.).] CIRRHOSIS OF THE LIVER 495 [694], PULMONARY EMPHYSEMA 2786 [638]
The Morbid Anatomy of Some of the Most Important Parts of the Human Body, 2nd ed. Walpole, NH: 1808. [In: Talbott JH. *A Biographical History of Medicine* (q.v.).] CHOLELITHIASIS 468 [449], CORONARY ARTERY DISEASE 614 [449]
The Morbid Anatomy of Some of the Most Important Parts of the Human Body. London: 1793. [Reprint: Birmingham, AL: Classics of Medicine Library; 1986.] CANCER OF THE STOMACH 414, CIRRHOSIS OF THE LIVER 494 [141-2], GASTRIC ULCER 1084 [87-8]

Baillou, Guillaume de.
Epidemiorum et Ephemeridium Libri Duo. Paris: 1740. [In: Major RH. *Classic Descriptions of Disease,* pp. 154,156 (q.v.).] DIPHTHERIA 773
On Rheumatism, 1642. [In: Ruhmann W. The earliest book on rheumatism. Barnard CC, translator. *Br J Rheum.* 1940;2:140-62.] RHEUMATOID ARTHRITIS 2909
Opera medica omnia. Venice: A. Jeremiam; 1734-36. [In: Major RH. *Classic Descriptions of Disease,* pp. 221-2 (q.v.).] RHEUMATISM 2907
Consultation CIX: concerning palpitation of the heart. In *Consiliorum medicinalium,* book II. Venice; 1735. [In: Major RH. *Classic Descriptions of Disease,* p. 439 (q.v.).] PERICARDITIS 2499
Quinta. In *Opera Omnia,* book II. Venice, 1736. [In: Major RH. *Classic Descriptions of Disease,* p. 219 (q.v.).] PERTUSSIS (WHOOPING COUGH) 2510

Baker, George. *An Essay Concerning the Cause of the Endemial Colic of Devonshire.* London: J. Hughs; 1767. [In: Major RH. *Classic Descriptions of Disease,* p. 348 (q.v.).] LEAD POISONING 1519

Baldwin, James. *The Fire Next Time,* 1963. New York: Dell; 1964:123-4. DEATH 675

Balfour, Thomas Graham. Letter to Charles West. [In: West C. *Lectures on the Diseases of Infancy and Childhood.* Philadelphia: Blanchard and Lea; 1860:596.] CLINICAL TRIALS 538

Balint, Michael. *The Doctor, His Patient, and the Illness.* New York: International Universities Press; 1957, p. 292. PATIENT-PHYSICIAN RELATIONS 2417

Banti, Guido. Splenomegaly with cirrhosis of the liver. *Sperimentale.* 1894;48:407-432. [In: Talbott JH. *A Biographical History of Medicine,* pp. 1145-6.] SPLENOMEGALY 3123

Banting FG, Best CH. The internal secretion of the pancreas. *J Lab Clin Med.* 1922;7:251-66. DIABETES MELLITUS 730

Banting, Frederick Grant.
Banting's notebook, October 31, 1920, 2:00 AM. *Arch Acad Med Toronto.* [In: Bliss M. *The Discovery of Insulin.* Chicago: University of Chicago Press; 1982, p. 50.] INSULIN 1456

In Hemingway E. "An absolute lie," says Dr. Banting of serum report. *The Toronto Star*. 11 Oct 1923 [Limited data]. INSULIN **1459**

Pancreatic extracts in the treatment of diabetes mellitus. *Canadian Med Assoc J*. 1922;12:141-6. INSULIN **1458**

The internal secretions of the pancreas. *Am J Physiol*. 1922;59:479. INSULIN **1457**

Barach, Alvan. [Recalled on his death, December 15, 1977]. [In: Simpson JB, *Contemporary Quotations*, p. 123 (q.v.).] MEDICAL CARE **1685**

Bárány, Robert. Localization in the cortex of the cerebellum. *Dtsch Med Wochenschr*. 1913;39:637-42. BÁRÁNY POINTING TEST **287**

Barbellion, Wilhelm Nero Pilatus.
A *Last Diary*. London: Hogarth Press; 1984, p. 347. SUFFERING **3181**
The Journal of a Disappointed Man. London: Chatto and Windus; 1919. [Reprint: London: Hogarth Press; 1984.] DEPRESSION **716** [89], MULTIPLE SCLEROSIS **2202** [274]

Barcroft, Joseph. Observations upon the effect of high altitude on the physiological processes of the human body, carried out in the Peruvian Andes, chiefly at Cerro de Pasco. *Phil Trans R Soc Lond B*. 1923;211:351-454. [In: Talbott JH. A *Biographical History of Medicine*, p. 969 (q.v.).] LUNG **1589**

Bard, Samuel. A *Discourse on the Duties of a Physician: Address to the First Graduating Class at the Medical School Established in Affiliation with What Was Then Known as King's College, New York*. New York: A&J Robertson; 1769. [In: Talbott JH. A *Biographical History of Medicine*, p. 356 (q.v.).] LEARNING **1522**

Barer M, Roos NP. Why are some people healthy and others not? *Prairie Med J*. 1996;66:30-1. MEDICAL CARE **1703**

Barnard, Christiaan Neethling. A human cardiac transplant: an interim report of a successful operation performed at Groote Schuur Hospital, Cape Town. *S Afr Med J*. 1967;41:1271-4. HEART SURGERY **1258**

Barnard, William George. The nature of the "oat-celled sarcoma" of the mediastinum. *J Path Bacteriol*. 1926;29:241-4. CANCER OF THE LUNG **404**

Barr ML, Bertram EG. A morphological distinction between neurons of the male and female, and the behaviour of the nucleolar satellite during accelerated nucleoprotein synthesis. *Nature*. 1949;163:676-7. BARR BODY **289**

Barsky A, Borus J. Somatization and medicalization in the era of managed care. *JAMA*. 1995;274(24):1931-4. SYMPTOMS **3249**

Bartlett E. An *Essay on the Philosophy of Medical Science*. Philadelphia: Lea & Blanchard; 1844, p. 154. STATISTICS **3140**

Bartlett, Elisha. An *Essay on the Philosophy of Medical Science*. Philadelphia: 1844. CLINICAL TRIALS **537**, MEDICINE **2096**, SYPHILIS **3262**

Bartoletti, Fabrizio. *Methodus in Dyspnoeain*, book IV, sect. IV, para. III. Bononiae: Heredes Evangelistae Sozzae; 1633, p. 383. CORONARY ARTERY DISEASE **608**

Basedow, Carl Adolph von.
Exophthalmus caused by hypertrophy of the connective tissue in the orbit [German]. *Wochenschr Ges Heilk*. 1840;6:197-204. [In: Clendening L. *Source Book of Medical History*, p. 519 (q.v.).] EXOPHTHALMOS **1024**
Exophthalmus caused by hypertrophy of the connective tissue in the orbit [German]. *Wochenschr Ges Heilk*. 1840;6:197-204. [In: Major RH. *Classic Descriptions of Disease*, p. 303 (q.v.).] HYPERTHYROIDISM **1362**
Exophthalmus caused by hypertrophy of the connective tissue in the orbit [German]. *Wochenschr Ges Heilk*. 1840;6:197-204. [In: Talbott JH. A *Biographical History of Medicine*, p. 1049 (q.v.).] HYPERTHYROIDISM **1363**

Basil the Great, Saint. *Homilies*, no. XIV, ch. 7. ALCOHOL **107**

Bassen FA, Kornzweig AL. Malformation of the erythrocytes in a case of atypical retinitis pigmentosa. *Blood*. 1950;5:381-7. ABETALIPOPROTEINEMIA (BASSEN-KORNZWEIG SYNDROME) **1**

Bassini, Edoardo. Nuovo metodo per la cura radicale dell' ernia inguinale. *Atti Congr Assoc Med Ital*. 1889;2:179-82. [In: Talbott JH. A *Biographical History of Medicine*, p. 1017 (q.v.).] HERNIORRHAPHY **1280**

Basta, Lofty L. A *Graceful Exit: Life and Death on Your Own Terms*. New York: Insight Books, Plenum Press; 1996. CARDIOLOGY **428** [209], DEATH **685** [preface], DYING **930** [9], MEDICAL EDUCATION **1802** [56], MEDICAL PRACTICE **1968** [48], MEDICAL TECHNOLOGY **2065** [34]

Bates, Mary Elizabeth. In Minney D. Mary Elizabeth Bates, MD. *Med Wom J*. 1948;55:30-1. INTERNSHIP **1466**, PATIENT-PHYSICIAN RELATIONS **2411**

Baum, Michael. Quack cancer cures or scientific remedies. *J R Soc Med.* 1996;89:543-7. ALTERNATIVE MEDICINE 130

Baxter, Daniel J. *The Least of These My Brethren: A Doctor's Story of Hope and Miracles on an Inner-City AIDS Ward.* New York: Harmony Books; 1997. DEATH 686 [58], MANAGED CARE 1622 [131], MEDICAL CARE 1704 [131]

Bayes, Thomas. An essay towards solving a problem in the doctrine of chances. *Philos Trans R Soc London.* 1763;53:370-418. STATISTICS 3131

Bayle, Gaspard Laurent. Recherches sur la phthisie pulmonaire. In: *Encyclopedie des Sciences Medicales.* Paris: 1838. [In: Major RH. *Classic Descriptions of Disease*, p. 73 (q.v.).] TUBERCULOSIS 3383

Bayliss WM, Starling EH. The movements and innervation of the small intestine. *J Physiol.* 1899;224:99-143. EXPERIMENTS 1034, INTESTINES 1469, 1470

Baynard, Edward. In Shorter E. *Doctors and Their Patients: A Social History.* New Brunswick, NJ: Transaction Publishers; 1991, p. 33. TREATMENT 3335

Bazelon, David L. *Equal Justice for the Unequal: Isaac Ray Lectureship Award Series of the American Psychiatric Association.* Chicago: University of Chicago Press; 1961. [In: Menninger K, Mayman M, Pruyser P. *The Vital Balance: The Life Process in Mental Health and Illness.* New York; 1963, p. 46.] PSYCHIATRISTS 2710

Bean, William Bennett.
Origin of the term "internal medicine". *N Engl J Med.* 1982;306:182-3. INTERNAL MEDICINE 1462
The department of internal medicine. *J Med Educ.* 1954;29:11. MEDICAL ECONOMICS 1711

Beard, George Miller.
Experiments with the "jumpers" or "jumping" Frenchmen of Maine. *J Nerv Ment Dis.* 1880;7:487-90. TOURETTE SYNDROME 3315
Neurasthenia, or nervous exhaustion. *Boston Med Surg J.* 1869;29:217-21. NEURASTHENIA 2245

Beaumont, William. *Experiments and Observations on the Gastric Juice and the Physiology of Digestion.* Plattsburgh; 1833. [In: McGovern JP, Roland CG (ed). *The Collected Essays of William Osler*, vol. III. Birmingham, AL: Classics of Medicine Library; 1985, p. 303.] SCIENCE 2950

Beauvoir, Simone de. *The Second Sex.* New York: Alfred A. Knopf; 1952. WOMEN 3470

Beck CS, Weckesser EC, Barry FM. Fatal heart attacks and successful defibrillation. *JAMA.* 1956;161:434-6. VENTRICULAR DEFIBRILLATION 3427

Becon, Thomas. *Catechism*, 1558. ALCOHOLISM 117

Beers, Clifford Whittingham. *A Mind That Found Itself: An Autobiography.* New York: Longmans, Green; 1908. PSYCHOSIS 2737 [81], SCHIZOPHRENIA 2935 [1]

Beethoven, Ludwig von.
Letter to Dr. F.G. Wegeler, June 29, 1801. Reprinted in Marek GR. *Beethoven: Biography of a Genius.* New York: Funk & Wagnalls; 1969, p. 208]. DEAFNESS 650
Letter to Dr. F.G. Wegeler, May 2, 1810. [In: *Beethoven's Letters.* Translated by Shedlock JS. New York: Dover; 1972, p. 970.] SUICIDE 3184

Behring E, Kitasato S. Ueber as Zustandekommen der Diptherie-Immunitat und der Tetanus-Immunitat bei Thieren. *Dtsch Med Wochenschr.* 1890;16:1113. ANTITOXINS 200

Behring, Emil Adolf von. The value of diphtheria serum [German]. *Dtsch Med Wochenschr.* 1893;19:415-8. [In: Talbott JH. A *Biographical History of Medicine*, p. 784 (q.v.).] DIPHTHERIA 776

Bell, Alexander Graham. The uses of radium. *Am Med.* 1903;6:261. RADIOTHERAPY 2820

Bell, Charles.
The Idea of a New Anatomy of the Brain. London: 1811. [Reprint: London: Dawsons of Pall Mall; 1966.] NERVOUS SYSTEM, 2237 [5-6], 2238 [22], THINKING 3292 [34-5]
On the motions of the eye, in illustration of the uses of the muscles and nerves of the orbit. *Philos Trans R Soc Lond.* 1823;113:166-86. BELL PALSY 293
On the nerves of the face: being a second paper on that subject. *Philos Trans R Soc London.* 1829;119:317-30. BELL PALSY 294
On the nerves: a view of their structure and function with the account of some experiments illustrative of their functions. *Phil Trans R Soc London.* 1821;111:398-424. [In: Kelly EC (ed). *Classics of Neurology.* Huntington, NY: Krieger; 1971, pp. 43-70.] NERVES 2229
On the nerves; giving an account of some experiments on their structure and functions, which lead to a new arrangement of the system. *Philos Trans R Soc London.* 1821;111:398-424. BELL PALSY 292

Bell, Joseph A. Pertussis prophylaxis with two doses of alum-precipitated vaccine. *Public Health Reports.* 1941;56(31):1535-46. CLINICAL TRIALS 546

Bellet, Paul S. Bedside presentations and patients' perceptions of their medical care [Letter]. *N Engl J Med.* 1997;337:714-5. PATIENT-PHYSICIAN RELATIONS 2453

INDIGESTION 1424, INSANITY 1453, LIFE 1542, LIVER 1560, MIND 2185, NARCOTICS 2217, PAIN 2323, PHRENOLOGY 2518, PHYSICIANS 2579, PLAGUE 2614, POISONS 2627, PRESCRIPTIONS 2670, SLEEPING SICKNESS (TRYPANOSOMIASIS) 3079, TRICHINOSIS 3360, TUBERCULOSIS 3393

Bigelow, Henry Jacob.

Boston Med Surg J. 1846;35:16. ANESTHESIA 157

Medical Education in America. Cambridge, MA: 1871. [In: Stevens R. *American Medicine and the Public Interest.* New Haven, CT: Yale University Press; 1971:36.] AMERICAN MEDICAL ASSOCIATION 137

Insensibility during surgical operations produced by inhalation. *Boston Med Surg J.* 1846;35:309-17. ANESTHESIA 158, PATENTS 2350

Bigelow, Jacob. *Nature in Disease.* Boston: 1854. MEDICAL PRACTICE 1926, MEDICINE 2098, TREATMENT 3344

Billingham RE, Brent L, Medawar PB. Actively acquired tolerance of foreign cells. *Nature.* 1953;172(4379):903-6. IMMUNOLOGY 1419

Billings, John Shaw.

An address on our medical literature. *Brit Med J.* 1881;2:262-8. WRITING 3491

Harvard Medical Association: annual dinner. *Boston Med Surg J.* 1894;131:136-42. CONTINUING EDUCATION 592

In Garrison FH. *John Shaw Billings: A Memoir.* New York: Putnam's; 1915, p. 17. EPILEPSY 979

On vital and medical statistics. *Med Rec.* 1889;36:589-601. STATISTICS 3147

Billings, Josh (Henry Wheeler Shaw).

Everybody's Friend, or; Josh Billing's Encyclopedia and Proverbial Philosophy of Wit and Humor. Hartford, CT: American Publishing Company; 1874. AGING 71 [242], MEDICINES 2142 [253], 2143 [279]

Works. New York: G.W. Carleton; 1881. DOCTORS 826

In: Cousins N. *Head First: The Biology of Hope.* New York: EP Dutton; 1989:125. HEALTH 1183

In: Day D. *Uncle Sam's Uncle Josh, or Josh Billings on Practically Everything Distilled from Josh's Rum-and-Tansy New England Wit.* Boston: Little, Brown; 1953:184. HEALTH 1182

Billroth, Christian Albert Theodor.

The Medical Sciences in the German Universities: A Study in the History of Civilization. Welch WH; translator. New York: Macmillan; 1924:43-9. PATIENT-PHYSICIAN RELATIONS 2389, 2390, PHYSICIANS 2571, RESEARCH 2858

Address to the Vienna Medical Society, 1881. [In: Nissen R. Billroth and cardiac surgery [Letter]. *Lancet.* 1963;2:250.] HEART SURGERY 1246

First successful pylorectomy for cancer [German]. *Wien Med Wochenschr.* 1881;31:161-5 [Translation by Brunschwig A and Simandl E reprinted in *Surg Gynecol Obstet.* 1951;92:375-9]. GASTRIC SURGERY 1083

In Rutkow IM. *The History of Surgery in the United States, 1775-1900.* San Francisco: Norman Publishing; 1988, p. xiii. HISTORY OF MEDICINE 1293

Bingel, Adolf. Über behandlung der diphtherie mit gewonlichem pferdeserum. *Deutsches Archiv für Klinische Medizin.* 1918;125:284-332. CLINICAL TRIALS 541

Binninger, Johann Nikolaus. *Observationum et Curationum Medicinalium.* Montbeliard: 1673. [In: Major RH. *Classic Descriptions of Disease,* p. 675 (q.v.).] HAY FEVER 1159

Bird, Brian. *Talking with Patients,* 2nd ed. Philadelphia: J.B. Lippincott; 1973:1. MEDICAL HISTORIES 1885

Black, Douglas Arthur Kilgour.

A Black look at the independent inquiry into inequalities in health. *J R Coll Phys.* 1999;33:148-9. POVERTY 2655

Evidence-free medicine. *Clin Med.* 2002;2:474-5. PHYSICIANS 2595

In: McLachlan G (ed). *Reviewing Practice in Medical Care: Steps to Quality Assurance.* London: Nuffield Provincial Hospitals Trust; 1981:ii. MEDICAL PRACTICE 1960

Medicine and the patient. In: *The Logic of Medicine.* London: Oliver & Boyd; 1968:2. MEDICAL CARE 1676

Blackall, John. *Observations on the Nature and Cure of Dropsies.* London: Longman; 1813. [In: Major RH. *Classic Descriptions of Disease,* pp. 576-7 (q.v.).] PROTEINURIA 2705

Blackmore, Richard. *A Treatise of the Spleen and Vapours.* London: 1725, p. xvi-xx. SPLEEN 3122

Blackwell, Barry. Drug therapy: patient compliance. *N Engl J Med.* 1973;289:249-52. PRESCRIPTIONS 2672

Blackwell, Elizabeth.

The Human Element in Sex, 1902. [In: *Essays in Medical Sociology.* New York: Arno Press; 1972:53.] SEX 3033

The Influence of Women in the Profession of Medicine [Address given at the opening of the winter session of the London School of Medicine for Women]. London: 1889. [In: *Essays in Medical Sociology,* vol. II. New York: Arno Press; 1972.] MEDICAL ETHICS 1829 [6], MEDICAL PROFESSION 1988 [5], PHYSICIANS 2574 [12], POVERTY 2654 [13], WOMEN IN MEDICINE 3474 [8-9], 3475 [9]

Blalock A, Taussig HB. The surgical treatment of malformations of the heart in which there is pulmonary stenosis or pulmonary atresia. *JAMA.* 1945;128:189-202. HEART SURGERY 1252

Blalock, Alfred.
Experimental hypertension. *Physiological Reviews.* 1940;20(2):159-93. HYPERTENSION 1353
Experimental shock: the cause of the low blood pressure produced by muscle injury. *Arch Surg.* 1930;20:959-96. SHOCK 3062

Blane, Gilbert.
Elements of Medical Logic, illustrated by practical proofs and examples, 2nd ed., 1819. MEDICAL EVIDENCE 1852
Observations on the Diseases Incident to Seamen, 1785. SCURVY 3018, STATISTICS 3133

Blaney JVZ. Valedictory address to the graduating class of Rush Medical College for Session 1853-1854. Chicago: 1854. SPECIALIZATION 3105

Bleuler, Eugen. *Dementia Praecox; or, the group of schizophrenias,* 1911. SCHIZOPHRENIA 2936, 2937

Bloche, M. Gregg. Clinical loyalties and the social purposes of medicine. *JAMA.* 1999;281(3):268-74. MEDICAL ETHICS 1849

Block K, Rittenberg D. On the utilization of acetic acid for cholesterol formation. *J Biological Chem.* 1942;145:625-36. CHOLESTEROL 474

Bloomfield, Arthur L. *A Bibliography of Internal Medicine: Communicable Diseases.* Chicago: University of Chicago Press; 1958, p. 94. SERUM THERAPY 3022

Blumberg BS, Alter HJ. A "new" antigen in leukemia sera. *JAMA.* 1965;191:541-6. AUSTRALIA ANTIGEN 270

Blumberg, Baruch S. In Manning PR and DeBakey L. *Medicine: Preserving the Passion.* New York: Springer-Verlag; 1987, p. 104. RESEARCH 2876

Blumgart, Herman L. Preparation for medical school and recruitment of candidates. *N Engl J Med.* 1964;271:238-42. MEDICAL PROFESSION 2010

Blundell, James. Observations of transfusion of blood. *Lancet.* 1829;2:321-24. BLOOD TRANSFUSION 318

Boccaccio, Giovanni. Preface to the Ladies. *The Decameron,* 1353. BUBONIC PLAGUE 354

Boe, François de le. *De Phthisis.* In *Opera Medica.* Amsterdami: 1679. [In: Major RH. *Classic Descriptions of Disease,* pp. 67-8 (q.v.).] TUBERCULOSIS 3372

Boeck, Caesar Peter Moeller. Multiple benign sarcoid of the skin. *J Cutan Genitourin Dis.* 1899;17:543-50. SARCOIDOSIS 2930

Boerhaave, Hermann. In *Boerhaave's Aphorisms: Concerning the Knowledge and Cure of Diseases.* Birmingham, AL: Classics of Medicine Library; 1986, p. 1. DISEASE 783

Bohr C, Hasselbalch K, Krogh A. The biological dependence of carbon dioxide tension of the blood on oxygen binding. *Scand Arch Physiol.* 1904;16:402-12. BOHR EFFECT 327

Bok, Derek. In *Realities of Medicine: September 9-13, 1985* [Conference pamphlet]. Chicago: University of Illinois College of Medicine at Chicago; 1985. MEDICAL PRACTICE 1961

Bombeck, Erma. Do you understand your doctor? [Syndicated column]. *Baton Rouge Morning Advocate.* 07 Sep 1981, p. 8D. PATIENT-PHYSICIAN RELATIONS 2434

Bondt, Jacob de. Certain miraculous works of nature which future medical researchers must investigate further [Latin]. In *Historia Naturalis et Medica Indias Orientalis,* book V, chap. 33. 1658, p. 85. [In: Carruba RW, Bowers JZ. The Western World's first detailed treatise on acupuncture: Willem ten Rhijne's de Acupunctura. *J Hist Med Allied Sci.* 1974;29:371.] ACUPUNCTURE 33

Bonet, Théophile. *A Guide to the Practical Physician* [Latin]. London: T. Flesher; 1684. [In: Talbott JH. *A Biographical History of Medicine,* p. 117 (q.v.).] PROGNOSIS 2695

Bonnett OT. *Why Healing Happens.* Aspen, CO: MacMurray & Beck; 1996:109. ILLNESS 1413

Bono, Edward de. *New Think: The Use of Lateral Thinking in the Generation of New Ideas.* New York: Avon Books; 1971. SCIENCE 2983 [132], 2984 [138]

Bontius, Jacobus. *An Account of the Diseases, Natural History, and Medicines of the East Indies,* 1769. BERIBERI 297

Borhani NO, Feinleib M, Garrison RT, et al. Genetic variation in blood pressure. *Acta Genet Med Gemellol.* 1976;25:137-44. HYPERTENSION 1358

Bornemeier WC. Presented before the Eleventh Annual Meeting and Teaching Seminar, International Academy of Proctology, N.Y.C., April 18, 1959. SPHINCTER ANI 3115

Bostock, John. Case of periodical affection of the eyes and chest. *Med-Chir Trans.* 1819;10:161. [In: Major RH. *Classic Descriptions of Disease,* pp. 677-8 (q.v.).] HAY FEVER 1160

Botallo, Leonardo. *De Catarrho Commentarius.* Paris: 1564. [In: Major RH. *Classic Descriptions of Disease,* p. 673 (q.v.).] HAY FEVER 1158

Bouillaud, Jean-Baptiste.
Traité Cliniques des Maladies du Coeur, 2nd ed, vol. 2. Paris: 1841. ENDOCARDITIS **959**
Traité Cliniques des Maladies du Coeur. Paris: 1835. [In: Major RH. *Classic Descriptions of Disease*, pp. 231-2 (q.v.).] RHEUMATIC HEART DISEASE **2906**
Clinical studies tending to refute Gall's opinion on the function of the cerebellum and to prove that this organ coordinates equilibrium and the ability to stand and walk. *Arch Med Gen*. 1827;15:225-47. CEREBELLUM **450**

Bouveret, Léon. Concerning essential paroxysmal tachycardia. *Rev Med*. 1889;9:753-93. PAROXYSMAL TACHYCARDIA **2347, 2348**

Bowditch, Henry Ingersoll. Letter to Olivia Bowditch, 14 October 1867. In: Bowditch VY, editor. *Life and Correspondence of Henry Ingersoll Bowditch*, volume 2. Boston: Houghton, Mifflin; 1902:146. MEDICAL BOOKS **1649**

Bowditch, Henry Pickering. Notes on the nature of nerve-force. *J Physiol (Lond)*. 1885;6:133-5. [In: Talbott JH. *A Biographical History of Medicine*, p. 946 (q.v.).] NERVES **2231**

Bowman, William. On the structure and use of the Malpighian bodies of the kidney, with observations on the circulation through that gland. *Philos Trans R Soc London*. 1842;132:57-80. [In: Fulton JF. *Selected Readings in the History of Physiology*, 2nd ed. Springfield, IL: Charles C. Thomas; 1966, pp. 357-60.] KIDNEY FUNCTION **1493**

Boyd, William. *A Textbook of Pathology*, 7th ed. Philadelphia: Lea & Febiger; 1961, p. 5. MEDICAL CARE **1674**

Boyle, Robert.
A continuation of new experiments physico-mechanical, touching the spring and weight of the air, and their effects. The second part, 1682. RESPIRATION **2888**
In Kaplan BB. *Divulging of Useful Truths in Physick*. Baltimore: Johns Hopkins University Press; 1993. BODY FLUIDS **324** [92], PHYSICIANS **2552** [125], RESPIRATION **2884** [85], SCIENCE **2939** [50], TREATMENT **3333** [138]

Brahmanic saying. MEDICAL CARE **1707,**

Brain, Russell. The need for a philosophy of medicine. *Lancet*. 1953;1:959-64. MEDICAL PRACTICE **1950**, MEDICINE **2118**

Brandeis, Louis D. *Business: A Profession*. Boston: Small, Maynard; 1925, p. 2. PROFESSIONS **2689**

Braodbent, Walter. An unpublished physical sign. *Lancet*. 1895;2:200-1. PERICARDITIS **2503**

Braun-Menendez E, Fasciolo JC, Leloir LF, Muñoz JM. The substance causing renal hypertension. *J Physiol*. 1940;98:283-98. HYPERTENSION **1354**

Brenner S, Jacob F, Meselson M. An unstable intermediate carrying information from genes to ribosomes for protein synthesis. *Nature*. 1961;190:576-81. MESSENGER RIBONUCLEIC ACID (MRNA) **2158**

Bridges, Robert. *The Testament of Beauty*. New York: Oxford University Press; 1930, p. 6. RESEARCH **2864**

Brierre de Boismont, Alexandre-Jacques-François. History of the rise, progress, ravages etc. of the blue cholera of India. *Lancet*. 1831;1:241-87. CHOLERA **470**, FLUID ELECTROLYTE DISORDERS **1056**

Bright, Richard.
Reports of Medical Cases, Selected with a View of Illustrating the Symptoms and Cure of Disease by a Reference to Morbid Anatomy, vol. 1. London: Logman, Rees, Orme, Brown & Green; 1827, pp. 2,3. [In: Talbott JH. *A Biographical History of Medicine*, p. 1037 (q.v.).] KIDNEY DISEASE **1490**
Address given at the commencement of a course of lectures on the practice of medicine. London, 1832. CLINICAL OBSERVATION **508**
Observations on jaundice; more particularly on that form of the disease which accompanies the diffused inflammation of the substance of the liver. *Guy's Hosp Rep*. 1836;1:604-37. LIVER DISEASE **1563**

Brodie, Benjamin Collins. Experiments and observations on the influence of the nerves of the eighth pair on the secretions of the stomach. *Trans R Soc Lond*. 1814;1:102-6. VAGOTOMY **3419**

Brody, Elaine M. Long-term care for the elderly: optimums, options, and opportunities. *J Am Geriatr Soc*. 1971;19:482-93. AGING **90**

Brody, Howard.
Stories of Sickness. New Haven: Yale University Press; 1987, p. 3. MEDICAL PRACTICE **1963**
The lie that heals: the ethics of giving placeboes. *Ann Intern Med*. 1982;97:112-8. PLACEBOS **2612**

Bronowski, Jacob. *Science and Human Values*. New York: Harper & Row; 1965:60-1. SCIENCE **2979**

Brook, Robert H. Practice guidelines and practicing medicine. *JAMA*. 1989;262:3027-30. JUDGMENT **1475**, MEDICAL CARE **1697**

Brower, Daniel R.
In Devine ET (ed). The medical profession and social reform. *Bull Am Acad Med.* 1902;6:76-91. MEDICAL PROFESSION **1991**
The treatment of acute insanity in a general hospital. *JAMA.* 1906;47:83-5. PSYCHIATRY **2718**
Traumatic insanity and its medico-legal relations. *Chicago Med Examiner.* 1879;39:609-15. [In: Beatty WK. Daniel Roberts Brower: neurologist, psychiatrist, and medico-legal expert. Part II. *Proc Inst Med Chicago.* 1988;41:124-8.] INSANITY **1452**

Browne, John. A remarkable account of a liver, appearing glandulous to the eye. *Philos Trans R Soc London.* 1685;15:1266-8. [In: Major RH. *Classic Descriptions of Disease*, p. 693 (q.v.).] CIRRHOSIS OF THE LIVER **493**

Browne, Thomas.
Hydriotaphia or Urne Buriall. London: 1658. [Reprinted in Endicott NJ (ed). *The Prose of Sir Thomas Browne.* New York: New York University Press; 1968:282.] DEATH **658**
Religio Medici. London: 1643. Translated by Greenhill WA. London: Macmillan; 1926. AGING **60** (part I, sect. 42) [66], ANATOMY **148** (part I, sect. 36), DEATH **656** (part I, sect. 44) [69-70], **657** (part II, sect. 9) [85], LIFE **1537** (part II, sect. 11) [115], MEDICAL PROFESSION **1977** (part II, sect. 9) [113], PRENATAL LIFE **2665** (part I, sect. 39) [63], SEX **3027** (part II, sect. 9) [110-1], SLEEP **3072** (part II, sect. 12) [118]

Brownlee, John. *Germinal Vitality: A Study of the Growth of Nations as an Instance of a Hitherto Undescribed Factor in Evolution.* Glasgow: Carter & Pratt; 1908 [Limited data]. EPIDEMICS **967**

Brown-Séquard, Charles Edouard. Recherches expérimentales sur la physiologie et la pathologie des capsules surrénales. *Arch Gen Med.* 1856;2:385,572. ADRENAL GLANDS **43**

Broyard, Anatole.
Intoxicated by my illness. In: *Intoxicated by My Illness and Other Writings on Life and Mortality: A Posthumous Collection of Essays.* New York: Clarkson N. Potter; 1992. PATIENT-PHYSICIAN RELATIONS **2447**
The patient examines the doctor. In: *Intoxicated by My Illness and Other Writings on Life and Mortality: A Posthumous Collection of Essays.* New York: Clarkson N. Potter; 1992. DOCTORS **861** [53], MEDICAL CARE **1699** [57], PATIENT-PHYSICIAN RELATIONS **2448** [43]

Bruecke, Ernst Wilhelm von. In Krebs HA. Excursion into the boarderland of biochemistry and philosophy. *Johns Hopkins Hosp Bull.* 1954;95:45-51. TELEOLOGY **3271**

Brunton, Thomas Lauder. On the use of nitrite of amyl in angina pectoris. *Lancet.* 1867;2:97-8. ANGINA PECTORIS **183**

Bruyère, Jean de la. In Dana CL. Evil spoken of physicians. *Proc Charaka Club.* 1902:1;90. PATIENT-PHYSICIAN RELATIONS **2376**

Bryce, James. Speech given at a dinner honoring General William Crawford Gorgas, chief U.S. medical officer at the construction of the Panama Canal, March 23, 1914. [In: Strauss MB (ed). *Familiar Medical Quotations*, p. 300 (q.v.).] MEDICAL PROFESSION **2002**

Buchan, William. In: *Domestic Medicine: or, a treatise on the prevention and cure of diseases by regimen and simple medicines*, 1798. HYPOCHONDRIA **1368**, HYSTERIA **1399**, LEECHES **1530**, PATIENT-PHYSICIAN RELATIONS **2382**, PREVENTIVE MEDICINE **2676**

Buckman, Robert. *How To Break Bad News: A Guide for Health Care Professionals.* Baltimore: Johns Hopkins University Press; 1992. MEDICAL CARE **1700** [9], MORTALITY **2198** [21]

Bucknill, John Charles. *The Address of John Charles Bucknill, MD, President of the Association of Medical Officers of the Asylums and Hospitals for the Insane, at the General Meeting held at the Freemason's Tavern, London, July 5, 1860.* Exeter: 1860 [Limited data]. PSYCHIATRISTS **2709**

Budd, William.
Memorandum on the nature and the mode of propagation of phthisis. *Lancet.* 1867;2:451-2. TUBERCULOSIS **3384**
On the fever at the clergy orphan asylum. *Lancet.* 1856;2:617. [In: Bloomfield AL, *Communicable Diseases*, p. 7 (q.v.).] TYPHOID FEVER AND TYPHUS **3408**

Buddha. *A Buddhist Bible.* Goddard D; editor. Boston: Beacon Press; 1994:23. LIFE **1536**

Buerger, L. Thrombo-angiitis obliterans; a study of the vascular lesions leading to presenile spontaneous gangrene. *Am J Med Sci.* 1908;136:567-80. THROMBOANGIITIS OBLITERANS (BUERGER DISEASE) **3297**

Burgdorfer W, Barbour AG, Hayes SF, et al. Lyme disease: a tick-borne spirochetosis? *Science.* 1982;216:1317-9. LYME DISEASE **1596**

Burgess, Anthony. *You've Had Your Time.* London: Heinemann; 1990. DYING **927**

Burkitt, Denis Parsons. A sarcoma involving the jaws in African children. *Br J Surg.* 1958-1959;46:218-23. BURKITT TUMOR (AFRICAN LYMPHOMA) 360

Burman, Michael S.
Arthroscopy of the knee joint. *J Bone Joint Surg Am.* 1934;16:255-68. ARTHROSCOPY 238
Arthroscopy or the direct visualization of joints: an experimental cadaver study. *J Bone Joint Surg Am.* 1931;13:669-95. [694]. ARTHROSCOPY 237

Burnet, Frank Macfarlane. Life's complexities: misgivings about models. *Australasian Ann Med.* 1969;4:363-7. GENETICS 1107

Burnet, Macfarlane. *Changing Patterns: An Atypical Autobiography.* London: William Heinemann; 1968:251-2. MEDICAL CARE 1678, SPECIALIZATION 3113

Burney, Fanny. Letter to Esther Burney, 1811. [In: Dally A. *Women under the Knife: A History of Surgery.* London: Hutchinson Radius; 1991:108.] MASTECTOMY 1642

Burnham, Walter. Extirpation of the uterus and ovaries for sarcomatous disease. *Nelson's Am Lancet.* 1854;8:147. HYSTERECTOMY 1397

Burns, Allan. *Observations on Some of the Most Frequent and Important Diseases of the Heart.* Edinburgh: 1809. [Reprint: New York: Hafner; 1964, p. 138.] CORONARY ARTERY DISEASE 615

Burton, Henry. On a remarkable effect upon the human gums produced by the absorption of lead. *Med-Chir Trans.* 1840;23:63. [In: Major RH. *Classic Descriptions of Disease,* p. 351 (q.v.).] LEAD POISONING 1520

Burton, Richard F. *Personal Narrative of a Pilgrimage to El-Madinah and Meccah,* vol. 1. Boston: Shepard, Clark and Brown Memorial Edition; 1858, pp. 53-4. MEDICAL PRACTICE 1928

Burton, Robert. *The Anatomy of Melancholy,* 1621. DEPRESSION 712, MAGICAL MEDICINE 1597, MEDICAL CARE 1654

Bush, Vannevar. [Letter]. *Bull N Y Acad Med.* 1971;47:1274-5. AGING 91

Butler, Joseph. *The Analogy of Religion,* 1736. STATISTICS 3130

Butler, Robert N.
Another reason to protect Medicare and Medicaid. *N Engl J Med.* 1996;334:794-6. AGING 100
Geriatrics and internal medicine. *Ann Intern Med.* 1979;91:903-8. AGING 94

Butt H, Snell A. The use of vitamin K and bile in treatment of the hemorrhagic diathesis in cases of jaundice. *Proc Staff Meetings Mayo Clinic.* 1938;13:74-80. VITAMIN K 3446

Buzzard, Farquhar. Preparation for medical practice. *Lancet.* 1933;2:820. MEDICAL HISTORIES 1878

Byar, David P. Randomized clinical trials: perspectives on some recent ideas. *N Engl J Med.* 1976;295:74-80. MEDICAL ETHICS 1843

Byford, William H.
A Treatise on the Chronic Inflammation and Displacements of the Unimpregnated Uterus. Philadelphia: Lindsay & Blakiston; 1864, p. 98. [In: Beatty WK. William Heath Byford: physician and advocate for women. *Proc Inst Med Chicago.* 1986;39:6-23.] PHYSICAL EXAMINATION 2523
The Practice of Medicine and Surgery Applied to the Diseases and Accidents Incident to Women. Philadelphia: 1865. [In: Beatty WK. William Heath Byford: physician and advocate for women. *Proc Inst Med Chicago.* 1986;39:6-23.] LEECHES 1531
Advantages of the prone position in examining the foetal circulation as a diagnostic sign of pregnancy. *Chicago Med J.* 1858;15:77-9. [79]. STETHOSCOPE 3171
Address delivered to the Woman's Medical College of Chicago, April 22, 1884. *Chicago Med Examiner.* 1884;48:561-74. [In: Beatty WK. William Heath Byford: physician and advocate for women. *Proc Inst Med Chicago.* 1986;39:6-23.] WOMEN IN MEDICINE 3473
The successful extirpation of an encephaloid kidney. *Trans Am Gynecol Soc.* 1880;5:71-9. ANTISEPSIS 199

Byrne GI. The challenge of defining disease [Letter]. *Science.* 2001;293(5536):1766. DISEASE 803

Byron, George Gordon. *Don Juan,* canto IV, stanza 52; 1819. ALCOHOL 113

Cabot, Richard C.
Social Service and the Art of Healing. New York: Moffat, Yard; 1909, pp. 4-8. ETHNIC STEREOTYPING 1002
The use of truth and falsehood in medicine: an experimental study. *Am Med.* 1903;5:344-4. PATIENT-PHYSICIAN RELATIONS 2400

Cade, John Frederick Joseph. Lithium salts in the treatment of psychotic excitement. *Med J Aust.* 1949;2:349-52. PSYCHOSIS 2740

Cadwalader, Thomas. *An Essay on the West-India Dry-Gripes to Which Is Added an Extraordinary Case in Physick.* Philadelphia: Benjamin Franklin; 1745. [In: Major RH. *Classic Descriptions of Disease,* p. 301 (q.v.).] OSTEOMALACIA **2299**

Cameron, H. Charles. Recollections of Lister. *Br Med J.* 1948;2:221-2. LISTER, JOSEPH **1553**

Campion, Edward W. Why unconventional medicine? *N Engl J Med.* 1993;328:282-3. [283]. ALTERNATIVE MEDICINE **129**

Camus, Albert.
The Plague, part V, 1947. PLAGUE **2615**
The myth of Sisyphus. In *The Myth of Sisyphus and Other Essays.* New York: Vintage; 1983:61. LIVING **1573**

Cannon WB, Fraser J, Hooper AN. Some alterations in distribution and character of blood in shock and hemorrhage. *JAMA.* 1918;70:526-31. SHOCK **3061**

Cannon, Walter Bradford.
The Wisdom of the Body. New York: W.W. Norton; 1932 [In the Introduction]. HOMEOSTASIS **1310**
In Beveridge WIB. *The Art of Scientific Investigation,* 3rd ed. New York: Vintage Press; 1958, p. 207. SCIENCE **2976**
The movements of the stomach studied by means of the Rontgen rays. *Am J Physiol.* 1898;1:359-82. GASTRIC FUNCTION **1081**
The opposition to medical research. *JAMA.* 1908;51:635-50. VIVISECTION **3452**

Cardano, Girolamo. *De malo recentiorum medicorum medendi usu libellus.* Venice: 1536. [In: Major RH. *Classic Descriptions of Disease,* p. 163 (q.v.).] TYPHOID FEVER AND TYPHUS **3405**

Carey, Mathew. *A Short Account of the Malignant Fever, Lately Prevalent in Philadelphia.* Philadelphia: 1793. YELLOW FEVER **3515**

Carlyle, Thomas. Chartism: critical and miscellaneous essays. In *The Works of Thomas Carlyle,* vol. 20. London: Chapman and Hall; 1899, p. 125. [In: New York: AMS Press; 1969.] STATISTICS **3139**

Carnochan, John Murray. *Contributions to Operative Surgery and Surgical Pathology,* preface. Philadelphia: 1857. [In: Rutkow IM, *The History of Surgery in the United States,* p. 35.] SURGERY **3221**

Carrel, Alexis. Transplantation in mass of the kidneys. *J Exp Med.* 1908;10:98-140. KIDNEY TRANSPLANTATION **1504**

Carr-Hill, R. Welcome? to the brave new world of evidence based medicine. *Soc Sci Med.* 1995;41:1467-8. MEDICAL EVIDENCE **1858**

Carson, James. *Essays, Physiological and Practical.* Liverpool: F.B. Wright; 1820. [In: Talbott JH. *A Biographical History of Medicine,* p. 495 (q.v.).] PNEUMOTHORAX **2625**

Carson, Rachel. *Silent Spring.* Boston: Houghton Mifflin; 1962:6. POLLUTION **2639**

Cartier, Jacques. In Hakluyt R. *The Principal Navigations,* 1600. [In: Major RH. *Classic Descriptions of Disease,* pp. 587-9 (q.v.).] SCURVY **3013**

Casal y Julian, Gaspar. *Historia Natural y Medica de el Principado de Asturias.* Translated by Rivera y Miranda R. Madrid: 1762. [In: Major RH. *Classic Descriptions of Disease,* p. 669 (q.v.).] PELLAGRA **2477**

Cassel, Christine K. The patient-physician covenant: an affirmation of Asklepios. *Ann Intern Med.* 1996;124:604-6. MANAGED CARE **1620**, MEDICAL CARE **1702**

Cassell, Eric J.
The Healer's Art: A New Approach to the Doctor-Patient Relationship. New York: Lippincott; 1976. DECISION MAKING **692** [16], ILLNESS **1406** [48], MEDICAL EDUCATION **1793** [44], SCIENCE **2989** [6-7]
The changing concept of the ideal physician. *Daedalus.* 1986;115:185-208. PATIENTS **2469**
Why should doctors read medical books? *Ann Intern Med.* 1997;127:576-8. TEXTBOOKS **3290**
[Book review]. *N Engl J Med.* 1995;332:1523. DOCTORS **863**

Castellani, Aldo. Trypanosoma in sleeping sickness: report of a paper given to the Royal Society. *Br Med J.* 1903;1:1218. SLEEPING SICKNESS (TRYPANOSOMIASIS) **3078**

Castello Branco Rodrigues, Joao de. *Curationum Medicinalium Centuriae Quator.* Basel: 1556. [In: Major RH. *Classic Descriptions of Disease,* pp. 558-9 (q.v.).] PURPURA **2794**

Castle, William Bosworth. Observations on the etiologic relationship of achylia gastrica to pernicious anemia. *Am J Med Sci.* 1929;78:748-64. PERNICIOUS ANEMIA **2509**

Cathell, Daniel Webster. *The Physician Himself and What He Should Add to His Scientific Acquirements.* Baltimore: 1882:174. [In: Holt N. The business of medicine: the professionalization-commercialization boundary in nineteenth-century medical practice. *Pharos.* 1998;61:32-7.] MEDICAL PRACTICE **1929**, PATIENT-PHYSICIAN RELATIONS **2392**

Celsus, Aulus Cornelius. *On Medicine.* CANCER 369 (book 5), HIPPOCRATES 1287 (book 1), MALARIA 1600 (book 3), PATIENT-PHYSICIAN RELATIONS 2365 (book 3), RECONSTRUCTIVE SURGERY 2836 (book 7), SURGEONS 3192 (book 3), TREATMENT 3329 (book 1)

Cervantes, Miguel de. *Don Quixote de la Mancha,* 1605; book 3, ch. 1. DEATH 655

Cesalpino, Andrea. *Quaestiones Medicae,* book II, question 17. Venice: 1593. [In: Foster M. Harvey and the Circulation of the Blood, lecture 2. *Lectures on the History of Physiology During the 16th and 18th Centuries.* Cambridge, England: Cambridge University Press; 1901, p. 34.] HEART 1227

Cesaric, Dobrisa. *Poems.* 1953 [Limited data]. PAIN 2326

Chadwick, James Reed. The value of the bluish coloration of the vaginal entrance as a sign of pregnancy. *Trans Am Gynecol Soc.* 1887;11:339-418. PREGNANCY 2660

Chain EB, Florey HW, Gardner AD, et al. Penicillin as a chemotherapeutic agent. *Lancet.* 1940;2:226-8. PENICILLIN 2481

Chalmers, Thomas Clark.
Ann N Y Acad Sci. 1993;703:122 [Limited data]. MEDICAL EDUCATION 1799
In Maguire J. Doctors making decisions. *Harvard Publ Health Rev.* Spring-Summer 1992. CLINICAL TRIALS 558
In Spencer S. Thomas C. Chalmers: faculty profile. *Healthy News.* 1984;4:2. CLINICAL TRIALS 554, 555

Chang Y, Cesarman E, Pessin MS, et al. Identification of herpesvirus-like DNA sequences in AIDS-associated Kaposi's sarcoma. *Science.* 1994;266:1865-6. KAPOSI SARCOMA 1477

Chapin, Charles V. *How to Avoid Infection.* Cambridge, MA: Harvard University Press; 1917:61-2. HYGIENE 1345

Charaka.
Charaka Samhita. Jamnagar, India: Shree Gulabkunverba Ayurvedic Society; 1949;5:326. [In: Menon IA, Haberman HF. The medical students' oath of ancient India. *Med Hist.* 1969;13:295-9. Also see: Etziony MB. *The Physician's Creed: An Anthology of Medical Prayers, Oaths and Codes Written and Receited by Medical Practitioners Through the Ages.* Springfield, IL: Charles C Thomas; 1973.] MEDICAL ETHICS 1813, 1814
In Singh M. Oaths, codes, ethics and the essence of medicine: a time for resurrection. *Natl Med J India.* 1997;10:190-3. PATIENT-PHYSICIAN RELATIONS 2366

Charcot, Jean-Martin.
Clinical Lectures on Diseases of the Nervous System. Paris: 1880. [In: Talbott JH. A *Biographical History of Medicine,* p. 825-6 (q.v.).] MULTIPLE SCLEROSIS 2201
Leçons du mardi. Paris: 1889 [Translation by Goetz CD. In: *Charcot the Clinician: The Twenty Lessons.* New York: Raven Press; 1987:175]. CLINICAL OBSERVATION 512, RESEARCH 2860
Lectures on the Diseases of the Nervous System Delivered at La Salpetriere. London: The New Sydenham Society; 1881. POLIOMYELITIS 2635 [136], 2636 [129-30]
Tuesday's Lessons. Vienna; 1892. In: Charcot. *The Complete Psychological Works of Sigmund Freud,* vol. III. London: The Hogarth Press and The Institute of Psycho-Analysis; 1962:13. MEDICAL EPISTEMOLOGY 1808
Charcot's disease, amyotrophic lateral sclerosis: A case of glossolabial laryngeal paralysis [Lecture of February 28, 1888]. [In: Goetz CG, translator. *Charcot the Clinician: The Tuesday Lectures.* New York: Raven Press; 1987:175.] DOCTORS 828
In Daudet A. *In the Land of Pain.* Barnes J; translator. London: Jonathan Cape; 2002:23. PATIENT-PHYSICIAN RELATIONS 2394
In Fere C. Charcot et son oeuvre. *Rev Deux Mond.* 1929;122:410-24. CLINICAL RESEARCH 529

Chargaff E. Chemical specificity of nucleic acids and mechanism of their enzymatic degradation. *Experientia (Basel).* 1950;6:201-9. DEOXYRIBONUCLEIC ACID (DNA) 706

Charles, Sara C. *Realities of Medicine: September 9-13, 1985.* [Conference pamphlet]. Chicago: The University of Illinois College of Medicine at Chicago; 1985. MALPRACTICE 1617

Chekhov, Anton. Letter to A.S. Suvorin, September 11, 1888. [In: *Letters of Anton Chekhov.* Translated by Heim MH. New York: Harper & Row; 1973, p. 106.] MEDICAL PROFESSION 1987

Chen K-H, Murray GF. Truths and untruths in village Haiti: an experiment in Third World survey research. In Marshall JF, Polgar S (eds). *Culture, Natality, and Family Planning.* Carolina Population Center: University of North Carolina at Chapel Hill; 1976, p. 241-62. RESEARCH 2870

Chen Shih-kung. *An Orthodox Manual of Surgery,* 1618. [Translated in T'ao Lee. Medical ethics in ancient China. *Bull Hist Med.* 1943;13:268-77.] MEDICAL ETHICS 1815

Cheselden, William. *The Anatomy of the Human Body,* 1756. ARTERIOSCLEROSIS 232

Chesterton, Gilbert Keith.
Preface to Dickens, David Copperfield, 1911. MARRIAGE **1638**
In McClenahan JL. Remarks to incoming Fellows, presented at the College of Physicians of Philadelphia, June 22, 1995. *Trans Studies Coll Phys Philadelphia.* 1995;17:164-8. HEALTH **1187**
Mr H.G. Wells and the Giants. In *Heretics*. London: 1905. HEALTH **1186**

Chevers, Norman. Observations on the diseases of the orifice and valves of the aorta. *Guy's Hosp Rep.* 1842;7:387-442. AORTIC SUBVALVULAR STENOSIS **202**, PERICARDITIS **2502**

Cheyne, George. *The English Malady; or, a treatise on nervous diseases of all kinds.* London: 1733. EMOTIONAL DISORDERS **952**, PSYCHIATRY **2713**

Cheyne, John. A case of apoplexy in which the fleshy part of the heart was converted into fat. *Dublin Hosp Rep.* 1818;2:216-23. CHEYNE-STOKES RESPIRATION **457**

Childs, Barton. A logic of medicine. In Scriver CR, Beaudet AL, Sly WS, Valle D (eds). *The Metabolic and Molecular Bases of Inherited Disease*, 7th ed. New York: McGraw-Hill; 1995. DISEASE **802** [229], DOCTORS **862** [231]

Choo Q-L, Kuo G, Weiner AJ, et al. Isolation of a cDNA clone derived from a blood-borne non-A, non-B viral hepatitis genome. *Science.* 1989;244:359-62. HEPATITIS **1274**

Chung-Ching, Chang. In Wong KC, Lien-Teh W. *History of Chinese Medicine: Being a Chronicle of Medical Happenings in China from Ancient Times to the Present Period.* Tietsin: Tietsin Press; 1932, p. 46. DIAGNOSIS **731**

Churchill, James Morss. *Cases Illustrative of the Immediate Effects of Acupuncturation in Rheumatism, Lumbago, Sciatica, Anomalous Muscular Diseases, and in Dropsy of the Cellular Fluid: Selected from Various Sources and Intended as an Appendix to the Author's Treatise on the Subject.* London: Callow & Wilson; 1828, pp. 1,17,18. ACUPUNCTURE **34**

Churchill, Winston S.
The Gathering Storm. The Second World War, vol. 1. Boston: Houghton Mifflin; 1948:421. NAPS **2214**
In Reynolds Q. *By Quentin Reynolds.* New York: McGraw-Hill; 1963:225. ALCOHOL **115**

Cicero.
De divinatione, book II, sect. XXV. PATIENT-PHYSICIAN RELATIONS **2364**
De finibus, nos. 1,13. In Adler MJ, Doren CV (eds). *Great Treasury of Western Thought.* New York: R.R. Bowker; 1977, p. 1147. MEDICINE **2077**

Citois, François. *De Novo et Populari apud Pictones Dolore Colico Bilioso Diatriba.* Augustorii Pictonum: Antonium Mesnier; 1616. [In: Major RH. *Classic Descriptions of Disease*, p. 339 (q.v.).] LEAD POISONING **1516**

Clark, Alonzo. In Savitz HA. *A Jewish Physician's Harvest.* New York: Ktav Publishing House; 1979. [In: Altshule M. (Book review). *N Engl J Med.* 1980;302:415.] PATIENTS **2459**

Clark-Kennedy AE.
In Kelly M. The tempestuous winds of fashion. *Arch Intern Med.* 1962;110:283-9. PATIENTS **2467**
Value judgments in medical practice. *J R Coll Phys Lond.* 1970;5:5-12. MEDICAL CARE **1680**

Cleary J, Carbone PB. Pharmacologic management of cancer pain. *Hosp Pract.* 1995;30:41-9. MEDICAL PRACTICE **1965**

Cleaveland, Clif. *Sacred Space: Stories from a Life in Medicine.* Philadelphia: American College of Physicians; 1998. MANAGED CARE **1624** [xvi], MEDICAL CARE **1705** [xix]

Cleaveland, Ruzha. Doctor discontent [Letter]. *N Engl J Med.* 1999;340(8):651. MEDICAL PROFESSION **2019**

Clement III. In Alexandrov AV, Bladin CF, Meslin EM, Norris JW. Do-not-resuscitate orders in acute stroke. *Neurology.* 1995;45:634-40. AGING **56**

Clendening, Logan. *Source Book of Medical History.* New York: Paul B. Hober; 1942.

Coates, Albert E.
Clinical lessons from prisoner of war hospitals in the Far East, Burma and Siam. *Med J Aust.* 1946;1:753-60. WARTIME MEDICINE **3456**
The practice of surgery in Japanese prison camp hospitals in Burma and Siam. *Surgery.* 1946;19:743-7. PEPTIC ULCER **2491**

Cochrane, Archibald Leman.
Effectiveness and Efficiency: Random Reflections on Health Services. London: Nuffield Provincial Hospitals Trust; 1972. CLINICAL TRIALS **550** [68-9], **551** [24], **552** [7], DIAGNOSIS **753** [35-6], MEDICAL ECONOMICS **1712** [1], **1713** [85], MEDICAL EVIDENCE **1856** [20-1], TESTS **3278** [43], TREATMENT **3355** [31], WRITING **3508** [4]
One Man's Medicine: An Autobiography of Professor Archie Cochrane. London: The Memoir Club; 1989, p. 158. CLINICAL TRIALS **556**

1931-1971: A critical review with particular reference to the medical profession. In *Medicines for the Year 2000*. London: Office of Health Economics; 1979, pp. 1-11. CLINICAL TRIALS **553**

Code, Charles F. Reflections on histamine, gastric secretion, and the H2-receptor. *N Engl J Med.* 1977;296:1459-62. GASTRIC ACID SECRETION **1078**

Codman, Ernest Amory. *A Study in Hospital Efficiency as Demonstrated by the Case Report of the First Five Years of a Private Hospital.* Boston: 1916. [In: Joint Commission for the Accreditation of Health Care Organizations; 1996.] MEDICAL AUDIT **1648**, REFORM **2843** [Dedication]

Cohlan, Sidney Q. Excessive intake of vitamin A as a cause of congenital anomalies in the rat. *Science.* 1953;117:535-6. VITAMIN A **3434**

Cohn, Ferdinand Julius. *Bacteria: The Smallest of Living Organisms*, 1872. BACTERIA **276**

Cohnheim, Julius Friedrich. *Vorlesungen über Allgemeine Pathologie.* Berlin: Hirschwald; 1877:24. [In: Major RH. *Classic Descriptions of Disease*, p. 467 (q.v.).] CORONARY ARTERY DISEASE **617**

Coit, Henry L. In Rogers FB. *Help Bringers: Versatile Physicians of New Jersey.* New York: Vantage Press; 1960:122. CHILDREN **460**

Coleridge, Samuel Taylor. *Table Talk.* [In: Strauss MB (ed). *Familiar Medical Quotations*, p. 217 (q.v.).] MEDICAL CARE **1659**, PATIENT-PHYSICIAN RELATIONS **2385**

Colles, Abraham.
Practical Observations on the Venereal Diseases, and on the Use of Mercury. 1837. [In: *Medical Classics*, vol. 4. Baltimore: Williams & Wilkins; 1939-40, p. 10.] SEXUALLY TRANSMITTED DISEASES **3057**
Footnote in: Stokes W. *The Diseases of the Heart and the Aorta.* Hodges and Smith; 1854:265. CONGESTIVE HEART FAILURE **577**
On the fracture of the carpal extremity of the radius. *Edinburgh Med Surg J.* 1814;10:182-6. [In: Kelly EC, *Medical Classics*, vol. 4, pp. 1038-42.] COLLES FRACTURE **565**

Collin, V. *Sound Analogous to the Creaking of New Leather* [French]. Paris: Didot le Jeune; 1824, p. 44. [In: Major RH. *Classic Descriptions of Disease*, p. 444 (q.v.).] PERICARDITIS **2501**

Collip, James Bertram. The extraction of a parathyroid hormone which will prevent or control parathyroid tetany and which regulates the level of blood calcium. *J Biol Chem.* 1925;63:395-438. PARATHYROID GLANDS **2337**

Colomb MR. *De re anatomica [On Anatomy]*, book XV; 1559. [In: Coppola ED. The discovery of the pulmonary circulation: a new approach. *Bull Hist Med.* 1957;31:47-77.] PULMONARY CIRCULATION **2781**

Colombat, Marc. *Traité des Maladies des Femmes et de l'Hygiène Spéciale de leur Sexe.* Paris: 1838. [In: Dally A. *Women Under the Knife: A History of Surgery.* London: Hutchinson Radius; 1991, pp. 92-3.] MASTURBATION **1644**

Colombo, Matteo Realdo. *De re Anatomica Libri.* Venice: 1559. [In: Major RH. *Classic Descriptions of Disease*, p. 699 (q.v.).] GALLSTONES **1073**

Colwell NP. *Medical Education 1913-14: Report of Commissioner of Education*, 1914:207. MEDICAL LICENSURE **1908**

Combe, James Scarth. History of a case of anaemia. *Trans Med-Chir Soc Edinb.* 1824;1:193-8. [In: Major RH. *Classic Descriptions of Disease*, pp. 531-2.] PERNICIOUS ANEMIA **2506**

Committee for the Standardization of Blood Pressure Readings. Standardization of methods of measuring the arterial blood pressure: a joint report of the committees appointed by the Cardiac Society of Great Britain and Ireland and the American Heart Journal. *Br Heart J.* 1939;1:261-7. BLOOD PRESSURE **314**

Commoner, Barry.
The Closing Circle: Nature, Man, and Technology. New York: Alfred A. Knopf; 1971, p. 189. SCIENCE **2982**
Peering at peer review. *Hosp Pract.* 1978;13:25-29. PEER REVIEW **2475**

Comroe, Julius, Jr. Publish and/or perish. *Am Rev Respir Dis.* 1976;113:561-5. PUBLISHING **2770**

Conant, James Bryant. *Science and Common Sense.* New Haven, CT: Yale University Press; 1951: 44. SCIENCE **2987**

Conference of the Medical Royal Colleges and their Faculties in the United Kingdom. Diagnosis of brain death: statement issued by the honourary secretary of the Conference of the Medical Royal Colleges and their Faculties in the United Kingdom. *Br Med J.* 1976;2:1187-8. BRAIN DEATH **347**

Confucius. In Brallier JM. *Medical Wits and Wisdom: The Best Medical Quotations from Hippocrates to Groucho Marx.* Philadelphia: Running Press; 1993, p. 241. TREATMENT **3324**

Conn, Jerome W. Presidential address. Part II: Primary aldosteronism: a new clinical syndrome. *J Lab Clin Med.* 1955;45:3-17. ALDOSTERONE **125**

Connolly, Cyril. *The Unquiet Grave*, part I; 1945 [orig. published under the pseudonym Palinurus]. OBESITY **2282**

Crenshaw, Theresa. *Men, Women, Sex, and AIDS*. NBC-TV Interview. 13 Jan 1987. SEXUALLY
TRANSMITTED DISEASES 3060

Creutzfeldt, Hans Gerhard. Über eine eigenartige herdformige erkrankung des zentralnervensystems.
Zeitschr Gesamte Neurol Psychiatrie. 1920;57:1-18. [In: Rottenberg DA, Hochberg FH. *Neurological
Classics in Modern Translation*. New York: Hafner Press; 1977, pp. 97-112.] CREUTZFELDT-JAKOB
DISEASE 639

Crichton, Michael. [Book review of "In My Clinical Experience"]. *N Engl J Med*. 1971;285:1491. CLINICAL
EXPERIENCE 505

Crick FHC, Burnett L, Brenner S, Watts-Tobin RJ. General nature of the genetic code for proteins.
Nature. 1961;192:1227-32. GENETIC CODE 1094

Crick, Francis Harry Compton. On protein synthesis. *Symp Soc Exp Biol*. 1958;12:138-63. PROTEIN 2701

Croatian proverbs. AGING 103, BREAST FEEDING 351, DENTAL HEALTH 700, 701, DYING 932, HEALTH
1209, 1210, ILLNESS 1414, MAGICAL MEDICINE 1598, NUTRITION 2278, PEPTIC ULCER 2494,
PHYSICIANS 2596, PREVENTIVE MEDICINE 2686, TOXINS 3319

Crohn BB, Ginzburg L, Oppenheimer GD. Regional ileitis; a pathologic and clinical entity. *JAMA*.
1932;99:1323-9. CROHN DISEASE 642

Cronin, Archibald Joseph. *The Citadel*. Boston: Little, Brown; 1965, p. 364. MEDICAL PROFESSION 2008

Croone, William. *On the Reason of the Movement of the Muscles*, 1667. MUSCLE 2211

Crosby, William H. They don't use multiple-choice tests to license airline pilots. *Forum Med*. 1980;3:467-
90. PATIENT-PHYSICIAN RELATIONS 2433

Cruveilier, Jean. *Anatomie Pathologique du Corps Humain*. Paris: 1829-1842. [In: Major RH. *Classic
Descriptions of Disease*, p. 688 (q.v.).] GASTRIC ULCER 1085, PEPTIC ULCER 2487

Culpeper, Nicholas.
A *Directory for Midwives, or a Guide for Women in Their Conception, Bearing, and Suckling Their
Children*. London: 1660. CLITORIS 561 [22], OVARIES 2307 [29], PENIS 2484 [20], SEX 3028 [68],
TESTES 3274 [11]

In Chance B. Nicholas Culpeper: student in physick and astrologie. *Ann Med Hist*. 1931;3:394-403. [In:
Coope R (ed). *The Quiet Art*, p. 175 (q.v.).] MEDICAL ETHICS 1818

Cumings, John Nathaniel. The copper and iron content of brain and liver in the normal and in hepatolenticular degeneration. *Brain*. 1948;71:410-5. HEPATOLENTICULAR DEGENERATION (WILSON
DISEASE) 1276

Curie P, Curie MS. A new radioactive substance contained in pitchblende. *C R Acad Sci*. 1898;127:175-8.
[In: Talbott JH. *A Biographical History of Medicine*, p. 998 (q.v.).] POLONIUM 2641

Curie P, Curie MS, Bemont G. A new highly radioactive substance contained in pitchblende. *C R Acad
Sci*. 1898;127:1215-7. RADIUM 2822

Curling, Thomas Blizzard.
On acute ulceration of the duodenum, in cases of burn. *Med-Chir Trans*. 1842;7:260-81. [In: Talbott JH.
A Biographical History of Medicine, p. 570 (q.v.).] CURLING ULCER 644

Two cases of absence of the thyroid body, and symmetrical swellings of fat tissue at the sides of the
neck, connected with defective cerebral development. *Med-Chir Trans*. 1850;33:303. [In: Major RH.
Classic Descriptions of Disease, pp. 283-4 (q.v.).] HYPOTHYROIDISM 1390

Currie, Edwina. *The Observer*, 15 February 1987. ACQUIRED IMMUNE DEFICIENCY SYNDROME (AIDS) 30

Cushing, Harvey.
The Life of William Osler. Volume II. Oxford: Clarendon Press; 1925:229. DEATH 670

William Osler, the Man. In *Consecratio Medici and Other Papers*. Boston: Little, Brown; 1928, p. 98.
OSLER, WILLIAM 2297

Letter to Dr. Henry Christian, 20 November 1911. SURGERY 3231

Psychiatrists, neurologists, and the neurosurgeon. In *Neurological Biographies and Addresses*, foundation
vol. London: Oxford University Press; 1936, pp. 30-1. MEDICAL PROFESSION 2007

The basophil adenomas of the pituitary body and their clinical manifestations (pituitary basophilism).
Bull Johns Hopkins Hosp. 1932;50:137-95. CUSHING SYNDROME 645

The humanizing of science. *Science*. 1935;81:137-55. RESEARCH 2865, SOCIAL WELFARE 3101,
TREATMENT 3352

Cutler EC, Levine SA. Cardiotomy and valvulotomy for mitral stenosis: experimental observations and
clinical notes concerning an operated case with recovery. *Boston Med Surg J*. 1923;188:1023-7.
HEART SURGERY 1250

Cutler EC, Levine SA, Beck CS. The surgical treatment of mitral stenosis: experimental and clinical studies. *Arch Surg*. 1924;9:689-821. ATRIAL FIBRILLATION 263

Da Costa, Jacob M.
Address to the Harvard Medical Alumni Association, June 27, 1893. Boston: G.H. Ellis; 1893. [In: Talbott JH. *A Biographical History*, pp. 1134-5 (q.v.).] MEDICAL EDUCATION **1752**
In Manning PR, DeBakey L. *Medicine: Preserving the Passion.* New York: Springer-Verlag; 1987, p. 31. LEARNING **1524**

Da Costa, John Chalmers.
Suicide. Address to the American Philosophical Society, October 7, 1910. [In: *Selections from the Papers and Speeches of John Chalmers da Costa.* Philadelphia: WB Saunders; 1931.] MENSTRUATION **2152**, SUICIDE **3186, 3187**
The Old Jefferson Hospital [Address given at the opening of Jefferson Medical College Hospital, Philadelphia, June 7, 1907]. In: *Selections from the Papers and Speeches of John Chalmers da Costa.* Philadelphia: WB Saunders; 1931:218-9. MEDICAL PROGRESS **2022**
The trials and triumphs of the surgeon. *N Y Med J.* 1915;15:709-18. CHARACTER **454**, EXPERIENCE **1029**, MEDICAL PROFESSION **2003**, PATIENT-PHYSICIAN RELATIONS **2404**, SURGEONS **3204**

Dailey UG, Grant WS. Vasovesiculitis simulating acute appendicitis. *Med J Rec.* 1924;119(Suppl):147-8. RECTAL EXAMINATION **2839**

Dailey, Ulysses Grant.
The future of medicine. *J Natl Med Assoc.* 1916;8:175-9. PUBLISHING **2763**
Until the doctor comes. *Chicago Defender* 02 Jan 1943. [In: Beatty WK. Ulysses Grant Dailey: surgeon, teacher, and ambassador. *Proc Inst Med Chicago.* 1985;38:140-51.] PATIENT-PHYSICIAN RELATIONS **2410**

Dale, Henry Hallett. Nomenclature of fibres in the autonomic nervouse system and their effects. *J Physiol.* 1933;80:10P-11P. NERVOUS SYSTEM **2242**

Dalton, John Call Jr. Address to the College of Physicians and Surgeons, New York, c. 1855. [In: Talbott JH. *A Biographical History of Medicine*, p. 631 (q.v.).] MEDICAL PROFESSION **1983**

D'Amato, Cintio. *On the Correct Method of Making Incisions in Veins of the Hand, and on Their Treatment* [Italian], ch. XIX. Venice; 1669. [Translation by Smith JF reprinted in Fayette, MO: Hooker Scientific Library, Central College; 1940. [In: Clendening L. *Source Book of Medical History*, pp. 286-7 (q.v.).] BLOODLETTING **323**

Dan, Bruce B. In Lyons RD. Scientists find even mild exercise prolongs life. *New York Times.* 27 Jul 1984, p. B7. EXERCISE **1022**

Dane DS, Cameron CH, Briggs M. Virus-like particles in serum of patients with Australia-antigen associated hepatitis. *The Lancet.* 1970;1(7649):695-8. DANE PARTICLE **647**

Daniel, Samuel. *The Queenes Arcadia*, 1606. SYNDROME **3251**

Darwin, Charles.
Autobiography. Edited by Barlow N. New York: Harcourt, Brace; 1959, p. 137. THINKING **3293**
The Descent of Man, 1871, chapter 5. MEDICAL CARE **1660**
The Origin of Species. London; 1859. [In: *Great Books of the Western World*, vol. 49. Chicago: Encyclopaedia Britannica; 1952, p. 243]. LIFE **1539**
The Variation of Animals and Plants Under Domestication, vol. 2. New York: D. Appleton; 1897, pp. 372-3. INFECTIOUS DISEASE **1434**
In Darwin F (ed). *The Life and Letters of Charles Darwin*, vol. 1. 1888. [In: New York: Appleton-Century-Crofts; 1959, p. 83]. SCIENCE **2963**
Letter to Charles Lyell, 1859. [In: Darwin F, editor. *The Life and Letters of Charles Darwin*, volume 1. New York: Basic Books; 1959:524.] RESEARCH **2853**
Letter to Henry Fawcett. [In: *More Letters of Charles Darwin: a record of his work in a series of hitherto unpublished letters.* Darwin F, editor. New York: D. Appleton; 1903; letter 133, volume 1, p. 195.] HYPOTHESIS **1385**

Daudet, Alphonse. *In the Land of Pain.* Barnes J; translator. London: Jonathan Cape; 2002:19. PAIN **2321**

Davidoff, Frank. Time. *Ann Intern Med.* 1997;127:483-5. MEDICAL ECONOMICS **1726**

Davidoff, Leo M. Migraine. In Pinner M, Miller BF (eds). *When Doctors Are Patients.* New York: WW Norton; 1952:97-8. MIGRAINE **2170**

Davies, Robertson.
Can a Doctor Be a Humanist? [The David Coit Gilman lecture given at Johns Hopkins Medical School, November 18, 1984]. [In: *The Merry Heart.* Toronto: McClelland & Stewart; 1996.] MEDICINES **2144** [92], PATIENT-PHYSICIAN RELATIONS **2438** [107-8], **2439** [95], SCIENCE **2996** [98], WISDOM **3463** [105]
The Cunning Man. Toronto: McClelland & Steward; 1994. DEATH **682** [95], ENVIRONMENT **964** [259-60], GERIATRICS **1115** [438-9], HYSTERIA **1400** [431], MEDICAL PRACTICE **1964** [413], PATIENTS **2470** [164-5], WISDOM **3464**

Davison, Wilburt C. In Barnes RH. You have a good sense of humor; you should be a doctor. *Pharos.* Fall 1991, p. 28. TEXTBOOKS **3289**

Day, Hughes W. Preliminary studies of an acute coronary care unit. *Lancet.* 1963;83:53-5. CORONARY CARE UNITS **634**

DeBakey ME. A surgical perspective. *Ann Surg.* 1991:213;499-531. [526-7]. SURGERY **3245**

Defoe, Daniel. *A Journal of the Plague Year,* 1722. BUBONIC PLAGUE **358**

Dekkers, Frederik. *Exercitationes Medicae Practicae circa Medendi Methodum.* Leyden: 1673. [In: Major RH. *Classic Descriptions of Disease,* p. 572 (q.v.).] PROTEINURIA **2702**

DeLillo, Don. *White Noise.* New York: Penguin Books; 1986. PATIENT-PHYSICIAN RELATIONS **2440** [75-6], **2441** [77]

Derbes, Vincent J. Psoriasis. *Ration Drug Ther.* 1981;15:1-6. DERMATOLOGY **721**

Descartes, René. *A Discourse on Method,* part VI. 1637. [In: *A Discourse on Method and Selected Writings.* Translated by Veitch J. New York: Dutton; 1951, p. 54.] MEDICINE **2087**

DeVita VT, Serpick AA, Carbone PP. Combination chemotherapy in the treatment of advanced Hodgkin's disease. *Ann Intern Med.* 1970;73:881-95. HODGKIN DISEASE **1305**

D'Herelle FH. Sur une microbe invisible antagoniste des bacilles dysentérique. *Comptes Rendus Acad Sci.* 1917;165:373-5. BACTERIOPHAGE **280**

Diamond, Louis Klein. Replacement transfusion as a treatment of erythroblastosis fetalis. *Pediatrics.* 1948;2:520-4. ERYTHROBLASTOSIS FETALIS **997**

Diamond, Seymour. Healthtalk: a pain in the head. *The New York Times.* 28 Dec 1979, p. D5. MIGRAINE **2173**

Dicke WK, Weijers HA, van de Kamer JH. Coeliac disease. Part II: The presence in wheat of a factor having a deleterious effect in cases of coeliac disease. *Acta Paediatr.* 1953;42:34-42. CELIAC DISEASE **446**

Dickens, Charles. *The Pickwick Papers,* ch. 30, 1837. MEDICAL STUDENTS **2059**

Dickinson, Emily.
Pain - has an element of blank -, 1862. PAIN **2318**
Surgeons must be very careful, 1859. SURGERY **3222**

Dickinson, Frances. *The Gynecologic Consideration of the Sexual Act.* Chicago; 1900. [In: Beatty WK. Francis Dickinson: ophthalmologist and flier. *Proc Inst Med Chicago.* 1985;38:10-5.] SCIENCE **2967**

Dickinson, William Howship. Notes of four cases of intermittent haematuria. *Lancet.* 1865;1:568-9. [In: Major RH. *Classic Descriptions of Disease,* p. 595 (q.v.).] PAROXYSMAL HEMOGLOBINURIA **2344**

Didache, or the Teaching of the Twelve Apostles. 2:2. In: Ancient Christian Writers: The Works of the Fathers in Translation. Kleist JA, translator. Westminster, MD: The Newman Press; 1948:16. ABORTION **5**

Didion, Joan. In bed. In *The White Album.* New York: Simon & Schuster; 1979, p. 171. MIGRAINE **2172**

Dinnerstein, Dorothy. *The Mermaid and the Minotaur: Sexual Arrangements and Human Malaise.* New York: Harper & Row; 1976:188. DEPENDENCY **711**

Dioscorides, Pedanius. *De Materia Medica.* c. 77. [In: Gunther RT (ed). *The Greek Herbal of Dioscorides.* New York: Hafner Publishing; 1968.] SALICYLATES **2924**

Disraeli, Benjamin.
The Young Duke, 1831. MARRIAGE **1636**
Attributed. STATISTICS **3145**
Speech, June 23, 1877. HEALTH **1181**

Dobson, Matthew. Experiments and observations on the urine in a diabetes. *Med Observations Inquiries.* 1776;5:298. [In: Major RH. *Classic Descriptions of Disease,* p. 257 (q.v.).] DIABETES MELLITUS **726**

Dochez, Alphonse Raymond. *P&S Quarterly.* Jun 1966, vol. 2, p. 18. RESEARCH **2869**

Dock, George. Some notes on the coronary arteries. *Med Surg Reporter.* 1896;75:1. [In: Major RH. *Classic Descriptions of Disease,* pp. 469-70 (q.v.).] CORONARY ARTERY DISEASE **619**

Dock, William.
In Weisse AB. *Conversations in Medicine: The Story of Twentieth-Century American Medicine in the Words of Those Who Created It.* New York: New York University Press; 1984. CORONARY ARTERY DISEASE **630** [33-4], DIURETICS **806** [20], PULMONARY EMBOLISM **2785** [28], THIOURACIL DRUGS **3295** [31]
Korotkoff's sounds. *N Engl J Med.* 1980;302:1264-6. DISCOVERY **777**
Medical Grand Rounds. New York: Morrisania City Hospital; 1968 [Unpublished]. OBSTETRICS **2287**
Medical Grand Rounds. New York: Morrisania City Hospital; 1970 [Unpublished]. RARE DISEASES **2823**

Dodrill FD, Hill E, Gerisch R. Some physiologic aspects of the artificial heart problem. *J Thorac Surg.* 1952;24:134-50. HEART SURGERY **1254**

Doll WRS, Hill AB. Smoking and carcinoma of the lung: preliminary report. *Br Med J.* 1950;2:739-48. SMOKING **3096**

Donné, Alfred. De l'origine des globules du sang, de leur mode de formation et de leur fin. *Comptes rendus de l'Académie des Sciences.* 1842;14:166-8. [In: Wintrobe MM. *Blood: Pure and Elegant: A Story of Discovery, of People, and of Ideas.* New York: McGraw-Hill; 1980:550. Also in: Spaet TH. Platelets: the blood dust. [Limited data.] PLATELETS (THROMBOCYTES) **2617**

Donne, John.
Devotions upon Emergent Occasions, 1624. ILLNESS **1401**, PATIENT-PHYSICIAN RELATIONS **2373**
Sermon XX. DISEASE **781**

Dormandy TL. In praise of peroxidation. *Lancet.* 1988:2:1126-8. NATURE **2224**

Dorsey, John Syng. *Elements of Surgery: For the Use of Students,* preface. Philadelphia: Edward Parker & Kimber & Conrad; 1813. [In: Rutkow IM, *The History of Surgery in the United States,* p. 4.] SURGERY **3219**

Douglas CG, Haldane JS, Henderson Y, Schneider EC. Physiological observations made on Pike's Peak, Colorado, with special reference to adaptation to low barometric pressures. *Philos Trans R Soc London B Biol Sci.* 1913;203:185-318. BALLISTOCARDIOGRAPHY **284**

Douglass, William. *A Summary, Historical and Political, of the Present State of the British Settlements of North America,* vol. 2. Boston; 1755. AMERICAN MEDICINE **138**, MEDICAL PRACTICE **1919**

Dover, Thomas. *The Ancient Physician's Legacy to his Country,* 5th ed. London: 1733. [In: Talbott JH. *A Biographical History of Medicine,* p. 169 (q.v.).] PUBLISHING **2757**

Dowell, Greensville. *A Treatise on Hernia: With a New Process for Its Radical Cure, and Original Contributions to Operative Surgery, and New Surgical Instruments,* preface. Philadelphia: D.G. Brinton; 1876. [In: Rutkow IM, *The History of Surgery in the United States,* vol. 1, p. 71 (q.v.).] HERNIAS **1279**

Doyle, Arthur Conan.
A Scandal in Bohemia. In: *The Adventures of Sherlock Holmes,* 1892. MEDICAL EVIDENCE **1854**
Behind the Times. In: *Round the Red Lamp,* 1894. DOCTORS **832**
The Romance of Medicine. In: *Round the Red Lamp,* 1894. CONSULTATION **587**, DOCTORS **831**, MEDICAL CARE **1662**, MEDICAL EDUCATION **1753**, **1754**
The Surgeon Talks. In: *Round the Red Lamp,* 1894. MEDICAL PROFESSION **1989**, **1990**

Drinker P, McKhann CF. The use of a new apparatus for the prolonged administration of artificial respiration. Part I: A fatal case of poliomyelitis. *JAMA.* 1929;92:1658-60. POLIOMYELITIS **2637**

Druez G. Un nouveau cas d'acantrocytose: dysmorphie érythrocytaire congenitale ave rétinite, troubles nerveux et stigmates dégénératifs. *Rev Hematol.* 1959;14:3-11. ACANTHOCYTOSIS **21**

Drummond, Jack Cecil.
Note on the role of the antiscorbutic factor in nutrition. *Biochem J.* 1919;13:77-80. VITAMIN C (ASCORBIC ACID) **3442**
The nomenclature of the so-called accessory food factors (vitamins). *Biochem J.* 1920;14:660. VITAMINS **3448**

Dryden, John. *Epistle to John Driden of Chesterton,* 1700. EXERCISE **1018**

Drzic, Marin. *Tirena.* 1549. [In: Kekez J. *Svaki je Kamen da se Kuca Gradi.* Osijek: Publishing Center of the Open University; 1990. Limited data.] PHYSICIAN HEALTH **2534**

Dubos, René Jules.
Man Adapting. New Haven, CT: Yale University Press; 1965. ACADEMIC HEALTH CENTERS **17** [447], POLLUTION **2640** [196-220]
Man, Medicine, and Environment. New York: Frederick A. Praeger; 1968. ADAPTATION **37** [85], **38** [87-8], DISEASE **792** [13-4], **793** [67], ENVIRONMENT **961** [85], **962** [94], **963** [41], ENVIRONMENTAL ILLNESS **965** [82], EVOLUTION **1011** [85], GENETICS **1106** [37-8], HEALTH **1198** [61], HUMANS **1338** [43], MEDICAL CARE **1679** [103], MEDICAL ETHICS **1840** [106], MEDICAL PRACTICE **1953** [66], **1954** [66], MEDICAL RESEARCH **2032** [105], MEDICAL SERVICES **2055** [103], MEDICINE **2122** [53], PHYSICIANS **2588** [94], PREVENTIVE MEDICINE **2680** [98], **2681** [93], PSYCHOSOMATIC MEDICINE **2745** [65]
Mirage of Health. Garden City, NY: Doubleday; 1959:230. HUMANS **1336**
The White Plague: Tuberculosis, Man, and Society. Boston: Little, Brown; 1952, p. 196-225. TUBERCULOSIS **3404**
Man versus environment. *Ind Med Surg.* 1961;30:369-73. DISEASE **790**
The three faces of medicine. *Bull Am Coll Phys.* 1961;2:162-6. HEALTH **1196**

Duchenne, Guillaume Benjamin Amand.
De l'electrisation localisée et de son application à la physiologie et la pathologie et à la therapeutique, 1855. POLIOMYELITIS **2632**

Recherches sur la paralysie musculaire pseudohypertophique, ou paralysie myosclérosique. *Arch Gen Med.* 1868;1:5-25, 179-209, 305-21, 421-43, 552-88. PSEUDOHYPERTROPHIC MUSCULAR DYSTROPHY (DUCHENNE MUSCULAR DYSTROPHY) **2706**

Duffy, Daniel F. Dialogue: the core clinical skill. *Ann Intern Med.* 1998;128:139-41. MEDICAL EDUCATION **1806**

Dumas, Alexandre. *The Count of Monte Cristo,* 1845, chapter 81. DEATH **662**, PHYSICIANS **2567**

Duncan, Allan. *Medicine, Madams and Mounties: Stories of a Yukon Doctor,* 1947. Vancouver: Raincoast Books; 1989 [reprint]. DEATH **673**

Dundas, David. An account of a peculiar disease of the heart. *Med-Chir Trans.* 1809;1:37. ANGINA PECTORIS **181**

Dunlop, E.E. Surgical treatment of dysenteric lesions of the bowel among allied prisoners of war in Burma and Thailand. *Br Med J.* 1946;1:124-7. WARTIME MEDICINE **3457**

Dunne, Peter Finley. Christian science. In *Mr. Dooley's Opinions.* New York: R.H. Russell; 1901, p. 9. NURSES **2269**

Dupuytren, Guillaume. In Paillard A, Marx M. Permanent retraction of the fingers. *Clinical Lectures on Surgery.* Translated by Doane AS. New York: Collins & Hannay Publishers; 1833, pp. 14-25. DUPUYTREN CONTRACTION **900**

Durant, Thomas M. *Temple Univ Med Cent Bull.* 1961;7:4 [Limited data]. CONTROVERSY **604**

Duroziez, Paul Louis.

Pure mitral stenosis [French]. *Arch Med Gen.* 1877;30:32-54,184-97. [In: Talbott JH. A *Biographical History of Medicine,* p. 1116 (q.v.).] MITRAL STENOSIS **2194**

The intermittent double femoral murmur in aortic insufficiency. *Arch Gen Med.* 1861;17:417-43. AORTIC VALVE REGURGITATION **212**

Duvall, Evelyn Millis. *Love and the Facts of Life.* New York: Association Press; 1967:168. SEX **3040**

Earle, Charles Warrington.

Chicago Med Recorder. 1891;2:347. ALCOHOLISM **122**

Report of the special committee on antiseptic obstetrics. *Trans Illinois State Med Soc.* 1888;38:154-75. ABORTION **9**

Simple but efficient medication in pediatrics. *Arch Pediatr.* 1891;8:17-23. [In: Beatty WK. Charles Warrington Earle: soldier, optimist, and hard worker. *Proc Inst Med Chicago.* 1990;43:124-42.] TREATMENT **3347**

The opium habit: a statistical and clinical lecture. *Chicago Med Rev.* 1880;2:442-6. RESPONSIBILITY **2894**

Ebstein, Wilhelm. *The Regimen to be Adopted in Cases of Gout.* London: JA Churchill; 1885:1-3. [In: Porter R, Rousseau GS. *Gout: The Patrician Malady.* New Haven, CT: Yale University Press; 1998:186.] GENETICS **1098**

Egeberg, Roger. AMAgrams. *JAMA.* 1969;210:2335. PEER REVIEW **2473**

Ehrenreich, Barbara.

Food worship. In *Worst Years of Our Lives.* New York: Pantheon; 1990, p. 20. EXERCISE **1023**

Welcome to Cancerland. *Harper's Magazine,* September 2001. CANCER OF THE BREAST **401** [52], **402** [48]

Ehrlich, Paul.

Closing Notes on Experimental Chemotherapy of Spirilloses. Berlin: J. Springer; 1910. [In: Talbott JH. A *Biographical History of Medicine,* p. 992 (q.v.).] PUBLIC HEALTH **2753**, SYPHILIS **3266**

A method for staining the tubercle bacillus [German]. *Dtsch Med Wochenschr.* 1882;8:269-70. [In: Brock TD (ed). *Milestones in Microbiology.* Englewood Cliffs, NJ: Prentice Hall; 1961, p. 119.] TUBERCULOSIS **3388**

Die Wertbestimmung des Diphtherieheilserums und deren theoretische Grundlagen. *Klinisches Jahrbuch.* 1897;6:299-326. [In: Tanford C, Reynolds J. *Nature's Robots: A History of Proteins.* Oxford: Oxford University Press; 2001:176.] ANTIBODIES **196**

On immunity, with especial reference to the relations existing between the distribution and the action of antigens. In *Harben Lectures,* lecture 1. London; 1908. [In: Clendening L. *Source Book of Medical History,* p. 418 (q.v.).] IMMUNITY **1416**

Einstein, Albert. In Maslow AH. *Motivation and Personality,* 2nd ed. New York: Harper & Row; 1970, p. 154. SCIENCE **2978**

Einthoven, Willem. The galvanometric registration of the human electrocardiogram, likewise a review of the use of capillary-electrometer in physiology. *Arch Ges Physiol.* 1903;99:472-80. [In: Willius FA, Keys TE, *Cardiac Classics*, p. 723 (q.v.).] ELECTROCARDIOGRAPHY **946**

Eisenberg, Leon. In: Markel H. So what's a responsible sun worshiper to do? *New York Times.* 2002;Aug 25:1,3. SCIENCE **3004**

Ekbom, Karl-Axel.

Asthenium crurum paraesthetica ("irritable legs"): a new syndrome consisting of weakness, sensation of cold and nocturnal paresthesia in the legs, responding to a certain extent to treatment with Priscol and Doryl. *Acta Med Scandinavica.* 1944;118:197-209. RESTLESS LEG SYNDROME **2900**

Restless legs: a clinical study. *Acta Med Scandinavica Suppl.* 1945;158:1-123. RESTLESS LEG SYNDROME **2901**

Eliot, George. *Middlemarch*, 1871. AUTOPSIES **271** [ch. 45], DOCTORS **824** [ch. 10], MEDICAL PROFESSION **1986** [ch. 16]

Eliot, Thomas Stearns. Whispers of immortality, 1920. DEATH **669**

Elkinton JR, Graham, JR. Forty-five years of migraine: observations and reflections "from the inside" by a physician-patient. *Cephalalgia.* 1985;5:185-95. MIGRAINE **2174**

Elkinton, J. Russell. When do we let the patient die? *Ann Intern Med.* 1968;68(3):695-9. MEDICAL ETHICS **1839**

Ellard, John. Emotional reactions associated with death. *Med J Aust.* 1968;1:979-83. PATIENT-PHYSICIAN RELATIONS **2423**

Elvehjem CA, Madden RJ, Strong FM, Woolley DW. The isolation and identification of the anti-black tongue factor. *J Biol Chem.* 1938;123:137-49. VITAMIN B$_{12}$ (CYANOCOBALAMIN) **3440**

Emanuel, Elliott. [Letter]. *CMAJ.* 1969;101:175. PSYCHIATRY **2719**

Emerson, Ralph Waldo. Work and days. In *Society and Solitude*, ch. 8. 1870. [In: Boston: Houghton, Mifflin; 1904, p. 158.] SCIENCE **2961**

Epstein, Joseph. Taking the bypass. *New Yorker.* 1999;Apr 12:61. SURGERY **3246**

Erasmus, Desiderius.

In Praise of the Healing Arts, 1518. MEDICINE **2083**

In poor health. *Colloquies*, 1518. PHYSICIANS **2545**

The funeral. *Colloquies*, 1518. DYING **903**

Erikson, Erik H. *Insight and Responsibility.* New York: W.W. Norton; 1964, pp. 236-7. HIPPOCRATES **1288**

Esmarch, Johann Friedrich August von. The art of bloodless operation [German]. *Samm Klin Vortr.* 1873;58:373-84. [In: Talbott JH. A *Biographical History of Medicine*, pp. 672-3 (q.v.).] ESMARCH BANDAGE **999**

Esquirol, Jean-Étienne-Dominique.

Des Maladies Mentales. Paris: 1838. DEMENTIA **698**

De la hypémanie ou mélancholie. In: *Des maladies mentales.* Paris: 1838. [In: Shorter E. A *History of Psychiatry: From the Era of the Asylum to the Age of Prozac.* New York: John Wiley & Sons; 1997:29.] MANIC-DEPRESSIVE ILLNESS **1629**

Euripides. *Electra*, ll. 426-9. FEES **1047**

Evans HM, Bishop KS. On the existence of a hitherto unrecognized dietary factor essential for reproduction. *Science.* 1922;56:650-1. VITAMIN E **3445**

Evelyn, John. Diary. BREAST FEEDING **350** [24 Aug. 1688], MALARIA **1601** [27 Jan. 1658], SURGERY **3214** [3 May 1650], **3215** [24 March 1672]

Ewing, James. Diffuse endothelioma of bone. *Proc N Y Pathol Soc.* 1921;21:17-24. EWING SARCOMA **1014**

Fabricius, Hieronymus.

De Venarum Ostiolis, 1603. VEINS **3423**

Surgical Works. Lyons: 1649. UMBILICAL VESSELS **3410**

Falloppio, Gabrielle. In Fulton JF. *Selected Readings in the History of Physiology.* Springfield, IL: Charles C. Thomas, 1966. [In: Talbott JH. A *Biographical History of Medicine*, pp. 67-8.] FALLOPIAN TUBES **1037**

Fallot, Étienne-Louis-Arthur. Contribution to the pathologic anatomy of morbus caeruleus (cardiac cyanosis). *Marseilles Med.* 1888;25:418-20. [In: Willius FA, Keys TE, *Cardiac Classics*, p. 689 (q.v.).] CONGENITAL HEART DISEASE (TETRALOGY OF FALLOT) **576**

Fanconi G, von Albertini A, Zellweger H. Osteopathia acidotica pseudorachitica. *Helvetica Paediatrica Acta.* 1948;2:95-112. DE TONI-FANCONI-VON ALBERTINI-ZELLWEGER SYNDROME **649**

Fleck, Ludwik. *Genesis and Development of a Scientific Fact*. Chicago: University of Chicago Press; 1979:27 [Translation of 1935 German edition]. SCIENCE **2975**

Fleming, Alexander.
Chemotherapy: Yesterday, Today, and Tomorrow. Cambridge: Cambridge University Press; 1946:36. ANTIBIOTICS **195**
On the antibacterial action of cultures of a penicillium, with special reference to their use in the isolation of B. influenzae. *Br J Exp Path*. 1929;10:226-36. PENICILLIN **2480**

Fletcher J, Chapman G, Jonson B, Massinger P. *The Bloody Brother*, 1630. ALCOHOL **109**

Fletcher, Joseph. *Morals and Medicine*. Princeton, NJ: Princeton University Press; 1954:37. PATIENTS **2466**

Flexner, Abraham.
Medical Education in the United States and Canada: A Report to the Carnegie Foundation for the Advancement of Teaching, bulletin 4. New York: The Carnegie Foundation; 1910. [In: Birmingham, AL: Classics of Medicine Library; 1990.] AMERICAN MEDICINE **139** [20], ANATOMY **153** [63], AUTOPSIES **272** [66], **273** [66], CLINICAL OBSERVATION **519** [92], CONTINUING EDUCATION **595** [57], DOGMATISM **873** [156], MEDICAL CARE **1666** [26], MEDICAL EDUCATION **1762** [x], **1763** [xi], **1764** [56], **1765** [17], **1766** [18-9], **1767** [xiii], **1768** [60-1], **1769** [57], **1770** [102], **1771** [56-7], **1772** [93], MEDICAL EVIDENCE **1855** [65], MEDICAL PROFESSION **1998** [xiii-iv], MEDICAL SCHOOLS **2034** [ix], **2035** [349], **2036** [xi], **2037** [xii], MEDICAL STUDENTS **2061** [57], MEDICAL WORKFORCE **2067** [14], **2068** [xiv], MEDICINE **2109** [156], PHYSIOLOGY **2602** [63], PUBLIC HEALTH **2752** [19], RURAL MEDICINE **2920** [16], **2921** [44], SCIENCE **2968** [157], WOMEN IN MEDICINE **3479** [178-9]
Medical Education: A Comparative Study. New York: Macmillan; 1925. [In: Wartman W. *Medical Teaching in Western Civilization: A History Prepared from the Writings of Ancient and Modern Authors*. Chicago: Year Book Medical Publishers; 1961.] MEDICAL EDUCATION **1777** [220-1], **1778** [227-8], MEDICAL PRACTICE **1941** [216-7], RESEARCH **2863** [220-1]

Flint, Austin.
A *Treatise on the Principles and Practice of Medicine; designed for the use of practitioners and students of medicine*, 5th ed, "revised and largely re-written." Philadelphia: Henry C. Leas's Son & Company; 1881:92. VULNERABILITY **3454**
A clinical lecture on anaemia, delivered at the Long Island College of Medicine. *Am Med Times*. 1860;1:181-8. MURMURS **2209**, PERNICIOUS ANEMIA **2507**, RESEARCH **2854**
On cardiac murmurs. *Am J Med Sci*. 1862;44:29-54. AUSTIN FLINT MURMUR **269**

Flourens, Pierre (Marie Jean-Pierre Flourens). *Recherches expérimentales sur les propriétés du système nerveux, dans les animaux vertébrés*, 1824. CEREBELLUM **449**

Foligno, Gentile da. In Donati M. *De Medica Historia Mirabili Libri Sex*. Mantua: 1586. [In: Major RH. *Classic Descriptions of Disease*, p. 696 (q.v.).] GALLSTONES **1074**

Forlanini, Carlo. A contribution to the surgical therapy of phthisis. Ablation of the lung? Artificial pneumothorax? [Italian] *Gazzetta Osp Clin Milano*. 1882;68:537. [In: *Tubercle*. 1934-5;16:61-87.] TUBERCULOSIS **3387**

Forrow L, Blair BG, Helfand I, et al. Accidental nuclear war: a post-Cold War assessment. *N Engl J Med*. 1998;338:1326-31. NUCLEAR WAR **2266**

Forssmann, Werner Theodor Otto. Die Sondierung des Rechten Herzens. *Klin Wochenschr*. 1929;8:2085-7. [In: Keys TE, Key JD, *Classics of Cardiology*, pp. 36-44 (q.v.).] CATHETERIZATION **441**

Foster GC, Baghdiantz A, Kumar MS, et al. Thyroid origin of calcitonin. *Nature*. 1964;202(4939):1303-5. CALCITONIN **367**

Foster, Gerald S. Case records of the Massachusetts General Hospital. *N Engl J Med*. 1977;296:617-23. GASTROENTEROLOGY **1086**

Foster, Michael. In Rolleston HD. *The Cambridge Medical School: a Biographical History*. Cambridge, England: Cambridge University Press; 1932, pp. 87-8. TEXTBOOKS **3288**

Fothergill, John.
Further account of the angina pectoris. *Med Observations Inquiries*. 1776;5:252. [In: Major RH. *Classic Descriptions of Disease*, p. 460 (q.v.).] CORONARY ARTERY DISEASE **610**
Remarks on that complaint commonly known under the name of the sick head-ache. *Med Observations Inquiries*. 1777-84;6:103-37. [In: Fox RH. *Dr. John Fothergill and His Friends: Chapters in Eighteenth Century Life*. London: Macmillan; 1919, pp. 61-2.] MIGRAINE **2167**

Foucault, Michel. The birth of the clinic. In Rothman DJ, Marcus S, Kiceluk SA (eds). *Medicine and Western Civilization*. New Brunswick, NJ: Rutgers University Press; 1995, p. 379. MEDICAL EDUCATION **1782**

Fox, E.L. A case of myxoedema treated by taking extract of thyroid by the mouth. *Br Med J*. 1892;2:941. [In: Bloomfield AL, *Selected Diseases*, pp. 191-2 (q.v.).] HYPOTHYROIDISM **1395**

On cocaine. In: *The Cocaine Papers*. Translated by Edminster SA. Vienna: Dunquin Press; 1963:60. COCAINE 562

On the psychical mechanism of hysterical phenomena: preliminary communication, 1893. [In: *The Standard Edition of the Complete Psychological Works of Sigmund Freud*, vol. 2. London: The Hogarth Press; 1955.] PSYCHOANALYSIS 2727 [17], 2728 [11], 2729 [6]

The dissolution of the Oedipus complex. [In: *The Standard Edition of the Complete Psychological Works of Sigmund Freud*, vol. 19. Translated by James Strachey. London: The Hogarth Press; 1961.] EMOTIONAL GROWTH 953 [173], GENETICS 1103 [174]

Friedman MH, Lapham ME. A simple, rapid procedure for the laboratory diagnosis of early pregnancies. *Am J Obstet Gynecol.* 1931;21:405-10. [In: Speert H. *Obstetric and Gynecologic Milestones.* New York: Macmillan; 1958:245.] PREGNANCY TESTS 2662

Fröhlich A, von Frankl-Hochwart L. Contribution to the knowledge of the effects of hypophysin (pituitrins), on the sympathetic and autonomic nervous systems. *Arch Exp Path.* 1910;63:347-56. PITUITRIN 2606

Fröhlich, Alfred. Ein fall von tumor der hypophysis cerebri ohne akromegalie. *Wien Klin Rdsch.* 1901;15:883-6. [In: Major RH. *Classic Descriptions of Disease*, pp. 331-3.] FRÖHLICH SYNDROME (DYSTROPHIA ADIPOSOGENITALIS) 1066

Fukuda K, Straus SE, Hickie I, et al. The chronic fatigue syndrome: a comprehensive approach to its definition and study. *Ann Intern Med.* 1994;121:953-9. CHRONIC FATIGUE SYNDROME 480

Fuller, Thomas.
Gnomologia, 1732. ALCOHOLISM 119
The Holy State and the Profane State. 1642. [In: Stevenson B. *The Home Book of Quotations*, 4th ed. New York: Dodd, Mead; 1944, p. 50.] PHYSICIANS 2551

Funk, Casimir.
J State Med. 1912;20:341-8. VITAMINS 3447
On the chemical nature of the substance which cures polyneuritis in birds induced by a diet of polished rice. *J Physiol Lond.* 1911-12;43:395-400. VITAMIN B$_1$ (THIAMINE) 3435

Gaertner LP. Letter to Louis E. Schmidt, April 1929. MEDICAL CARE 1670

Galabin, Alfred L. On the interpretation of cardiographic tracings, and the evidence which they afford as to the causation of the murmurs attendant upon mitral stenosis. *Guy's Hosp Rep.* 1875;20:261-314. HEART BLOCK 1239

Galbraith, John Kenneth. In Cassidy J. Profile: Height of eloquence. *The New Yorker.* 30 Nov 1998, vol. 74, pp. 70-5. AGING 101

Galen.
Complete Works. Translated by Reedy. Ann Arbor: University of Michigan; 1968. CANCER 370, CANCER OF THE BREAST 390
De Tumoribus.. CANCER 371
Hygiene. Translated by Green RM. Springfield, IL: Charles C Thomas; 1951. BREAST FEEDING 349 [24], INFANTS 1426 [28], METABOLISM 2159 [7], MOTHER AND CHILD 2199 [29], PREVENTIVE MEDICINE 2675 [5]
On Anatomical Procedures. ANATOMY 144
On Medical Experience, ch. 7. Translated by Walzer R, Frede M. In *Three Treatises on the Nature of Science.* Indianapolis: Hackett; 1985, p. 59. STATISTICS 3127
On Nerves, Veins, and Arteries. In Smith ES (ed). *Galen on Nerves, Veins, and Arteries: A Critical Edition and Translation from the Arabic.* Madison: University of Wisconsin; 1969. CIRCULATION 486 [188], 487 [160-1], NERVES 2228 [113]
On Protecting the Health, book V. [In: *Sleep Thieves: An Eye-Opening Exploration into the Science and Mysteries of Sleep.* New York: The Free Press; 1996, p. 205.] PHYSICIAN HEALTH 2533
On Respiration and the Arteries, chs. 1,5. Translated by Furley DJ, Wilkie JS. Princeton, NJ: Princeton University Press; 1984, pp. 81,133. RESPIRATION 2883
On the Affected Parts, book I, ch. 2. DIAGNOSIS 732 [book I, ch. 2], 733 [book I, ch. 5], EPILEPSY 972 [book III, ch. 9], ERRORS 994 [book V, ch. 2], MEDICAL EDUCATION 1736 [book IV, ch. 1], PATHOGENESIS 2351 [book I, ch. 2], SPINAL CORD 3119 [book III, ch. 14]
On the Humour. In Adler MJ, Van Doren C (eds), *Great Treasury of Western Thought.* New York: R.R. Bowker; 1977, p. 1155. MEDICAL CARE 1653
On the Pulse. In Clendening L. *Source Book of Medical History.* New York: Harper & Bros.; 1942:42-4. CIRCULATION 488

On the Sects for Beginners, ch. 1. In *Three Treatises on the Nature of Science*. Translated by Walzer R, Frede M. Indianapolis, IN: Hackett; 1985. MEDICINE **2079** [ch. 1, p. 3], **2080** [ch. 3, p. 5]

On the Usefulness of the Parts of the Body. [In: Fulton JF (ed). *Selected Readings in the History of Physiology*. Springfield, IL: Charles C Thomas; 1930.] HEART **1225** [42], SPINAL CORD **3120** [592]

In Strauss MB (ed). *Familiar Medical Quotations*, p. 492 (q.v.). DRUGS **878**

Gallo RC, Salahuddin SZ, Popovic M, et al. Frequent detection and isolation of cytopathic retroviruses (HTLV-III) from patients with AIDS and at risk for AIDS. *Science*. 1984;224:500-3. [502]. ACQUIRED IMMUNE DEFICIENCY SYNDROME (AIDS) **29**

Galton, Francis.

Inquiries into Human Faculty and Its Development. London: Macmillan; 1883. [In: New York: AMS Press; 1973:33.] STATISTICS **3146**

The history of twins as a criterion of the relative powers of nature and nurture. *J Anthropol Inst Great Britain Ireland*. 1876;5:391-406. [In: Galton DJ, Dalton CJ. Francis Galton: his approach to polygenic disease. *J R Coll Phys Surg*. 1997;31:570-3.] GENETICS **1097**

Galvani, Luigi. Part four: Conjectures and some conslusions. In: *Commentary on the Effects of Electricity on Muscular Motion*. Green RM; translator. Cambridge, MA: Elizabeth Licht; 1953:60. NERVOUS SYSTEM **2235**

Garland, Joseph.

Shattuck Lecture: The proper study of mankind. *N Engl J Med*. 1964;270:1137. WRITING **3504**

The patient hires his doctor. In *The Doctor's Saddle-Bag*. Boston: [Published privately]; 1930, pp. 12-6. QUACKERY **2808**

Garrett HE, Dennis EW, DeBakey ME. Aortocoronary bypass with saphenous vein graft; seven-year follow-up. *JAMA*. 1973;223:7;792-4. HEART SURGERY **1256**

Garrod, Alfred Baring.

A *Treatise on Gout and Rheumatic Gout (Rheumatic Arthritis)*, 3rd ed. London: Longman's, Green; 1876. [In: Talbott JH. A *Biographical History of Medicine*, p. 1085 (q.v.).] GOUT **1145**

The Nature and Treatment of Gout and Rheumatic Gout, 2nd ed. London: Walton & Maberly; 1863, p. 98. [In: Porter R, Rousseau GS. *Gout: The Patrician Malady*. New Haven, CT: Yale University Press; 1998, p. 176.] GOUT **1146**

Observations on certain pathological conditions of the blood and urine in gout, rheumatism, and Bright's disease. *Med-Chir Trans*. 1848;31:83-97. [In: Talbott JH. A *Biographical History of Medicine*, p. 1084 (q.v.).] GOUT **1144**

Garrod, Archibald Edward. The chemistry of the species and of the individual. In *Inborn Errors of Metabolism*. London: Henry Frowde and Hodder & Stoughton; 1923. GENETICS **1100** [3], **1101** [10]

Garth, Samuel. *The Dispensary*, canto VI, 1699. MEDICINE **2089**, TUBERCULOSIS **3373**

Gascoyne-Cecil, Robert Arthur Talbot, Marquess of Salisbury. Letter to Lord Lytton, Viceroy of India, June 15, 1877. [In: Jones S. In the genetic toyshop. *The New York Review of Books*. April 1998, vol. 23, no. 45, pp. 14-6.] DOCTORS **825**

Gates, Frederick Taylor. *Chapters in My Life*. New York: Free Press; 1977:180-2. OSLER, WILLIAM **2298**

Gauss KF. In Beveridge WIB. *The Art of Scientific Investigation*, 3rd ed. New York: Vintage Press; 1958, p 200. SCIENCE **2954**

Gavarret, Louis-Dominique-Jules. *Principes généraux de statistique médicale, ou, développement des règles qui doivent à son emploi*, Paris: Bechet jeune & Labé; 1840:116-7. CLINICAL TRIALS **536**

Gay, John. *Fables, part I. The Sick Man and the Angel*, 1727. MEDICAL FEES **1868**

Gaylin W, Cass LR, Pelligrino ED, et al. Doctors must not kill. *JAMA*. 1988;259:2139-40. PHYSICIAN ASSISTED SUICIDE **2530**

Gee, Samuel. *Medical Lectures and Aphorisms*. London: Smith, Elder; 1902, p. 227. MEDICINE **2104**

Geiger, H Jack. A Life in Social Medicine. In: Bassuk EL, Carman RW (eds). *The Doctor Activist: Physicians Fighting for Social Change*. New York: Plenum; 1996:25. MEDICINE **2136**

Gendron, Claude Deshais. In Shimkin MB. Gendron's enquiries into the nature, knowledge, and cure of cancers. *Cancer*. 1956;9:645-7. QUACKERY **2800**

George, David Lloyd. Speech to the House of Commons. London, 1912. [In: Abse D. *Doctors and Patients*. Oxford: Oxford University Press; 1984:29.] RURAL MEDICINE **2922**

Gerbec, Marko. *Appendix ad Epheridum Academiae Caesaro-Leopoldino-Carolinae Naturae Curiosum in Germania: Centuria VII et VIII*. Nuremberg: 1719. [In: Major RH. *Classic Descriptions of Disease*, p. 354 (q.v.).] HEART BLOCK **1234**

Gerhard, William Wood. On the typhus fever, which occurred at Philadelphia in the spring and summer of 1836. *Am J Med Sci*. 1837;19-20:289-322. [In: Major RH. *Classic Descriptions of Disease*, pp. 186-7 (q.v.).] TYPHOID FEVER AND TYPHUS **3407**

Gross J, Pitt-Rivers RV. 3:5:3'-Triiodothyronine. Part 1: Isolation from thyroid gland and synthesis. *Biochem J.* 1953;53:645-50. THYROID GLAND **3305**

Gross, Samuel David. *Autobiography of Samuel D. Gross, MD.* Philadelphia: 1887. [Reprint: New York: Arno Press; 1972.] SURGEONS **3202** [172], VIVISECTION **3451** [97], WRITING **3492** [138], **3493** [73], **3494** [141]

Gross, Samuel Weissell. *A Practical Treatise on Impotence, Sterility, and Allied Disorders of the Male Sexual Organs,* preface. Philadelphia: 1881. [In: Rutkow IM. *The History of Surgery in the United States,,* vol. 1. San Francisco: Norman Publishing; 1988:344.] INFERTILITY **1438**

Grotjahn, Alfred's physician father. Dedication inscribed on September 28, 1896 in a casebook given to his son Alfred Grotjahn, MD. In Weindling P. Medical practice in imperial Berlin: the casebook of Alfred Grotjahn. *Bull Hist Med.* 1987;61:391-410]. MEDICAL HISTORIES **1873**

Gruber, Howard E. The origin of *The Origin of Species* [Review of Eiseley LE. *Darwin and the Mysterious Mr. X: New Light on the Evolutionists*]. *The New York Times Book Review.* 22 Jul 1979, p. 7. SCIENCE **2988**

Grundy HM, Simpson SA, Tait JF. Isolation of a highly active mineralocorticoid from beef adrenal extract. *Nature.* 1952;169:795-6. ALDOSTERONE **124**

Guitry, Sacha. *Elles et Toi,* 1948. ADULTERY **49**

Gull WW, Anstey E. In J. Russell Reynolds (ed). *A System of Medicine,* vol. 2. London: Macmillan; 1868, p. 293. HYPOCHONDRIA **1370**

Gull, William Withey.
A *Collection of the Published Writings,* vol. 2. London: New Sydenham Society; 1896. DOCTORS **833** [viii], MEDICINE **2103** [lix]

Memoir. In *A Collection of the Published Writings of William Withey Gull.* London: The Sydenham Society; 1896, p. xxiii. GENETICS **1099**, PATIENT-PHYSICIAN RELATIONS **2396**

Anorexia nervosa (apepsia hysterica, anorexia hysterica). *Trans Clin Soc Lond.* 1874;7:22-8. ANOREXIA NERVOSA **191**

On a cretinoid state supervening in adult life in women. *Trans Clin Soc London.* 1873;7:180-5. HYPOTHYROIDISM **1391, 1392**

The address in medicine delivered before the Annual Meeting of the British Medical Association at Oxford. *Lancet.* 1968;2:171-6. ANOREXIA NERVOSA **190**

Gullen, William. *First Lines of the Practice of Physic, with practical and explanatory notes by John Rotheram.* Philadelphia: 1792. PERITONITIS **2505**

Guy de Chauliac.
La grande chirurgie de M. Guy de Chauliac. Tournons; 1619. [In: Major RH. *Classic Descriptions of Disease,* p. 89 (q.v.).] BUBONIC PLAGUE **355**

In Brennan WA. *Guy de Chauliac (AD 1363), On wounds and Fractures.* Chicago: W.A. Brennan; 1923, on page preceding index. SURGEONS **3197**

Gye, William Ewart. The aetiology of malignant new growth. *Lancet.* 1925;2:109-17. CANCER **381**

Haberlandt, Ludwig. Über Hormonale Sterilisierung des Weiblichen Tierkoerpers. *Münchener Medizinische Wochenschrift.* 1921;68:1577-8. CONTRACEPTION **601**

Hagstrom, Warren O. *The Scientific Community.* New York: Basic Books Publishers; 1965, pp. 12-23. PUBLISHING **2767**

Haines, Andrew. Working together to reduce poverty's damage. *Br Med J.* 1997;314:529-30. HEALTH GAPS **1213**

Haldane JS, Douglas CG, Henderson Y, Schneider EC. Physiological observations made on Pike's peak, Colorado, with special reference to adaptation to low barometric pressures. *Phil Trans R Soc Lond B.* 1913;203:185-318. LUNG **1588**

Haldane JS, Priestly JG. The regulation of the lung-ventilation. *J Physiol.* 1905;21:225-66. RESPIRATION **2891**

Haldane, John Scott.
Mechanism, Life, and Personality. London: 1914. [In: Talbott JH. *A Biographical History of Medicine,* p. 958 (q.v.).] GENETICS **1102**

Respiration. New Haven, CT: Yale University Press; 1922:viii. RESEARCH **2861**

The therapeutic administration of oxygen. *Br Med J.* 1917;1:181-3. OXYGEN THERAPY **2310**

Hales, Stephen. *Statical Essays: containing Haemastaticks; or, an account of some hydraulick and hydrostatical experiments made on the blood and blood-vessels of animals,* vol. 2, 1733. BLOOD PRESSURE **309**, PULMONARY CIRCULATION **2783**

Hale-Wight, W. Thomas Hodgkin. *Guy's Hosp Rep.* 1924;74:117-36. LARYNGOSCOPE **1513**

Haley RW, Kurt TL, Hom J. Is there a Gulf War syndrome? Searching for syndromes by factor analysis of symptoms. *JAMA*. 1997;277:215-22. GULF WAR SYNDROME **1156**

Hall, Arthur. *Practitioner* 1941. [In: Coope R (ed). *The Quiet Art*, p. 16 (q.v.).] MEDICAL PRACTICE **1946**

Hall, Marshall. On the reflex function of the medulla oblongata and medulla spinalis. *Philos Trans R Soc London*. 1833;123:635-65. NERVOUS SYSTEM **2239**, REFLEX ACTION **2842**

Halle John.
   In Daniels AM. The last explorers [Review of Nuland SB, *Wisdom of the Body*, and Bodanis D, *The Secret Family*]. *Times Literary Supplement*. 30 Jan 1998, no. 4948, p. 36. SURGEONS **3199**
   In *Goodly Doctrine and Instruction*. 1916 [Published privately]. CONSULTATION **586**

Haller, Albrecht von. *Opuscula Pathologica*. Lausanne: 1755. [In: Major RH. *Classic Descriptions of Disease*, p. 408 (q.v.).] PERICARDITIS **2500**

Halsted, William Stewart. The results of operations for the cure of cancer of the breast performed at the Johns Hopkins Hospital from June 1889 to January 1894. *Ann Surg*. 1894;20:497-555. CANCER OF THE BREAST **397**

Hamburger, Jean. In Wolstenholme GEW, O'Connor M (eds). *Ethics in Medical Progress: Ciba Foundation Symposium*. Boston, MA: Little, Brown; 1966, pp. 137-8. MEDICAL ETHICS **1838**

Hamilton, Alice. *The American Scholar*. 1938. [In: Amster, LJ. Gentlewoman explorer in the dangerous trades. *Hosp Pract*. 1986;21:206-54.] INDUSTRIAL MEDICINE **1425**

Hamilton, Walton H. In *Realities of Medicine: September 10-14, 1984* [Conference pamphlet]. Chicago: University of Illinois College of Medicine; 1984. MEDICAL SERVICES **2053**, MEDICINE **2115**

Hammer, Adam. Ein fall von thrombotischen verschlusse einer der Kranzarterien des herzens. *Dtsch Med Wochenschr*. 1878;28:97-102. CORONARY ARTERY DISEASE **618**

Hammond, William A. Miryachit: a newly described disease of the nervous system, and its analogs. *N Y Med J*. 1884;39:191-2. TOURETTE SYNDROME **3318**

Hammurabi. *The Code of Hammurabi.*. Translated by King LW. Accessed 14 Jul 1999 at http://www.yale.edu/lawweb/avalon/hamframe.htm. MEDICAL FEES **1861** [law 217], **1862** [law 221], **1863** [law 215], **1864** [law 216], **1865** [law 206]

Hardison, Joseph E. Sounding Board. To be complete. *N Engl J Med*. 1979;300:193-4. MALPRACTICE **1615**, MEDICAL CARE **1689**, TESTS **3279**, **3280**

Hargraves MM, Robinson H, Morton R. Presentation of two bone marrow elements: the "tart" cell and the "L. E." cell. *Proc Staff Meeting Mayo Clinic*. 1948;23(2):25-8. LUPUS ERYTHEMATOSUS **1593**

Harington, John. *The Metamorphosis of Aiax: A New Discourse of a Stale Subject*, 1596. BOWEL MOVEMENTS **332**, UROSCOPY **3416**

Harley, George. On intermittent haematuria; with remarks upon its pathology and treatment. *Med-Chi Trans*. 1865;48:161-73. [In: Talbott JH. *A Biographical History of Medicine*, p. 1118 (q.v.).] PAROXYSMAL HEMOGLOBINURIA **2343**

Harmon, Albert V. *Large Fees and How To Get Them: A Book for the Private Use of Physicians*. Chicago: W.J. Jackman; 1911. DOCTORS **837** [37,41], **838** [166], MEDICAL EDUCATION **1773** [17],

Harrell, George T. *J Med Educ*. 1958;33:217. [In: Fred HL. Learning medicine. *South Med J*. 1988;81:422-3.] CONTINUING EDUCATION **597**

Harris, Seale. *Woman's Surgeon: The Life Story of J. Marion Sims*. New York: Macmillan; 1950. pp. 243-52. INFERTILITY **1439**

Harrison, Tinsley R.
   Principles of Internal Medicine. Philadelphia: Blakiston; 1950. PATIENT-PHYSICIAN RELATIONS **2414** [5], PHYSICIANS **2582** [1], **2587** [7]
   Severe angina pectoris: considerations of surgical and medical management. *JAMA*. 1973;223:1022-6. TREATMENT **3356**

Hartmann, Heinz. *Psychoanalysis and Moral Values*. New York: International Universities Press; 1960, pp. 54-6. SCIENTISTS **3008**

Harvey, William.
   An Anatomical Treatise on the Movement of the Heart and Blood in Animals, 1628. ANATOMY **146**, CIRCULATION **489**, **490**, HEART **1228**, **1229**
   Anatomical Exercitations, Concerning the Generation of Living Creatures. London: 1653. [In: Birmingham, AL: Classics of Medicine Library; 1991, preface.] RESEARCH **2852**
   In Asher R. *Richard Asher Talking Sense*. Baltimore: University Park Press; 1972, p. 40. DOGMATISM **871**
   In Dock G. Some notes on the coronary arteries. *Med Surg Reporter*. 1896;75:1. [In: Major RH. *Classic Descriptions of Disease*, p. 468 (q.v.).] CORONARY ARTERY DISEASE **609**

Haserick JR, Lewis LA, Bortz DW. Blood factor in acute disseminated lupus erythematosus: 1. Determination of gamma globulin as specific plasma fraction. *Am J Med Sci*. 1950;219:660-3. LUPUS ERYTHEMATOSUS **1594**

Hilton, John. *Rest and Pain: A Course of Lectures on the Influence of Mechanical and Physiological Rest in the Treatment of Accidents and Surgical Diseases, and the Diagnostic Value of Pain*. London: George Bell & Sons; 1892. PAIN 2319 [500], 2320 [499], REFERRED PAIN 2840 [222-3], REST 2897 [3], SYNOVIAL MEMBRANE 3252 [467]

Hinshaw HC, Feldman WH. Streptomycin in treatment of clinical tuberculosis: a preliminary report. *Proc Staff Meetings Mayo Clinic*. 1945;20:313-8. TUBERCULOSIS 3400, 3401

Hippocrates.

Aphorisms. In Adams F (ed). *The Genuine Works of Hippocrates*. London: 1849. [In: Birmingham, AL: Classics of Medicine Library; 1985.] EMPYEMA 958 [738], GOUT 1127 [757], 1128 [757], 1129 [756], MEDICAL PRACTICE 1915 [697], OBESITY 2279 [713], PROGNOSIS 2691 [762], TREATMENT 3328 [293], TUBERCULOSIS 3368 [738], URINARY TRACT CALCULUS 3414

Aphorisms, 2.3 (IV:109). Loeb Classical Library. Cambridge, MA: Harvard University Press. SLEEP 3071

Aphorisms, 3.24-31 (IV:131-5). Loeb Classical Library. Cambridge, MA: Harvard University Press. AGING 53

Aphorisms, 7.87 (IV:217). Loeb Classical Library. Cambridge, MA: Harvard University Press. SURGERY 3211

Aphorisms, no. 38. CANCER 368

Breaths (I. Referenced by Plutarch in *Aitia romana*, 291c). [In: Jouanna J. *Hippocrates*. DeBevoise MB, translator. Baltimore: Johns Hopkins University Press; 1999:352.] MEDICAL PRACTICE 1913

Decorum, ch. 14 (II:297. Loeb Classical Library. Cambridge, MA: Harvard University Press). NON-COMPLIANCE 2261

Decorum, ch. 7. Loeb Classical Library. Cambridge, MA: Harvard University Press. PATIENT-PHYSICIAN RELATIONS 2362

Fourteen Cases of Disease. CHEYNE-STOKES RESPIRATION 456

Of the Epidemics. In Adams F (ed). *The Genuine Works of Hippocrates*. London: 1849. [In: Birmingham, AL: Classics of Medicine Library; 1985.] MEDICAL PRACTICE 1914 [360], MUMPS 2203 [100-1]

On Airs, Waters, and Places, ch. 1-2 (I:127). Loeb Classical Library. Cambridge: Harvard University Press. [In: Jouanna J. *Hippocrates*. DeBevoise MB, translator. Baltimore: Johns Hopkins University Press; 1999:212.] LIFE STYLE 1549

On Ancient Medicine. In Adams F (ed). *The Genuine Works of Hippocrates*. London: 1849. [In: Birmingham, AL: Classics of Medicine Library; 1985.] ERRORS 993, MEDICINE 2073 [162], 2074 [164], RESEARCH 2850

On Ancient Medicine, ch. 2 (I:27-29). Loeb Classical Library. Cambridge: Harvard University Press. [In: Jouanna J. *Hippocrates*. DeBevoise MB, translator. Baltimore: Johns Hopkins University Press; 1999:253.] MALPRACTICE 1611

On Fractures. In Adams F (ed). *The Genuine Works of Hippocrates*. London: 1849. [In: Birmingham, AL: Classics of Medicine Library; 1985.] BONE SETTING 328

On Hemorrhoids. HEMORRHOIDS 1267, PAIN 2315

On Injuries of the Head. In Adams F (ed). *The Genuine Works of Hippocrates*. London: 1849. [In: Birmingham, AL: Classics of Medicine Library; 1985.] NERVOUS SYSTEM 2232 [464], PNEUMONIA 2623 [313-36], SKULL FRACTURE 3070 [376]

On Joints, ch. 46 (III:293). Loeb Classical Library. Cambridge, MA: Harvard University Press. SPINAL CORD 3118

On Sterile Women. [In: Jouanna J. *Hippocrates*. DeBevoise MB, translator. Baltimore: Johns Hopkins University Press; 1999:173.] PREGNANCY 2656

On Surgery (III:63). Loeb Classical Library. Cambridge: Harvard University Press. SURGERY 3209

On Surgery. In Adams F (ed). *The Genuine Works of Hippocrates*. London: 1849. [In: Birmingham, AL: Classics of Medicine Library; 1985, p. 474.] SURGERY 3212

On the Articulations. In Adams F (ed). *The Genuine Works of Hippocrates*. London: 1849. [In: Birmingham, AL: Classics of Medicine Library; 1985, p. 648.] TREATMENT 3326

On the Sacred Disease. In Adams F (ed). *The Genuine Works of Hippocrates*. London: 1849. [Reprint: Huntington, NY: Krieger; 1972.] EPILEPSY 969 [353], 970 [347]

Physicians, ch. 5 (VIII:307). Loeb Classical Library. Cambridge, MA: Harvard University Press. SURGERY 3210

Precepts. In: *Hippocrates*, volume I. Loeb Classical Library. Cambridge, MA: Harvard University Press; 1995. FEES 1048, HEALING 1163 [313], MEDICAL CARE 1650 [319], MEDICAL PRACTICE 1911, PATIENT-PHYSICIAN RELATIONS 2361 [319]

Preliminary Discourse. In Adams F (ed). *The Genuine Works of Hippocrates*. London: 1849. [In: Birmingham, AL: Classics of Medicine Library; 1985, p. 18.] PROGNOSIS 2694

Regimen, ch. 58 (IV:345). Loeb Classical Library. Cambridge, MA: Harvard University Press. SEX 3024

The Book of Prognostics. In Adams F (ed). *The Genuine Works of Hippocrates.* London: 1849. [In: Birmingham, AL: Classics of Medicine Library; 1985.] BOWEL MOVEMENTS 331 [243], DELIRIUM 696 [238], EMPYEMA 957 [248-9], PHYSICAL EXAMINATION 2519 [235-5], PROGNOSIS 2690 [234], 2692 [252], 2693 [251]

The Hippocratic Oath. In Temkin O, Temkin CL (eds). *Selected Papers of Ludwig Edelstein.* Baltimore: Johns Hopkins University Press; 1967, p. 6. ABORTION 4

The Law, ch. 1. In Adams F (ed). *The Genuine Works of Hippocrates.* London: 1849. [In: Birmingham, AL: Classics of Medicine Library; 1985.] MEDICAL EDUCATION 1735 [785], MEDICINE 2075 [784], PHYSICIANS 2539

The Oath. In Adams F (ed). *The Genuine Works of Hippocrates.* London: 1849. [In: Birmingham, AL: Classics of Medicine Library; 1985, p. 779.] MEDICAL ETHICS 1812

The Physician, ch. 1. Translated by Jones WHS. [In: Fabre J. *The Hippocratic Doctor: Ancient Lessons for the Modern World.* London: Royal Society of Medicine; 1997:8.] PHYSICIAN HEALTH 2532

In *Latin Proverbs.* [Reichert HG. *Unvergangliche Lateinische Spruchweisheit: Urban und Human.* Wiesbaden: Panorama Verlag. MEDICAL PRACTICE 1912

In Basta LL. *A Graceful Exit: Life and Death on Your Own Terms.* New York: Insight Books, Plenum Press; 1996, p. 227. TREATMENT 3325

In Beck T. *Hippokrates Erkenntnisse.* Jena; 1907. [In: Major RH. *Classic Descriptions of Disease,* pp. 147-8 (q.v.).] TETANUS 3285

In Collinge W. *The American Holistic Health Association Complete Guide to Alternative Medicine.* New York: Warner Books; 1996, p. 266. MEDICAL CARE 1652

In Lloyd GER, *Hippocratic Writings.* Harmondsworth, England: Penguin Books; 1978. DISEASE 778 [264], LIVING 1565 [209], MEDICAL CARE 1651 [94], TREATMENT 3327 [266]

In Peterson WF. *Hippocratic Wisdom.* Springfield, IL: Charles C Thomas Publishers; 1946, p. 62. PLEURITIS 2622

Hirschcowitz BI, Curtiss LE, Peters CW, Pollard HM. Demonstration of the new gastroscope, the "fiberscope." *Gastroenterology.* 1958;35:50-3. GASTROSCOPY 1089

Hirschsprung, Harald. Stuhletragheit Neugeborener in folge von Dilatation und Hypertrophie des Colons. *Jahrb Kinderheilk.* 1888;27:1-7. [In: Roed-Peterson K, Erichsen G. The Danish pediatrician Harald Hirschsprung. *Surg Gynec Obst.* 1988;166:181-5.] HIRSCHSPRUNG DISEASE 1290

His, Wilhelm Jr.
Nutrition therapy of gout. *Post-Graduate.* 1910;25:23-40. [In: Talbott JH. A *Biographical History of Medicine,* p. 1165 (q.v.).] GOUT 1149

The activity of the embryonic human heart and its significance for the understanding of the heart movement in the adult. *Arb Med Klin Leipzig.* 1893;14-49. [In: *J Hist Med.* 1949;4:289-318.] ATRIOVENTRICULAR BUNDLE 264

Hodes ME, Rohn RJ, Bond W. Effect of a plant alkaloid, vincaleukoblastine, in humans. *J Lab Clin Med.* 1959;54:826. VINBLASTINE 3429

Hodge, Hugh Lenox. *Foeticide, or criminal abortion; a lecture introductory to the course on obstetrics, and diseases of women and children,* Philadelphia: 1839. ABORTION 8

Hodgkin AL, Huxley AF. Action potentials from inside a nerve fibre. *Nature.* 1939;144:710-1. NEUROTRANSMISSION 2253

Hodgkin, Thomas.
Lectures on the Morbid Anatomy of the Serous and Mucous Membranes, 1836. APPENDICITIS 222

On some morbid appearances of the absorbent glands and spleen. *Med-Chir Trans.* 1832;17:68-114. [In: Talbott JH. A *Biographical History of Medicine,* p. 1043 (q.v.).] HODGKIN DISEASE 1302

On the retroversion of the valves of the aorta. *Lond Med Gaz.* 1828-9;3:433-43. AORTIC VALVE REGURGITATION 208, 209

Hoefer, Wolfgang. *Hercules Medicus sive Locorum Communium Liber.* Nuremberg; 1675. [In: Major RH. *Classic Descriptions of Disease,* p. 282 (q.v.).] HYPOTHYROIDISM 1388

Hoffman, Felix. *Journal,* 10 August 1897. Bayer Leverkusen Archives. [In: Jeffreys D. *Aspirin: The Remarkable Story of a Wonder Drug.* New York: Bloomsbury; 2004:70.] ASPIRIN (ACETYLSALICYLIC ACID) 244

Hofmeister, Franz. Über Bau und Gruppierung der Eiweisskörper. *Ergebnisse der Physiologie.* 1904;1:759-802. [In: Teich M, Needham DM. A *Documentary History of Biochemistry, 1770-1940.* Leicester: Leicester University Press; 1992:792.] AMINO ACIDS 141

Hollister JH. Cook EP, Hamilton JL. Report on drugs and medicines. *Trans Ill State Med Soc.* 1873;23:118-29. CONTINUING EDUCATION **591**

Hollister, John Hamilcar.

Memories of Eighty Years: Auto-sketches, Random Notes, and Reminiscences. Chicago: 1912. FAMILY DOCTORS **1044** [73], MEDICAL PROFESSION **1981** [49-50]

Cholera. *JAMA.* 1885;4:564-71. GERM THEORY **1116**

The physician and his journals [Editorial]. *JAMA.* 1889;13:420-1. MEDICAL JOURNALS **1897**

The revision of medical writing. *North Am Pract.* 1893;5:125-6. MEDICAL JOURNALS **1898**

Holmes, Bayard. The hospital problem. *JAMA.* 1906;47:320. HOSPITALS **1322**

Holmes GP, Kaplan JE, Gantz NM, et al. Chronic fatigue syndrome: a working case definition. *Ann Intern Med.* 1988;108:387-9. CHRONIC FATIGUE SYNDROME **477**

Holmes, Gary P. Defining the chronic fatigue syndrome. *Rev Infect Dis.* 1991;12(Suppl 1):S53-5. CHRONIC FATIGUE SYNDROME **479**

Holmes, Oliver Wendell.

Border Lines of Knowledge in Some Provinces of Medical Science [Introductory lecture given to the Medical Class of Harvard University, November 6, 1861]. [In: *Medical Essays by Oliver Wendell Holmes.* Birmingham, AL: Classics of Medicine Library; 1987, p. 265.] DRUGS **888**

Currents and Counter-Currents in Medical Science [Address to the Massachusetts Medical Society Annual Meeting, May 30, 1860]. [In: *Medical Essays by Oliver Wendell Holmes.* Birmingham, AL: Classics of Medicine Library; 1987.] DRUGS **886, 887,** MEDICAL PROFESSION **1984,** MEDICINE **2099,** PATIENT-PHYSICIAN RELATIONS **2387,** PRESCRIPTIONS **2667, 2668**

Our Hundred Days in Europe, 1887. AGING **72,** SURGERY **3226**

Over the Teacups, 1892. AGING **73, 74,** DOCTORS **829,** DYING **911,** HOMEOPATHY **1308,** KNOWLEDGE **1508,** NUTRITION **2276,** SPECIALIZATION **3107**

Scholastic and Bedside Teaching. [Address to the medical class of Harvard University, November 6, 1867]. [In: *Medical Essays by Oliver Wendell Holmes.* Birmingham, AL: Classics of Medicine Library; 1987, p. 291.] KNOWLEDGE **1507**

The Autocrat of the Breakfast Tabl,e 1892. ARGYRIA **230,** LIFE **1538,** SCIENCE **2955,** VISION **3430**

The Professor at the Breakfast Table, 1892. MEDICAL EVIDENCE **1853,** PRESCRIPTIONS **2669,** SCIENCE **2956**

The Young Practitioner [Valedictory address to the graduating class of Bellevue Hospital College, March 2, 1871]. [In: *Medical Essays by Oliver Wendell Holmes.* Birmingham, AL: Classics of Medicine Library; 1987.] ILLNESS **1404,** MEDICAL CARE **1661,** MEDICAL SUPERSTITIONS **2063,** NOMENCLATURE **2257,** PHYSICIANS **2570**

Rip Van Winkle, MD, canto II. In *Complete Poetical Works,* 1893. DOCTORS **830**

The contagiousness of puerperal fever. *N Engl Q J Med.* 1843;1:503-30. [In: *Medical Essays by Oliver Wendell Holmes.* Birmingham, AL: Classics of Medicine Library; 1987.] PUERPERAL FEVER **2778** [128-9], **2779** [103]

Homans J. *Three Hundred and Eighty-Four Laparotomies for Various Diseases.* Boston: N. Sawyer; 1887. [In: Rutkow IM, *The History of Surgery in the United States,* p. 96.] SURGERY **3225**

Home, Everard. Life of John Hunter. In Hunter J. *Treatise on the Blood: Inflammation and Gunshot Wounds.* Philadelphia; 1796. [In: Major RH. *Classic Descriptions of Disease,* pp. 461-2 (q.v.).] CORONARY ARTERY DISEASE **611**

Homer.

The Iliad. ALCOHOL **105** [book VI], MILITARY MEDICINE **2176** [book XI]

The Odyssey, book XVII. PHYSICIANS **2538**

Hooke, Robert.

Micrographia, or some physiological descriptions of minute bodies made by magnifying glasses with observations and inquiries thereupon, 1665. Facsimile reprint. New York: Dover Publications; 1966:115. CELLS **447**

An account of an experiment by M. Hooke, of preserving animals alive by blowing through their lungs with bellows. *Philos Trans R Soc London.* 1666;1:539-40. ARTIFICIAL RESPIRATION **239,** RESPIRATION **2885**

Hooker, Joseph Dalton. Letter to Charles Darwin, January 1865. [In: Huxley L (ed). *The Life and Letters of Sir Joseph Dalton Hooker,* vol. 2. London: John Murray; 1918, p. 72.] NOMENCLATURE **2255**

Hope, James. *A Treatise on the Diseases of the Heart.* London: 1839. AORTIC VALVE MURMURS **204,** AORTIC VALVE REGURGITATION **211,** HEART FAILURE **1243,** HEART SOUNDS **1245,** MITRAL REGURGITATION **2188,** PULMONARY STENOSIS **2790**

Hopkins, Frederick Gowland. Lecture given in 1913. [In: Needham J, Baldwin E (ed). *Hopkins and Biochemistry*. Cambridge, England: Heffer; 1949:155.] ENZYMES **966**

Hopkins HH, Kapany NS. A flexible fibrescope, using static scanning. *Nature*. 1954;173:39-41. FIBEROSCOPY **1055**

Horner, Johann Friedrich. A form of ptosis [German]. *Klin Augenheilk*. 1869;7:193-8. [In: Talbott JH. A *Biographical History of Medicine*, p. 704 (q.v.).] HORNER SYNDROME **1314**

Horsley, Victor Alexander Haden.H. On the function of the thyroid gland. *Proc R Soc Lond*. 1885;38:5-7. THYROID GLAND **3302**

Hounsfield, Godfrey Newbold. Computerized transverse axial scanning (tomography). Part 1: Description of system. *Br J Radiol*. 1973;46:1016-22. RADIOLOGY **2817**

House of Delegates, American Medical Association. Proceedings of the AMA House of Delegates Proceedings 220:144. (June 1970). Quoted in: 410 U.S. 113. Supreme Court of the United States. Roe, et al. v. Wade, District Attorney of Dallas County. Footnote 39. ABORTION **12**

House of Lords. *Sidaway v. Governors*. AC 871 [Law Reports, Appeal Cases, Third Series, England and Wales]; 1985. [In: Marks P. The evolution of the doctrine of consent. *Clin Med*. 2003;3(1):45-7.] MEDICAL CARE **1693**

Houston, Charles S. Acute pulmonary edema of high altitude. *N Engl J Med*. 1960;263:478-9. HIGH-ALTITUDE MEDICINE **1285**

Howard, John. In Wilson E. *The History of the Middlesex Hospital*. London: 1845. CASE RECORDS **433**

Howell WH, Holt LE. Two new factors in blood coagulation: heparin and pro-antithrombin. *Am J Physiol*. 1918-19;47:328-41. HEPARIN **1273**

Huang Ti Nei Ching Su Wen. *The Yellow Emperor's Classic of Internal Medicine*. Translated by Veith I. Berkeley: University of California Press; 1970. AGING **52**, HEALTH **1168**, PREVENTIVE MEDICINE **2674**

Hudson, Robert P. *Disease and Its Control: The Shaping of Modern Thought*. Westport, CT: Greenwood Press; 1983. DISEASE **798** [x], **799** [x], SUICIDE **3189** [4]

Huebner RJ, Jellison WL, Pomerantz C. Rickettsialpox: a newly recognized rickettsial disease. Part 1: Isolation of the etiological agent. *Public Health Rep*. 1946;61:1605-14. RICKETTSIALPOX **2917**

Huebner RJ, Todaro GJ. Oncogenes of RNA tumor viruses as determinants of cancer. *Proc Natl Acad Sci*. 1969;64:1087-94. ONCOGENES **2291**

Huggins CB, Hodges CV. Studies on prostatic cancer. Part I: The effect of castration, of estrogen, and of androgen injection on serum phosphatases in metastatic carcinoma of the prostate. *Cancer Res*. 1941;1:293-7. CANCER OF THE PROSTATE GLAND **410**

Hughes SG, Wagner GS, Swaim MW. Dr. Stead on doctoring: advice to emerging physicians. *Pharos*. 1998;61:20-2. QUACKERY **2810**

Hughes, M. Louis. Undulant (Malta) fever. *Lancet*. 1896;2:238-9. BRUCELLOSIS **352**

Hume, David. *An Enquiry Concerning Human Understanding. Part One. Of Miracles*, 1748. MIRACLES **2186**

Humphry, George M. The Hunterian oration. *Br Med J*. 1879;1:259-64. [In: Talbott JH. A *Biographical History of Medicine*, p. 1006 (q.v.).] MEDICAL EDUCATION **1749**

Hunt R, Taveau RdM. On the physiological action of cholin derivatives and new methods for detecting cholin. *BMJ*. 1906;2(2399):1788-91. ACETYLCHOLINE **22**

Hunt WE, Wooley CF. The pulsatile pain of acute aortic dissection: a neurosurgeon's personal experience. *Am Heart J*. 1996;132:1267-8. AORTIC DISSECTION **201**

Hunter, Charles. A rare disease in two brothers. *Proc R Soc Med*. 1917;10, Sect Dis Child; 104-16. HUNTER'S SYNDROME **1342**

Hunter, John.
  A *Treatise on the Blood, Inflammation, and Gun-Shot Wounds*. London: 1794. [In: Birmingham, AL: Classics of Medicine Library; 1982.] INFLAMMATION **1440** [249], REST **2896** [212]
  Of Poisons. In *The Complete Works of John Hunter, F.R.S*. Philadelphia: 1841. CANCER **376** [376-85], CANCER OF THE BREAST **394** [380]
  Letter to Edward Jenner, August 2, 1775. MEDICAL RESEARCH **2024**, SCIENCE **2943**

Hunter, Kathryn Montgomery. *Doctor's Stories: The Narrative Structure of Medical Knowledge*. Princeton, NJ: Princeton University Press; 1991. EVIDENCE **1007** [81], MEDICAL HISTORIES **1887** [82]

Hunter, Richard. *Psychiatry and Neurology* [President's address, 1972]. [In: *Proc R Soc Med*. 1973;66:359-64.] PSYCHIATRY **2722**

Hunter, William.
  The Anatomy of the Human Gravid Uterus Exhibited in Figures, preface. Birmingham, England: John Baskerville; 1774. [In: Birmingham, AL: Classics of Medicine Library; 1980. Limited data.] MEDICAL ILLUSTRATION **1894**

In Andrews HR. William Hunter and his work in midwifery. *Br Med J*. 1915;191:277-82. ANATOMY 150, DYING 906

Huntington, George. On chorea. *Med Surg Rep*. 1872;26:317-21. [In: Talbott JH. *A Biographical History of Medicine*, p. 851 (q.v.).] HUNTINGTON CHOREA 1343

Hurst, Arthur. In Coope R (ed). *The Quiet Art*, p. 79 (q.v.).] PRESCRIPTIONS 2671

Hurst, J. Willis.

Organ language. In *Essays from the Heart*. New York: Raven Press; 1995, p. 78. CLINICAL CHEMISTRY 502

Pretense. In *Essays from the Heart*. New York: Raven Press; 1995, p. 82. MEDICAL HISTORIES 1889

Hutchinson, John. Of the capacity of the lungs, and on the respiratory functions, with a view of establishing a precise and easy method of detecting disease by the spirometer. *Med-Chir Trans*. 1846;29:137. RESPIRATION 2890, SPIROMETRY 3121

Hutchinson, Jonathan.

Case of arteritis in the temporal arteries. *Archives of Surgery*, vol. 1; 1890. TEMPORAL ARTERITIS 3273

Clinical lecture on heredito-syphilitic struma: and on the teeth as a means of diagnosis. *Br Med J*. 1861;1:515-7. SYPHILIS 3263

Hutchison, Robert.

[Letter to the Editor.] *BMJ*. 1953;1:671. MEDICAL PRACTICE 1949

Br Med J. 1953;1:671 [Limited data]. MEDICAL PRACTICE 1945

The chemistry of the thyroid gland and the nature of its active constituent. *J Physiol*. 1896;20:474-96. THYROID GLAND 3303

Huth, Edward Janavel.

Irresponsible authorship and wasteful publication. *Ann Intern Med*. 1986;104:257-8. PUBLISHING 2772

Science, information systems, and the future of medical practice. *Pharos*. 1986;49:2-5. MEDICINE 2133

What has become of the cuspidor? *Ann Intern Med*. 1964;60:163-4. SMOKING 3097

Hutten, Ulrich von. *De Morbo Gallico*. Almayn, Germany: 1519. Translated by Daniel Turner. London: 1730. [In: Major RH. *Classic Descriptions of Disease*, p. 34.] SYPHILIS 3256

Huxham, John.

Observations on the Air and Epidemic Diseases Together with a Short Dissertation on the Devonshire Colic. London: 1759, p. 5. [In: Major RH. *Classic Descriptions of Disease*, pp. 341-2 (q.v.).] LEAD POISONING 1518

A method for preserving the health of seamen in long cruises and voyages. In *An Essay on Fevers*. London; 1757. [In: Major RH. *Classic Descriptions of Disease*, p. 648 (q.v.).] SCURVY 3017

Huxley, Aldous.

Human potentialities. In *The Humanist Frame*. London: George Allen & Unwin; 1961, p. 424. ENVIRONMENT 960

In Coren S. *Sleep Thieves: An Eye-Opening Exploration into the Science and Mysteries of Sleep*. New York: The Free Press; 1996, p. 175. SLEEP 3075

Huxley, Julian. The crowded world. In *Essays of a Humanist*. London: Chatto & Windus; 1964, p. 249. POPULATION CONTROL 2649

Huxley, Thomas Henry. The connection of the biological sciences with medicine. In: *Science and Culture*, 1881. MEDICAL EDUCATION 1750, MEDICINE 2101

Hyams, Kenneth C. Developing case definitions for symptom-based conditions. *Epidemiol Rev*. 1998;20:148-56. CHRONIC FATIGUE SYNDROME 482

Hyde, Edward, Earl of Clarendon. *The Life of Edward, Earl of Clarendon, Lord High Chancellor of England and Chancellor of the University of Oxford, containing an account of the Chancellor's life from his birth to the Restoration in 1660*. Oxford: 1759. ANGINA PECTORIS 176, PROSTATISM 2699

Imhotep. In *Ebers Papyrus*. Translated by Bryan CP. London: Garden City Press; 1930:135. CIRCULATION 485

Ingelfinger, Franz J.

Arrogance. *N Engl J Med*. 1980;303:1507-11. MEDICAL EDUCATION 1792, PATIENT-PHYSICIAN RELATIONS 2432

Journal ventures that flopped. *N Engl J Med*. 1976;295:727-9. WRITING 3510

Ingram, Vernon Martin. Gene mutations in human haemoglobin: the chemical difference between normal and sickle cell haemoglobin. *Nature*. 1957;180:326-8. SICKLE CELL DISEASE 3066

Institute of Medicine. Executive summary. In *Marijuana and Medicine: Assessing the Science Base*. Washington, DC: National Academy Press; 1999, pp. 3-4. MARIJUANA 1633

Jennett, W. Bryan. Is the teaching ward round obsolete? *Proc R Soc Medicine.* 1969;62:848. MEDICAL EDUCATION **1785**

Jensen EV, Jacobson HI, Smith S, et al. The use of estrogen antagonists in hormone receptor studies. *Gynecol Invest.* 1972;3(1):108-23. CANCER OF THE BREAST **399**

Jerome, Jerome K. *Three Men in a Boat: To Say Nothing of the Dog,* ch. 1. 1899. [Reprint: New York: Time-Life Books; 1964, p. 2.] HYPOCHONDRIA **1372**

Jewett, Sarah Orne. *A Country Doctor,* 1884. MEDICAL PRACTICE **1930**, PHYSICIANS **2572**

Johannsen, Wilhelm Ludwig. *Am Naturalist.* 1911;45:132. GENES **1092**

John of Arderne.

De arte phisicale et de cirurgia. Translated by Power D. London: John Bale; 1922. CANCER OF THE RECTUM **411**

On the Behaviour of a Leech. c. 1400. [In: Coope R (ed). *The Quiet Art,* p. 42 (q.v.).] READING **2826**

John of Mirfield.

Brevarium bartomolomaei. 1393. [In: Bennion E *Antique Medical Instruments.* Berkeley, CA: Sotheby Parke Bernet/University of California Press; 1979, p. 16.] MEDICAL FEES **1867**

In Aldridge HR (ed). *Johannes de Mirfield of St. Bartholomew's, Smithfield: His Life and Works.* Cambridge, England: Cambridge University Press; 1936, p. 69. CONSCIOUSNESS **579**

Johnson, Horton A. Diminishing returns on the road to diagnostic certainty. *JAMA.* 1991;265:2229-31. TESTS **3283**

Johnson, Samuel.

The Idler. no. 17; 1758. VIVISECTION **3450**

Lives of the Poets. Akenside, 1781. PHYSICIANS **2562**

Lives of the Poets. Collins, 1781. DEPRESSION **714**

Lives of the Poets. Garth, 1781. PHYSICIANS **2563**

Diary entry, April 14, 1770. NARCOTICS **2216**

In Boswell J. *The Life of Samuel Johnson,* 1791. AGING **68**

Letter to Bennet Langton, September 24, 1783. [In: Littlejohn D (ed). *Dr. Johnson: His Life in Letters.* Englewood Cliffs, NJ: Prentice-Hall; 1965, p. 203.] GOUT **1137**, SARCOCELE **2928**

Letter to Dr. Richard Brocklesby, August 16, 1784. [In: Boswell J. *The Life of Samuel Johnson.* London: Oxford University Press; 1957, p. 1340.] PATIENT-PHYSICIAN RELATIONS **2379**

Letter to Edmund Hector, March 7, 1776. In Redford B (ed). *The Letters of Samuel Johnson,* vol 2. Princeton, NJ: Princeton University Press; 1992, p. 301. ILLNESS **1402**

Letter to Mrs. Thrale, June 19, 1783. [In: Littlejohn D (ed). *Dr. Johnson: His Life in Letters.* Englewood Cliffs, NJ: Prentice-Hall; 1965, pp. 196-7.] STROKES **3178**

Letter to Mrs. Thrale, December 27, 1783. VISITORS **3431**

Jokanovic, Vladimir. In Loknar V. *Croatian Medical Quotations* [Limited data]. PHYSICIANS **2598**

Jonas, H. Philosophical reflections on experimenting with human subjects. *Daedalus.* 1969;98:219-47. PATIENT-PHYSICIAN RELATIONS **2424**

Jones HB. Papers in chemical pathology: Lecture III. *Lancet.* 1847;2:88. BENCE JONES PROTEINURIA **295**

Jones, John. *Plain, concise, practical remarks on treatment of wounds and fractures; to which is added, a short appendix on camp and military hospitals; principally designed for the use of young military surgeons in North America,* 1775. SURGEONS **3200**, SURGERY **3217**, **3218**

Jones KL, Smith DW. Recognition of the fetail alcohol syndrome in early infancy. *Lancet.* 1973;2:999. FETAL ALCOHOL SYNDROME **1050**

Jones KL, Smith DW, Ulleland CN, Streissguth AP. Pattern of malformation in offspring of chronic alcoholic mothers. *Lancet.* 1973;1:1267-71. FETAL ALCOHOL SYNDROME **1051**

Jones R, Lodge OJ. The discovery of a bullet lost in the wrist by means of the roentgen rays. *Lancet.* 1896;1:476-7. RADIOLOGY **2816**

Jonsen, Albert R. Do no harm. *Ann Intern Med.* 1978;88:827-32. MEDICAL CARE **1687**

Jordan, Sara Murray. First lady of the Lahey Clinic. *Reader's Digest,* Oct 1958, pp. 67-71. HEALTH **1194**, COSMETIC SURGERY **637**

Joseph, Carol L. Small sacrifices. On being a doctor. *Ann Intern Med.* 1994;121:2;143. WOMEN IN MEDICINE **3481**

Jouanna, Jacques. *Hippocrates.* DeBevoise MB, translator. Baltimore: Johns Hopkins University Press; 1999:129. MEDICAL ETHICS **1848**

Journal of the American Medical Association's Committee on Human Studies. A definition of irreversible coma: report of the ad hoc committee of the Harvard Medical School to examine the definition of brain death. *JAMA.* 1968;205:337-40. DEATH **676**

Ketelaer, Vincent. *Commentarius Medicus de Apthis Nostratibus seu Belgarum Sprouw.* Amsterdam: 1715. [In: Major RH. *Classic Descriptions of Disease,* pp. 657-9.] SPRUE **3124**

Keynes, John Maynard. *Essays in Biography,* 1933. THINKING **3294**

Khanolkar VR, Sanghvi LD, Rao KCM. Smoking and chewing of tobacco in relation to cancer of the upper alimentary tract. *Br Med J.* 1955;1:1111-4. TOBACCO **3313**

Kierkegaard, Søren. In Basta LL. *A Graceful Exit: Life and Death on Your Own Terms.* New York: Insight Books, Plenum Press; 1996:239. DYING **908**

Kimmelstiel P, Wilson C. Intercapillary lesions in the glomeruli of the kidney. *Am J Pathol.* 1936;12:83-98. KIDNEY DISEASE **1491**

King, Albert Freeman Africanus.A. Insects and disease: mosquitos and malaria. *Popular Science Monthly* Sep 1883, vol. 23, pp. 644-58. [In: Major RH. *Classic Descriptions of Disease,* p. 117 (q.v.).] MALARIA **1605**

King, Thomas Wilkinson. Observations on the thyroid gland. *Guy's Hosp Rep.* 1836;1:429-56. THYROID GLAND **3301**

Kinglake, Alexander W. *Eothen, or Traces of Travel Brought Home from the East.* London: 1844. QUARANTINE **2811**

Kingsley, Sidney. *Men in White,* act 1, scene IV. New York: Covici, Friede; 1933, p. 66. DOCTORS **847**

Kinsey AC, Pomeroy WB, Martin CE. *Sexual Behavior in the Human Male.* Philadelphia: W.B. Saunders; 1948, p. 660. HOMOSEXUALITY **1311**

Kipling, Rudyard. A Doctor's Work. In *A Book of Words,* 1908. MEDICAL PRACTICE **1938**

Kircher, Athanasius.
Naturliche und Medicinalische Durchgrundung der Laidigen Ansteckenden Sucht und so Genanten Pestilentz. Augsburg: 1680, p. 39. [In: Major RH. *Classic Descriptions of Disease,* pp. 96-7 (q.v.).] BUBONIC PLAGUE **357**

Scrutinium Physico-medicum Contagiosae, luis quae Pestis Dicitur. Rome: 1658. [In: Major RH. *Classic Descriptions of Disease,* p. 11 (q.v.).] INFECTIOUS DISEASE **1433**, MICRO-ORGANISMS **2161**

Kirkes, William Senhouse. On some of the principal effects resulting from the detachment of fibrinous deposits from the interior of the heart, and their mixture with the circulating blood. *Med-Chir Trans.* 1852;35:281-324. CEREBRAL EMBOLISM **451**, EMBOLISM **947**

Kirklin, John. *Time.* 03 May 1963. SURGERY **3243**

Kitzhaber, John. In: Lamm RD. Doctor Kitzhaber/Governor Kitzhaber. *Pharos.* 2000;63(3):8-10. MEDICAL ECONOMICS **1733**

Klein, G. The role of gene dosage and genetic transpositions in carcinogenesis. *Nature.* 1981;294:313-8. RESEARCH **2872**

Klemperer P, Pollack AD, Baehr G. Diffuse collagen disease; acute disseminated lupus erythematosus and diffuse scleroderma. *JAMA.* 1942;119:4;331-2. COLLAGEN VASCULAR DISEASE **564**

Klinefelter HF, Reifenstein EC, Albright F. Syndrome characterized by gynecomastia, aspermatogenesis without A-Leydigism, and increased excretion of follicle-stimulating hormone. *J Clin Endocrinol.* 1942;2:615-27. KLINEFELTER SYNDROME **1506**

Klinefelter, Harry. What's wrong with the R/O concept. *Resident Staff Phys.* 1973;19:33-5. DIAGNOSIS **754**

Knight, James A. Moral growth in medical students. *Theor Med.* 1995;16:265-80. MEDICAL EDUCATION **1800**

Knights Hospitallers of St. John of Jerusalem. In Hume E. *The Medical Works of the Knights Hospitallers of St. John of Jerusalem.* Baltimore: The Johns Hopkins Press, 1940. PATIENT-PHYSICIAN RELATIONS **2370**

Knowles, John H. Experts, enclaves, and the public interest. *Conn Med.* 1966;30:743. MEDICAL PROFESSION **2011**

Koch, Robert. Die aetiologie der tuberculose. *Berl Klin Wochenschr.* 1882;19:212-30. [In: Koch R. *Medical Classics,* vol 2. Baltimore: Williams and Wilkins; 1937-38.] CAUSATION (ETIOLOGY) **444** [116], TUBERCULOSIS **3389** [861,880], **3390** [877]

Koch, Theodore. Conferenz zur erörterung der cholerafrage. *Berlin Klin Wocchenschr.* 1884;21:477,493 [Translation reprinted in *Br Med J.* 1884;2:403,453. As cited in Bloomfield AL, *Communicable Diseases,* p. 25 (q.v.)]. CHOLERA **473**

Kocher, Emil Theodor. Postoperative results of extirpation of the thyroid [German]. *Arch Klin Chir.* 1883;29:254-337. [In: Talbott JH. *A Biographical History of Medicine,* pp. 1013-4 (q.v.).] HYPOTHYROIDISM **1394**

Kolff WJ, Berk HTJ. The artificial kidney: a dialyser with a great area. *Acta Med Scand.* 1944;117:121-34. KIDNEY ARTIFICIAL **1487**

Letter to his cousin Christophe, 16 April 1810. In Huybrechts-Riviere C. *Correspondence des Laennec des Annees 1808 a 1815 d'Apres le Fonds Rouxeau de Nantes*, no. 2463. Universite de Nantes; 1980, pp. 69-70. DEATH **661**

Letter to his cousin Meriadec, 24 April 1820 [In: Duffin J. *To See With a Better Eye*, p. 241 (q.v.).] AUSCULTATION **268**

Letter to his cousin Meriadec, 8 June 1821. [In: Duffin J, *To See with a Better Eye*, p. 240 (q.v.).] EDUCATION **939**

Letter to his father, c. 1813. [In: Duffin J. *To See with a Better Eye: A Life of R.T.H. Laennec*. Princeton, NJ: Princeton University Press; 1998:347.] PATHOLOGY **2354**

Letter to his uncle Guillaume Laennec, 14 April 1816. [In: Duffin J. *To See with a Better Eye: A Life of R.T.H. Laennec*. Princeton, NJ: Princeton University Press; 1998:105.] DOCTORS **823**

Manuscript of *Musée Laennec*. c. 1821. [In: Duffin J. *To See with a Better Eye: A Life of R.T.H. Laennec*. Princeton, NJ: Princeton University Press; 1998:233.] SCIENCE **2945**

Memoire sur auscultation. In *Academie des Sciences*, 1818. [In: Duffin J. *To See with a Better Eye: A Life of R.T.H. Laennec*. Princeton, NJ: Princeton University Press; 1998:138.] TUBERCULOSIS **3379**

Laforet, Eugene G. The hopeless case. *Arch Intern Med*. 1963;112:314-25. HOPELESS CASES **1313**

Lampedusa, Guiseppe di. *The Leopard*. Translated by Colquhoun A. New York: Pantheon; 1960, p. 262. DEATH **674**

Lancisi, Giovanni Maria. *De Motu Cordis et Aneurysmatibus*. Rome: 1728. SYPHILIS **3259**

Landsteiner K, Wiener AS. An agglutinable factor in human blood recognized by immune serum for Rhesus blood. *Proc Soc Exp Biol Med N Y*. 1940;43:223. BLOOD GROUPS **308**

Lanfrancho of Milan. In Garrison FH. *An Introduction to the History of Medicine*, 4th ed. Translated by Huth EJ. Philadelphia: W.B. Saunders; 1929, p. 155. SURGEONS **3194**

Lang, Andrew. In Strauss MB (ed). *Familiar Medical Quotations*, p. 568 (q.v.). STATISTICS **3151**

Langdon LO, Toskes PP, Kimball HR. Future roles and training of internal medicine subspecialists. *Ann Intern Med*. 1996;124:686-91. INTERNAL MEDICINE **1463**

Lange, Johannes. *Medicinalium Epistolarum Miscellanea*. Basel: 1554. ANEMIA **154**

Langone, John. *Harvard Med: The Story Behind America's Premier Medical School and the Making of America's Doctors*. New York: Crown; 1995, p. 158. PATIENT-PHYSICIAN RELATIONS **2449**

Langstaff, George. Cases of fungus haematodes, with observations. *Med-Chir Trans*. 1817;8:272-305. CANCER OF THE PROSTATE GLAND **407**

Laplace, Pierre-Simon. *Philosophical Essay on Probabilities [Essai philosophique sur les probabilités]*, 1825. CLINICAL TRIALS **533**, STATISTICS **3134**, VACCINATION **3417**

Larkin, Phillip. Aubade. In *Collected Poems*. New York: Farrar, Straus & Giroux; 1989. DEATH **679**

Larrey, Dominique Jean. *Memoirs of Military Surgery and Campaigns of the French Armies*. Translated by Hall RW. Baltimore: Joseph Cushing; 1814, p. 28. [In: Birmingham, AL: Classics of Medicine Library; 1987, p. 28.] MILITARY MEDICINE **2179**

Larson, Leonard. Statement to the Senate Finance Committee, June 27, 1960. AGING **85**

Lasagna, Louis. *The Doctors' Dilemmas*. New York: Harper & Row; 1962:290. AGING **86**, LIFE **1547**

Latham, Peter Mere.

A *Word or Two on Medical Education*, 1864. [In: Martin R (ed). *The Collected Works of Dr. P.M. Latham*, vol II. London: The New Sydenham Society; 1878, p. 560.] MEDICAL EDUCATION **1746**

General Remarks on the Practice of Medicine, 1836. [In: Martin R (ed). *The Collected Works of Dr. P.M. Latham*, vol. 2. London: The New Sydenham Society; 1878.] DRUGS **884** [376], EXPERIENCE **1027** [466]

In Bean WB (ed). *Aphorisms from Latham*. Iowa City: Prairie Press; 1962. CLINICAL OBSERVATION **509** [90], DIAGNOSIS **739** [101], MEDICAL PRACTICE **1922** [26], **1924** [22], MEDICAL PROFESSION **1982** [19], PATIENT-PHYSICIAN RELATIONS **2386** [101], PATIENTS **2456** [101], PSYCHOSOMATIC MEDICINE **2744** [56]

In Martin R (ed). *The Collected Works of Dr. P.M. Latham*. London: The New Sydenham Society; 1878. DIAGNOSIS **740** [vol I; lecture XIV; p. 173], MEDICAL PRACTICE **1923** [II; II; 23], MURMURS **2207** [I; II; 17], **2208** [I; II; 3]

Latta, Thomas. In Lewins R. Injection of saline solutions in extraordinary quantities into the veins in cases of malignant cholera. *Lancet*. 1831-32;2:243-4. FLUID THERAPY **1058**

Lauterbur, Paul Christian. Image formation by induced local interactions: examples employing nuclear interactions: examples employing nuclear magnetic resonance. *Nature*. 1973;242:190-1. RADIOLOGY **2818**

Laveran, Alphonse. De la nature parasitaire des accidents, de l' impaludisme. *C R Acad Sci*. 1881;93:627. [In: Bloomfield AL, *Communicable Diseases*, p. 348 (q.v.).] MALARIA **1604**

Lavoisier, Antoine-Lavoisier. *Experiments on Animal Respiration and the Changes Occuring When Air Passes Through the Lungs*, 1777. RESPIRATION **2889**

Leacock, Stephen. *How To Be a Doctor*. 1911. [In: Leacock S. *Literary Lapses*. Toronto: McClelland and Stewart; 1993, pp. 36-7.] TREATMENT **3350**

Lederberg, Joshua. Sloppy research extracts a greater toll than misconduct. *Scientist*. 1995;9(4):13. RESEARCH **2879**

Leeuwenhoek, Anton von.
Den Waaragtigen Omloop des Bloeds; 65th Missive [to the Royal Society]; 1688. CAPILLARIES **420**
Letter to Lambert Velthuysen, July 11, 1679. In *The Collected Letters of Anton van Leeuwenhoek*. Amsterdam: Swets & Zeitlinger; 1939. GOUT **1131**
Observations communicated to the publisher in a Dutch letter of the 9th of October 1676. *Phil Trans R Soc London*. 1677;12:821-31. MICROSCOPE **2162**

Lehmann HE, Hanrahan GE. Chlorpromazine: new inhibiting agent for psychomotor excitement and manic states. *AMA Arch Neurol Psychiatry*. 1954;71:227-37. WRITING **3501**

Lehmann, Jörgen. Para-aminosalicylic acid used in the treatment of tuberculosis. *Lancet*. 1946;1:15-6. TUBERCULOSIS **3402**

Leibniz, Gottfried. *Leibniz Selections*. Wiener P; editor. New York: Charles Scribnerís Sons; 1951:82-3, chapter 2. STATISTICS **3129**

Lejumeau, Jacques-Alexandre. *Memoire sur l'Auscultation, Appliquee a l'Etude de la Grossesse*. Paris: 1822. FETAL HEART **1052**, PREGNANCY **2658**

Leoniceno N. *Libellus de Morbo Gallico*. Venice: 1535. [In: Major RH. *Classic Descriptions of Disease*, p. 16.] SYPHILIS **3253**

Lettsom, John. *On Himself*. 1780. [In: Stevenson B, *The Home Book of Quotations*, 4th ed, p. 468.] PHYSICIANS **2560**

Lever, John Charles Weaver. Cases of puerpural convulsions, with remarks. *Guy's Hosp Rep*. 1843;2:495-517. ECLAMPSIA **937**

Levi-Montalcini, Rita. *In Praise of Imperfection: My Life and Work*. Attardi L; translator. New York: Basic Books; 1988:5. RESEARCH **2877**

Levin P, Burnham L, Katzin EM, Vogel P. The role of iso-immunization in the pathogenesis of erythroblastosis fetalis. *Am J Obstet Gynecol*. 1941;42:925-37. ERYTHROBLASTOSIS FETALIS **996**

Levine, Rachmiel. Lecture to New York Diabetes Association, *ca.* 1970. FAT **1046**

Lewis, Aubrey J. Melancholia: a clinical survey of depressive states. *J Ment Sci*. 1934;80:277-378. CAUSATION (ETIOLOGY) **445**

Lewis, Denslow.
Clinical lecture on obstetrics and gynecology. *Chicago Clin Rev*. 1894;4:118-33. CASES **436**
Letter to George Henry Cleveland, August 14, 1896. [In: Beatty WK. Denslow Lewis: gynecologist, teacher, and gadfly. Part I. *Proc Inst Med Chicago*. 1989;42:8-20.] WRITING **3495**
Mutilating operations in obstetric practice: clinical lecture on obstetrics and gynaecology. *Clinical Review*. 1900;12:12-26. OBSTETRICS **2286**
Obstetric manipulation: clinical lecture on obstetrics and gynaecology. *Clin Rev*. 1900;11:414-32. OBSTETRICS **2285**
The best method of teaching gynecology. *JAMA*. 1896;27:618-21. MEDICAL PRACTICE **1932**
The gynecologic consideration of the sexual act. *Trans Section Obstet Dis Women Am Med Assoc*. 1899;453-68. [In: Beatty WK. Denslow Lewis: gynecologist, teacher, and gadfly. Part II. *Proc Inst Med Chicago*. 1989;42:32-6.] SEX **3032**, SEX EDUCATION **3046**
The limitation of the venereal diseases. *Med-Legal J*. 1903;23:83-90. SEX **3034**, WOMEN **3468**
The social evil. *Buffalo Med J*. 1906;62:249-57. MEDICINE **2106**
The study of obstetrics-concealed haemorrhage [Clinical lecture on obstetrics and gynaecology]. In *Obstetric Clinic*. Chicago: Colegrove; 1900, p. 5. [In: 1903, p. 5.] MEDICAL EDUCATION **1756**
What should be the policy of the State toward prostitution? *Med Rec*. 1895;46:651-53. [In: Beatty WK. Denslow Lewis: gynecologist, teacher, and gadfly. Part III. *Proc Inst Med Chicago*. 1989;42:85-92.] PROSTITUTION **2700**

Lewis IJ, Sheps CG. *The Sick Citadel: The American Academic Medical Center and the Public Interest*. Cambridge, MA: Oelgeschlager, Gunn & Hain; 1983, p. 157. PSYCHOSOCIAL MEDICINE **2742**

Lewis T, Rothschild MA. The excitatory process in the dog's heart. *Philos Trans R Soc London*. 1915;206:181-226. [In: Talbott JH. A *Biographical History of Medicine*, p. 1169 (q.v.).] HEART **1231**

Lewis, Thomas.
Clinical Disorders of the Heart Beat. London: Shaw and Sons; 1912:72. ATRIAL FIBRILLATION **261** [72], **262** [71], PULSUS ALTERNANS **2792** [108], **2793** [108],
Clinical Science: Illustrated by Personal Experiences. London: Shaw and Sons; 1934, p. 179. CLINICAL TRIALS **544**, STATISTICS **3155** [179]

Auricular fibrillation and its relationship to clinical irregularity of the heart. *Heart*. 1910;1:306-72. ATRIAL FIBRILLATION **260**

Auricular fibrillation: a common clinical condition. *Br Med J*. 1909;2:1528. ATRIAL FIBRILLATION **259**

Reflections upon reform in medical education. *Lancet*. 1944;1:619-21. NOMENCLATURE **2258**

The value of quinidine in cases of auricular fibrillation and methods of studying the clinical reaction. *Am J Med Sci*. 1922;163:781-94. EMBOLISM **949**

Leyden, Ernst von.
About fatty heart. *Zeitschrift für Klinische Medizin*. 1882;5:1-25. [In: Talbott JH. *A Biographical History of Medicine*, p. 1126 (q.v.).] OBESITY **2281**

Contribution to our knowledge about bronchial asthma. *Archiv Path Anat*. 1872;54:325. ASTHMA **252**

Lidz, Theodore. The adolescent and his family. In Caplan G, Lebovici S (eds). *Adolescence: Psychosocial Perspectives*. New York: Basic Books; 1969:109. ADOLESCENCE **40**

Liley, Albert William. Intrauterine transfusion of foetus in haemolytic disease. *Br Med J*. 1963;2:1107-9. FETAL TRANSFUSION **1053**

Lind, James. *A Treatise on the Scurvy*, 1753. [Stewart CP, Guthrie D (eds). *Lind's Treatise on Scurvy*. Edinburgh: Edinburgh University Press; 1953.] MEDICAL EVIDENCE **1850** [7], SCURVY **3015**, [90-1], **3016** [149-50]

Lipkin, Mack. A suggestion for teaching the care of patients. *N Engl J Med*. 1985;313:122. PUBLISHING **2771**

Lipkin, Mack, Jr. Sisyphus or Pegasus? The physician interviewer in the era of corporatization of care. *Ann Intern Med*. 1996;124:511-3. MANAGED CARE **1621**

Lister, John. By the London Post: Christmas books. *N Engl J Med*. 1975;292:467-9. DRUGS **896**

Lister, Joseph.
Letter to his father. 1854. [In: Coope R (ed). *The Quiet Art*, p. 69 (q.v.).] SURGEONS **3201**

On a new method of treating compound fractures, abscess, etc., with observations on the conditions of suppuration. *Lancet*. 1867;1:326-9. ANTISEPSIS **197**

On the antiseptic principle in the practice of surgery. *Lancet*. 1867;2:353-6, 668-9. ANTISEPSIS **198**

On the early stages of inflammation. *Philos Trans R Soc London*. 1858;2:645. [In: *The Collected Papers of Joseph Lister*, vol. 1. Birmingham, AL: Classics of Medicine Library; 1979, p. 209.] INFLAMMATION **1441**

Liston, Robert. [Letter]. *Lancet*. 1847;1:8. ANESTHESIA **160**

Little, William John. Course of lectures on the deformities of the human frame: lecture VIII. *Lancet*. 1843-4;1:318-20. ASPHYXIA NEONATORUM **242**

Llewellyn, Richard Llewellyn Jones.
Aspects of Rheumatism and Gout: Their Pathogeny, Prevention, and Control. London: William Heinemann Medical Books; 1927:6-7. BIORHYTHMS **302**

Gout. London: W. Heinemann; 1920, p. 36. GOUT **1147**

Lloyd, Ian. Official Record, House of Commons, 23 April 1990, cols. 96-8. [In: Franklin S. *Embodied Progress: A Cultural Account of Assisted Conception*. London: Routledge; 1997, p. 205.] GENETICS **1111**

Locke, John. Letter to Richard Morton, 20 January 1693. [In: Dewhurst K. *John Locke (1632-1704), Physician and Philosopher: A Medical Biography with an Edition of the Medical Notes in His Journals*. London: Wellcome Historical Medical Library; 1963, p. 310.] MEDICAL PRACTICE **1917**

Lodge, David. *Therapy*. New York: Penguin Books; 1996, p. 5. COMPASSION FATIGUE **569**

Loeb L, Bassett RB. Effect of hormones of anterior pituitary on thyroid gland in the guinea pig. *Proc Soc Exp Biol Med*. 1929;26:860-2. THYROID-STIMULATING HORMONE **3306**

Long, Crawford Williamson.
Trans Georgia Med Surg Assoc. 1853. ANESTHESIA **164**

An account of the first use of sulphuric ether by inhalation as an anesthetic in surgical operations. *South Med Surg J*. 1849;5:705-13. ANESTHESIA **162**

Long, Perrin H. *Resident Phys*. 1964;10:75-6. WOMEN IN MEDICINE **3480**

Longcope, Warfield T.
In Manning PR and DeBakey L. *Medicine: Preserving the Passion*. New York: Springer-Verlag; 1987, p. 199. PATIENT-PHYSICIAN RELATIONS **2445**

Methods and medicine. *John Hopkins Hosp Bull*. 1932;50:4-20. LIVING **1572**

Louis, Pierre-Charles-Alexandre.
Anatomical, Pathological, and Therapeutic Researches on the Yellow Fever of Gibraltar of 1828. Translated by Shattuck GC Jr. Boston: Charles C. Little & James Brown; 1839:117. YELLOW FEVER **3517**

Essay on Clinical Instruction. Translated by Martin P. London: S. Highley; 1834, pp. 26-8. STATISTICS **3136**

Recherches anatomiques, pathologiques et therapeutiques sur la maladie connue sous les noms de gastro-enterite. Paris: Bailliere; 1829, p. vii. [In: Bloomfield AL, *Communicable Diseases*, p. 5 (q.v.).] SCIENCE **2947**

Researches on Phthisis, 2nd ed. London: Sydenham Society; 1844, p. 278. [In: Birmingham, AL: Classics of Medicine Library; 1986, p. 278.] LIBIDO **1535**

Researches on the Effects of Bloodletting in Some Inflammatory Diseases, and on the Influence of Tartarized Antimony and Vesication in Pneumonitis. Translated by Putnam CG. Boston: 1836. [In: Birmingham, AL: Classics of Medicine Library; 1986.] CLINICAL EPIDEMIOLOGY **503** [64-5], CLINICAL RESEARCH **527** [96-7]

Inscription on a photograph sent to Dr. Henry I. Bowditch, 1872. [In: Middleton WS. A biographic history of physical diagnosis. *Ann Med Hist*. 1924;6:426-51.] RESEARCH **2857**

Louyer-Villermay, Jean-Baptiste. Observations pour Servir a l'Histoire des Inflammations de l'Appendice du Caecum [Observations of Use in the Inflammatory Conditions of the Cecal Appendix]. *Arch Gen Med*. 1824;5:246-50. APPENDICITIS **221**

Lowe CR. Occupational medicine and epidemiology. Presidential address. *Proc R Soc Med*. 1974;67:643-6. SCIENCE **2986**

Lowenstein, Jerome. *The Midnight Meal and Other Essays About Doctors, Patients, and Medicine*. New Haven, CT: Yale University Press; 1997. DIAGNOSIS **756** [57], MEDICAL ECONOMICS **1727** [9], MEDICAL EDUCATION **1804** [17], PATIENT-PHYSICIAN RELATIONS **2451** [22]

Lower, Richard.

A Treatise on the Heart on the Movement and Colour of the Blood and on the Passage of the Chyle into the Blood, 1669. Translated by Franklin KJ; 1932. [In: Birmingham, AL: Classics of Medicine Library; 1989.] BLOOD TRANSFUSION **317** [174-6], BRAIN **339** [92-3], PERICARDIAL FLUID **2498** [38], PERICARDIUM **2504** [5-6], PHARMACOLOGY **2512** [172], PULMONARY CIRCULATION **2782** [165-6], RESPIRATION **2886** [170]

De catarrhis, 1672. Hunter R, MacAlpine I; translators. London: Dawson's of Pall Mall; 1963. CATARRH **440** [4], NOMENCLATURE **2254** [3], PITUITARY TUMORS **2605** [8], VENIPUNCTURE **3425** [12-3]

An account of the experiment of transfusion practiced upon a man in London. *Philos Trans R Soc London*. 1667;1:557-64. BLOOD TRANSFUSION **316**

Lowy, Frederick. Health maintenance organizations in Canada: some ethical considerations. *CMAJ*. 1988;139:105-9. MEDICAL ETHICS **1845**

Loxterkamp, David. Hearing voices: how should doctors respond to their calling? *N Engl J Med*. 1997;335:1992-3. MANAGED CARE **1623**

Lu G-D, Needham J. *Celestial Lancets: A History and Rationale of Acupuncture and Moxa*. Cambridge: Cambridge University Press; 1980:6. ACUPUNCTURE **36**

Lucas, Frank Laurence. *The Greatest Problem and Other Essays*. New York: Macmillan; 1961. POPULATION CONTROL **2647** [320-1], **2648** [300]

Lucas WP. *The Modern Practice of Pediatrics*. [In: Coope R (ed). *The Quiet Art*, p. 145 (q.v.).] TRUTH **3366**

Lucretius (Titus Lucretius Carus). *On the Nature of Things*, book IV. DREAMS **874**

Ludmerer, Kenneth M. *Learning to Heal: The Development of American Medical Education*. New York: Basic Books; 1985. FRENCH MEDICINE **1067** [30], PHYSICIANS **2591** [280]

Ludwig, Carl Friedrich Wilhelm.

Quarterly Review, 2nd ed. Leipzig: C.F. Winter; 1858. [In: Talbott, A *Biographical History of Medicine*, pp. 609-10 (q.v.).] MOLECULAR BIOLOGY **2196**

Nieren und harnbereitung. In *Handwörter der Physiologie*, vol. 2. Braunschweig; 1842-53, pp. 637-8. [In: Fulton JF. *Selected Readings in the History of Physiology*, 2nd ed. Springfield, IL: Charles C Thomas; 1966, pp. 360-1.] KIDNEY FUNCTION **1494**

Luria SE, Anderson TF. The identification and characterization of bacteriophages with the electron microscope. *Proc Natl Acad Sci*. 1942;28(4):127-30. BACTERIOPHAGE **281**

Luther, Martin. *Of Sicknesses and of the Causes Thereof*. c. 1566. [Translation by Hazlitt W reprinted in *The Table-Talk of Martin Luther*. Philadelphia: The Lutheran Publication Society; 1868, p. 383]. HEALTH **1172**, PHYSICIANS **2548**

Lydston, George Frank.

Stricture of the Urethra. Chicago: 1893. [In: Beatty WK. G. Frank Lydston: urologist, author, and pioneer transplanter. *Proc Inst Med Chicago*. 1990;43:35-69.] MEDICAL EDUCATION **1751**

An organized profession. *N Y Med J*. 1904;79:649-51. PATIENT-PHYSICIAN RELATIONS **2401**

Muscle building as illustrated by the modern Samson, Sandow. *JAMA*. 1893;21:419-22. EXERCISE **1020**, **1021**

Sex mutilations in social therapeutics, with some of the difficulties in the application of eugenics to the human race. *N Y Med J*. 1912;95:677-85. BIRTH **305**

Sexual neurasthenia and the prostate. *Med Rec.* 1912;81:218-20. QUACKERY **2807**

The indications for and the technique of prostatectomy. *N Y Med J.* 1904;80:249-54. MEDICAL JOURNALS **1900**

The training school fake and its victims. *N Y Med J.* 1904;79:1198-200. NURSING **2274**

Lyly, John. *Euphues and His England*, 1580. ALCOHOLISM **118**

Macallum AB. The inorganic composition of the blood in vertebrates and invertebrates, and its origin. *Proc R Soc London.* 1910;B82:602-24. BODY FLUIDS **325**

Macaulay, Thomas Babington. *History of England*, chapter 20, 1848. SMALLPOX **3081**

MacCallum WG, Voegtlin C. On the relation of tetany to the parathyroid glands and to calcium metabolism. *J Exp Med.* 1909;11:118-51. PARATHYROID GLANDS **2336**

MacIntyre, William. Case of mollities and fragilitas ossium. *Medico-Chemical Society Transactions.* 1850;33:211-32. MULTIPLE MYELOMA **2200**

Mackay, Ian R. In Manning PR, DeBakey L. *Medicine: Preserving the Passion.* New York: Springer-Verlag; 1987, p. 172. MEDICAL RECORDS **2023**

Mackenzie J, Orr J. *Principles of Diagnosis and Treatment in Heart Affections*, 3rd ed. London: Humphrey Milford;1926:189-90. HYPERTENSION **1349**

Mackenzie, James.

Angina Pectoris. London: 1923. [In: Talbott JH. A *Biographical History of Medicine*, p. 1152 (q.v.).] CORONARY ARTERY DISEASE **621**

The Study of the Pulse. Edinburgh: 1902. BLOOD PRESSURE **312**, EXTRASYSTOLES **1035, 1036**, SPHYGMOGRAPH **3116** [preface]

In Froude H (ed). *Diseases of the Heart*, 3rd ed, chap. 30. London: Oxford University Press; 1913. ATRIAL FIBRILLATION **257, 258**

In Willius FA, Dry TJ. A *History of the Heart and the Circulation.* Philadelphia: W.B. Saunders; 1948, p. 350. MEDICAL EDUCATION **1776**

The inception of the rhythm of the heart by the ventricle. *Br Med J.* 1904;1:529-36. ATRIAL FIBRILLATION **256**

MacLagan, Thomas John. The treatment of acute rheumatism by salicin. *Lancet.* 1876;1:342-3. SALICYLATES **2925**

Maclean, Norman. *Young Men and Fire.* Chicago: University of Chicago Press; 1992, p. 296. COMPASSION **568**

MacLeod, Sheila. *The Art of Starvation.* London: 1981. ANOREXIA NERVOSA **192**

MacWilliam, John Alexander. Cardiac failure and sudden death. *Br Med J.* 1889;1:6-8. VENTRICULAR FIBRILLATION **3428**

Maddox, John. In O'Donnell M. The toxic effect of language on medicine. *J R Coll Phys Lond.* 1995;29:525-9. MEDICAL JOURNALS **1907**

Maddrey WC, Boitnott JK. Hepatitis induced by isoniazid and methyldopa. *Hosp Pract.* 1975;10:119-25. ADVERSE DRUG EFFECTS **51**

Maeder, Thomas. Wounded healers. *Atlantic Monthly.* 1989;263:37-47. PSYCHIATRISTS **2712**

Magendie, François. Experiences sur les fonctions des racines des nerfs rachidiens. *J Physiol Exp Path.* 1822;2:276-9. [In: Fulton JF. The Historical Contribution of Physiology to Neurology. *Science, Medicine, and History: Essays on the Evolution of Scientific Thought.* Underwood EA (ed). New York: Oxford University Press; 1953, p. 541.] NERVES **2230**

Mahoney JF, Arnold RC, Harris A. Penicillin treatment of early syphilis: a preliminary report. *Venereal Dis Inf.* 1943;24:355-7. SYPHILIS **3267**

Maimonides, Moses.

Daily Prayer of a Physician Before Visiting a Sick Man, 1863. [In: Kagan SR. Maimonides' prayer. *Ann Med Hist.* 1938;10:429-32.] MEDICAL PROFESSION **1975**

Regimen of Health, 1198. EXERCISE **1017**

In Minkin JS. *The World of Moses Maimonides, with Selections from His Writings.* New York: Thomas Yoeseloff; 1957, pp. 149-50. MEDICAL PROFESSION **1974**

In Rosner F, Munter S. *The Medical Aphorisms of Moses Maimonides.* New York: Yeshiva University Press; 1970. ADOLESCENCE **39** [vol. 1, treatise 3], SEX **3026** [vol. 2, treatise 17]

Main TF. The ailment. *Br J Med Psychol.* 1957;30:129-45. PATIENT-PHYSICIAN RELATIONS **2418**

Major, Ralph H. *Classic Descriptions of Disease, with Biographical Sketches of the Authors*, 2nd ed. Springfield, IL: Charles C Thomas; 1939.

Malgaigne, Joseph-François. *Advice on the Choice of a Library*, 1905. [In: Rogers FB. *JAMA.* 1968;204:141-4.] BOOKS **330**, HEALTH **1188**, READING **2832, 2833**

Malpighi, Marcello. In Hayman JM Jr. Malpighi's "Concerning the structure of the kidneys." *Ann Med Hist.* 1925;7:242-63. KIDNEY **1479**

Malthus, Thomas Robert. *An Essay on the Principle of Population,* chapter 1, 1798. POPULATION CONTROL **2646**

Mandeville, Bernard. *The Fable of the Bees,,* vol. II, dialogue V, 1729. PAIN **2317**

Mann, George V.
Challenging some sacrosanct beliefs about diet and nutrition. *Resident Staff Phys.* 1977;23:88-95. MEDICAL EVIDENCE **1857**
Diet-heart: end of an era. *N Engl J Med.* 1977;297:644-50. PEER REVIEW **2474**

Mann T, Keilin D. Sulphanilamide as a specific inhibitor of carbonic anhydrase. *Nature.* 1940;146(3692):164. CARBONIC ANHYDRASE INHIBITORS **424**

Mann, Thomas.
Joseph the Provider. New York: Alfred A. Knopf; 1944:39. WRITING **3498**
The Magic Mountain. Translated by Lowe-Porter HT. New York: Alfred A. Knopf; 1927, p. 532. DYING **915**
The Confessions of Felix Krull, Confidence Man. New York: Alfred A. Knopf; 1955:38. PHYSICIANS **2585**

Mannes, Marya. Of time and the woman. *Psychosomatics.* 1968;9:8. AGING **89**

Manning PR, DeBakey L. *Medicine: Preserving the Passion.* New York: Springer-Verlag; 1987 [Precedes first chapter]. DOCTORS **860**

Mansfield, Katherine. [Journal entry written as she was dying of tuberculosis]. [In: Dubos R, *Man Adapting,* p. 351 (q.v.).] HEALTH **1190**

Manu P, Lane TJ, Matthews DA. The frequency of the chronic fatigue syndrome in patients with symptoms of persistent fatigue. *Ann Intern Med.* 1988;109:554-6. CHRONIC FATIGUE SYNDROME **478**

Marchand FJ. Über arteriosclerose (atherosclerose); 1904. [In: Pickering G. Language: the lost tool of learning in medicine and science. Lancet. 1961;2:115-9.] ATHEROSCLEROSIS **253**

Mare, Walter de la. *Winged Chariot,* 1951. AGING **83**

Marfan, Antoine. *Bulletin of the Medical Society of Paris.* 1896;13:220-6. MARFAN SYNDROME **1630**

Marie, Pierre.
Essays on Acromegalia. London: Adlard & Son; 1891:28. ACROMEGALY **32**
De l'osteo-arthropathie hypertrophiante pneumique. *Revue de Médecine.* 1890;10:1-36. [In: Jouanna J. *Hippocrates.* DeBevoise MB, translator. Baltimore: Johns Hopkins University Press; 1999:297.] HYPERTROPHIC OSTEOARTHROPATHY (DIGITAL HIPPOCRATISM) **1366**
Sur la nature et sur quelques-uns des symptomes de la maladie de basedow. *Archives de Neurologie.* 1883;6:79. TREATMENT **3345**

Marine D, Lenhart CH. Relation of iodin to the structure of human thyroids: relation of iodin and histologic structure to diseases in general; to exophthalmic goiter; to cretinism and myxedema. *Arch Intern Med.* 1909;4:440-93. THYROID GLAND **3304**

Markowitz, Jacob.
A series of over 100 amputations of the thigh for tropical ulcers. *J R Army Med Corps.* 1946;86:159-70. WARTIME MEDICINE **3458**
Experiences with cholera in a jungle camp in Thailand. *J R Army Med Corps.* 1946;86:150-8. HYGIENE **1346**
Transfusion of defibrinated blood in P.O.W. camps at Chungkai and Nakom Paton, Thailand. *J R Army Med Corps.* 1946;86:189-97. WARTIME MEDICINE **3459**

Markowski, B. Some experiences of a medical prisoner of war. *Br Med J.* 1945;2:361-363. WARTIME MEDICINE **3455**

Marriott HL, Kekwick A. Continuous drip blood transfusion: with case records of very large transfusions. *Lancet.* 1935;1:977-81. BLOOD TRANSFUSION **321**

Marsac. Phélippeaux: Notice biographique et bibliographique sur Philippe Le Goust, médecin du XVIIe siècle, lue à la séance générale de la Société des archives historiques de la Saintonge et de l'Aunis, le 12 mars, par le Dr. Phélippeaux (de Saint Savinien). *Arch Tocol.* 1879;6:304-20. [In: Speert H. *Obstetric and Gynecologic Milestones,* new ed. New York: Parthenon; 1996:515.] PREGNANCY **2657**

Marshall BJ, Warren JR. Unidentified curved bacilli in the stomach of patients with gastritis and peptic ulceration. *Lancet.* 1984;1:1311-4. PEPTIC ULCER **2493**

Marshall, Barry J. Unidentified curved bacilli on gastric epithelium in active chronic gastritis [Letter]. *Lancet.* 1983;1:1273-5. PEPTIC ULCER **2492**

Martial (Marcus Valerius Martialis).
Epigrams I, 30. SURGEONS **3193**
Epigrams I, 47. DOCTORS **808**
Epigrams VI, 53. PHYSICIANS **2543**
Epigrams X, 47. DEATH **651**

Marusic M, Petrovecki M, Petrak M, Marusic A. *Introduction to Medical Research*. Zagreb: Medicinska naklada; 2000:33. PHYSICIANS **2592**

Marusic, Matko.
[Personal communication to a contributor]. 1982. LIVING **1577**
[Personal communication to a contributor]. 1988. SCIENCE **2997**
Frauds of paramedicine. *Acta Facultatis Medicae Zagrabiensis*. 1986;27:57-75. PHYSIOLOGY **2604**
Hypocritical humanism. *Lijecnicki Vjesnik*. 1990;112:201. STETHOSCOPE **3172**
Physiologic foundations of life, death and the disease. *Lijec Vjesn*. 1987;109:93-5. EVOLUTION **1013**
Slobodna Hrvatska, znanost i znanstveni kriteriji. In Polsek D (ed). *Visible and Invisible Academia* [Croatian]. Zagreb: Institut drustvenih znanosti Ivo Pilar; 1998, pp. 47-56. PUBLISHING **2774**

Marx, Karl. *Economic and Philosophical Manuscripts of 1844*. New York: International Publishers; 1964, p. 111. HUMANS **1333**

Masters WH, Johnson VE. *Human Sexual Response*. Boston: Little, Brown; 1966, p. 188. PENIS **2486**

Mather, Cotton. *The Angel of Bethesda*, 1724. [Jones GW (ed). Barre, MA: American Antiquarian Society and Barre Publishers; 1972.] ARTHRITIS **235** [79-80], BIRTH **304** [238], CONSTIPATION **581** [276], DIET **760** [17], EPILEPSY **975** [83], GOUT **1133** [69], HEMORRHOIDS **1268** [220], IRON-DEFICIENCY ANEMIA **1472** [234], JAUNDICE **1473** [191], OBESITY **2280** [283], PAIN **2316** [54], PHYSICIANS **2555** [43], RICKETS **2916** [276], SCURVY **3014** [83], SEXISM **3049** [233], SEXUALLY TRANSMITTED DISEASES **3055** [83], SMOKING **3090** [307], **3091** [303], TUBERCULOSIS **3374** [180], URINARY TRACT CALCULUS **3415**, WOMEN **3465**

Matthaei JH. Nirenberg MW. Characteristics and stabilization of DNAase-sensitive protein synthesis in *E. coli* extracts. *Proc National Academy Sciences*. 1961;47:1580-8. DEOXYRIBONUCLEIC ACID (DNA) **709**

Maugham, W. Somerset.
Of Human Bondage, chapter 55, 1915. MEDICAL PROFESSION **2004**
The Moon and Sixpence, chapter 1, 1919. PSYCHOANALYSIS **2730**

Maxwell, James Clerk. *The Scientific Letters and Papers of James Clerk Maxwell*. Volume 1. Cambridge: Cambridge University Press; 1990:675-9. COLOR VISION **566**

Maynow, John. *De Rachitide*, 1668. [In: Aterman K. Extrarenal nephroblastomas. *J Cancer Res Clin Oncol*. 1989;115:409-17.] WRITING **3488**

Mayo CH, Hendricks WA. Carcinoma of the right segment of the colon. *Ann Surg*. 1926;83:357-63. CANCER **382**

Mayo, Charles Horace.
Univ Toronto Med J. April 1928. MEDICAL PRACTICE **1943**
Address to the Clinical Congress of the American College of Surgeons, Boston, October 9, 1928 [Limited data]. PHYSIOLOGY **2603**
Educational possibilities of the National Medical Museum in the standardization of medical training. *JAMA*. 1919;73:411-3. HEALTH POLICY **1215**, MEDICAL CARE **1667**
President's address. *Collected Papers of the Mayo Clinic and Mayo Foundation*. 1905-1909, p. 601-4. MEDICINE **2108**
Preventive medicine. *Texas State J Med*. 1928;24:403-5. PUBLIC HEALTH **2754**
Problems in medical education. *Collected Papers of the Mayo Clinic and Mayo Foundation*. 1926;18:1093-102. SCIENCE **2973**
Splenomegaly. *Collected Papers of the Mayo Clinic and Mayo Foundation*. 1935;27:555-66. SURGERY **3235**
The examination, preparation, and care of surgical patients. *Lancet*. 1916;36:1-4. CLINICAL OBSERVATION **520**
The influence of pain and mortality in modern medical practice. *Proc Interstate Postgraduate Med Assoc North Am*. 19 Oct 1931, pp. 245-8. PAIN **2324**
The old and the new in prostatic surgery. *Ann Surg*. 1934;100:883-6. AGING **81**

Mayo, William J.
[Discussion of Keys TT. *The Medical Books of William Worrall Mayo: Pioneer Surgeon of the American Northwest*]. *Collected Papers of the Mayo Clinic and Mayo Foundation*. 1938;30:938-43. PHYSICAL EXAMINATION **2528**
An address on the relation of the basic medical sciences to surgery. *CMAJ*. 1927;17:652-7. MEDICAL PROFESSION **2006**
Chronic duodenal ulcer. *JAMA*. 1915;64:2036-40. PEPTIC ULCER **2490**
In the time of Henry Jacob Bigelow. *JAMA*. 1921;77:597-603. EXPERIENCE **1030**
Master surgeons of America: Frederic S. Dennis. *Surg Gynecol Obstet*. 1938;67:535-6. SURGERY **3239**

Radical operations on the stomach with especial reference to mobilization of the lesser curvature. *Surg Gynecol Obstet.* 1923;36:447-53. TESTS **3276**

The aims and ideals of the American Medical Association [Address given at the 66th Annual Meeting of the National Education Association, Minneapolis, July 1-6, 1928]. *Proc Natl Educ Assoc.* 1928;66:158-63. MEDICINE **2113**

The economic relation of the university system to the development of a social democracy. *Collected Papers Mayo Clinic Mayo Foundation.* 1933;25:1105-7. MEDICAL EDUCATION **1779**

The preliminary education of the clinical specialist. *Collected Papers of the Mayo Clinic and Mayo Foundation.* 23;1931:1001-5. MEDICINE **2114**

Mayow, John. *Tractatus quinque medico-physici.* Oxford: 1674. [In: Talbott JH. *A Biographical History of Medicine,* p. 146.] RESPIRATION **2887**

McBurney, Charles.
Experience with early operative interference in cases of disease of the vermiform appendix. *N Y Med J.* 1889;50:676-84. APPENDICITIS **225**

The incision made in the abdominal wall in cases of appendicitis, with a description of a new method of operating. *Ann Surg.* 1894;20:38-43. APPENDICITIS **226**

McCance RA, Widdowson EM. In Ashwell M (ed). *A Scientific Partnership of 60 Years.* London: British Nutrition Foundation; 1993, p. 65. RESEARCH **2878**

McCance, Robert A. Practice of experimental medicine [President's address, 1950]. [In: *Proc R Soc Med.* 1951;44:189-94.] RESEARCH **2867**

McClenahan, John L.
X-ray Technician. 1961;32:498 [Limited data]. MEDICAL PRACTICE **1951**
1993 [Limited data]. HOSPITALS **1329**
Aphorism. 1964 [Limited data]. PLACEBOS **2611**
Something about symptoms. *Med Affairs.* 1982;3:8-12. DIAGNOSIS **749**

McClenahan WU. *G.P.* Philadelphia: Dorrance; 1974. CONVALESCENCE **605** [127], MEDICAL MARRIAGES **1909** [85], MEDICAL PRACTICE **1957** [129], PATIENT-NURSE RELATIONS **2360** [5], RESUSCITATION **2902** [114]

McCollum EV, Davis M. The necessity of certain lipids in the diet during growth. *J Biol Chem.* 1913;15:167-75. VITAMIN A **3433**

McCollum EV, Simmonds N, Becker JE, Shipley PG. Studies on experimental rickets. Part XXI: An experimental demonstration of the existence of a vitamin which promotes calcium deposition. *J Biol Chem.* 1922;53:293-312. VITAMIN D **3444**

McCord, May Kennedy. In Randolf V. *Ozark Superstitions.* New York: Dover Publications; 1964. [Reprinted as *Ozark Magic and Folklore.* New York: Dover Publications; 1984;126.] WARTS **3460**

McCully, Kilmer S. Vascular pathology of homocysteinemia: implications for the pathogenesis of arteriosclerosis. *Am J Pathol.* 1969;56(1):111-28. ARTERIOSCLEROSIS **233**

McDade JE, Shepard CC, Fraser DW. Legionnaires' disease: isolation of a bacterium and demonstration of its role in other respiratory disease. *N Engl J Med.* 1977;297:1197-203. LEGIONNAIRES DISEASE **1532**

McDermott, Walsh. Education and general medical care. *Ann Intern Med.* 1982;96:512-7. RESEARCH **2873**

McDowell E. Three cases of extirpation of diseased ovaria. *Eclectic Repertory Anal Rev.* 1817;7:242-4. SURGERY **3220**

McGoon, Dwight C. *Ecstasy, a Basis for Meaning in the World.* [In: Hurst JW. *Essays from the Heart.* New York: Raven Press; 1995, p. 10.] PATIENT-PHYSICIAN RELATIONS **2454**

McGrigor, James. *The Autobiography and Services of Sir James McGrigor.* London: Longman, Green, Longman & Roberts; 1861. [In: Talbott JH. *A Biographical History of Medicine,* p. 435 (q.v.).] MILITARY MEDICINE **2180**

McHugh, Paul R. What's the story? *Am Scholar.* 1995;64:191-203. CASE HISTORIES **432**

McIlhany JL, Shaffer JW, Hines EA. The heritability of blood pressure: an investigation of 200 twin pairs using the cold pressor test. *Johns Hopkins Med J.* 1975;136:57-74. HYPERTENSION **1357**

McKeown, Thomas.
The Role of Medicine: Dream, Mirage, or Nemesis? [Rock Carling Monograph]. London: Nuffield Provincial Hospitals Trust; 1976. [In: Princeton, NJ: Princeton University Press; 1979, p. 178.] MEDICINE **2126**

A historical appraisal of the medical task. In McLachlan G, McKeown T (eds). *Medical History and Medical Care: A Symposium of Perspectives.* London: Oxford Univerisity Press; 1971, p. 48. MEDICAL CARE **1683**

McKevitt C, Morgan M. Illness doesn't belong to us. *J R Soc Med.* 1997;90:491-5. PHYSICIAN HEALTH **2535, 2536**

Merton, Thomas.
  Conjectures of a Guilty Bystander. Garden City, NY: Doubleday; 1966:203. SUICIDE **3188**
  The Sign of Jonas: The Journal of Thomas Merton. New York: Harcourt Brace; 1953. DOCTORS **851** [302], INSOMNIA **1455** [43-4]

Meynert, Theodore. *Klinische Vorlesungen über Psychiatrie.* Vienna: Braumuller, 1890, p. v. [In: Shorter E. A *History of Psychiatry: From the Era of the Asylum to the Age of Prozac.* New York: Wiley; 1997, p. 77.] PSYCHIATRY **2717**

Mibelli, Vittorio. A new form of keratosis: angiokeratoma. *C R Cong Int Derm Syph.* 1890;89-91. ANGIOKERATOMA **186**

Miescher, Johann Friedrich. Ueber die Chemische Zusammensetzung der Eiterzellen. In: Hoppe-Seyler F; editor. *Medicinisch-chemische Untersuchungen.* Berlin: Verlag von August Hirschwald; 1871, Heft 4:441-60. Pages 453, 458. DEOXYRIBONUCLEIC ACID (DNA) **703**

Milkman, Louis Arthur. *Multiple Spontaneous Idiopathic Symmetrical Fractures* [Paper read before the American congress of Radiology, Chicago, Illinois, September 25-28, 1933]. [In: *Am J Roentgenol.* 1934;32:622-34.] OSTEOMALACIA **2300**

Mill, John Stuart. Inaugural address given at the University of St. Andrews, St. Andrews, Scotland, February 1, 1867. In Mill JS. *Dissertations and Discussions,* vol 4. 1868, p. 335. [In: *Collected Works of John Stuart Mill,* vol. XXI. Toronto, Canada: University of Toronto Press; 1963, p. 218.] MEDICAL EDUCATION **1747**

Miller BJ, Gibbon JH Jr, Gibbon MH. Recent advances in the development of a mechanical heart and lung apparatus. *Ann Surg.* 1951;134:694-708. HEART SURGERY **1253**

Miller H. The recognition of neurotic illness. *Practitioner.* 1947;159:128-35. [128]. SPECIALIZATION **3111**

Miller, George E. "Teaching and learning in medical school" revisted. *Med Educ.* 1978;12(5)[Supplement: Innovations in medical education: Proceedings pf the 1977 Conference of the Association for Medical Education in Europe]:120-5. MEDICAL EDUCATION **1790**

Miller, Henry George.
  Then and Now [Inaugural Marden lecture given at the Royal Free Hospital, November 1971] [Limited data]. MEDICAL CARE **1681**
  Accident neurosis. *Br Med J.* 1961;1:992-8. LITIGATION **1558**
  Henry Millerisms. *World Neurol.* 9 April 1968, p. 8. DIAGNOSIS **751**, DIZZINESS **807**, EPILEPSY **980**, HEADACHE **1161**,   PAIN **2328**, PREVENTIVE MEDICINE **2679**, SIGMOIDOSCOPY **3067**
  In McLachlan G, McKeown T (eds). *Medical History and Medical Care.* London: Oxford University Press for the Nuffield Provincial Hospital Trust; 1971:224. HEALTH **1199**
  New doctors' dilemmas. *Encounter.* 1969;32:25-34. HEALTH POLICY **1216**
  Psychiatry: medicine or magic? *Br J Hosp Med.* 1970;3:122-6. PSYCHIATRY **2720**, **2721**, PSYCHOSOMATIC MEDICINE **2746**
  The charm of neurology. *Br Clin J.* Oct 1974, pp. 435-7. NEUROLOGY **2252**

Miller TG, Abbott, WO. Intestinal intubation: practical technique. *Am J Med Sci.* 1934 May;187:595-9. MILLER-ABBOTT TUBE **2183**

Miller, William Ian. Journal: Ann Arbor, December 1997. *American Scholar.* 1998;67:143-6. SEX **3045**

Mills JS. *Ann Intern Med.* 1972;77:570. LIFE STYLE **1551**

Milton, John. *Paradise Lost,* 1667, book XI, lines 538-46. AGING **61**

Mindererus, Raymund. *Medicina Militaris, or a Body of Military Medicines Experimented,* 1620. GONORRHEA **1125**, MILITARY MEDICINE **2177** [16-7]

Minkowski, Oskar. Lecture given to medical students in Breslau, Germany. 1923. [In: Bliss M. *The Discovery of Insulin.* Chicago: University of Chicago Press; 1982, p. 169.] INSULIN **1460**

Minot GR, Murphy WP. Treatment of pernicious anemia by a special diet. *JAMA.* 1926;87:470-6. PERNICIOUS ANEMIA **2508**

Misaurus, Philander [pseudonym]. *The Honour of the Gout,* 1720. [In: Porter R, Rousseau GS. *Gout: The Patrician Malady.* New Haven, CT: Yale University Press; 1998:72.] DOCTORS **816**

Mitchell JRA. Review of *Cecil Textbook of Medicine. Lancet.* 1982;2:744-5. WRITING **3512**

Mitchell, Silas Weir.
  Circumstance. New York: Century; 1901. [In: Talbott JH. A *Biographical History of Medicine,* p. 421 (q.v.).] PATIENT-PHYSICIAN RELATIONS **2398**
  Doctor and Patient, 3rd ed. Philadelphia: 1889. [In: Talbott JH. A *Biographical History of Medicine,* p. 420 (q.v.).] CLINICAL OBSERVATION **513**
  Dr. North and His Friends. New York: Century; 1900, pp. 456-7. PHYSICIANS **2577**
  Fat and Blood and How To Make Them. Philadelphia: J.B. Lippincott; 1877, p. 27. NEURASTHENIA **2246**
  The Birth and Death of Pain, 1896. ANESTHESIA **166**, PAIN **2322**

Morgan, Thomas Hunt. *The Theory of the Gene.* New Haven, CT: Yale University Press; 1926. GENETICS 1104 [351], 1105 [25]

Morgan, William Keith C. The annual fiasco (American style). *Med J Aust.* 1969;2:923-5. SCREENING 3012

Moroney MJ. *Facts from figures.* Baltimore: Penguin Books; 1951, p. 3. STATISTICS 3157

Morris CDW. Acetylsalicylic acid and platelet stickiness [Letter]. *Lancet.* 1967;1(7484):279-83. ASPIRIN (ACETYLSALICYLIC ACID) 246

Morris, Robert Tuttle. *Doctors Versus Folks.* Garden City, NY: Doubleday Page; 1915:158. PATIENT-PHYSICIAN RELATIONS 2405

Morrissey JF, Barreras RF. Drug therapy: antacid therapy. *N Engl J Med.* 1974;290:550-4. PRESCRIPTIONS 2673

Morrow, Prince Albert. *A System of Genito-Urinary Diseases, Syphilology, and Dermatology,* preface. New York: D. Appleton; 1893-4. [In: Rutkow IM, *The History of Surgery in the United States,* vol. 1, p. 353.] SPECIALIZATION 3109

Moss, N. Henry. Superspecialization: a surgeon's view, health affairs. *Med Affairs.* Summer 1973, pp. 6-8. MEDICAL PRACTICE 1955

Mosso, Angelo. *Fatigue.* Translated by Drummond M, Drummond WB. New York: 1915. PSYCHOSIS 2738

Mott, Valentine. *Pain and Anaesthetics: An Essay Introduction to a Series of Surgical and Medical Monographs,* 2nd ed. Washington, DC: McGill and Witherow; 1863:11. SURGERY 3223

Moynihan, Berkeley George Andrew.
Duodenal Ulcer. Philadelphia: WB Saunders; 1910, pp. 122-3. PEPTIC ULCER 2488
The Pathology of the Living and Other Essays, preface. Philadelphia: WB Saunders; 1910, p. 6. PATHOPHYSIOLOGY 2359, PREVENTIVE MEDICINE 2677
In Bevan PG. Berkeley Moynihan. *J Med Biography.* 1993;1:76-82. PATIENTS 2462, SURGERY 3237, 3238

Mr Tut-Tut. *One Hundred Proverbs.* Yutang L, editor. *The Wisdom of China and India.* New York: Random House; 1942:1094. HEALTH 1175

Müller, Johannes.
Über den Feinern Bau und die Formen der Krankhaften Geschwulste, lief 1. Berlin: G. Reimer; 1838. [In: Rather LJ, Rather P, Frerichs JB. Rather LJ, Rather P, Frerichs JB. *Johannes Müller and the Nineteenth-Century Origins of Tumor Cell Theory.* Canton, MA: Science History Publications; 1986:93-9.] CANCER 377
Handbuch der Physiologie des Menschen [Elements of Physiology], 1834-40. NERVOUS SYSTEM 2240
Inaugural lecture as docent of physiology at University of Bonn, October 19, 1824. [In: Kruta VJE. *Purkyne Physiologist: A Short Account of His Contributions to the Progress of Physiology.* Prague: Academia; 1969:20.] SCIENCE 2946

Mullis K, Faloona F, Scharf S, et al. Specific enzymatic amplification of DNA in vitro: the polymerase chain reaction. *Cold Spring Harbor Symposium on Quantitative Biology.* 1986;51(Pt 1):263-73. POLYMERASE CHAIN REACTION (PCR) 2645

Mumford, E. *From Students to Physicians.* Cambridge, MA: Harvard University Press; 1970, p. 158. MEDICINE 2123

Munthe, Axel. *The Story of San Michele.* New York: EP Dutton; 1929:33. COLITIS 563

Murphy, Edmond A. Clinical genetics: some neglected facets. *N Engl J Med.* 1975;292:458-62. MEDICAL PRACTICE 1958

Murphy, John Benjamin.
Organized medicine: its influence and its obligations. *JAMA.* 1911;57:1-9. CONTINUING EDUCATION 596
Resection of arteries and veins injured in continuity (end-to-end suture) experimental and clinical research. *Med Rec.* 1897;51:73-88. VASCULAR SURGERY 3422
Students' clinics at opening of session this year. In *The Surgical Clinics of John B. Murphy, MD,* vol. 2. Philadelphia: WB Saunders; 1913:1061-5. MEDICAL EDUCATION 1775

Murray, George Redmayne. The life-history of the first case of myxoedema treated by thyroid extract. *Br Med J.* 1920;1:359-60. HYPOTHYROIDISM 1396

Murrell, William. Nitroglycerine as a remedy for angina pectoris. *Lancet.* 1879;1:80-1. ANGINA PECTORIS 184

Nash, Ogden. I yeild to my learned brother, or Is there a candlestick maker in the house? In *The Face is Familiar: The Selected Verse of Ogden Nash.* Boston: Little, Brown; 1940, p. 8. MEDICAL PROFESSION 2009

Neel, James V. The inheritance of sickle cell anemia. *Science.* 1949;110:64-6. SICKLE CELL DISEASE 3064

Neeson, Stella. Mysticism lost. *JAMA.* 1975;232:374-6. BELIEF 291

Osler G. Letter to Katherine Cushing, 15 August 1903. Cushing Papers, Sterling Library, Yale University, Reel 157, Series IV, Box 198, Folders 55-60, Katherine Crowell Cushing correspondence; 1897-1940. POST-PARTUM CARE **2652**

Osler, William.

After Twenty-five Years [Address given at the McGill University, September 21, 1899]. [In: *Aequanimitas, with Other Addresses to Medical Students, Nurses, and Practitioners of Medicine*. Birmingham, AL: Classics of Medicine Library; 1987.] LITERATURE **1554** [213], MEDICAL EDUCATION **1755** [210-1], WORK **3482** [213]

Books and Men [Remarks made at the opening of the new building of the Boston Medical Library, January 12, 1901]. [In: *Aequanimitas with Other Addresses to Medical Students, Nurses, and Practitioners of Medicine*, 3rd ed. Philadelphia: Blakiston; 1932.] HISTORY OF MEDICINE **1295** [212-3], MEDICAL HISTORIES **1874** [212-3],

Books and Men [Remarks made at the opening of the new building of the Boston Medical Library, January 12, 1901]. [In: *Aequanimitas, with Other Addresses to Medical Students, Nurses, and Practitioners of Medicine*. Birmingham, AL: Classics of Medicine Library; 1987, p. 221.] MEDICAL PRACTICE **1933**

Books and Men [Remarks made at the opening of the new building of the Boston Medical Library, January 12, 1901]. [In: *Boston Med Surg J*, 17 Jan 1901.] BOOKS **329** [2], READING **2829** [3], **2830** [3]

British Medicine in Greater Britain, 1897. [In: *Aequanimitas, with Other Addresses to Medical Students, Nurses, and Practitioners of Medicine*, 3rd ed. Philadelphia: Blakiston; 1932, p. 168.] HUMANITIES **1331**

Chauvinism in Medicine [Address given at the Canadian Medical Association, Montreal, September 17, 1902]. [In: *Aequanimitas, with Other Addresses to Medical Students, Nurses, and Practitioners of Medicine*, 3rd ed. Philadelphia: Blakiston; 1932.] DOCTORS **834** [267], MEDICAL PROGRESS **2021** [266]

Chauvinism in Medicine [Address given at the Canadian Medical Association, Montreal, September 17, 1902]. In *Montreal Med J*. 1902;31:684-99. DOGMATISM **872**, HISTORY OF MEDICINE **1296**

Chauvinism in Medicine [Address given at the Canadian Medical Association, Montreal, September 17, 1902]. [In: McGovern JP, Roland CG (eds). *The Collected Essays of Sir William Osler*, vol. 1. Birmingham, AL: Classics of Medicine Library; 1985.] MEDICAL PRACTICE **1935** [301], MEDICAL PROFESSION **1992** [279], MEDICINE **2105** [154], NATIONALISM **2218** [286],

Counsels and Ideals: Selected Aphorisms, 1906. [In: Birmingham, AL: Classics of Medicine Library; 1985, p. 171.] DOCTORS **835**

Ephemerides, 1895. [In: *Montreal Med J*. 1896;24:518-22.] DIAGNOSIS **743**, MEDICAL CARE **1663**

Internal Medicine as a Vocation [Address given at the New York Academy of Medicine, October 19, 1897]. [In: *Aequanimitas, with Other Addresses to Medical Students, Nurses, and Practitioners of Medicine*, 3rd ed. Philadelphia: Blakiston; 1932.] CHAUVINISM **455** [135], TRAVEL **3320** [136]

Internal Medicine as a Vocation [Address given at the New York Academy of Medicine, October 19, 1897]. [In: McGovern JP, Roland CG (ed). *The Collected Essays of Sir William Osler*, vol. II. Birmingham, AL: Classics of Medicine Library; 1985, p. 151.] PHYSICIANS AND THE PRESS **2599**

Nurse and Patient, c. 1900. [In: *Aequanimitas, with Other Addresses to Medical Students, Nurses, and Practitioners of Medicine*. Birmingham, AL: Classics of Medicine Library; 1987, p. 163.] NURSES **2268**

Remarks on Specialism, 1892. In Camac CNB (ed). *Counsels and Ideals and Selected Aphorisms*. New York: Houton, Mifflin; 1905, p. 183. [In: Birmingham, AL: Classics of Medicine Library; 1985, p. 183.] SPECIALIZATION **3108**

Teacher and Student, 1892. [In: *Aequanimitas, with Other Addresses to Medical Students, Nurses, and Practitioners of Medicine*. Birmingham, AL: Classics of Medicine Library; 1987.] ERRORS **995** [21-43], TEACHERS **3268** [79]

Teaching and Thinking, 1895. [In: *Aequanimitas with Other Addresses to Medical Students, Nurses, and Practitioners of Medicine*, 3rd ed. Philadelphia: Blakiston; 1932.] DRUGS **889** [125], TEACHERS **3269** [128]

The Army Surgeon [Address given at the closing exercises of the Army Medical School, Washington, DC, February 28, 1894]. [In: *Aequanimitas, with Other Addresses to Medical Students, Nurses, and Practitioners of Medicine*. Birmingham, AL: Classics of Medicine Library; 1987.] CLINICAL OBSERVATION **514** [111], DIAGNOSIS **742** [103-20], **746** [299], LEARNING **1525** [111-2], MEDICAL SOCIETIES **2058** [117]

The Fixed Period, 1905. In McGovern JP, Roland CG (eds). *The Collected Essays of Sir William Osler*, vol. 1. Birmingham, AL:Classics of Medicine Library; 1985:397-9. AGING **76**

The Functions of a State Faculty [President's address given at the 99th Annual Session, Baltimore, April 27, 1897]. [In: Cushing H. *The Life of Sir William Osler*, vol. 1. Oxford: Clarendon Press; 1925, p. 447.] PHYSICIANS **2575**

The Functions of a State Faculty [President's address given at the 99th Annual Session, Baltimore, April 27, 1897]. In McGovern JP, Roland CG (eds). *The Collected Essays of Sir William Osler*, vol. II. Birmingham, AL: Classics of Medicine Library; 1985, p. 128. HISTORY OF MEDICINE **1294**

The Hospital as a College, 1903. [In: *Aequanimitas, with Other Addresses to Medical Students, Nurses, and Practitioners of Medicine*. Birmingham, AL: Classics of Medicine Library; 1987, p. 331.] MEDICAL EDUCATION **1760**

The Influence of Louis on American Medicine, 1897. In McGovern JP, Roland CG (eds). *The Collected Essays of Sir William Osler*, vol. III. Birmingham, AL: Classics of Medicine Library; 1985, p. 193. STATISTICS **3148**

The Leaven of Science [Address given at the opening of the Wistar Institute of Anatomy and Biology of the University of Pennsylvania, May 21, 1894]. [In: *Aequanimitas, with Other Addresses to Medical Students, Nurses, and Practitioners of Medicine*, 3rd ed. Philadelphia: Blakiston; 1932, p. 95.] EVOLUTION **1010**

The Leaven of Science [Address given at the opening of the Wistar Institute of Anatomy and Biology of the University of Pennsylvania, May 21, 1894]. [In: McGovern JP, Roland CG (eds). *The Collected Essays of Sir William Osler*, vol. 1. Birmingham, AL: Classics of Medicine Library; 1985, p. 61.] SCIENCE **2964**

The Master-word in Medicine [Address given to undergraduates at the medical school of the University of Toronto, October 1, 1903]. [In: *Aequanimitas, with Other Addresses to Medical Students, Nurses, and Practitioners of Medicine*, 3rd ed. Philadelphia: Blakiston; 1932.] EQUANIMITY **989** [368], WORK **3483** [356-7],

The Master-word in Medicine [Address given to undergraduates at the medical school of the University of Toronto, October 1, 1903]. [In: *Aequanimitas, with Other Addresses to Medical Students, Nurses, and Practitioners of Medicine*. Birmingham, AL: Classics of Medicine Library; 1987.] MEDICAL PROFESSION **1993** [387], **1994** [387], READING **2831** [384],

The Master-word in Medicine [Address given to undergraduates at the medical school of the University of Toronto, October 1, 1903]. In *The Master-word in Medicine*. Baltimore: John Murphy; 1903, pp. 29-30. MEDICAL PRACTICE **1936**

The Student Life [Farewell address given to American and Canadian Medical students, 1892]. [In: *Aequanimitas, with Other Addresses to Medical Students, Nurses, and Practitioners of Medicine*, 3rd ed. Philadelphia: Blakiston; 1932.] EDUCATION **941** [400], LIVING **1570** [404-5], MEDICAL STUDENTS **2060**, PATIENT-PHYSICIAN RELATIONS **2402** [405], WORK **3484** [400-1]

The Student Life [Farewell address given to American and Canadian Medical students, 1892]. [In: McGovern JP, Roland CG (eds). *The Collected Essays of Sir William Osler*, vol. II. Birmingham, AL: Classics of Medicine Library; 1985.] MEDICAL HISTORIES **1877** [431], TRUTH **3365** [258]

A bed-side library for medical students. *Johns Hopkins Med Bull*. 1919;341:217-18. LITERATURE **1556**

A study of death [unpublished manuscript]. In: *Bibliotheca Osleriana*. Montreal: McGill-Queen's University Press; 1969(7644):19. [In: Golden RL. Sir William Osler: humanistic thanatologist. *Omega: Journal of Death and Dying*. 1997-8;36(3):241-58.] DYING **913**

A way of life. In *A Way of Life and Selected Writings of Sir William Osler*. New York: Dover; 1958, p. 239. LIVING **1571**

Address to the Ontario Medical Association, Toronto, June 3, 1909. *Canada Lancet*. 1909;42:899-912. [In: *The Collected Essays of Sir William Osler*, vol II. Birmingham, AL: Classics of Medicine Library; 1985, p. 364.] DOCTORS **836**

Aequanimitas [valedictory address given at the University of Pennsylvania, May 1, 1889]. In: *Aequanimitas*, 1932. EQUANIMITY **987**, **988**, HUMANS **1334**, PATIENT-PHYSICIAN RELATIONS **2393**, TRUTH **3364**

An account of certain organisms occurring in the liquor sanguinis. *Proc R Soc Lond*. 1874;22:391-8. PLATELETS (THROMBOCYTES) **2618**, THROMBOCYTES (BLOOD PLATELETS) **3298**

Aneurysm of the abdominal aorta. *Lancet*. 1905;2:1089-96. MEDICAL ERROR **1810**

Chronic cyanosis, with polycythemia and enlarged spleen: a new clinical entity. *Am J Med Sci*. 1903;126:187-201. POLYCYTHEMIA **2644**

Chronic infectious endocarditis. *Quart J Med*. 1909;2:219-30. BACTERIAL ENDOCARDITIS **278**

Harvard Medical Association: annual dinner. *Boston Med Surg J*. 1894;136-42. WOMEN IN MEDICINE **3478**

Address to the Abernethian Society. 1885. [In: Ross JR. Your patient and you. *St. Bartholomew Hosp J*. 1950;54:50-8.] DIAGNOSIS **741**

On a form of chronic inflammation of bones (osteitis deformans). *Med-Chir Trans*. 1877;42:37-63. [In: Talbott JH. *A Biographical History of Medicine*, p. 1080 (q.v.).] PAGET DISEASE OF THE BONE (OSTEITIS DEFORMANS) **2313**

On disease of the mammary areola preceding cancer of the mammary gland. *St Bart Hosp Rep*. 1874;10:87-9. [In: Talbott JH. *A Biographical History of Medicine*, p. 1079 (q.v.).] PAGET DISEASE OF THE NIPPLE **2314**

Paget, Stephen.
The Surgery of the Chest. Bristol: John Wright & Company; 1896:121. HEART SURGERY **1247**

The discipline of practice. In *Confessio Medici*. New York: Macmillan; 1909, p. 83. MEDICAL CARE **1665**

Paige, Leroy Robert "Satchel". *Maybe I'll Pitch Forever*. Garden City, NY: Doubleday; 1962:227. HEALTH **1197**

Palmer, Walter L. Gastroenterology, internal medicine, and the general practitioner. *Gastroenterology* 1947;9:119. [In: *Ann Intern Med*. 1993;118:387.] MEDICINE **2116**

Pancoast, Joseph. *A Treatise on Operative Surgery; Comprising a Description of the Various Processes of the Art, Including All the New Operations*. Philadelphia: Carey & Hart; 1846. ACUPUNCTURE **35** [28], RECONSTRUCTIVE SURGERY **2838** [348]

Papanicolaou GN, Traut HF. The diagnostic value of vaginal smears in carcinoma of the uterus. *Am J Obstet Gynecol*. 1941;42:193-206. CANCER OF THE UTERUS **417**, PAPANICOLAOU (PAP) SMEAR **2332**

Paré, Ambroise.
The Apology and Treatise Containing the Voyages Made into Divers Places. Translated by Packard FR. New York: Paul B. Hoeber; 1921; pp. 12, 28, 163. CLINICAL TRIALS **530**

The Collected Works of Ambroise Paré. London: 1634. [Reprint: Pound Ridge, NY: Milford House; 1968.] ADULTERY **48** [book 25], SYPHILIS **3258** [book 19]

The Workes of That Famous Chirurgion Ambroise Paré. Paris: 1575; London: 1649. ANEURYSM **168**, BUBONIC PLAGUE **356**, PLEURISY **2620**

In Hamby WB. *The Case Reports and Autopsy Records of Ambroise Paré*. Springfield, IL: Charles C Thomas; 1960. CANCER OF THE BREAST **393**, CANCER OF THE LIP **403**

In Keynes G (ed). *The Apologie and Treatise of Ambroise Paré*, part 1. London: Falcon Educational Books; 1951:21. HEALING **1165**

Paracelsus (Theophrastus Bombastus von Hohenheim).
Das Zweite Buch der Grossen Wundarznei, foreword. 1536. MEDICINE **2084**

De Generatione Stultorum.. HYPOTHYROIDISM **1386**

Doctors and Patients. Translated by Abse D. Oxford, England: Oxford University Press; 1984. DOCTORS **811**

Seven Defensiones: The Reply to Certain Calumniations of His Enemies. In Temkin CL. *Four Treatises of Theophratus von Hohenheim, called Paracelsus* Baltimore: Johns Hopkins University Press; 1941. DRUGS **879** [22], EXPERIENCE **1025** [29]

Ens Dei. In *Volumen Medicinae Paramirum, c.* 1520 [Translation by Leidecker KF reprinted in *Supplements to the Bulletin of the History of Medicine*, no. 11. Baltimore: Johns Hopkins University Press; 1949:61]. PHYSICIANS **2546, 2547**

Spitalbuch [Preface. Volume VII, page 374] In: *Sämtliche werke*. Sudhoff K, Mathiessen W; editors. München, Berlin: O.W. Barth, R. Oldenbourg; 1923-33. [Translated in Pagel W, Rattansi P. Vesalius and Paracelsus. *Med Hist*. 1964;8:309-28.] SURGEONS **3198**

Pardee, Harold Ensign Bennett. An electrocardiographic sign of coronary artery obstruction. *Arch Intern Med*. 1920;26:244-57. CORONARY ARTERY DISEASE **628**

Parent-Duchatelet AJB. *De la Prostitution dan la Ville de Paris*, 2nd ed. Paris: 1837. [In: Speert H. *Obstetric and Gynecologic Milestones*. New York: Macmillan; 1958:229-30.] PREGNANCY **2659**

Parisé, Reveille. *La Gazette Médicale*. 1851;29. [In: Löwy I. The Polish School of Philosophy of Medicine: from Tytus Chalubinski (1820-1889) to Ludwik Fleck (1896-1961). Dordrecht: Kluwer Academic Publishers; 1990:85.] MEDICINE **2097**

Park WH, Bullowa JGM, Rosenbluth MB. The treatment of lobar pneumonia with refined specific antibacterial serum. *JAMA*. 1928;91:1503-8. CLINICAL TRIALS **542**

Parkinson D. Concussion. *Mayo Clin Proc*. 1977;52:492-6. CONCUSSION **572**

Parkinson, James. *Essay on the Shaking Palsy*. London: 1817. [In: Birmingham, AL: Classics of Medicine Library; 1986.] MEDICAL SCIENCE **2043** [i], PARKINSONISM **2339** [8-9], **2340** [1], **2341** [3,6,8]

Queckenstedt, Hans Heinrich Georg. Diagnosis of compression of the spinal cord. *Dtsch Z Nervenheilk.* 1916;55:325-33. [In: Talbott JH. *A Biographical History of Medicine,* p. 983 (q.v.).] QUECKENSTEDT TEST **2812**

Quincke, Heinrich Irenaeus.
Acute circumscribed edema of the skin. *Monat Prakt Dermatol.* 1882;1:129-31. ANGIONEUROTIC EDEMA (QUINCKE DISEASE) **187**
Observations on capillary and venous pulse. *Berlin Klin Wocehnschr.* 1868;5:357. [In: Willius FA, Keys TE, *Cardiac Classics,* p. 569 (q.v.).] AORTIC VALVE REGURGITATION **213**, CAPILLARY PULSE **423**
Vagus stimulation in man [German]. *Klin Wochenschr.* 1871;8:349-52. [In: Talbott JH. *A Biographical History of Medicine,* p. 1133 (q.v.).] CAROTID SINUS **430**

Quine, William Edward.
[Discussion.] *Trans Ill State Med Soc.* 1894;44:564. MEDICAL TESTIMONY **2066**
The ideals and the practices of the medical profession. *Ill Med J.* 1905;7:530. MEDICAL PROFESSION **1996**

Qureshi, Bashir. [Book review of Jones L, Sidell M. *The Challenge of Promoting Health: Exploration and Action*]. *J R Soc Med.* 1997;90:705. HEALTH **1207**

Rabelais, François. *Gargantua and Pantagruel,* 1532, book 1, chapter 41. ALCOHOLISM **116**, MEDICAL PROFESSION **1976**

Radlauer, Steven. High-roller physicians [Letter]. *The New York Times.* 05 Nov 1986, p. A30. PATIENT-PHYSICIAN RELATIONS **2443**

Ramón y Cajal, Santiago.
Chacharas de café [Chatting Over Coffee] . Madrid: 1920. [In: Current comment: a Spanish medical philosopher. *JAMA.* 1921;76:595.] AGING **80**, FAMILIES **1039**, HUMANS **1335**, INTELLIGENCE **1461**, MEDICAL FEES **1869**
In Craigie EH, Gibson WC. *The World of Ramón y Cajal: With Selections from His Nonscientific Writings.* Springfield, IL: Charles C Thomas; 1968. AGING **82** [256], DEATH **671** [156], DYING **916** [155], RELIGION **2847** [266], TREATMENT **3351** [169]

Ramazzini, Bernardino. *De Moribus Artificum Diatriba,* 1713. [Translation by Wright WC. In: Birmingham, AL: Classics of Medicine Library; 1983.] OCCUPATIONAL MEDICINE **2288** [11], **2289** [13], PATIENT-PHYSICIAN RELATIONS **2377** [13]

Ramsey, Paul.
Fabricated Man: The Genetics of Ethics Control. New Haven, CT: Yale University Press; 1970:123. MEDICAL ETHICS **1841**
The Patient as Person: Explorations in Medical Ethics. New Haven, CT: Yale University Press; 1970:xi. PATIENT-PHYSICIAN RELATIONS **2425**

Ranchin, François. *Opuscula Medica.* Lyon: 1627. [In: Freeman JT. Francois Ranchin, contributor of an early chapter in geriatrics. *J Hist Med.* 1950;5:422-31.] GERIATRICS **1113**

Raynaud, Maurice. *De l'Asphyxie Locale et de la Gangrene Symetrique des Extremites [On Local Asphyxia and Symmetrical Gangrene of the Extremities].* Paris: 1862. [In: *Selected Monographs.* Translated by Barlow T. London: New Sydenham Society; 1888, pp. 31-2.] RAYNAUD PHENOMENON **2824**, **2825**

Razis, Dennis V. A new role for medicine. *J R Soc Med.* 1994;87:190-2. POPULATION CONTROL **2651**

Récamier, Joseph-Claude-Anthelme. *Récherches sur le Traitement du Cancer, par la Compressions Méthodique Simple ou Combinée, et Sur l'Histoire Génénerale de la MIme Maladie.* Paris: Gabon; 1829. [In: Shimkin MB, *Contrary to Nature: Cancer,* p. 112 (q.v.).] CANCER METASTASIS **389**

Recklinghausen, Friedrich von. *Multiple Fibromas of the Skin and Multiple Neuromas* [German]. Berlin: A. Hirschwald; 1882. [In: Talbott JH. *A Biographical History of Medicine,* p. 691 (q.v.).] NEUROFIBROMATOSIS **2249**

Reed, Walter.
Med Rec. 1901;60:6-10. YELLOW FEVER **3521**
Etiology of yellow fever: an additional note. *JAMA.* 1901;36:431-40. YELLOW FEVER **3520**

Refsum, Sigvald Bernhard. Heredopathia atactica polyneuritiformis, a familial syndrome not hitherto described. *Acta Psychiatr Neurol Scand Suppl.* 1946;38:1-303. REFSUM'S DISEASE **2844**

Rehberg, Poul Brandt. Studies on kidney function. Part I: The rate of filtration and reabsorption in the human kidney. *Biochem J.* 1926;20:447-82. KIDNEY FUNCTION **1496**

Rehn, Ludwig. Penetrating cardiac wounds and cardiac suture [German]. *Arch Klin Chir.* 1897;55:315-29. [In: Keys TE, Key JD. *Classics of Cardiology,* vol. 3. Malabar, FL: Robert E. Krieger Publishing; 1983, p. 36-44.] HEART SURGERY **1248**

Reid, Thomas. *Inquiry into the Human Mind on the Principles of Common Sense*, 4th ed. London: T. Cadell; 1785. [In: Brookes DR (ed). *A Critical Edition*, ch. 6, sec. 24. University Park, PA: Pennsylvania State University Press; 1997, p. 202.] TREATMENT 3337

Reik, Theodor.
Psychology of Sex Relations. New York: Farrar & Rinehart; 1945, p. 144. SEX 3039
The Many Faces of Sex: Observations of an Old Psychoanalyst. New York: Farrar, Straus & Giroux; 1966. AGING 88 [64], PSYCHIATRISTS 2711 [55]

Reil, Johann Christian. *Beitrag zu den Prinzipien für Jede Zukünstige Pharmakologie*, 1797. [In: Jeffreys D. *Aspirin: The Remarkable Story of a Wonder Drug.* New York: Bloomsbury; 2004:37.] PHARMACOLOGY 2513

Reinhardt, Uwe E. Wanted: a clearly articulated social ethic for American health care. *JAMA.* 1997;278:1446-7. HEALTH POLICY 1222

Reiter, Hans Conrad. Previously unknown spirochetal infection (spirochetal arthritis). *Dtsch Med Wochenschr.* 1916;42:1535-6. [In: Talbott JH. *A Biographical History of Medicine*, p. 803 (q.v.).] REITER SYNDROME 2845

Relman, Arnold S.
As companies buy hospitals, treatment of poor is debated. *The New York Times.* 25 Jan 1985 , p. A1. MEDICAL ECONOMICS 1718
Economic considerations in emergency care: what are hospitals for. *N Engl J Med.* 1985;312:372-373. HOSPITALS 1327
More on the Ingelfinger rule. *N Engl J Med.* 1988;318:1125-6. PUBLISHING 2773
Practicing medicine in the new business climate. *N Engl J Med.* 1987;316:1150-1. PATIENT-PHYSICIAN RELATIONS 2444
The new medical-industrial complex. *N Engl J Med.* 1980;303:963-70. MEDICAL ECONOMICS 1714

Renard, Jules. *Journal*, 1887. DREAMS 875

Rendu, Henri-Jules-Marie. Repeated epistaxis in a patient having small cutaneous and mucous membrane angiomas. *Gazette Hop* 1896;69:1322-3. [In: Talbott JH. *A Biographical History of Medicine*, pp. 1137-8 (q.v.).] HEREDITARY HEMORRHAGIC TELANGIECTASIA 1278

Restak, Richard. *Brainscapes: An Introduction to What Neuroscience Has Learned About the Structure, Function, and Abilities of the Brain.* New York: Hyperion; 1995, p. 91. BRAIN 346

Reverdin, Jaques-Louis. Accidents consecutifs à l'ablation totale du goitre. *Rev Med Suisse Romande.* 1882;2:539. [In: Bloomfield AL, *Selected Diseases*, p. 186 (q.v.).] HYPOTHYROIDISM 1393

Rexroth, Kenneth. Introduction. In: Lawrence DH. *Selected Poems.* New York: Penguin Books; 1980:22-3. DEATH 680

Rhazes.
De Variolis et Morbillis Commentarius [A Treatise on the Small-pox and Measles]. London: G Bowyer; 1776. [In: *Medical Classics*, vol. 1. Baltimore: Williams and Wilkins; 1939-40, pp. 27-8.] SMALLPOX 3080
In Maimonides M. *The Preservation of Youth: Essays on Health.* Translated by as-Sihha FT [Limited data]. PATIENT-PHYSICIAN RELATIONS 2369

Richards, Alfred Newton. The nature and mode of regulation of glomerular function. *Am J Med Sci.* 1925;170:781-803. KIDNEY 1482

Richards, Dickinson Woodruff. *Trans Assoc Am Phys.* 1962;75:1-10. CLINICAL OBSERVATION 524

Richards, Peter. *Learning Medicine: An Informal Guide to a Career in Medicine.* London: BMJ Publishing Group; 1985. DOCTORS 859 [9-10], LEARNING 1528 [84], MEDICAL EDUCATION 1794 [11], MEDICAL PROFESSION 2013 [9-10], 2014 [13]

Richerand, Anseleme-Balthasar. *Historie des progrès récens de la chirurgie*, 1825. [In: Tröhler U. To improve the evidence of medicine: arithmetic observation in clinical medicine in the eighteenth and early nineteenth centuries. *Hist Phil Life Sci.* 1988;10(Supp):31-40.] CLINICAL TRIALS 534

Rickes EL, Brink NG, Koniusky FR, et al. Crystalline vitamin B$_{12}$. *Science.* 1948;107:396-7. VITAMIN B$_3$ (NICOTINAMIDE) 3436

Ricketts, Maura N. Is Creutzfeldt-Jakob disease transmitted in blood? *CMAJ.* 1997;157:1367-70. CREUTZFELDT-JAKOB DISEASE 640, 641

Ricord, Philippe. *A Practical Treatise on Venereal Diseases.* Paris: 1838. GONOCOCCAL OPHTHALMIA 1122, SYPHILIS 3260, 3261

Riehl G, Paltauf R. Tuberculosis verrucosa cutis. *Vierteljahr-Schrift für Dermatologie und Syphilologie.* 1886;13:19-48. [In: Talbott JH. *A Biographical History of Medicine*, pp. 1103-4 (q.v.).] TUBERCULOSIS 3391

Riehl, Gustav. The therapy of deep burns. *Wien Klin Wochenschr.* 1925;38:833-4. BURN THERAPY 361

Riesman, David. Deceased diseases. *Ann Med Hist.* 1936;8:160-7. DISEASE 786

Riis, Jacob. *How the Other Half Lives.* 1901. [In: Ott K. *Fevered Lives: Tuberculosis in American Culture Since 1870.* Cambridge, MA: Harvard University Press; 1996, p. 132.] SANITATION 2927

Rilke, Maria Rainer. On poverty and death. *Das Stunden-Buch*, 1905 [Translation by Barrows A, Macy J. *The Book of Hours.* New York: Riverhead Books; 1996, p. 131]. DYING 914

Rimmer, William. In: Bartlett TH. *The Art Life of William Rimmer: Sculptor, Painter, and Physician.* Boston: James R. Osgood; 1890:146. ANATOMY 152

Riverius, Lazarus. *The Practice of Physick, in Seventeen Several Books.* Translated by Culpeper N. London; 1668. [In: Major RH. *Classic Descriptions of Disease*, p. 516 (q.v.).] PURPURA 2795

Robertson, Douglas Argyll. On an interesting series of eye symptoms in a case of spinal disease, with remarks on the action of belladonna on the iris, etc. *Edin Med J.* 1869;14:696-708. ARGYLL ROBERTSON PUPIL 229

Robitzek EH, Selikoff IJ. Hydrazine derivatives of Isonicotinic acid (Rimifon; Marsilid) in the treatment of acute progressive caseous-pneumonic tuberculosis: a preliminary report. *Am Rev Tuberc.* 1952;65:402-28. TUBERCULOSIS 3403

Rochefoucauld, François, Duc de la. *Moral Reflections, Sentences, and Maxims*, 1678 [fifth edition]. AGING 62-65, HEALTH 1177, SUFFERING 3180

Rochoux, Jacques André. *Bulletin de l'Academie Nationale de Medicine.* 1836;1:533. TREATMENT 3343

Rodenhauser, Paul. On creativity and medicine. *Pharos.* 1996;59:2-6. MEDICAL EDUCATION 1803

Roesler, Hugo. *Temple Univ Med Center Bull.* 1960;7:4 [Limited data]. HUMANS 1337, PHILOSOPHY 2516

Roger, Henri-Louis. Clinical researches on the congenital communication on the two sides of the hearts by failure of occlusion of the interventricular septum [French]. *Bull Acad Natl Med.* 1879;8:1074-94. [In: Willius FA, Keys TE, *Cardiac Classics*, p. 635 (q.v.).] CONGENITAL HEART DISEASE (ROGER DISEASE) 574

Rogers, David E. Some observations on having a coronary. *The Pharos.* 1986;49:12-4. CORONARY ARTERY DISEASE 631, 632

Roget, Peter Mark. *Animal and Vegetable Physiology, Considered with Reference to Natural Theology* London: 1834. [In: Talbott JH. *A Biographical History of Medicine*, p. 405 (q.v.).] EVOLUTION 1009

Rollo, John. A Short Account of the Royal Artillery Hospital at Woolwich; with Some Observations on the Management of Artillery Soldiers, Respecting the Preservation of Health. Addressed to the officers of the regiment, and dedicated to the Master-General and Board of Ordinance; 1801. [In: Chalmers I, Tröhler U. Helping physicians to keep abreast of the medical literature: *Medical and Philosophical Commentaries*, 1773-1795. Ann Intern Med. 2000;133(3):238-42.] MEDICAL EDUCATION 1744

Romano, John. *JAMA.* 1961;78:741-7 [Limited data]. MEDICAL PRACTICE 1952

Ronsard, Pierre de. In Vogel K. What is time? *Proc Charaka Club.* 1947;11:37-56. DEATH 652

Röntgen, Wilhelm Conrad.

In Glasser O. *Wilhelm Conrad Röntgen and the Early History of the Roentgen Rays.* Springfield, IL: Charles C Thomas; 1934. EXPERIMENTS 1033 [74], SCIENTISTS 3005 [100], UNIVERSITIES 3411 [100]

On a new kind of rays. *Nature.* 1896;53:274-6. [In: Keys TE, Keys JD. *Classics of Cardiology*, vol. 3. Malabar, FL: Robert E. Krieger Publishing; 1983, pp. 4-6.] RADIOLOGY 2815

Root, Eliza H. Change of climate for the tubercular. *Woman Med J.* 1904;14:269-71. TUBERCULOSIS 3392

Rose, Michael.

In Gladwell M. The new age of man [Interview of Michael Rose]. *The New Yorker.* 30 Sep 1996, vol 72, no. 29, pp. 56-67. LIVING 1580

The objective tangent. *Lancet.* 1977;2:1340-2. MEDICAL CARE 1686

Rosen, George. *A History of Public Health.* New York: MD Publications; 1958, p. 25. PUBLIC HEALTH 2755

Rosenau, Milton. *Preventive Medicine and Hygiene.* New York: Appleton; 1927, p. 172. TUBERCULOSIS 3398

Rosenberg CE, Golden J (eds). *Framing Disease: Studies in Cultural History.* New Brunswick, NJ: Rutgers University Press; 1992. p. xiii. DISEASE 800

Rosenberg, Charles E.

The Care of Strangers: The Rise of America's Hospital System. New York: Basic Books; 1987. HEALTH POLICY 1219 [352], HOSPITALS 1328 [11], MEDICAL CARE 1695 [351], MEDICAL ECONOMICS 1719 [352], 1720 [350], 1721 [351]

The Cholera Years: The United States in 1832, 1849, and 1866. Chicago: University of Chicago Press; 1962, p. 5. DISEASE 791

Why care about the history of medicine? Introduction to *Explaining Epidemics, and Other Studies in the History of Medicine.* Cambridge: Cambridge University Press; 1992:5. HISTORY OF MEDICINE 1297

Rutty, John. *A Chronological History of the Weather and Seasons on the Prevailing Diseases in Dublin.* London: Robinson & Roberts; 1770. [In: Major RH. *Classic Descriptions of Disease*, p. 234 (q.v.).] RELAPSING FEVER **2846**

Ryle, John Alfred. Clinical sense and clinical science. *Lancet.* 1939;1:1083-7. CLINICAL OBSERVATION **523**

Rynd, Francis. Description of an instrument for the subcutaneous introduction of fluids in affections of the nerves. *Dublin Q J.* 1861;32:13. [In: Clendening L. *Source Book of Medical History*, p. 420.] FLUID THERAPY **1059**

Sabouraud, Raymond Jacques Adrien. *Elementary Manual of Regional Topographical Dermatology.* Paris: Mason; 1905. [In: Talbott JH. *A Biographical History of Medicine*, p. 1111 (q.v.).] RINGWORM (TINEA CAPITIS) **2919**

Sachs, Bernard Parney. On arrested cerebral development, with special reference to its cortical pathology. *J Nervous Mental Dis.* 1887;14:541-53. AMAUROTIC FAMILIAL IDIOCY (TAY-SACHS DISEASE) **134**

Sackett DL, Richardson WS, Rosenberg W, Haynes RB.
Evidence-Based Medicine: How To Practice and Teach Evidence-Based Medicine. New York: Churchill Livingstone; 1997, p. 2. MEDICAL EVIDENCE **1859**
Evidence-Based Medicine: How To Practice and Teach Evidence-Based Medicine. New York: Churchill Livingstone; 1997, p. 2. MEDICAL EVIDENCE **1860**

Sacks, Oliver W.
Awakenings. New York: Summit Books; 1987, p. 26. MEDICINE **2125**
Migraine. Los Angeles: University of California Press; 1992, p. 234. MEDICAL HISTORIES **1884**
The Man Who Mistook His Wife for a Hat. New York: Summit Books; 1985, p. 105. HUMANS **1339**
In Clemons W. Listening to the lost. *Newsweek.* 29 Aug 1984. [In: *Migraine.* Los Angeles: University of California Press; 1992, p. 234.] MIGRAINE **2171**

Sagan, Carl. *Broca's Brain: Reflections on the Romance of Science.* New York: Random House; 1979, p. 14. BRAIN **344**

Sakel, Manfred Joshua. Schizophreniebehandlung mittels insulin-hypoglykamie sowie hypoglykamischer schocks. *Wien Med Wschr* 1934;84(45):1211-14 [Translation by Wortis J reprinted in *Amer J Psychiatry.* 1937;93:829-41]. PSYCHOSIS **2739**

Saliceto, Gulielmus de. *Liber in Scientia Medicinali.* Placentiae: Johannes Petrus de Ferratis; 1476. [In: Major RH. *Classic Descriptions of Disease*, pp. 570,2 (q.v.).] KIDNEY DISEASE **1489**

Salk, Jonas. Studies in human subjects on active immunization against poliomyelitis. Part I: A preliminary report of experiments in progress. *JAMA.* 1953;13:1081-98. POLIOMYELITIS **2638**

Salt HB, Wolf OH, Lloyd JK, et al. On having no beta-lipoprotein: a syndrome comprising abetalipoproteinemia, acanthocytosis, and steatorrhea. *Lancet.* 1960;2:325-9. ABETALIPOPROTEINEMIA (BASSEN-KORNZWEIG SYNDROME) **2**

Samter M, Beers RF. Intolerance to aspirin: clinical studies and consideration of its pathogenesis. *Ann Intern Med.* 1968;68:975-83. ASPIRIN IDIOSYNCRASY SYNDROME **248**

Sandström, Ivar Victor. On a new gland in man and several mammals [German]. *Uppsala Lakareforenings Forhandlingar.* 1879-80;15:441-71. [In: Talbott JH. *A Biographical History of Medicine*, pp. 937-8 (q.v.).] PARATHYROID GLANDS **2335**

Sanger, Margaret.
Motherhood in Bondage. New York: Brentano's; 1928. CONTRACEPTION **602** [293], LOVE **1585** [323-4]
Woman and the New Race. New York: Brentano's; 1920. SEX **3037** [168], WOMEN **3469** [225]

Sarngadharan MG, Popovic M, Bruch L, et al. Antibodies reactive with human T-lymphotropic retroviruses (HTLV-III) in the serum of patients with AIDS. *Science.* 1984;224:506-8. ACQUIRED IMMUNE DEFICIENCY SYNDROME (AIDS) **28**

Sauerbruch, Ernst Ferdinand. Die beeinflussung von lungenerkrankungen durch kunstliche lahmung des zwerchfells (phrenikotomie). *Munch Med Wochenschr.* 1913;60:625-6. [In: Talbott JH. *A Biographical History of Medicine*, p. 1036 (q.v.).] TUBERCULOSIS **3395**

Sauvages, François Boissier de. *Nosologie methodique*, vol. 7. Lyon; 1772, p. 12. [In: Foucault M, *Madness and Civilization: A History of Insanity in an Age of Reason.* New York: Pantheon Books; 1965, p. 85.] PSYCHOSIS **2736**

Scarlett, Earle P.
In Sickness and in Health: Reflections on the Medical Profession. Roland CG (ed). Toronto: McClelland & Stewart; 1972. AGING **92** [220], DOCTORS' WIVES **870** [20-1], DOCTORS **857** [xvii], DYING **922** [223], GUILLOTINE **1155** [33], HEALTH **1200** [179], **1201** [179], MEDICAL STUDENTS **2062** [3], PHILOSOPHY **2517** [xvi], PHYSICIANS **2589** [12-3], PUBLISHING **2768** [101], WRITING **3509** [102],

Interview. In Bobey N. The ram's horn: the commonplace book of Dr. Earle Parkhill Scarlett. *Ann R Coll Phys Surg Canada.* 1997;30:292-5. WRITING **3511**

Schatz A, Bugie E, Waksman SA. Streptomycin, a substance exhibiting antibiotic activity against gram-positive and gram-negative bacteria. *Proc Soc Exp Biol Med.* 1944;55:66-9. STREPTOMYCIN **3176**

Schaudinn F, Hoffmann E. Vorläufiger bericht über das vorkommen von spirochaeten in syphilitschen krankheitsprodukten und bei papillomen. Arbeiten aus dem Kaiserlichen Gesundheitsamte. 1905;22:527-34. SYPHILIS **3264**

Schiebinger, Londa. *Nature's Body: Gender in the Making of Modern Science.* Boston: Beacon Press; 1993. SCIENCE **3000** [3], **3001** [114]

Schindler, Rudolf. Die diagnostische Bedeutung der Gastroskopie. *Munchen Med Wochenschr.* 1922;69:535-7. GASTROSCOPY **1088**

Schmidt, Marcia C. Diagnosis of rheumatic disease: tests and traps. *Hosp Pract.* 1984;19:82e-82r. TESTS **3282**

Scholander, Per Frederik. Analyzer for accurate estimation of respiratory gases in one-half cubic centimeter samples. *J Biol Chem.* 1947;167:235-50. RESPIRATORY GASES **2893**

Schönlein, Johann Lucas. Peliosis rheumatica. In *Allgemeine und Specielle Pathologie und Therapie,* 3rd ed., vol. 3. Herisau, Switzerland; Literatur-Comptoir; 1837, pp. 48-9. [In: Talbott JH. A *Biographical History of Medicine,* pp. 504-5 (q.v.).] HENOCH-SCHÖNLEIN PURPURA **1271**

Schoolman, Harold M.
Sounding board. The role of the physician as a patient advocate. *N Engl J Med.* 1977;296:103-5. RESPONSIBILITY **2895**
The role of the physician as a patient advocate. *N Engl J Med.* 1977;296:103-5. DECISION MAKING **691**

Schroeder, Steven A. The medically uninsured: will they always be with us? *N Engl J Med.* 1996;334:1130-3. HEALTH POLICY **1220, 1221,** MEDICAL ECONOMICS **1724**

Schwann, Theodor. Über das Wesen des Verdauungsprocesses. *Arch Anat Physiol Wissensch Med.* 1836;90-138. [In: *Selected Readings in the History of Physiology,* 2nd ed. Translated by Fulton JF, Wilson LG. Springfield, IL: Charles C Thomas; 1966, pp. 190-2.] DIGESTION **766**

Schwartz, William B. The effect of sulfanilamide on salt and water excretion in congestive heart failure. *N Engl J Med.* 1949;240:173-7. CARBONIC ANHYDRASE INHIBITORS **425**

Scott, Walter. In Lockhart JG. *Memoirs of the Life of Sir Walter Scott,* 1838. POLIOMYELITIS **2629**

Seidelman, William E. Medical selection: Auschwitz antecedents and effluent. *Int J Health Serv.* 1991;21:401-15. EUGENICS **1003**

Sells, Arthur Lytton. *Oliver Goldsmith: His Life and Works.* London: George Allen & Unwin; 1974, pp. 109-10. MEDICAL PRACTICE **1956**

Selye, Hans.
Newsweek. 31 March 1958. [In: Simpson JB, *Contemporary Quotations,* p. 187 (q.v.).] HEALTH **1193**
The Stress of Life. New York: McGraw-Hill, 1956, p. vii. STRESS **3177**

Selzer, Richard.
Liver. In *Mortal Lessons: Notes on the Art of Surgery.* New York: Simon & Schuster; 1976, p. 64. LIVER **1561**
Speech to the University of Dallas, 1984. [In: Anderson CM. *Richard Selzer and the Rhetoric of Surgery.* Carbondale: Southern Illinois University Press; 1989, p. 46.] NATURE **2223**
The corpse. In *Mortal Lessons: Notes on the Art of Surgery.* New York: Simon & Schuster; 1976, p. 136. DEATH **678**
The surgeon as writer [Speech to the Humanities Symposium, Dalhousie University, 1991] [Limited data]. SURGEONS **3208**

Semmelweis, Ignaz Phillip. *The Etiology, the Concept, and the Prophylaxis of Childbed Fever,* vol II. Vienna: C.A. Hartleben's Verlags-Expedition, 1861. [In: *Medical Classics,* vol. 5. Baltimore: Williams and Wilkins; 1940-41, p. 533.] INFECTION **1428**

Senapati, Asha. The clinical section: a special case for case reports. *J R Soc Med.* 1996;89:95. CASE REPORTS **435**

Seneca.
Epistles, first century AD. ALCOHOL **106,** TREATMENT **3330**
In Nuland SB. *How We Die: Reflections on Life's Final Chapter.* New York: Alfred A. Knopf; 1994:151. SUICIDE **3182**

Sennert, Daniel. *De Febribus,* book IV. Venice: 1641. [In: Major RH. *Classic Descriptions of Disease,* p. 199 (q.v.).] SCARLET FEVER **2931**

Servetus, Michael. *Christianismi Restitutio,* 5th ed, 1553. [In: Osler W. Michael Servetus. *John Hopkins Hosp Bull.* 1910;21:1-11.] LUNG **1587,** PULMONARY CIRCULATION **2780**

Service, Robert William. The Battle of the Bulge. In: *More Collected Verse of Robert Service*. New York: Dodd, Mead; 1953:8-9. OBESITY **2283**

Seuss, Dr (Theodore Geisel). *You're Only Old Once!*. New York: Random House; 1986. MEDICAL CARE **1694**

Shakespeare, William.
  As You Like It, 1598. AGING **59**
  Coriolanus, 1608. INFECTION **1427**
  Hamlet, 1600. SUICIDE **3183**
  Henry IV, Part II, 1597. IMPOTENCE **1422**
  Julius Caesar, 1599. EPILEPSY **974**
  Macbeth, 1606. ALCOHOL **108**, CAESAREAN SECTION **362**, CONFIDENTIALITY **573**, CONSULTANTS **583**, MEDICINE **2086**, PSYCHOTHERAPY **2747**
  Richard II, 1595. EUTHANASIA **1004**
  Richard III, 1592. DEFORMITY **694**, RABIES **2813**
  Romeo and Juliet, 1594. MIGRAINE **2165**

Shapiro, Eugene. Blame old age, not Medicare. *New York Times*. 3 Jan 1985:A21. AGING **96**

Sharpey-Schafer, Edward Albert. Description of a simple and efficient method of performing artificial respiration in the human subject especially in cases of drowning. *Med-Chir Trans*. 1904;87:609-14. ARTIFICIAL RESPIRATION **240**

Shattuck, George Cheyne Jr. In Louis PCA. *Anatomical, Pathological, and Therapeutic Researches on the Yellow Fever of Gibraltar of 1828*. Translated by Shattuck GC Jr. Boston: Charles C. Little and James Brown; 1839, p. xii. [In: Bloomfield AL, *Communicable Diseases*, p. 492.] STATISTICS **3138**

Shaw, George Bernard.
  Misalliance, preface; 1914. PATIENT-PHYSICIAN RELATIONS **2403**
  The Doctor's Dilemma. [Play first produced in 1906 and first published in 1908. The "Preface on Doctors" was first published in 1911.] ANIMAL RESEARCH **189**, BELIEF **290**, DECISION MAKING **690**, DOCTORS **839-45**, EXPERIENCE **1028**, HEALTH **1189**, HEALTH POLICY **1214**, LONGEVITY **1582**, MALPRACTICE **1613**, MEDICAL ETHICS **1830**, MEDICAL JOURNALS **1901**, MEDICAL PRACTICE **1939**, MEDICAL PROFESSION **1999-2001**, MEDICAL SERVICES **2052**, MEDICINE **2110**, PATIENTS **2460**, PLACEBOS **2610**, PROFESSIONS **2688**, PUBLIC INFORMATION **2756**, QUACKERY **2806**, SURGERY **3229, 3230**, TREATMENT **3349**

Sheehan, Harold Leeming.
  Post-partum necrosis of the anterior pituitary. *J Pathol Bacteriol*. 1937;45:189-214. HYPOPITUITARISM **1383**
  Simmonds's disease due to post-partum necrosis of the anterior pituitary. *Q J Med*. 1939;8(n.s.):277-309. HYPOPITUITARISM **1384**

Shem, Samuel. *The House of God*. New York: Richard Marek Publishers; 1978, p. 376. CARDIAC ARREST **426**, FEVER **1054**, MEDICAL CARE **1688**, NEEDLE ASPIRATION **2226**

Sherrington, Charles Scott.
  The Endeavour of Jean Fernel. Cambridge: Cambridge University Press; 1946:142. RESEARCH **2866**
  The central nervous system. In: Foster M. A *Text-book of Physiology*, 7th ed. London: 1897. SYNAPSE **3250**

Sherwood T. Science in radiology. *Lancet*. 1978;1:594-95. [594]. STATISTICS **3163**

Shimkin, Michael B. *Contrary to Human Nature: Cancer*. Washington, DC: Department of Health, Education and Welfare; 1977.

Shorb, Mary Shaw. Activity of vitamin B_{12} for the growth of *Lactobacillus lactis*. *Science*. 1948;107:397-8. VITAMIN B_3 (NICOTINAMIDE) **3437**

Shorter, Edward.
  A History of Psychiatry: From the Era of the Asylum to the Age of Prozac. New York: Wiley; 1997. NEURASTHENIA **2248** [130], PSYCHIATRY **2725** [109], **2726** [160], PSYCHOANALYSIS **2733** [170], **2734** [153], PSYCHOTHERAPY **2749** [144], PSYCHOTROPIC DRUGS **2750** [255]
  Doctors and Their Patients: A Social History. New Brunswick, NJ: Transaction Publishers; 1991. ALTERNATIVE MEDICINE **128** [12], MALPRACTICE **1618** [11], MEDICINE **2134** [259]
  The Making of the Modern Family. New York: Basic Books; 1975. FAMILIES **1040**, SEX **3041**
  Sucker-punched again! Physicians meet the disease-of-the-month syndrome [Editorial]. *J Psychosom Res*. 1995;39:115-8. CHRONIC FATIGUE SYNDROME **481**

Shrady, George Frederick.
  A plea for the specialist. *Med Rec*. 1885;27:183. SPECIALIZATION **3106**
  Medical authorship. *Medical Record*. 1867;2:445-6. PUBLISHING **2760**

Siegler, Mark. Falling off the pedestal: What is happening to the traditional doctor-patient relationship? *Mayo Clin Proc.* 1993;68:461-7. MEDICAL ECONOMICS **1723**

Siena, Cherubino da. *Regole della vita matrimoniale, circa* 1450. [In: Sweeney C. The truth about sex at any given moment. *New York Times Magazine.* 1999;18:114-5.] MARRIAGE **1635**

Sigerist, Henry E.
Classics of medicine. In *The University at the Crossroads: Addresses and Essays.* New York: Henry Schuman; 1946, p. 100. MEDICAL RESEARCH **2031**

In Falk LA. Medical sociology: the contributions of Dr. Henry E. Sigerist. *J Hist Med Allied Sci.* 1958;13:214-28. MEDICAL SERVICES **2054**

In Marti-Ibanez F (ed). *Henry E. Sigerist on the History of Medicine.* New York: MD Publications; 1960, p. 111. PHYSICIANS **2586**

The university at the crossroads. In *The University at the Crossroads: Addresses and Essays.* New York: Henry Schuman; 1946. EDUCATION **942** [62-3], **943** [77]

Sigurdsson B, Gudmundsson KR. Clinical findings six years after outbreak of Akureyri disease. *Lancet.* 1956;1:766-7. CHRONIC FATIGUE SYNDROME **476**

Sill, Edward Rowland. *An Adage from the Orient,* 1887. ALCOHOLISM **121**

Simmonds, Morris. Ueber hypophysisschwund mit tödlichem ausgang. *Deutsche Medizinische Wochenschrift.* 1914;40:322-3. HYPOPITUITARISM **1382**

Simon, Gustav. Exstirpation einer Niere am Menschen. *Deutsche Klinik.* 1870:22:137-8. KIDNEY SURGERY **1502**

Simpson, Alexander. Superinvolution of the uterus. *Edinburgh Med J.* 1883;28(Part 2):961-8. HYPOPITUITARISM **1381**

Simpson, James Beasley (ed). *Contemporary Quotations.* New York: Galahad Books; 1964.

Simpson, James Young.
Account of a New Anaesthetic Agent for a Substitute for Sulphuric Ether. Edinburgh: 1847. ANESTHESIA **161**

Answer to the religious objections advanced against the employment of anaesthetic agents in midwifery and surgery. In *Anaesthesia, or the Employment of Chloroform and Ether in Surgery, Midwifery, etc.* Philadelphia: Lindsay & Blakiston; 1849:110. ANESTHESIA **163**

Simpson, Michael A. A mythology of medical education. *Lancet.* 1974;3:399-401. PUBLISHING **2769**

Sims, James Marion. On vaginismus. *Trans Obstet Soc London.* 1862;3:356-67. VAGINISMUS **3418**

Singer, Isaac Bashevis. Jachid and Jechidah. In: *Collected Stories: Gimpel the Fool to The Letter Writer.* New York: Library of America; 2004:398-405. LIFE **1548**

Singer K, Fisher B, Perlstein MA. Acanthrocytosis: a genetic erythrocytic malformation. *Blood.* 1952;7:577-91. ACANTHOCYTOSIS **20**

Sippy, Bertram Welton. Gastric and duodenal ulcer; medical care by an efficient removal of gastric juice corrosion. *JAMA.* 1915;64:1625-30. PEPTIC ULCER **2489**

Sjögren, Henrik. Zur kenntnis der Keratoconjunctivitis sicca (Keratitis filiformis bei Hypofunction der Tramendrüsen). *Acta Ophth.* [Suppl II] 1933;1-151. [Translated in A new conception of kerato-conjunctivitis sicca. Hamilton JB, translator. *Australasian Med.* 1943:97.] SJÖGREN SYNDROME **3069**

Skoda, Josef. *Abhandlung über Perkussion und Auskultation.* Vienna; 1839. [In: Major RH. *Classic Descriptions of Disease,* p. 612.] PHYSICAL EXAMINATION **2522**

Skrabanek, Petr. Preventive medicine and morality. *Lancet.* 1986;1:143-4. AGING **97**, PREVENTIVE MEDICINE **2683**, **2684**

Slye, Maud. Cancer and heredity. *Ann Intern Med.* 1928;12:951-76. CANCER **383**

Small, William. In Hull G. William Small, 1734-1775: No publications, much influence. *J R Soc Med.* 1997;90:102-5. MEDICAL PRACTICE **1920**, **1921**

Smith, Adam. *The Wealth of Nations,* book I. New York: Modern Library; 1937, p. 105. MEDICAL PROFESSION **1980**

Smith, Fred M. The ligation of coronary arteries with electrocardiographic study. *Arch Intern Med.* 1918;22:8-27. CORONARY ARTERY DISEASE **626**

Smith, Homer William.
From Fish to Philosopher. Boston: Little, Brown; 1959:2. KIDNEY **1486**

Lectures on the Kidney. Lawrence: University of Kansas Press; 1943, p. 3. KIDNEY **1483**

The Physiology of the Kidney. New York: Oxford University Press; 1937, pp. 58-61. KIDNEY FUNCTION **1498**

On a proper knowledge of man. In *Proceedings of the Charaka Club,* vol. XII. Hastings House Publishers; 1985, p. 35. CONSCIOUSNESS **580**

Renal physiology between two wars. In *Lectures on the Kidney.* Lawrence: University of Kansas Press; 1943. KIDNEY **1485** [75], KIDNEY FUNCTION **1500** [77]

Smith, Joel P. Depression: darker than darkness. *The American Scholar*. 1997;66:495-9. DEPRESSION 719
Smith, Sydney.
In Lady Holland. *Memoir of Sydney Smith*, 1855, vol. I, ch. 11. MARRIAGE 1637
In Virgin P. *Sydney Smith*. London: Harper; 1994:277. GOUT 1143
Smith, Theobold. Letter to Dr. Krumbhaar. *J Bacteriol*. 1934;27:19-20. MEDICAL RESEARCH 2030
Smollett, Tobias. *Humphry Clinker*, 1771. AGING 67 [letter of Matthew Bramble, 26 October], EXERCISE 1019 [letter of Matthew Bramble, 26 October], MIND 2184 [letter of Matthew Bramble, 14 June]
Smyth, Harley S. Technology and human worth. *Ann R Coll Phys Surg Canada*. 1982;15:405-6. ABORTION 15
Snow, Charles Percy.
Human care. *JAMA*. 1973;225:617-21. HOSPITALS 1324
The Status of Doctors. Lecture given to the Royal Society of Medicine, London, May 18, 1966. Text in *Proc R Soc Med*. 1967;60:153-6. WRITING 3506
Snow, John. *On the Mode of Communication of Cholera*, 1849. [In: Clendening L. *Source Book of Medical History*, p. 469 (q.v.).] CHOLERA 472
Socrates. Plato, *Phaedo*. MEDICAL FEES 1866
Soemmerring, Samuel Thomas von.
Abbildungen und Beschreibungen Einiger Misgeburten. Mainz: 1791. ACHONDROPLASIA 23
De Morbis Vasorum Absorbentium Corporis Humani. Frankfurt: 1795. [In: Shimkin MB, *Contrary to Nature: Cancer*, p. 94 (q.v.).] SMOKING 3092
Solimena M, Folli F, Denis-Donini S, et al. Autoantibodies to glutamic decarboxylase in a patient with stiff-man syndrome, epilepsy, and type I diabetes mellitus. *N Engl J Med*. 1988;318:1012-20. STIFF-PERSON SYNDROME (STIFF-MAN SYNDROME) 3174
Solly, Samuel. In Abse D. *Doctors and Patients*. Oxford, England: Oxford University Press; 1984, p. 93. SEXUALLY TRANSMITTED DISEASES 3058
Solomon, Andrew. Anatomy of melancholy. *The New Yorker*. 12 Jan 1998, vol. 73, no. 42, pp. 46-61. DEPRESSION 720
Solzhenitsyn, Alexander. *Cancer Ward*. New York: Modern Library; 1968, p. 143. MIRACLES 2187
Sontag, Susan. *Illness as Metaphor*. New York: Farrar, Straus & Giroux; 1978. DISEASE 796 [58], 797 [55], ILLNESS 1408 [56-7], 1409 [3]
Soranus of Ephesus. *Gynecology*. Temkin O; translator. Baltimore: Johns Hopkins University Press; 1956. CONCEPTION 571 [35], MENSTRUATION 2148 [17]
Soros G, Madrick J. The international crisis: an interview. *New York Review of Books*. 1999;46(1):36-7,38,40. DEATH 687
Soros, George. In Ramirez A. Soros giving $15 million for program on medical ethics and money. *The New York Times*. 15 Apr 1999, p. B12. MEDICAL ECONOMICS 1732
Souttar, Henry Sessions. The surgical treatment of mitral stenosis. *Br Med J*. 1925;2:603-6. HEART SURGERY 1251
Spallanzani, Lazzaro. In Coope R (ed). *The Quiet Art*, 1958, p. 4 (q.v.).] SCIENCE 2944
Spence, James. *The Need for Understanding the Individual as a Part of the Training and Functions of Doctors and Nurses* [Address delivered at a conference on mental health held in March 1949]. [In: *The Purpose and Practice of Medicine: Selections from the Writings of Sir James Spence*. London: Oxford University Press; 1960, pp. 273-4.] MEDICAL PRACTICE 1948
Spens, Thomas. History of a case in which there took place a remarkable slowness of the pulse. *Med Commentaries*. 1793;7:458-65. [In: Major RH. *Classic Descriptions of Disease*, pp. 358-9 (q.v.).] HEART BLOCK 1236
Sperry, Roger W. Some effects of disconnecting the cerebral hemispheres [Nobel lecture]. *Science*. 1982;217(4566):1223-6. BRAIN 345
Spies TD, Vilter CF, Koch MB, Caldwell MH. Observations of the anti-anemic properties of synthetic folic acid. *Southern Med J*. 1945;38:707-9. FOLIC ACID 1064
Spilker, Bert. *Guide to Clinical Trials*. New York: Raven Press; 1991, p. 836. CLINICAL TRIALS 557
Spiro, Howard.
Duodenal ulcer disease. *Hosp Pract*. 1985;20:70a-70z. GASTROENTEROLOGY 1087
What is empathy and can it be taught? *Ann Intern Med*. 1992;116:843-6. EMPATHY 955, 956, EQUANIMITY 990, MEDICAL EDUCATION 1798, MEDICAL HISTORIES 1888, MEDICAL SCHOOLS 2042
Spock, Benjamin. *The Common Sense Book of Baby and Child Care*. New York: Duell, Sloan & Pearce; 1946:4. CHILDREN 461
Sprengel, Kurt. Preface. In: *Neue litterarische nachrichten für aertze, wundaertze und naturforscher*, 1786. [In: Kronick DA. *A History of Scientific and Technical Periodicals: The Origins and Development of the Scientific and Technological Press, 1665-1790*, 2nd ed. Metuchen, NJ: Scarecrow Press; 1976:197.] PUBLISHING 2758

The Works of Thomas Sydenham, MD, 3rd ed, vol. 1. Translated by Latham RG. London: Sydenham Society; 1848-1850. [In: Birmingham, AL: Classics of Medicine Library; 1979.] MEDICAL EDUCATION **1740** [4], MEDICAL HISTORIES **1871** [14], MEDICAL PROFESSION **1978** [25], MEDICINE **2088** [11], PATIENT-PHYSICIAN RELATIONS **2375** [25]

The Works of Thomas Sydenham, MD, 3rd ed, vol. 2. Translated by Latham RG. London: Sydenham Society; 1848-1850. [In: Birmingham, AL: Classics of Medicine Library; 1979:182.] CLINICAL OBSERVATION **506**

The Works of Thomas Sydenham, MD. Translated by Latham RG. London: Sydenham Society; 1848-1850. [In: Birmingham, AL: Classics of Medicine Library; 1979.] {Limited data.] DISEASE **782**

Tractatus de Podagra et Hydrope. London: 1683. [Reprinted as On gout. In: *The Works of Thomas Sydenham, MD*, 3rd ed, vol. 2. Birmingham, AL: Classics of Medicine Library; 1979:124-5.] GOUT **1132**

Febris scarlatina [On the scarlet fever]. In *Observationes Medicae*. London: 1676. [In: *The Works of Thomas Sydenham, MD*, 3rd ed., vol. 2. Birmingham, AL: Classics of Medicine Library. 1979, p. 242.] SCARLET FEVER **2932**

In Coope R (ed). *The Quiet Art*. London: E&S Livingstone; 1958. SERVICE **3023** [251], TREATMENT **3334** [129]

In Strauss MB (ed). *Familiar Medical Quotations*, p. 494 (q.v.). HUMOR **1341**

Sylvius, Jacobus. *Opera Medica*. Geneva: 1635. ANATOMY **147**

Szasz, Thomas. *The Second Sin*. New York: Anchor Press; 1973. PSYCHOSIS **2741**

Szent-Györgyi, Albert. Observations on the function of perioxidase systems and the chemistry of the adrenal cortex: description of a new carbohydrate derivative. *Biochem J.* 1928;22:1387-409. VITAMIN C (ASCORBIC ACID) **3443**

Talbor, Robert. *The English Remedy, or Talbor's Wonderful Secret*. London: 1682, p. 1. [In: Major RH. *Classic Descriptions of Disease*, p. 114 (q.v.).] MALARIA **1602**

Talbott, John Harold. *A Biographical History of Medicine: Excerpts and Essays on the Men and Their Work*. New York: Grune and Stratton; 1970.

Tallis, Raymond. The reluctance to trust in trust. [Review of Wier R (ed). *Physician-Assisted Suicide*. Bloomington: Indiana Univerity Press; 1997.] *Times Literary Supplement.* 30 Jan 1998, no. 4948, pp. 6-7. DECISION MAKING **693**, MEDICAL ETHICS **1847**

Taylor, Charles Fayette. *Infantile Paralysis and Its Attendant Deformities*. Philadelphia: Lippincott; 1867. [In: Bloomfield AL, *Communicable Diseases*, p. 410 (q.v.).] POLIOMYELITIS **2634**

Taylor, Robert L. *Mind or Body: Distinguishing Psychological from Organic Disorders*. New York: McGraw-Hill; 1982, p. 32. PSYCHIATRY **2723**

Temple LKF, McLeod RS, Gallinger S, Wright JG. Defining disease in the genomic era. *Science*. 2001;293(5531):807-8. DISEASE **804**

Tennyson, Alfred. In Nuland SB. *How We Die: Reflections on Life's Final Chapter*. New York: Alfred A. Knopf; 1994:86. DEATH **664**

Tenon, Jacques. *Memoirs on Paris Hospitals*, part 4, 1788. HOSPITALS **1320**

Tertullian (Quintus Septimius Tertullianus).
Apologetical Works and Minucius Felix Octavius. Translated by Daly EJ. New York: Fathers of the Church; 1950. ABORTION **7** [31-2], CONTRACEPTION **598** [32], MARRIAGE **1634** [24]

In *Latin Proverbs from Reichert, H.G., Unvergangliche Lateinische Spruchweisheit: Urban und Human*. Panorama Verlag; Wiesbaden [Limited data]. MEDICINE **2078**

Thacher, James. *An Essay on Demonology, Ghosts, and Apparitions*. Boston: Carter & Hendee; 1831. [In: Talbott JH. *A Biographical History of Medicine*, p. 366 (q.v.).] QUACKERY **2803**

Theodoric.
The Surgery of Theodoric, vol. 1. Translated by Campbell E, Colton J. New York: Appleton-Century-Crofts; 1960, p. 5. SURGEONS **3195**

The Surgery of Theodoric, vol. 2. Translated by Campbell E, Colton J. New York: Appleton-Century-Crofts; 1960. CANCER **375** [26], CANCER OF THE BREAST **392** [310],

Thiérry, François. Description d'une malade appelee mal de la rosa. *J Med-Chir Pharmacol.* 1755;2:337-46. [In: Major RH. *Classic Descriptions of Disease*, pp. 665-6 (q.v.).] PELLAGRA **2476**

Thomas, Dylan. Do not go gentle into that good night. Written in 1951. DYING **917**

Thomas, Hugh Owens. *Diseases of the Hip, Knee, and Ankle Joints with Their Deformities Treated by a New and Efficient Method*. Liverpool: T. Dobb; 1875. [In: Talbott JH. *A Biographical History of Medicine*, p. 709 (q.v.).] THOMAS HIP-SPLINT **3296**

Thomas, Lewis.

The Youngest Science. New York: Viking Press; 1983, p. 236. MEN **2145**

Alturism. *New York Times Magazine*. 4 July 1976, pp. 108-9. DISEASE **795**

Biostatistics in medicine [Editorial]. *Science*. 1977;198:675. STATISTICS **3162**

Hazards of science. In *The Medusa and the Snail: More Notes of a Biology Watcher*. New York: Viking; 1979. BIOLOGY **301** [73], TRUTH **3367** [74]

How to fix the premedical curriculum. In *The Medusa and the Snail*. New York: Viking; 1979, p. 137. MEDICAL EDUCATION **1791**

In time of plague. In *The Fragile Species*. New York: Macmillan Publishing; 1992, p. 48. HISTORY OF MEDICINE **1298**

Leech, leech, etc. In *The Youngest Science: Notes of a Medicine Watcher*. New York: Viking; 1983. MEDICAL TECHNOLOGY **2064** [60], PATIENT-PHYSICIAN RELATIONS **2437** [56]

Medical lessons from history. In *The Medusa and the Snail: More Notes of a Biology Watcher*. New York: Viking; 1979. MEDICINE **2127** [159], **2128** [166]

Notes of a biology watcher: facts of life. N Engl J Med. 1977;296:1462-4. EVOLUTION **1012**

Notes of a biology watcher: on cloning a human being. N Engl J Med. 1974;291:1296-97. GENETICS **1108**

Notes of a biology watcher: on probability and possibility. N Engl J Med. 1974;290:388-9. BRAIN **343**

Notes of a biology watcher: the health-care system. N Eng J Med. 1975;293:1245-6. HEALTH **1202, 1203,** MEDICAL CARE **1684,** MEDICALIZATION OF LIFE **2069**

Nurses. In *The Youngest Science: Notes of a Medicine Watcher*. New York: Viking; 1983, pp. 65-6. NURSES **2270**

The art and craft memoir. In *The Fragile Species*. New York: Macmillan Publishing; 1992, p. 25. HUMANS **1340**

Your very good health. In *Lives of a Cell: Notes of a Biology Watcher*. New York: Viking Press; 1974, p. 83. HUMAN BODY **1330**

Thomson, William, Lord Kelvin. *Popular Lectures and Addresses*, 1891-1894. [In: *Bartlett's Familiar Quotations*, 14th ed. Boston: Little, Brown; 1968:723.] SCIENCE **2965**

Thoreau, Henry David.

A Writer's Journal. Stapleton L (ed). New York: Dover Publications; 1960, p 21. HEALTH **1179**

Journal, 1851. DISEASE **784**

Journal, February 18, 1860. DRUGS **885**

Thorn GW, Engel LL, Eisenberg H. Treatment of adrenal insufficiency by means of subcutaneous implants of pellets of desoxycorticosterone acetate (a synthetic adrenal cortical hormone). *Bull Johns Hopkins Hosp*. 1939;64:155-66. [165-6]. ADRENOCORTICAL INSUFFICIENCY (ADDISON DISEASE) **47**

Thorn, George W. In Manning PR, DeBakey L. *Medicine: Preserving the Passion*. New York: Springer-Verlag; 1987, p. 103. CONSULTATION **590**

Thorp JM Jr, Wells SR, Bowes WA Jr, Cefalo RC. Integrity, abortion, and the pro-life perinatologist. *Hastings Center Report*. 1995;25(1):27-8. PATIENT-PHYSICIAN RELATIONS **2450**

Tilton, James. *Economical Considerations on Military Hospitals and the Prevention and Cure of Diseases Incident to an Army*. Wilmington (Delaware): J. Wilson; 1813. [In: Talbott JH. *A Biographical History of Medicine*, p. 431 (q.v.).] MILITARY MEDICINE **2178**

Tissot, Samuel Auguste David.

A Treatise on the Diseases Produced by Onanism. Lausanne: 1760. [Translation: New York: 1832.] MASTURBATION **1643**

About the Health of Learned People. Lausanne: 1769. [In: *Ann Intern Med*. 1993;118:882.] TOBACCO **3311, 3312**

Tizard, J.P.M. Donald Winnicott: the president's view of a past president. *J R Soc Med*. 1981;74:267-74. HEALTH **1204**

Todd, John W. Points of view. Cost and complexity of medicine. *Lancet*. 1968;2:823-7. TESTS **3277**

Toni, Giovanni de. Remarks on relations between renal rickets (renal dwarfism) and renal diabetes. *Acta Paediatr*. 1933;16:479-84. DE TONI-FANCONI-VON ALBERTINI-ZELLWEGER SYNDROME **648**

Too Kim. In Wylie A. Notes on the western regions [Translated from *Tsëen Han Shoo*, book 96, part 1]. *J R Anthropol Inst Great Britain Ireland*. 1881;10:20-73. [In: Clarke CRA. Three journeys to high altitude: medicine, Tibetan thangkas, and Sepu Kangri. *J R Coll Phys London*. 1999;33:78-84.] HIGH-ALTITUDE MEDICINE **1283**

Verghese, Abraham.
  My Own Country: A Doctor's Story of a Town and its People in the Age of AIDS. New York: Simon & Schuster; 1994. ACQUIRED IMMUNE DEFICIENCY SYNDROME (AIDS) 31 [67], RADIOLOGY 2819 [261]
  The physician as storyteller. *Ann Intern Med.* 2001;135(11):1012-7. PATIENTS 2472
Vesalius A. *The Fabric of the Human Body,* preface. 1543. [In: Clendening L. *Source Book of Medical History,* p. 128.] SPECIALIZATION 3103
Victoria, Queen. In: Bennion E. *Antique Medical Instruments.* Berkeley: University of California Press; 1979:15. ANESTHESIA 165
Vidal, Jean-Baptiste Emile. *Considerations on Chronic Primary Articular Rheumatism* [French]. Paris: Thesis; 1855. [In: Talbott JH. *A Biographical History of Medicine,* p. 1090 (q.v.).] RHEUMATOID ARTHRITIS 2910
Vieussens, Raymond.
  Traité nouveau de la structure et des causes de movement natural du coeur, 1715. AORTIC VALVE REGURGITATION 206
  In Herrick JB. *A Short History of Cardiology.* Charles C. Thomas; 1942, p. 43. MITRAL STENOSIS 2189
Vigevano, Guido da. *Anothomia Designata per Figuras,* 1345. ANATOMY 145
Vigo, Johannis de.
  Practica in Arte Chirurgia Copiosa. Rome: 1514. [In: Major RH. *Classic Descriptions of Disease,* p. 28.] SYPHILIS 3255
  Practica in Arte Chirurgica Copiosa. Rome: 1514. [In: Simpson JA, Weiner ESC. *The Oxford English Dictionary,* 2nd ed., vol. XI. Oxford: Clarendon Press; 1989:737.] TUBERCULOSIS 3370
Villemin, Jean-Antoine. *Etudes sur la Tuberculose; Preuves Rationelle et Experimentales de sa Specifite et Son Inoculabilite.* Paris: 1868. [In: Major RH. *Classic Descriptions of Disease,* p. 75 (q.v.).] TUBERCULOSIS 3385
Vinci, Leonardo da.
  Treatise on Painting, ch. 1. In *The Notebooks of Leonardo da Vinci.* Arranged and translated by Mac Curdy E. New York: Reynal & Hitchcock; 1958, p. 634. STATISTICS 3128
  In MacCurdy E. *The Notebooks of Leonardo da Vinci.* New York: Reynal & Hitchcock; 1938. ARTERIOSCLEROSIS 231 [127], HEART 1226 [128]
Virchow, Rudolf Ludwig Karl.
  Cellular Pathology as Based upon Physiological and Pathological Histology, 7th American ed. Translated by Chance F. New York: 1860. [In: Birmingham, AL: Classics of Medicine Library; 1978.] CELLULAR BASIS OF LIFE 448 [27], EMBOLISM 948 [204], THROMBOPHLEBITIS 3299 [201-2]
  Die Bindegewbsfrage. *Virchow Arch.* 1859;16:1-20. [In: Atterman K. Connective tissue: an eclectical historical review with particular reference to the liver. *Histochem J.* 1981;13:341-96.] CONNECTIVE TISSUE 578
  In Eisenberg L. Rudolf Ludwig Karl Virchow, where are you now that we need you? *Am J Med.* 1984;77:524-32. PUBLIC HEALTH 2751
  In Garrison FH. Medical proverbs. *Bull N Y Acad Med.* 1928;4:997-1005. WRITING 3496
  The morality of scientists. *Minerva.* Winter 1987, p. 512. MEDICAL JOURNALS 1899
  Weisses blut. *Neue Notizen Geb Natur Heilk.* 1845;36:151-6. [In: Major RH. *Classic Descriptions of Disease,* pp. 554-6 (q.v.).] LEUKEMIA 1534
Volkmann, Richard von. Ischemic paralysis and contractures [German] *Z Chir.* 1881;8:801-3. [In: Talbott JH. *A Biographical History of Medicine,* p. 1008 (q.v.).] VOLKMANN ISCHEMIC CONTRACTURES 3453
Voltaire. *Zadig,* 1747. QUACKERY 2802
Voorhees, Irving Wilson. Colds: their cause and cure. *Am Med.* 1917;12:125. INFECTION 1430

Wachter R, Goldman L. The emerging role of "hospitalists" in the American health care system. *N Engl J Med.* 1996;335(7):514-7. HOSPITALISTS 1318
Wakley, Thomas. In Sprigge SS. *The Life and Times of Thomas Wakley.* London: Longman Green; 1897, p. 76. MEDICAL JOURNALS 1895
Waldeyer-Hartz, Wilhelm. Paper (1888). [In: *Oxford English Dictionary,* 2nd ed. Volume III. Oxford: Clarendon Press; 1989:188.] CHROMOSOMES 475
Walker AM, Bott PA, Oliver J, McDowell MC. The collection and analysis of fluid from single nephrons of the mammalian kidney. *Am J Physiol.* 1941;134:580-95. KIDNEY 1484
Walker, Mary B. Treatment of myasthenia gravis with physostigmine. *Lancet.* 1934;1(5779):1200-1. MYASTHENIA GRAVIS 2212

The histological lesions produced by the tox-albumen of diphtheria. *Bull Johns Hopkins Hosp.* 1982;3:17-8. DIPHTHERIA 775

Wells, Herbert George. *The Salvaging of Civilization: The Probable Future of Mankind.* New York: Macmillan; 1922:42. INFORMED CONSENT 1445

Wells, William Charles.

On rheumatism of the heart. *Trans Soc Improvement Med Chir Knowledge.* 1810;111:372. [In: Major RH. *Classic Descriptions of Disease,* p. 228 (q.v.).] RHEUMATIC HEART DISEASE 2905

On the presence of the red matter and serum of blood in the urine of dropsy, which has not originated from scarlet fever. *Trans Soc Improvement Med-Chir Knowledge.* 1812;3:194-240. [In: Major RH. *Classic Descriptions of Disease,* pp. 574-5 (q.v.).] PROTEINURIA 2704

Wenger, Nanette K. In Charney P (ed). *Coronary Artery Disease in Women: What All Physicians Need To Know.* Philadelphia: American College of Physicians; 1999, pp. 3-4. CORONARY ARTERY DISEASE 633

Wepfer JJ. *Observationes anatomicae, ex cadaveribus eorum, quos sustulit apoplexia.* Schaffausen: J. C. Suteri; 1658. [In: Major RH. *Classic Descriptions of Disease,* p. 514-5.] SUBARACHNOID HEMORRHAGE 3179

Werlhof, Paul Gottlieb. *Disquisito Medica et Philologica de Variolis et Anthracibus.* Hanover: 1735. [In: Major RH. *Classic Descriptions of Disease,* p. 592 (q.v.).] PURPURA 2796

Wesley, John. *The Iliac Passion,* 1747. [London: Epworth Press; 1960:29-32.] ALCOHOL 112, CAFFEINE 364

West, Randolph. Activity of vitamin B_{12} in Addisonian pernicious anemia. *Science.* 1948;107:398. VITAMIN B_5 (PANTOTHENIC ACID) 3438

Wharton, Edith. Vesalius in Zante (1564). *North American Review.* 1902;175:625-31. DEATH 665

Whipple AO. Determining factors in the safety and success of present-day radical surgery. *Surgery.* 1949;25:169-177. [176]. SURGERY 3240

Whipple, George Hoyt. A hitherto undescribed disease characterized anatomically by deposits of fat and fatty acids in the intestinal and mesenteric lymphatic tissues. *Johns Hopkins Hosp Bull.* 1907;18:382-91. INTESTINAL LIPODYSTROPHY (WHIPPLE DISEASE) 1467

Whistler, Daniel. *Disputatio medica inauguralis, de morbo puerili Anglorum, quem patrio idomate indigenae vocant The Rickets.* Leyden: W. C. Boxii; 1645. [In: Major RH. *Classic Descriptions of Disease,* p. 651 (q.v.).] RICKETS 2914

Whitby, Lionel Ernest Howard. Chemotherapy of pneumococcal and other infections with 2-(p-aminobenzenesulphonamido) pyridine. *Lancet.* 1938;1:1210-2. SULFONAMIDES 3190

White, E.B. Letter of March 11, 1963. In *Letters of E.B. White.* New York: Harper & Row; 1976, p. 497. HOSPITALS 1323

White, Paul Dudley. *Patterns of Incidence of Certain Diseases Throughout the World: Opportunities for Research Through Epidemiology.* Washington, DC: U.S. Government Printing Office; 1959, p. 51. EPIDEMIOLOGY 968

Whitehead, Alfred North.

Dialogues of Alfred North Whitehead. Boston: Little, Brown; 1954:165. DOCTORS 849

J Electrocardiol. 1981;14:66 [Limited data]. SCIENCE 2977

Whytt, Robert.

An Essay on the Vital and Other Involuntary Motions of Animals. Edinburgh: Hamilton, Balfour & Neill; 1751, p. 314. PENIS 2485

An Essay on the Vital and Other Involuntary Motions of Animals. Edinburgh: Hamilton, Balfour & Neill; 1751, pp. 250-1. [In: Wilson KC. The reflex action: a contribution of physiology to neurology. *Pharos.* 1996;59:34-6.] REFLEX ACTION 2841

Wildavsky, A. Doing better and feeling worse: the political pathology of health policy. *Daedalus.* 1997;106:105-23. HEALTH POLICY 1218

Wilde, Oscar.

The Importance of Being Earnest, 1895. EDUCATION 940, HEALTH 1184

The Picture of Dorian Gray, 1891, ch. 19. AGING 75

Wilford, John Noble. Medicine men successful where science falls short. *The New York Times.* 07 Jul 1972, p. 33. MEDICAL ETHICS 1842, NATIVE AMERICAN MEDICINE 2219

Wilks, Samuel.

Abstract of a clinical lecture on pyaemia as a result of endocarditis. *Br Med J.* 1868;1:297. BACTERIAL ENDOCARDITIS 277

Cases of enlargement of the lymphatic glands and spleen (or Hodgkin's disease); with remarks. *Guy's Hosp Rep.* 1865;3:56-67. HODGKIN DISEASE 1303

Historical notes on Bright's disease, Addison's disease, and Hodgkin's disease. *Guy's Hosp Rep.* 1877;22:259-74. CLINICAL OBSERVATION 511, SCIENCE 2962

Williams RJ, Lyman CM, Goodyear GH, et al. Pantothenic acid, a growth determinant of universal biological occurrence. *J Am Chem Soc.* 1933;55:2912-27. VITAMIN B$_{12}$ (CYANOCOBALAMIN) **3441**

Williams, Tennessee. *Suddenly Last Summer,* 1957. AGING **84**

Williams, William Carlos.

Poem. 1963. In *Realities of Medicine: September 9-13, 1985* [Conference pamphlet]. Chicago: The University of Illinois College of Medicine; 1985. AGING **87**

The Autobiography of William Carlos Williams. New York: Random House; 1951, p. 360. PATIENT-PHYSICIAN RELATIONS **2415**

In Rosenthal ML (ed). *The William Carlos Williams Reader.* New York: New Directions; 1966, p. 307. MEDICINE **2117**

Letter to Dr. Coles. In Ballantyne J (ed). *Bedside Manners: An Anthology of Medical Wit and Wisdom.* London: Virgin Books; 1995, pp. 6-7. MEDICAL SCHOOLS **2038**

Willis, Thomas.

Cordials, 1675. In Dewhurst K. *Thomas Willis's Oxford Lectures.* Oxford: Sandford Publications; 1980:56-7. ALCOHOL **110**

Pharmaceutice rationalis, sive diatriba de medicamentorum operationibus in humano corpore. London: 1674. ASTHMA **250**, DIABETES MELLITUS **725**, ESOPHAGEAL TUBE FEEDING **1001**, PLEURISY **2621**

The Anatomy of the Brain and Nerves. London: 1664. NEUROLOGY **2250, 2251**

The Practice of Physick; or, the whole practical part of physick. London: 1684. CIRCLE OF WILLIS **483**, DEPRESSION **713**, MANIC-DEPRESSIVE ILLNESS **1627**, NARCOLEPSY **2215**, RESTLESS LEG SYNDROME **2898**

Treatise on Hysteria and Hypochondria. London: 1670. NERVOUS SYSTEM **2234**

Pain. In: Dewhurst K. *Thomas Willis's Oxford Lectures.* Oxford: Sandford Publications; 1980:68. DIGESTION **765**

Wakefulness. In: Dewhurst K. *Thomas Willis's Oxford Lectures.* Oxford: Sandford Publications; 1980:112-3. CAFFEINE **363**

Willius FA, Keys TE. *Cardiac Clasics.* St. Louis: C.V. Mosby; 1941.

Wills, Lucy. Treatment of "pernicious anaemia of pregnancy" and "tropical anaemia," with special reference to yeast extract as a curative agent. *Br Med J.* 1931;1:1059-64. FOLIC ACID **1063**

Wilms, Max. *Die Mischgeschwulste.* Leipzig: A. Georgi; 1899. [In: Shimkin MB, *Contrary to Nature: Cancer,* p. 147 (q.v.).] NEPHROBLASTOMA (WILMS TUMOR) **2227**

Wilson, Edward O. *On Human Nature.* Cambridge, MA: Harvard University Press; 1978. GENETICS **1109** [14], **1110** [17], SEX **3042** [141]

Wilson KH, Blitchington R, Frothingham R, Wilson JAP. Phylogeny of the Whipple's disease-associated bacterium. *Lancet.* 1991;338(8765):474-5. INTESTINAL LIPODYSTROPHY (WHIPPLE DISEASE) **1468**

Wilson, Logan. *The Academic Man: A Study in the Sociology of a Profession.* London: Oxford University Press; 1942:197. PUBLISHING **2765**

Wilson, Samuel Alexander Kinnier. Progressive lenticular degeneration: a familial nervous disease associated with cirrhosis of the liver. *Brain.* 1912;34:295-509. HEPATOLENTICULAR DEGENERATION (WILSON DISEASE) **1275**

Wilthauer J, Wohlgemut J. Über aspirine (acetylsalicylsäure). *Therapeutische Halbmonatshefte.* 1899;13:276. [In: Krantz JC. *Historical Medical Classics Involving New Drugs.* Baltimore: Williams & Wilkins; 1974:40.] ASPIRIN (ACETYLSALICYLIC ACID) **245**

Wiltshire, John. *Samuel Johnson in the Medical World: The Doctor and the Patient.* Cambridge, England: Cambridge University Press; 1991, p. 6. ILLNESS **1412**

Winnicott, Donald Woods. Psycho-somatic illness in its positive and negative aspects. *Int J Psychoanal.* 1966;47:510-6. HYPOCHONDRIA **1376, 1377**

Winterbottom, Thomas Masterman. *An Account of the Native Africans in the Neighborhood of Sierra Leone,* vol. 2. London: J. Hatchard & J. Mawman; 1803, pp. 29-30 [Major RH. *Classic Descriptions of Disease,* p. 235 (q.v.)]. SLEEPING SICKNESS (TRYPANOSOMIASIS) **3077**

Wintrobe, Maxwell M.

Blood, Pure and Eloquent. New York: McGraw-Hill Book; 1980, p. 720. CLINICAL OBSERVATION **525**

Med J St Joseph Hosp Houston. 1975;10:165. PHYSICAL EXAMINATION **2529**

In Weisse AB. *Conversations in Medicine: The Story of Twentieth-Century American Medicine in the Words of Those Who Created It.* New York: New York University Press; 1984. HEMATOLOGY **1261** [83], **1262** [91]

Wiseman, Richard. *Severall Chirurgical Treatises,* 2nd ed. London: 1686. ANEURYSM **170**

Withering, William. *An Account of the Foxglove and Some of Its Medical Uses, with Practical Remarks on Dropsy and Other Diseases*. London: 1785. [In: Birmingham, AL: Classics of Medicine Library; 1979.] DIGITALIS 768 [2], 769 [184,186], TREATMENT 3338 [xix]

Wolff, Harold G. *Stress and Disease*, 2nd ed. Springfield, IL: Charles C Thomas; 1968, p. viii. RESEARCH 2868

Wolff, Kaspar Friedrich. *Theoria Generationis*. Translated by Meckel JF. Halle; 1812. [In: Talbott JH. A *Biographical History of Medicine*, p. 288 (q.v.).] EMBRYOLOGY 951

Wollaston, William Hyde.
On cystic oxide, a new species of urinary calculus. *Philos Trans R Soc London*. 1810;100:223-30. CYSTINURIA 646
On gouty and urinary concretions. *Philos Trans R Soc London*. 1797;87:386-400. GOUT 1138

Woltman HW, Moersh FP. Progressive fluctuating muscular rigidity and spasm ("stiff-man" syndrome): report of a case and some observations in 13 other cases. *Mayo Clin Proc*. 1956;31:421-7. STIFF-PERSON SYNDROME (STIFF-MAN SYNDROME) 3173

Wood, Paul H.
Diseases of the Heart and Circulation, 3rd ed. Philadelphia: J.B. Lippincott; 1968, p. 1. MEDICAL HISTORIES 1880
An appreciation of mitral stenosis. *Br Med J*. 1954;1:1113-24. PULMONARY CIRCULATION 2784

World Health Organization.
Chronicle of the World Health Organization. 1947;1:13. HEALTH 1192
Effects of Nuclear War on Health and Health Services, 2nd ed. Geneva: World Health Organization; 1987. NUCLEAR WAR 2265

World Medical Association.
Declaration of Geneva. *World Medical Association Bulletin*. 1949;1:15. MEDICAL ETHICS 1834
Declaration of Helsinki: recommendations guiding physicians in biomedical research involving human subjects. *JAMA*. 1997;277:925-6. MEDICAL ETHICS 1837

Wright, Frank Lloyd. Frank Lloyd Wright talks of his art. *New York Times Magazine*. October 4, 1953. pp. 26-7,47. PHYSICIANS 2584

Wright, Lois (Lucy Waite).
Doctor Helen Rand. Chicago: Physician's Publishing; 1891:43. [In: Beatty WK. Lucy Waite: surgeon and free thinker. *Proc Inst Med Chicago*. 1992;45:52-8.] WOMEN IN MEDICINE 3476
Modern gynecology. *Am J Surg Gynecol*. 1901;14:169-70. SURGEONS 3203
Removal of the uterus in bilateral diseases of the appendages; report of cases. *Chicago Med Rec*. 1896;10:383-9. SURGERY 3227
The surgical situation. *Med Rec*. 1908;74:834-6. [835]. SURGERY 3228

Wylie, Norma. *Sharing the Final Journey: Walking with the Dying*. Hantsport, Nova Scotia: Lancelot Press; 1996 [Limited data]. ALZHEIMER'S DISEASE 133

Wyman HC. *Abdominal Surgery*, preface. Detroit: G.S. Davis; 1888. [In: Rutkow IM, *The History of Surgery in the United States*, p. 101.] RESEARCH 2859

Wynder EL, Graham EA. Tobacco smoking as a possible etiologic factor in bronchiogenic carcinoma: a study of six hundred and eighty-four proved cases. *JAMA*. 1950;143:329-36. SMOKING 3095

Wynder, Ernst L. In Shenker I. Doctors ponder way to shatter fatal illusions of immortality. *The New York Times*. 30 Sep 1975, p. 39. PREVENTIVE MEDICINE 2682

Yahr, Melvin D. Early recognition of Parkinson's disease. *Hosp Pract*. 1981;16:65-80. TREMOR 3358

Yalow, Rosalyn S. In Altman LK. *Who Goes First? The Study of Self-Experimentation in Medicine*. New York: Random House; 1987, p. 314. INFORMED CONSENT 1448

Yeo R. The grateful patient. *Gentlemen's Magazine*. 1732, vol. 2, p. 769. [In: Talbott JH. A *Biographical History of Medicine*, p. 200.] SURGERY 3216

Young, Edward. *Night Thoughts. Night I*, 1742. DEATH 659

Young, Hugh Hampton. The early diagnosis and radical cure of carcinoma of the prostate: being a study of 40 cases and presentation of a radical operation which was carried out in four cases. *Bull Johns Hopkins Hosp*. 1905;16:315-21. CANCER OF THE PROSTATE GLAND 409

Yourcenar, Marguerite. *Memoirs of Hadrian*. New York: Pocket Books; 1977:2. PATIENTS 2465

Zancariis, Albert de. In McVaugh MR. Bedside manners in the Middle Ages. *Bull Hist Med*. 1997;71:201-23. PATIENT-PHYSICIAN RELATIONS 2372

Ziegler, Ernst. *A Text-Book of Special Pathological Anatomy,* ch. XV. Translated by MacAllister D, Cattell HW. New York: Macmillan; 1897. pp. 143-5. OSTEOPOROSIS **2301**

Zimmer, George. Learning from our patients: one participant's impact on clinical trial research and informed consent. *Ann Intern Med.* 1997;126:892-7. CANCER **387**

Zimmer, Paul. *What Zimmer Would Be.* In *Family Reunion: Selected and New Poems.* Pittsburgh: University of Pittsburgh Press; 1983, p. 13. MEDICINE **2132**

Zinoffsky, Oscar. Über die Grösse des Hämoglobinmolecüls. *Zeitschrift für physiologische Chemie.* 1885;10:16-34. [Translated in Tanford C, Reynolds J. *Nature's Robots: A History of Proteins.* Oxford: Oxford University Press; 2001:2.] HEMOGLOBIN **1265**

Zinsser, Hans. *Rats, Lice, and History.* Boston: Little, Brown; 1963, pp. 13-4. INFECTIOUS DISEASE **1435, 1436**

Zoll, Paul Maurice. Resuscitation of the heart in ventricular standstill by external electric stimulation. *N Eng J Med.* 1952;247:768-71. PACEMAKERS **2311**

Zoller MJ, Smith M. Oligonucleotide-directed mutagenesis using M13-derived vectors: an efficient and general procedure for the production of point mutations in any fragment of DNA. *Nucleic Acids Research.* 1982;10(20):6487-500. DEOXYRIBONUCLEIC ACID (DNA) **710**

Zollinger RM, Ellison EH. Primary peptic ulcerations of the jejunum associated with islet cell tumors of the pancreas. *Ann Surg.* 1955;142:709-28. ZOLLINGER-ELLISON SYNDROME **3522**

Subject Index

In this contextual index of key words, cross-references direct readers to related entries in the index itself and to corresponding topic headings (SMALL CAPS) in the text. The numbers given are the quotation numbers.

A

Abdomen
  left side of a. greatly increased in size, 1533
  obstruction in a., 3323
  sprue attacks a., 3124
  tumidity of a. in ascites, 241
  very tumid and painful, 220
Abdominal
  general a. pain in appendicitis, 225
  inflammation of a. region, 2505
  sudden, severe a. pain, 224
Ablation
  of thyroid produces profound trouble, 1393
Abortifacient
  do not administer a., 1817
Abortion
  as paradox of medicine, 15
  authority of practitioner employed, 8
  do not kill by a., 5
  I will not give remedy, 4
  midwives have the power, 3
  rejoice, unfortunate husband, 6
Abscess
  deep-seated a., 223
  evacuate a. by expectoration, 958
  fecal a., 223
  in appendix, 219
  inflammation changes into a., 733
  sign of cancer is hot a., 392
Absence
  conspicuous by a., 3449
Absence of disease
  health more than a., 1200
  health not merely a., 1192
Absorb
  easier to buy books than a. them, 2835
Absorption

when a. is suspended, 471
Abstinence
  obstinate a., 2280
Abstract meaning
  do not search for a., 1574
Abstraction
  disease is a., 2467
Absurdity
  medical service is murderous a., 3230
Abuse
  children need care with a., 2918
  of psychiatrist, 2746
  of sexual functions, 3031
  sick employ physicians and a. them, 2376
  use of tobacco is a., 3311
Acanthosis
  red blood cells showed a., 2
Accepted
  children who are never quite a., 461
Access
  standards for medical school a., 1766
Accomplice
  apothecary is physician's a., 218
Accoucheur
  saves a. considerable time, 992
Accoucheurs
  specialty of a. to grave, 1006
Accuracy
  high standards of a., 1742
Accurate
  unambiguous and a. wording, 3499
Accusation
  of malpractice, 1613
Acetylcholine
  substance of extraordinary physiologic activity, 22
Acetylsalicylic acid
  hypersensitivity to, 247

life-threatening reactions to a., 248
Aches
  rheumatism is common name for a. and pains, 2908
Achievement
  problems in medical care not lack of a., 1682
  technical a. must not become out God, 1680
Acid
  acid treatment on tubercle bacilli, 3388
  free a. is essential in digestive action, 766
  gouty material is lithic a., 1138
  hexuronic a., 3443
  pantothenic a., 3438
  ulcer patients "milked" for a., 2491
Acid phosphatase
  prostate cancer with elevation of a., 410
Acidosis
  death is a., 668
Acoustics
  well-known fact in a., 3168
Acquired responses
  endless variety of a., 963
Act of god
  disease is a., 782
ACTH
  rheumatoid arthritis improved by a., 2912
Action
  reflex a., 2841, 2842
  surgeon is man of a., 3206
Action potential
  axons and a., 2253
Activism
  medicine not haven for a., 2017
Activity
  any a. can cause stress, 3177
Adaptable
  surgeon should be a., 3197

Adaptation
  to environment largely
    vanished, 1109
Adapted
  individual a. to environment,
    1191
Addicted
  reforming men who are a., 122
  to word "significant, 3510
Addiction
  to soft lead pencil, 3504
Adhesion
  in pericarditis, 2502
Adhesions
  of pericardium to body of
    heart, 2499
Admissions policies
  are root of trouble, 1791
  produce specialists and
    bioscientists, 1789
Admissions policy
  jettison a., 1792
  public consensus about, 1797
Adolescent
  sexual instinct in a., 3034
Adolescents
  cancer like gang of a., 386
Adrenal cortical hormone
  rheumatoid arthritis improved
    by a., 2912
Adrenal tumor
  removal of the a., 125
Adrenal tumors
  a. with polyglandular
    syndrome, 645
Adrenalectomized
  dogs, 47
Adrenergic receptors
  two distinct types of a., 44
Adultery
  infidelity is only link to
    husband, 49
  passion of a., 1817
Advance
  great a. of science, 2969
Adventures
  infectious disease as a., 1435
Adventurous
  aging man to become a., 92
Advertisement
  patent medicine a., 1372
Advertises
  any physician who a. cure is
    quack, 2805
Advice
  for medical student, 1746
  nearly always futile, 2417
  no right to intrude a., 2005
  sought to confirm, 589
Advocate
  decisions not made by patient
    a., 2895
  physician as patient's
    advocate, 1625
Affirmative

human understanding more
    excited by a. than negative,
    2851
Affront
  never resent a. by sick man,
    2378
African
  sarcoma of the jaws of A. chil-
    dren, 360
Africans
  afraid of sleeping sickness,
    3077
Age
  see also Old, Old age; AGING
  annual sigmoidoscopy after a.
    40, 3067
  discoveries made by a., not
    individual, 2962
  disease of persons of middle
    or advanced a., 494
  everyone is older than he
    thinks, 2665
  lends graces, 830
  may enter medicine at any a.,
    2004
  of retirement for surgeon,
    3232
  phthisis occurs between a.
    18-35, 3368
  surgeon should be of youthful
    a., 3192
  when cancer of breast occurs
    under age 40, 394
  wisdom and a., 3462
Aged
  prone to obesity, 2284
Aging
  all would live long, 66
  body first surrenders to old
    age, 58
  forsaking worship of goddess
    Longevity, 86
  indistinguishable from
    vegetation, 95
  long old age full of continual
    evils, 55
  must outlive thy youth, 61
  old men suffer difficulty
    breathing, 49
  penalized for crime, 93
  the best thing age can do, 71
  watching power vanish, 102
Agony
  of whole corpus, 678
Agree
  find another who will not a.,
    813
Air
  see also Respiration;
    RESPIRATION
  as great physician, 3351
  body composed of earth, fire,
    water, a., 779
  desiring to draw in all the a.
    possible, 249
  lung partially deprived of a.,
    2522

made of four elements, 1508
  rich in oxygen, 1588
Air cells
  enlarged in emphysema, 2786
Akuyreyri disease
  attack of a., 476
Albumin
  detected a. except with con-
    vulsions, 937
Albuminous urine
  dropsy connected with a.,
    1490
Albuminuria
  nephrotic edema and a., 1491
Alias
  articles written under a., 1905
Alimentary canal
  Curling ulcer of, 644
Allergic
  toxic and a. effects, 965
Allergy
  changed capacity for reaction,
    126
  common form of drug a., 247
Allopathy
  midway between a. and
    Christian Science, 127
Alone
  feel a. when suffering, 3181
  more a. than ever been, 1323
Alveolar air
  oxygen pressure and a., 1589
Amative propensities
  inquired about state of a.,
    1535
Amaurotic familial idiocy
  (Tay-Sachs disease)
  agenetic condition, 134
Ambulance
  flying a., 2179
American
  first A. herbal, 1277
  surgeon should be better
    qualified than European,
    3220
  will get drunk, shoot you, 643
Amino acids
  proteins arise by condensation
    of a., 141
Amputation
  bilateral a. of thigh, 3458
  in Buerger's disease, 3297
  of entire breast, 391
Amyl nitrate
  similarity existing between its
    general action and that of a.,
    184
  would probably produce the
    same effect, 183
Anachronism
  clinician as a., 1783
Analysis
  fairly accurate gas a., 307
  statistical a., 3157
Analytic
  science of medicine is a., 1950
Analyzed trial

aim of a. of medicine is
health, 2079
and science of medicine, 1942
application of a. of medicine,
1932
as great physician, 3351
consists of disease, patient,
and physician, 1914
delicate a. of handling ideas,
1450
doctoring is a. of curing
illness, 1939
enthusiasm for healing a.,
1742
familiar with a. and science of
past, 1293
glory of healing a., 2081
healing a.taught only in
hospitals, 1743
investigations into a. of
healing, 2088
is intuitive, 1950
is myself, 2953
life is short, a. long, 1915
limits of a., 3340
medicine as a., 3467
mysterious is source of all a.,
2978
nature doesn't always need
assistance of a., 3334
nearly abandoned a. of curing,
2134
oath to teach a. of medicine,
1812
of curing disease, 2098
of detachment, 1992
of domestic medicine, 2676
of engraving, 1894
of intimacy, 2445
of listening to patients, 2390
of observation, 518
of practice of medicine, 1940
of probability, 2123
old a. replaced by new science,
2107
power of a., 1981
practice of medicine is a.,
1936
progress of a. and science of
medicine, 274
psychoanalysis is to therapy as
expressionism is to a., 2734
surgery should be merciful a.,
3239
surgery should be work of a.,
3205
ten words comprising a., 3335
the writer's a., 3498
whole a. of medicine, 3326
Art of medicine, 1740
cannot be inherited, 2084
is valuable, 2077
not invented, 2073
to devise practical measures,
1953
to follow nature, 3337
Arterial blood

from sheep, 316
Arterial oxygen pressure
raising a., 1588
Arterial pressure, see also
HYPERTENSION
rise of mean a., 1348
to determine normal a., 312
Arterial tension
diminution occasioned in a.,
183
Arteries
arise from a. deep in muscles,
170
bounding up under skin,
635
cancer involved with a., 375
cephalic a., 483
lose power to propel blood,
232
pulsate and react forcefully,
212
similar to natural lining
membrane of a., 171
temporal a. inflamed, 3273
Arterioles
trouble localized to a., 2825
Artery
contraction of orifice of pulmonary a., 575
full of spiritous blood, 169
occlusive disease of coronary
a., 1256
periarteritis nodosa affliction
of a., 2497
pulmonary a., 2780
right middle cerebral a., 451
surgery on femoral a., 3422
Arthritis
of Lyme disease, 1595
rheumatoid a., 2562-2564
Articles
similarity of journal a., 1905
Artificial
heart, 1254
pneumothorax, 3387
respiration, 2637
Artist
doctor is a., 857
how much a. in doctors, 851
Arts
influence of medical school
on liberal a., 1791
love of the a., 1650
medicine most noble of a.,
2075
sciences that belong to healing a., 2043
Ascending aorta
and arteries arising from it,
210
Aspirin (acetylsalicylic acid)
a remedy for ague, 243
a. appears more satisfactory,
244
a. is now being tested for
usefulness, 244

effects of a. on platelet
stickiness, 246
Assertiveness
male adolescent's
instrumental a., 40
Assessment
clinical a. must be numerical,
548
Assimilated
event a. into substance of
being, 1031
Assimilative teacher
of wide learning, 1771
Assistant
physician as a., 2552
Asthma
as disease of heart, 1244
orthopnea is also called a.,
2296
Astray
some physicians went a. in
medicine, 2598
Asylums
public a. for maniacs, 2156
Atherosclerosis, see also
ARTERIOSCLEROSIS
degree of a. in coronary
arteries, 629
the name a. is not sufficient,
246
Athlete
pulmonary edema in a., 1285
Athletics
a. for health, 1021
Atmosphere
septic property of the a., 198
Atmospheric particles
the vitality of the a., 197
Atoms
limited number of chemical
a., 2196
Atrophied
a. body, 1022
Atrophy
do not let intellectual life a.,
1555
extreme a. of both kidneys,
1505
Attack
came one morning, 611
disease, not symptom, 3347
of fibrillation of auricles, 949
of malaria, 1604
of migraine, 2167
of paroxysmal tachycardia,
2077-2080
of periarteritis nodosa, 2497
symptoms of migraine a.,
2174
typical of occlusion of
coronary arteries, 628
Attacks
of purpura, 2797
paroxysmal a. of pain, 622
sprue a. abdomen, 3124
Attention
power of a., 1947

Competence
  boundaries of c., 2070
  compassion and c., 1800
Competency
  a modest c., 726
Competent
  motivation for remaining c.,
    2454
  no man c. unless practiced on
    self, 1751
Competition
  grant application for c., 1151
Complaints
  chronic somatic c., 482
  dust and soot of your c., 989
  hypochondriac c., 1369
  of old people, 1113
Complications
  excessive bedrest causes c.,
    2785
Compliment
  to be observer is greatest c.,
    512
Compound
  crystalline c., 3439
Compound E
  was laboratory jargon, 636
Compression, 918
  force blood out by c., 999
  of trachea by tumor, 173
Compromise
  practice of medicine as c.,
    1922
Compromising
  care to cost control, 1728
Compulsive behavior
  medical education requires c.,
    1803
Concentration
  accompanied by depression,
    1370
  is price for success, 3484
Concept
  of care, 1683
Conception
  best time for fruitful
    intercourse, 571
  is prevented, 599
  to overcome obstacles
    preventing c., 1439
Concretion
  gouty c., 1138
Conduct
  judging professional c., 1840
Confessor
  physician as c., 2572
Confidence
  in doctor, 2393
  increase c. in making decision,
    691
  science proceeds on basis of
    c., 2995
Confidentiality
  will not divulge what see or
    hear, 1812
Conflict
  anorexia is situated in c., 193

Conformity
  dull c. is crime against
    intelligence, 2517
  peer review rewards c., 2474
Confusion
  increases, 1509
Congenital defect, *see also*
    CONGENITAL HEART DIS-
    EASE
  hemolytic anemia dependent
    on c., 606
  incompatible with long life,
    574
Congestion
  of portal system, 2257
Congestive heart failure
  swelling of the
    hypochondrium, 577
Conjecture
  skillful c., 268
Conjugal act
  designed for begetting
    children, 603
Conjunctiva
  gonorrheal matter in c., 1122
Conjunctivitis
  in Reiter syndrome, 2845
Connective tissue
  disproportionate c. reaction,
    642
Consanguinous marriage
  offspring of a c., 20
Conscience
  at expense of c., 744
Conscientious
  mighty c. doctor, 838
Consciousness
  turns the face of c. away, 99
Consequences
  of success of medicine, 1695
Consolation
  ministry of c., 1997
Conspiracy
  medicalization of life not a c.,
    2070
  profession as c. against laity,
    2000
  to exploit suffering, 2001
  to hide shortcomings, 1613
Constitution
  in causation of disease, 780
  quarrel with c. for being sick,
    656
Consultation
  husband appears dead, 587
  practice of medicine derives
    from c., 1948
Consumption, *see* Tuberculosis;
    TUBERCULOSIS
Contact
  doctor of first c., 1678
  most important c., 1821
Contagion
  of syphilis, 3253, 3255, 3258
  of venereal disease, 3054
Contagions
  differences of c., 1432

Contagious
  plague is c. disease, 356
  puerperal fever is c., 2779
  typhoid fever is c., 3408
Contagiousness
  of bubonic plague, 355
Contamination
  of air, earth, rivers and sea,
    2639
Contemplation
  insomnia a form of c., 1455
Contraception
  c. is a sin, 602
  soft sponge is introduced, 600
Contract
  breach of c., 1821
  medical c. with patient, 2431
Contraction
  each c. appeared lengthened,
    208
  of orifice of pulmonary artery,
    575
Contradiction
  do not suffer gladly c., 2162
Contribution
  manuscript considered c.,
    2767
  of women to medicine, 3474
Control
  complete educational c., 1763
  over how I will die, 685
  taken for antibody treatment
    or c., 542
Control group
  serves to determine natural
    course of malady, 544
Control trial, *see also* CLINICAL
    TRIALS
  in c. attempt to systematize
    impressions, 544
Contusion
  skull fracture with c., 3070
Convention
  national psychiatric c., 2712
Conviction
  disease mistaken for religious
    c., 1424
Convince
  do experiment to c. yourself,
    2869
  you must c. me first, 690
Convulsion, *see also* Epilepsy,
    Fit; EPILEPSY
  epilepsy is c. of all parts of
    body, 972
  epileptic c. preceded paralysis,
    1516
Convulsions
  seize other side of body, 2232
Copper
  in hepatolenticular
    degeneration, 1276
Copulation
  gives delight in c., 561
Coronary artery
  occlusive disease of c., 1256

high level of d., 1960

Deduction
makes explicit information already there, 2994

Deductive
scientific method not d., 2980

Defecation
management of d. not aseptic, 1346

Defect
chief d. of education, 1779
developmental d. of heart, 574
intellectual d., 639

Defects
moral or physical d., 1820

Defense mechanism
how quickly the d. goes to work, 452

Deference
too great a d. to shame of patient, 2523

Deferral of death
as privilege of status, 1703

Deficiency
dietary d. causes pellagra, 2478, 2479

Definable illnesses
suffering from scientifically d., 482

Defining
difficulty in d. disease, 793

Definition
biological and social d., 791

Deformed
persons, 695
unfinished, 694

Deformity
limb presents considerable d., 565

Degeneration
apish d., 1335

Delirium
auricle passes into fibrillation or d., 262

Delivery
crisis in d. of care, 1682
of care is to do as much nothing as possible, 1688
of what we know, 1958
psychosis after d. of infant, 2653

Delusion
drugs are a d., 3349
succumbed to messianic d., 2005

Demand
increasing d. for medical care, 2055

Dementia
generalized d. progressed, 132
poverty, loneliness, incontinence, dependence, and d., 97

Dental
decay, 1060

Denture

remove d. before giving resuscitation, 2902

Deoxyribonucleic acid (DNA)
a chemical entity, 703
biologically active fraction, 705
desoxypentose nucleic acids, 706
full equipment of virulence, 704
genetic and non-genetics parts, 707
inhibition by DNAase, 709
mutations in DNA fragments, 710

Dependence
conflict over d. and autonomy, 193
poverty, loneliness, incontinence, d., and dementia, 97

Dependency
yearning to be guided, 711

Deportment
of hospital physicians, 2383

Depression
anxiety and d., 2724
healing d. with kindly word, 2748
hypochondria accompanied by d., 1370
of one's own spirits, 1373
that no one talks about, 605
universal Melancholy, 713

Derangement
mania is chronic d. of mind, 2735

Dermatitis
patch test for d., 2349

Desire
distinguishes ethics from science, 1833
for family, 1041
mistaken for love, 1586

Desoxycorticosterone acetate
crystalline d., 47

Destiny
future d. of human race, 2649
of physician, 2582

Detachment
art of d., 1992
first teach science, then d., 1798
much lauded, 990

Detail
attend to every d., 1736
enmeshed in exceptional d., 1969

Details
recital of endless d., 570

Detention
randomized caning and d., 550

Deterioration
intellectual d., 98

Development

professional d. and politics, 2124

Devil
created doctor, 717

Devils
hundred d. leap into my body, 116

Devotion
institution judged on d. of teachers, 2037

Diabetes
previous history of d., 1491
severe juvenile d. with ketosis, 1458
xanthoma with d., 3514

Diabetes insipidus
subdivision of diabetes, 723

Diabolical
physician shows three faces, including d., 2372

Diagnose
psychiatrists don't d. patients like other doctors, 2722

Diagnosis
announce d. like unfurling banner, 2374
don't expect d. on first visit, 2410
gastroscopy in d., 1088
great physician understands d., 1926
is giving name to disease, 2258
judgment lies at heart of d., 1706
of duodenal ulcer, 2490
of malignant disease of uterus, 417
plurality must not be posited without necessity, 735
quick d., 2392
temptation of machine-made d., 3276
what happens after d., 1957
will result of test change d., 3277

Diagnostician
physician as d., 1957

Dialogue
between literature and medicine, 1557

Dialysing-apparatus
artificial kidney is d., 1487

Dialysis
selection of patients for d., 1844
vivo d., 1488

Diamond
show glass from d., 454

Diarrheal discharge
in typhoid fever, 3408

Diastolic
pressure, 314

Didactic teaching
as hopelessly antiquated, 1768
clinical teaching as, 1772

Die, see also Death

Electrocardiogram
  changed on fourth day, 628
  with lesion there is definite e.,
    627
Electronic equipment
  impact on care, 634
Elements
  air made of four e., 1508
Elite group
  AIDS made us an e., 31
Elusive
  disease is e. entity, 800
Emaciated
  to the last degree, 190
Emancipation
  of medicine, 2105
Embarrassment
  medical history as e., 1298
Embolism
  mitral stenosis causes e., 2194
Embryo
  molded into a human form,
    950
Emergencies
  meet e. day after day, 1930
Emergency care
  steps to ensure e., 1327
Emetine
  was available only sporadically,
    3457
Emotion
  any e. can cause stress, 3177
  empathy is magical e., 955
  romantic e., 3036
Emotional
  disturbance in convalescence,
    296
  driven by e. hunger, 2712
  needs can affect course of
    disease, 2446
  support not easily quantified,
    1704
Emotional disorders
  the English malady, 952
Emotions
  evanescent and unconnected
    e., 697
  should be attended to, 2384
  surgeon must be anesthetized
    against e., 3208
Empathy
  listening and e., 1806
Emperor
  patient as e., 2465
Employee
  physician as e., 1710
Empyema
  pus in chest forms e., 3372
Encouragement
  of patient, 2386
Encyclopedic
  rather be humane than e.,
    2433
Endocarditis
  attacks of e., 202
Endocrine function
  in homosexual patient, 1312

Enema
  may take two days, 1329
Enemies
  diseases as e., 789
  have mankind for e., 871
  ignorance and disease as e.,
    787
Enemy
  cancer as e., 387
Energy
  reduced in depression, 719
Engineers
  suffer from lack of verbalism,
    3506
English
  tuberculosis is E. disease,
    3374
Englishmen
  doctors are just like other E.,
    839
Engraving
  art of e., 1894
Enrollment
  of women in medical school,
    3479
Enterprise
  science is great e., 2993
Enthusiasm
  as motive force of progress,
    2022
  of teachers, 2037
Environment
  alien e. of hospital, 2468
  changes in e., 2861
  individual adapted to e., 1191
  man is product of e., 961
  must understand e., 2463
  pollution of e., 2639, 2640
  seek fresh e., 1569
  that supports life, 1543
  true interior e., 2175
Environmental
  counter new e. threats, 961
  unpleasant effects of e. forces,
    37
Enzymes
  reactions are catalyzed by e.,
    966
Epidemic
  influenza e., 1442
  not all die during e., 780
  worst e. since Middle Ages,
    1444
Epigenesis
  theory of e., 951
Epilepsy, see also Convulsion,
    Convulsions, Fits
  body falls to the ground, 973
  slow pulse in e., 1235
  victims of e. may die, 1515
Epileptic convulsion
  preceded paralysis, 1516
Epileptic fits
  seized with e. and died, 1518
Epileptics
  turns e. into Ethiopians, 230
Epinephrine (adrenaline)

a small quantity suffices, 982
  blood-pressure raising
    principle, 984
  raises and supports blood-
    pressure, 983
Epistaxis
  hereditary hemorrhagic
    telangiectasia with e., 1278
Epstein-Barr virus syndrome
  chronic fatigue syndrome and
    E., 477
Equal
  man not born e., 1337
Equality
  of men and women, 3470
Equanimity
  as ideal, 1997
Equilibrium
  between tubercle bacillus and
    man, 3404
Equities
  many e. maximized in
    hospital, 1719
Equity
  system in which there is no e.,
    1730
Erection
  cannot will e. of penis, 2485
  of priapism, 2687
Erosion
  of mucosa in peptic ulcer,
    2487
Error, see also Mean
  chemical e., 1101
  made by young people, 1970
Eruption
  of tubercles on arms, 3514
  spontaneous e. of cancer, 389
  vesicular-papular e., 2917
Eruptions
  are reddish, 459
Erythema
  of lupus erythematosus, 1592
  painful nodular e., 278
Erythrocytic anomaly
  is not due to abnormal
    hemoglobin, 21
  with unusual type of
    "crenation", 20
Essence
  intimacy is e. relationship,
    2445
Estrogen
  for osteoporosis, 2302, 2305
  for prostate cancer, 410
Ether
  I tried the e. inhalation today,
    160
  was given to Mr. Venable, 164
Etherization
  in a state of e, 162
Ethical
  dilemmas, 693
  major e. principle, 554
  paralysis, 2065
  to do randomized clinical
    trial, 555

Ethics
  principles of medical e., 12
  tends to depreciate caring, 2051
Ethiopian
  black as an E., 48
Ethiopians
  turns epileptics into E., 230
Etiquette
  professional e., 519
Eunuchoidism
  patient with e. has impotence, 1380
Eunuchs
  gout in e., 1129
Evacuation
  disease relieved by natural e., 3341
  of wounded from battlefield, 2179
Evaluation
  peer review e., 2195-2197
Everyday life
  disregard knowledge from e., 692
Evidence
  we have arrived at e., 2857
Evil
  king's e., 3393
  remedies often worsen e., 3332
Evolution
  in e. species developed specialization, 1338
Exaggeration
  of doctor, 1610
Examination
  abolition of e., 1755
  case records of e., 433
  post-mortem e., 2357
  rectal e., 588
  vaginal e. failed completely, 3418
Examine
  pester doctors to e. them, 1376
Examined
  hypochondriacs fail to get e., 1377
Excellence
  definition of e., 1969
Excess
  all e. is ill, 111
Excitement
  manic e. from hashish, 1631
  nervous e., 1628
Excluded
  who is e. in science, 3000
Excrement
  is best soft and consistent, 331
Excretion
  urinary e. performed with ease, 3415
Excuse
  disease e. for vice, 2894
  for unnecessary tests, 3280

"I'd want it done" e., 1689
Exercise
  aim of e., 1053
  better to hunt in fields, 1018
  heart disease shows up during e., 1240
Exertion
  diseases caused by e., 3327
  persisting in e., 180
Exhaustion
  neurasthenia as nervous e., 2245
Existence
  destroy reason for e., 2002
Exotic
  psychiatry made to seem e., 2719
Expectations
  medical advances create rising e., 1679
  scientific medicine raises e., 1695
Expense
  government interference causes great e., 1667
Experience
  a benign e., 101
  does not come to all, 1525
  fallacious, 1915
  happenings that compose his life's e., 94
  illness transformed into e. of others, 1782
  "in my e." is phrase of prejudice or bias, 505
  intuition is inference from e., 1947
  is sole guide, 506
  may not be of equivalent e., 516
  medical practice learned only by e., 1940
  misled even by e., 2020
  physician hides behind e., 2592
  validated by science, 3000
  value of e., 514
Experienced clinician
  student should see e., 1785
Experiment, see also Medical science, Science; MEDICAL SCIENCE, SCIENCE
  comparative e., 539
  devising an e., 2856
  don't just think, try e., 2943
  essence of e. is comparison, 3160
  in pernicious anemia, 2509
  investigation and e., 2867
  is artificial, impatient, 2946
  more from observation than e., 2104
  put question to test of e., 526
  surgery is e. in bacteriology, 3238
  truth of discovery based on e., 2951

why not e., 2024
Experimental approach
  to questions of effectiveness, 556
Experimental medicine
  first requirement in e., 2026
Experimental method
  revolution e. effected, 2959
Experimentation
  medicine as e., 2127
Experimenting
  on myself, 441
Experiments
  disease creates e., 2603
  limits on e., 1827
  nature conducts gigantic e., 968
  never unsuccessful e., 2958
  on kidneys of frogs, 1482
  on lung-ventilation, 2891
  patients not subjects of e., 1826
  populations of e., 3149
Expert
  get one or two e. men, 586
  status of e. testimony, 2066
  surgeon should be e., 3197
Expertise
  must have clinical e., 1860
Experts
  never trust e., 825
Exploit
  conspiracy to e. suffering, 2001
Exploitation
  of injury, 1558
Explosion
  nuclear e., 2265
Expressionism
  psychoanalysis and e., 2734
Extract
  from pancreatic ducts, 1457
  of pancreas, 1458
  thyroid e., 1396
Extreme
  diseases, 3328
Extremities, see also Arm, Leg, Limb
  became blue, 2643
  coldness of e., 2691
  debility of lower e., 2628
  gangrene of four e., 2824
  in heart failure, 1241
  scleroderma affecting e., 3011
  very much too short, 23
Eye, see also OPHTHALMOSCOPY
  headache over e., 2167
  in Horner's syndrome, 1314
  tumor over e., 1863
  will remain awake, 3073
  wounds on left e. are incurable, 2802
Eyeball
  motion of the e., 293
Eyeballs
  apparently enlarged, 1361

blackwater f., 1607
can't find f., 1054
in pertussis, 2510
mild f. cease by fourth day,
    2693
no f. with purpura, 2794
of pneumonia, 2623
of Reiter syndrome, 2845
only cause of childbed f., 1428
puerperal f., 1429
relapsing f., 2846
rheumatic f., 2904
rheumatic f. in mitral
    stenosis, 2194
scarlet f., 2931
sign of burning f., 733
took to bed with acute f., 456
treatment of f., 3350
typhoid f., 2988-2992
undulant f., 352
with empyema, 957
with poliomyelitis, 2628, 2629
yellow f., 3092-3098
Fevers
    delirium in f., 696
    of malaria, 1600
    purple f., 1270
Fiber optics
    principle of f., 1089
Fibers
    common-sense nerve f., 3462
Fibrillate
    heart f., 428
Fibrillation
    of auricles, 949
Fibrin
    reached into coronary artery,
        618
Fibrinous
    structure apt to become
        hardened, 202
Field
    dry f. is essential in surgery,
        3236
Filament
    quartz f. in galvonometer, 946
Filtration rate
    glomerular f., 1499
Filtration theory
    in favor of f., 1496
Finger
    fails to recognize small pulse
        beat, 1035
    one f. in throat, 665
    touch f. with eyes shut, 287
Fingernail
    capillary pulse on f., 213
Fingers
    as musician f. strings of
        instrument, 3203
    become ex-sanguine, 2825
    Heberden nodes on f., 1259
    if tips of f. are falling off, 1076
    in Dupuytren's contracture,
        900
    in Trousseau sign, 3362
    keep f. at pulse, 1015

replace brains, 3237
Fire
    body composed earth, f.,
        water, air, 779
    life is like f., 3010
Fistula
    dog possesses gastric f., 767
Fit
    during sleep, 980
    first f. of asthma, 251
    of angina pectoris, 182
    preventive medicine tells ill
        person he is f., 2679
Fits, *see also* Epilepsy; EPILEPSY
    beginning in left foot, 978
    make patient fall down, 976
    of asthma, 250
    puerperal f., 937
    seized with epileptic f., 1518
Fixity
    of purpose, 2868
Flea bites
    purpura like f., 2794, 2795
    spots like f., 3405, 3406
Fleas
    on plague rat, 2613
Flesh
    melting of f. into urine, 724
    wasting away of f., 724
Flexibility
    of method, 2868
Fluid
    detecting f. in chest, 2520
    diet, 760
    from bends of loops of Henle,
        1501
    highly fetid f. in appendicitis,
        220
    in ascites, 241
    infusion of f., 361
    menstrual f., 2848
Fluid-electrolyte disorders
    blood in patients with cholera,
        1056
Fluid pressure
    in Queckenstedt test, 2812
Flux
    substances in animals in f.,
        2159
Focal glomerulonephritis
    (Berger-Hinglais disease)
    diffuse intercapillary deposits,
        1061
Follow-up
    long enough f., 1648
Food, *see also* Diet; NUTRITION
    as treatment for scurvy, 3014,
        3016, 3017
    for sick and healthy, 2278
    gout influenced by f., 1149
    medicine unnecessary if men
        ate proper food, 2073
    mixing subnitrate of bismuth
        with f., 1081
    particularly appetizing f., 765
    relationship of ulcer to, 2488

special f. for pernicious
    anemia, 2508
vitamins in, 3014-3029
Food industry
    as surrogate physician, 1202
Foods
    wholesome f., 763
Fool
    make f. of self, 1899
    physician who treats self is f.,
        2578
Fool's paradise
    cast out of f., 953
Foolishness
    becomes wisdom, 2021
Fools
    characteristic of f., 1386
    some suffer f. gladly, 2710
Foot
    pain in f., 998
Forbidding
    subject of marital sexuality is
        f., 3041
Forces
    cosmic f., 671
    cultural f., 1106
    environmental f., 37
    market f., 1220
Forehead
    is without motion, 294
Foreskin
    of penis, 2484
Foretell
    function of consultant is to
        f., 1776
Forever
    do not try to live f., 1582
    heart does not stop f., 1226
Forgetfulness
    complete f., 697
Forms
    endless f. most beautiful and
        wonderful, 1539
    fill out a few f., 1694
Fortune
    physician as plaything of f.,
        2562
Fortune tellers
    treat those professing cure as
        f., 845
Foundation
    medicine's moral f., 1701
Foxglove
    active herb no other than f.,
        768
    given in large doses, 769
Fracture
    Thomas splint for f., 3296
    ununited f., 523
Fractures
    treating f. and dislocations,
        328
France
    syphilis in F., 3257
Freckles
    defined as disease, 799
Freed man

pays physician, 1864
Freedom
from disease, 792
patient ought to have f., 2428
French disease
syphilis as F., 3254
Frenchman
will drink himself to death,
643
Frog
as arch-martyr to science, 168
proclaiming he is learned
physician, 2799
Frogs
collection of urine in f., 1482
experiments on kidneys of f.,
1482
Fun
medicine in f., 1183
Functioning
aging person's f., 90
Functions
human and animal f., 1333
Futile treatment
to attempt f. displays
ignorance, 3325
Future
anticipations for the f., 38
competent to aid progress in
f., 1293
given sense of f., 2981
in f. will have clarification of
problems of sex and love,
3039
its f. is behind it, 80
live neither in past nor f.,
3482
pain has no f. but itself, 2318
past and f. absorbed by
present, 720

G

Gallbladder
cholecystography of g., 467
cholelithiasis of g., 468
Gallic aneurysm
known by signs of venereal
disease, 3259
Galvanometer
composed of filament, 946
Gamble
those who g. with men's lives,
1445
Gambling
ask doctor to stop g. with your
life, 2443
Gangrene
compromised the appendix,
221
in Buerger's disease, 3297
of four extremities, 2824
penicillin for, 2481
Gap
bridge uncomfortable g., 756

Garrodian ideal
in thinking, 862
Gastric fistula
dog possesses g., 767
Gastric function
free muriatic acid, 1080
Gastric juice
appears at fistula, 767
protect ulcer from g.
corrosion, 2489
Gastric lavage
in appendicitis, 227
Gastric ulcer
peptic ulcer differentiated
from g., 2488
Gastritis
gastroscopy in diagnosis of g.,
1088
Gauge
index of the pressure g., 311
Gender, *see* Man, Men,
Woman, Women; WOMEN
Gene
assumption g. is constant,
1104
g. of avian sarcoma virus, 384
Generalization
is risk of cancer researcher,
2872
Generation
keep pace only with our g., 88
Generosity
open-hearted g., 92
Genes
chromosome view of inheritance, 1093
members of each pair of g.,
1105
proposed the terms gene and
genotype, 1092
Genetic code
a group of three bases, 1094
Genetic differences
in blood pressure, 1358
Genetic disease
sickle cell anemia, 3064
Genetic material
copying mechanism for g., 708
Genetics
pea hybrids form egg and
pollen cells, 1095
several varieties of a group of
plants, 1096
Genital
brain is appendage of g.
glands, 2731
Genius
eccentricities of g., 2059
Genome
map of human g., 1111
Genomics
newly developing discipline of
mapping/sequencing, 1112
Gentle
surgeon should be g., 3195
surgery should be g., 3239
Geometric ratio

population increases in g.,
2646
Geometry
what g. is to the astronomer,
150
Germ-cell
each g. contains, 1105
Germ-plasm
nuclear g., 1102
Germ theory
attempting to extend g., 1429
Germans
received no blood from g.,
3455
Gestation
gain few extra weeks of g.,
1052
Gift
able physicians are g. of God,
2548
g. of children, 460
manuscript as g., 2767
of life, 2366
science is noble g., 2952
scientific discipline is g., 2964
Girl
father loves g. above all, 953
what g. needs through life,
3471
Girls
need to know consequences of
intercourse, 3046
Gland
thyroid g., 2899-2901
Glanders
tuberculosis analogous to g.,
3385
Glands
absorbent glands enlarged,
414
around base of heart, 2504
brain is appendage of genital
g., 2731
cancer attacks conglomerate
g., 376
discovered in kidneys, 1479
liver consisted of parts of g.,
493
lymph g. in Hodgkin's disease,
1302, 1303
of Peyer, 3407
Glandular bodies
betwixt stomach and spleen
were two g., 413
Glandular nature
kidneys of g., 1478
Glans
is extreme part of the penis,
2484
Globules
so few g. in the blood, 156
Glomerular clearance
substance suitable for
measuring g., 1498
Glomerular filtration rate
possible to precisely measure
g., 1499

tendency to report only i.
cases harmful, 1900
to approach i. of medical
practice, 1954
Idealist
scientist as i., 3005
Ideals
of profession tend to demoralization, 2068
three personal i., 1997
university is place for
cultivation of i., 3411
Ideas
all i. originate in brain, 3292
alternation of isolated i., 697
delicate art of handling i.,
1450
has few or no i., 698
I have two fixed i., 76
may prove wrong, 3002
pathological i., 2728
vague preconceived i., 873
Identity
physician's illness link to i.,
2535
Idiosyncrasy
of physician, 2388
Ignorance
confess i., 3490
fight against i. and quackery,
746
greater i., greater dogmatism,
872
is enemy of human race, 787
life is word that means i.,
3432
look to statistics to avoid i.,
3139
man's i. is private property,
2063
of men, 3050
physician's i. is threat, 877
state of medicine worse than
total i., 2095
to attempt futile treatment
displays i., 3325
to confess i. is wiser, 743
use probabilities in direct proportion to your i. of individual, 3165
Ignorant
not so bad being i., 3367
of true cause, 993
science teaches us to be i., 2972
Ignorant physicians
are satanic spirits, 2547
Ileum
disease of terminal i., 642
Meckel diverticulum in i.,
1647
Ill
doctors can't afford to be i.,
869
doctors fall i., 868
forbid doing i. to be one's
neighbor, 1032

preventive medicine tells i.
person he is fit, 2679
too i. to see doctor, 922
Illegible
writing even more i. than
most doctors, 2671
Illness, see also Sickness;
ILLNESS
as qualification for entry to
medical school, 1794
at termination of i., 971
belongs to patients link to r.,
2536
care for people not i., 1677
in doctor's family, 2756
misbalance is i., 442
not to be encouraged, 1184
physician, 2250-2255
role of physician in i. and
health, 1707
so-called mental i., 2716
too strong for available
remedies, 3325
way i. has befallen him, 734
Illnesses
ready receiver for i., 1212
suffering from definable i.,
482
Illumination
uses statistics as support, not
i., 3151
Illusion
laymen's i. about science,
2990
Images
spend most of day dealing
with i. of people, 2819
Imaginary
flouted as i. conditions, 2807
trouble is i., 838
Imagination
failure of i. in scientific
inquiry, 2875
not of human i. but of human
curiosity, 114
Immobility
incontinence, i., instability
and intellectual
deterioration, 98
Immortal
in a sense i., 1107
Immortality
Joseph Guillotin achieved
type of i., 1155
Immovable
in heart failure, 1242
Immune sera
rabbit i., 308
Immunity
of rabbits and mice, 200
to tuberculosis, 3398
Immunology
power to react
immunologically, 1419
Impairments
self-reported i., 480
Imperialism

modern medical i., 1731
Imperturbability
liable to be misinterpreted,
987
quality patient wants in
doctor is i., 2393
Impossible
margin of the i., 1713
Impostors
ignorant and unprincipled i.,
2803
Impotence
desire outlives performance,
1422
he does not have virile
greenness, 1421
lifelong i., 1380
Impression
truth as i., 2400
Improvement
smallpox vaccination as most
important i., 3086
Improvements
in American and European
surgery, 3220
in heart disease is persistent,
251
Inability
to speak, 216
Incision
scream lasted during making
of i., 1642
Inclination
beware to let own i. be known
too much, 2609
Incompetence
prosthesis for i., 899
Incontinence
immobility, i. , instability, 98
poverty, loneliness, i., 97
Incurable
fails only in i. cases, 878
give the disease up for i., 739
Indecisions
hide you i., 2398
Independence
madness defined as
intellectual i., 1453
Independent
women are becoming i., 3468
Indifference
perfect i. toward objects once
held ear, 698
Indignation
against quacks, cults, and
cranks, 2808
Indisposition
had long suffered under an I.,
176
Indisputable
evidence, 1008
Individual
accept homosexual i., 1311
anecdotes represent
particularity of i., 1887
at birth i. destined to die,
1103

girls need to know conse-
quences of i., 3046
indulgence of sexual i., 3026
is unlawful and wicked, 599
menstruation provoked by i.,
2199
promiscuous i. with the
female sex, 3030
venereal disease from sexual
i., 3054
Interdependent
medical profession is i., 3114
Interest
in humanity, 2408
patient's fear of doctor losing
i., 2440
physician has i. in people,
2587
Interesting
paper short enough to be i.,
3500
Interests
many i. to be served, 1719
put patient's i. ahead of own,
863
Interference
with important public health
questions, 3003
Interior environment
provides physical needs, 2175
Intern
quality i. should develop, 2416
what it takes to be i., 2590
Internal medicine
a joint educational committee
in i., 136
first written use of term, 1462
surgery is salvation of i., 3235
training for obstetrician is i.,
2287
Internists
distinguish themselves, 135
Interrogation
of patient, 431
Interstitial nephritis
bruit heard in i., 1071
Interventricular septum
deficiency in i., 575
Interview
prescription signals end to i.,
2672
Intestinal lipodystrophy
(Whipple disease)
search by computer for similar
rRNA sequences, 1468
Intestinal mucosa
showed enlarged villi, 1467
Intestinal obstruction
pancreatitis confounded with
i., 2331
Intestinal symptoms
in purpura, 2797
Intestine
stenosis. of lumen of i., 642
Intestines
sprue affecting, 3125
Intimacy

avoid i. with patients, 1819
doctor and patient have
peculiar i., 2445
Intimidation
inartistic professions threaten
by i., 2688
Intolerance
cursed spirit of i., 2218
Intolerant
attitude of mind, 455
Intra-abdominal
radiologist from i. problem,
1086
Intractable pain
in carcinoma, 2328
Intraocular pressure
increase in i., 1118
Intuition
strive for i., 1947
Intuitions
primitive i. to do right thing,
693
Intuitive
art of medicine is i., 1950
public loves doctor to appear
i., 2392
Inulin
polysaccharide i. fulfills specifications, 1498
Invented
medicine i. for sake of sick,
2074
medicine not i. if we used
proper regimen, 2073
Inventions
no place for new i., 2852
Investigation
and practice are one in spirit,
1941
medical profession has
responsibility for i. and
experiment, 2867
methods of i., 2855
Investigators
not always good teachers,
3269
Investment
good-will returns to i., 1717
Iridology
naturopathy, i., reflexology,
and the like, 128
Irishman
will die of hypertension, 643
Iron
in hepatolenticular
degeneration, 1276
Irregular
breathing was i., 457
Irregularity
complete i. of heart, 260
Islands of Langerhans
furnish secretion to blood,
729
Iso-immunization
of Rh- mother, 996
Isolate

women i. themselves from
intellectual life, 3466
Isonicotinic acid
tuberculosis treated with
derivatives of i., 3403
Italy
syphilis in I., 3253, 3254, 3257
typhoid fever in I., 3406
Itching
acute i. and smarting, 1160

J

Jail
practice of medicine worse
than j., 1921
Japan
acupuncture in, 33
Japanese
practice borrowed from the J.,
35
Jaundice
from inflammation of liver,
1563
white j., 1472
Jaw
in tetanus, 2883-2885
Jealous
she must never be j., 870
Jerking pulse
j. in aortic valve regurgitation,
211
Joint
gout attacking j., 1145
pain in j. of great toe, 1139
Reiter syndrome affecting j.,
2845
Joints
arthritis is general pain in all
j., 234
arthroscopy for study of j., 237
in rheumatoid arthritis,
2562-2564
rheumatoid spondylitis
affecting j., 2913
rickets affecting j., 2914, 2915
Journal of American Medical
Association
says in two thousand words,
1906
trustees and editor of J., 1896
Journalism
medical j., 1897
Journals
good writing in j. is rare, 3499
statistics somewhat like old
medical j., 3147
Journey
to break the monotony of
medical practice, 137
Joy
in creation of life, 3475
Judge
doctors not less virtuous than
j., 1830

Male, *see also* Man, Men
  adolescent's instrumental
    assertiveness, 40
  childhood lasts longer for m.
    than female, 2145
  disease generally attacks
    persons of the m. sex, 180
  every m. shall be circumcised,
    492
  homosexual experience, 1311
Males
  power to generate ceases in
    m., 54
Malformation
  cyanosis result of cardiac m.,
    576
Malignant
  fever, 3515
  so-called m. hypertension,
    1350
Malpighian bodies
  separate from blood the
    watery portion, 1493
Malpractice
  errors and want of skill are
    manifest, 1611
Man, *see also* Male, Men
  adolescent years of m., 39
  after a m. has taken wine, 110
  decaying old m., 56
  essential quality as m., 2465
  grows old, 52
  homeopathic physician as
    education m., 1307
  how to cure a disease thanhow
    to make a m., 149
  is not the disease, 2396
  is product of environment,
    962
  keen and ambitious m., 185
  proper study of mankind is
    m., 3020
  takes a drink, 121
  unique characteristics of m.,
    38
Mandate
  of medicine, 2137
Mandible
  dislocation of m., 805
Mania
  in m., improvement with
    lithium, 2740
  models of m. are infinite,
    2735
Maniacs
  public asylums for m., 2156
Manic-depressive illness
  a melancholy disposition
    growing worse, 1627
  hereditary transmission of
    mania, 1629
Manipulations
  such m. interfere with natural
    selective processes, 1011
Mankind
  proper study of m. is man,
    3020

Manners
  forms of bad m., 2413
Manometer
  mercury in the m. drops, 313
Manure
  seeds flourish in m., 1048
Manuscript
  as gift, 2767
  spent hours on m., 3492
Marfan syndrome
  elongation of the bones, 1630
Market forces
  health care changes from m.,
    1220
Marketplace
  discipline of m., 1719
Marmite
  in m. is curative agent, 1063
Marriage
  it destroys one's nerves to be
    amiable, 1636
  m. resembles a pair of shears,
    1637
  monogamous erotic
    relationships, 1639
  offspring of a consanguinous
    m., 20
  respect each other's
    personality and privacy, 1640
  the devil knows how to do so
    much, 1635
  you cannot lose your heart
    and have it, 1638
Mastectomy
  when radical m. is only
    treatment available, 398
Master
  arithmetic is bad m. but good
    servant, 528
Materia medica
  if m. sunk to bottom of sea,
    885
Maternity
  qualities of m., 2574
Mathematical
  certainty only when can apply
    m. sciences, 3128
  replacement for sensible
    thought, 3161
Mathematicians
  more m. in hospitals in future,
    3113
Mathematics
  application of m. is aim of
    science, 2960
Mean
  probably error of m., 3153
Meaning
  give disease a m., 797
  inquiring into m. of things,
    2517
Measles
  typhoid fever different from,
    3405
Measure
  to know something is be able
    to m. it, 2965

Meat
  portion of king's m., 560
Meatus
  auditory m. in Valsalva
    maneuver, 3420
Mechanic
  use as many instruments as
    m., 1931
Medical advances
  create rising expectations,
    1679
Medical books
  physician without m., 330
  reading only m. makes dull
    man, 2832
  remain long useful, 1649
Medical care
  a blind man with a club, 1662
  a physician should trace back,
    1658
  each problem should have its
    own plan, 1675
  learning to talk to his
    patients, 1699
  the Bolam principle, 1693
  the science of medicine, 1690
  treating the person rather
    than the disease, 1672
  utmost skill to save the life,
    1660
Medical decisions, *see also*
    DECISION MAKING
  scientific basis of m., 1475
Medical economics
  accountability is inescapable,
    1733
  nominally altruistic sciences
    as medicine, 1734
Medical education, *see also*
    Education
  confidence in the unreserved
    treatment, 1744
  healthy scepticism [sic] which
    medical training induces,
    1754
  keep confidence inviolate,
    1753
  obtain a firm grasp of the
    great truths, 1750
  reward them for compliance
    rather than independence,
    1790
  the vestibule of m., 153
Medical ethics
  a double ethical standard,
    1839
  a man of serious conscience,
    1841
  a moral enterprise, 1846
  cherish a feeling of deep
    responsibility, 1825
  consecrate my life to the
    service of humanity, 1834
  duties implied by clinical
    fidelity, 1849
  physicians should be ever
    ready, 1815

are commonly affected with
scirrhous livers, 496
Bacchus hath drowned more
m., 119
born in the same year, 72
capable and sensible m., 1747
carcinoma of lung in m. from
smoking, 3095, 3099
previous healthy, homosexual
m., 27
reforming m. who are
addicted, 122
sixteen cases, all in m., 1476
where m. sit and hear each
other groan, 70
women find it easier than m.
to grow old, 74
worship at temple of god
Stomach, 228
Mendelian lines
spontaneous cancer
transmitted along m., 383
Meningococcus
sulfonamides for m., 3190
Menopause
medicalizing m., 2056
menstruation ceases and the
uterus begins to shrink,
2147
Menses
gout after m. stopped, 1127
Menstrual blood
flows from liver to womb, 154
Menstrual discharge
appears in females, 3025
ceases in females, 54
Menstrual fluid, classed as
"prime matter", 2848
Menstruation
dividing the asexual child
from the sexual female,
2155
first appears around the
fourteenth year, 2148
indicates her greenness, 2149
provoked by intercourse, 2199
see that red banner unfurl and
morn, 2154
Mental
five m. powers, 2236
great influence of m. distress,
2744
true m. physician, 2709
Mental cruelty
three ways of m., 2412
Mental misery
compatible with health, 1198
Mental state
distinct change in m., 1391
Mentors
questions about values of his
m., 41
Merchants
physicians act like m., 1951
Merciful
surgery should be m. art, 3239
Mercurials

m. as diuretic, 806
Merit
papers vary greatly in m., 1896
Messenger ribonucleic acid
(mRNA)
is not the intermediate carrier,
2158
system of regulation, 2157
Metabolism
instability of nuclein m., 1147
the quantity of carbonic acid
exhaled, 2160
Metal
radioactivity of m., 2641
Metamorphosis
of hospital, 1326
Metaphysics
root of medicine in m., 2125
Method
flexibility of m., 2868
hope rests on continuation of
m., 3452
investigation and practice are
one in m., 1941
numerical, see Numerical
method
numerical m., 3148
of research, 2855, 2858
reliance on laboratory m.,
3275
research m. will dominate
teaching, 2863
revolution experimental m.
effected, 2959
scientific m. not deductive,
2980
statistical m., see Statistics;
STATISTICS and related
topics
to ascertain superiority of
treatment, 3136
Method of Bouillaud
m. consists of application of
blister, 770
Methods
new m. of cure, 3339
newer m. of treatment are
good, 3324
Mice
destroy the m. and rats, 357
Microscope
ovary seen in m., 2309
Middleman
doctor as m., 2144
Migraine
head be suddenly seized with
pain, 2163
m. stems from black bile,
2163
Military medicine
worth a troop of other men,
2176
Milk
did not coagulate, 1079
mother's m., 349
Miller-Abbott tube
a new apparatus, 2183

Millionaires
system considers m. and
paupers, 1670
Mind
assumed gentle, placid
indifference, 1391
blanks at total emptiness, 679
cancer also state of m., 385
casts off rebelliously, 87
chance favors prepared m.,
777
cultivate quiet m., 991
dependent on condition of
body, 2087
developing memory rather
than m., 1779
distraction of m., 2736
dulls the noble m., 105
excitement of m., 1628
giving whole m. to patient,
1947
great anxiety of m., 1451
highest faculties of m., 509
if his m. grows torpid, 68
if m. not satisfied, body
cannot be cured, 1653
in what respects their body
and m. will eventually fail, 63
inquiring, analytical m., 860
intolerant attitude of m., 455
languished under depression
of m., 714
likes a strange idea, 452
mania is chronic derangement
of m., 2735
minister to diseased m., 2747
need alert m. in examination
of patient, 2529
pain as uncomfortable frame
of mind, 2323
sound m., 1169
tasks burden most
sophisticated of m, 1961
travel expands m., 3321
trinity of body , heart, m.,
1188
truly scientific m., 2974
vigorous and cultivated m.,
1983
will not relinquish old age if
m. is sound, 3182
Minerals
radioactivity of, 2641
Ministry
of consolation, 1997
Miracles
no testimony is sufficient,
2186
Misbalance
of constitution, 442
Miscreants
encouraged by heedless
multitude, 2803
Misery
abodes of pain and m., 1038
mental m. compatible with
health, 1198

the animal spirits being brought from the head, 2234

there is present in animals an electricity, 2235

transmit their messages to the central n.s. in a very simple way, 2243

two kinds of chemical transmission, 2242

Neuralgia
relief of n., 1059

Neuritis
psychic disorder with n., 1509

Neurologic diseases
incessant studies on major n., 2860

Neurologic injury
in Gulf War veterans, 1156

Neurologist
tends to turn to psychotherapy, 2007

Neurology
exact knowledge of the Muscles, 2250

psychiatry is n. without signs, 2721

what is found under microscope is called n., 2725

Neuromuscular activity
self-serving n., 580

Neurosis
switch from psychosisto n. as object of study, 2726

Neutrality
preserving of, 24

regulation, 25

New science
clinical epidemiology is name of n., 504

New
complaint had to be discovered, 563

publish notes on anything n., 521

unafraid of the n., 2974

Newborn
each n. has right to be wanted, 464

Night
death comes at n., 918

Nitrate of amyl
similarity existing between its general action and that of n., 184

Nitrate
of amyl, 184

of silver, 230

Nitrogen mustard
in Hodgkin's disease, 1304

Nobel awards
for discovery of insulin, 1459

Nodule
bluish-red, moderately firm n., 1476

Noise
dreams may be just n., 876

Nomenclature, *see also* Name
pseudo-science consists of n., 1853

system of n., 985

word vitamin acceptable n., 3448

Noncompliance
lie about the taking of things prescribed, 2261

Noncognitive
cognitive and n. disciplines, 3245

Normal state
to feel tired, harassed, 1199

Nose
breath enters the n., 2881

cancer attacks n., 376

Nose bleeds
telangiectasia with n., 1278

Nosocomial infection
inbred disease of hospitals, 2262

Nosology
clear and precise definitions of disease, 2264

new diseases with terrifying names, 2264

Nostril
has no motion, 294

Note
make a n. at the time, 434

Note-taking
value of n., 1877

Nothing
do as much n. as possible, 1688

there is simply n., 683

Nourishment
disturbance of n. of heart, 618

my soul's n., 57

Nuclear
germ-plasm, 1102

Numbers
prove something true, 3163

Numerical method
application of n. to medicine, 3152

some misled by term n., 3138

to get accurate knowledge, 3148

Nuremberg Code
consent of subject absolutely essential in N., 1446

Nurse
as part of army of quiet workers, 1994

marriage of n. and physician, 1909

night duty n., 1665

past is good n., 1295

patient-nurse relations, 2360

puerperal fever carried by n., 2779

Nursing
those n. abstain from sex relations, 2199

Nurture

nature prevails over n., 1097

Nutrition, *see* Diet, Food;
NUTRITION
inmost phenomena of n., 2275

Nystagmus
horizontal n., 287

in multiple sclerosis, 2201

O

Oat-celled tumor
of lung, 404

Obesity
I never missed a meal, 2283

in Frohlich syndrome, 1066

o. is a mental state, 2282

Object
investigation and practice are one in o., 1941

Object lesson
medicine as o., 2103

Objectivity
in science must be built, 3001

Obligation
ethical o., 1836

physician obligated to patient only, 2424

to keep in touch with science, 2031

Oblivion
is not to be hired, 658

Obscene
sexual instinct in adolescent is o., 3034

Observation
and experiment have gathered facts, 498

as first requirement in experimental medicine, 2026

by nurses, 2271, 2272

can't learn by o., 1799

experience and o. are too much neglected, 1919

fight through thickets of erroneous o., 2987

first degree of value set on clinical o., 507

foundation of medicine is reason and o., 2090

impulsive insanity has no foundation in scientific o., 1452

increase power of o., 1885

is simple, indefatigable, 2946

know more from o. than experiment, 2104

medicine founded on o., 2099

of clinical facts, 499

of retina, by ophthalmoscopy, 2293

operative skill not gained by o., 3241

physician cannot remain outside observed events, 2580

those who devote themselves to o., 2947

Observations
sound scientific t. to correlate o., 1028

Observer
difference between o. and experimenter, 2855

Obsessed
with health, 1203

Obsession
medicine as magnificent o., 2015

Obstetrics
cures are achieved in o., 1965

Obstruction
excretion of bile meets with o., 1473

gallbladder, 1069

in abdomen, 3323

in coronary system, 627

manifestations of coronary o., 625

mitral o., 1150

of liver and spleen, 33

pancreatitis confounded with intestinal o., 2331

Obvious
scientist not content to stop at o., 2973

Occlusion
attack typical of o. of coronary arteries, 628

Occlusive disease
of coronary artery, 1256

Occult cancer
better not to apply treatment to o., 368

Occupation
of looking after machines, 2064

profession distinguished from, 2689

Occupations
having two o. instead of none, 1987

Offense
of scientist is to declare true what is not, 2991

Oil
is congealed candy, 1046

Old, *see also* Age, Old age; AGING, GERIATRICS
complains of o. people, 1113

death relieves world of o. men, 660

exchange new diseases for o., 794

family doctor, 1044

good o. family doc, 1045

man in sense immortal, 1107

men must die, 668

physician, 890

seek o. physician, 2596

when a man grows o., 52

young feel sorrows more sharply than o., 672

Old age, *see also* Age, Longevity, Old; AGING, GERIATRICS, LONGEVITY
death which comes with o., 902

doubt may condemn one to premature o., 2847

merely extend life in o., 1572

of physician is happiest periods, 2570

premature o., 107

rides triumphant, 911

should burn and rave, 917

will not relinquish o. if mind is sound, 3182

Old man
knows exceptions to rules, 1661

Old people
put o. to bed, 81

Older
everyone is o. than thinks, 2665

Omission
errors of o., 3344

Operation, *see also* Surgery; SURGERY
every o. is experimental, 3352

intubation such practical and successful o., 1471

one stage o. for lung cancer, 405

patient most important person at o., 2462

Operations
pain of surgical o., 157

performed one or more o. annually, 162

Ophthalmoscopy
optic nerve is distinguished, 2292

Opiate
an unlocked door in prison of identity, 2217

Opinion
active interchange of p., 2046

as form of evidence, 1856

difference of o. between physicians, 1708

has succumbed to messianic delusion, 2005

no o. formulates whole truth in sciences, 2959

public o. about physicians, 1767

we often differed in o., 1824

Opium
for pain and spasms in sstomach, 2216

Opportunities
for women have increased, 3479

Optical unit
fiberoptic o., 1055

Optimism
outrageous o., 2128

Oranges
for scurvy, 3014, 3016, 3017

Order
logical o. for scientific paper, 3505

Organ
brain is most public o., 343

brain is uniquely human o., 342

each o. speaks its own language, 502

exhibiting damaged function, 732

heart is tough o., 1233

periarteritis nodosa affecting, 2497

spleen, 3122

that no longer function, 674

Organic lesions
on same plane as surgical diseases, 738

Organic mechanism
life as o., 1543

Organism
power of human o., 1330

Organized being
observe o. as a whole, 2759

Organized medicine
resist non clinicians running HMOs, 1910

Organs
brain is master of the o., 339

cancer appears in all o., 377

heterogeneous involvement of various o., 564

more o. are described, more we fail to grasp meaning of system of self, 3021

Orifice
coronary artery completely occluded at o., 619

left auricoventricular o., 202

Orthopaedics
to understand the Title of Orthopaedia, 2295

Os sacrum
in myositis ossificans, 2213

Oslerian ideal
in practice, 862

Ossific disease
of aortic opening, 215

Ossification
of coronary arteries, 614

of mitral valve, 2191

Ossified
heart with o. coronary arteries, 615

Ossifying
matter flows out of bones, 232

Osteoporosis
change in bone mineral mass, 2306

that category of decreased bone mass, 2304

Others

returned from German clinics,
140
sacred mission on earth, 2567
the Glory of accidental
success, 2554
wear stethoscopes primarily in
cafeterias, 3172
welcome over all the wide
earth, 2538
where p. gather, opinions
gather likewise, 584
who had treated the greated
number, 2540
women p., 3051-3060
worthlessness of most
medicines, 2556
Physick
Apollo was god of p., 2091
is not learned at universities,
1738
Physiognomy
as art of determining
character, 453
of disease, 510
Physiologist
domains closed to p., 529
Physiology
as biological science, 1769
cannot explain pathology by
p. alone, 2045
in p. no discovery is useless,
2048
owes more to medicine, 2104
physician without p. and
chemistry, 3348
Piles
women subject to p., 1269
Pineal tumors
with polyglandular syndrome,
645
Pity
in women, 3475
Placebos
accompanied by a charm,
2607
Plague
havoc of p. has been rapid,
3081
Planet
love the whole p., 960
Plant
ginseng as restorative p., 1117
Plantar reflex
disturbance of p., 275
Plastic surgery, 2837
Plate
show gold from p., 454
Platelets
pale granular masses, 2618
show incessant diversity in the
blood, 2617
Pleasant
how p. to die, 906
to rise in the morning, 91
Pleasure
bride should experience p.,
3032

sexual p. in women, 3033
to practice medicine, 2546
Pleasures
health is greatest p., 1171
Plethoric persons
blood of p., 2642
Pleurisy
acupuncture for, 33
in p. inflammation produces
empyema, 958
Plutarch
shown path of resignation,
646
Pneumonia
as captain of men of death,
1591
Pneumothorax
artificial p. in phthisis, 3387
Pocks
break out, 459
Poet
medical student resembles p.,
2060
Poetry
make rule to read p. once a
week, 3293
true p. of life, 1570
Poison
differentiates p. from remedy,
879
poison for rats and mice, 357
soluble p. diffused through
body, 775
spiritous liquors are a certain,
though slow, p., 112
Poisonous
all substances are p., 879
Poisons
and harmful dust brought
under control, 1425
and medicines sometimes
same, 888
in English a deadly poison,
2627
Mr. Henbane, the toxicologist,
2626
Policies
admissions p. are root of
trouble, 1791
admissions p. to medical
school, 1789
Policy
setting editorial p., 1902
to provide medical care to
soldier, 2180
Poliomyelitis
a certain kind of paralysis,
2630
an abrupt, sudden beginning,
2635
atrophy of the anterior
cornua, 2636
partial paralysis shows itself,
2632
suffered from the humidity
and cold, 2633
Political

poverty is basically a
p. problem, 2655
Politician
cardinal qualities of p., 2011
lazy doctor becomes p., 2003
Politicians
in p. overstrain is common,
2738
Politics
professional development and
p., 2124
Polymerase chain reaction
(PCR)
alternative method for
synthesis, 2645
Polyneuritis
due to lack of substance in
diet, 3435
Polypharmacy
p. is prosthesis, 899
Polyposis
gastroscopy in diagnosis of p.,
1088
Poor, see also Poverty; POVERTY
argument on behalf of p.
medical school, 2036
demands of p. public, 1214
disease is fate of p., 788
doctor is dangerous, 843
doctors should be advocates
of p., 2655
gout not disorder of p., 1135
gratuitous services to p., 2051
superfluous doctor is
p. doctor, 2067
views p. with contempt, 663
Portal system
congestion of p., 2257
Position
Trendelenburg p., 3359
Positive
false p. result of test, 3279
Positive health
question concept of, 1199
Post-graduate study
characteristic of profession,
593
Post-HIV era
Creutzfeldt-Jakob disease in,
641
Post-menopausal
osteoporosis a p. condition,
2303
Post-mortem examination
evidence from living
outweighs p., 2359
learning from p., 2357
Post-operative treatment
as essential as operation, 3234
Post-partum care
take the advice of a strong
woman, 2652
Posture
in heart failure, 1241, 1243
Potential
axons and action p., 2253
Poverty

Procreation, *see* Intercourse,
Sex; SEX
Procreative
sex must be p. to be
enjoyable, 3045
Profession
attitude of medical p. toward
standards, 1767
education constantly
discussed by p., 1752
honest practice of ., 1816
ideals of p. tend to
demoralization, 2068
keep p. abreast of times, 596
medicine more than p., 2015
now practiced in world
dominated by business,
2053
p. not only technologists, 854
post-graduate study
characteristic of p., 593
reform p., 2843
specialization of medical p.,
2736-2746
that neglects humanities,
1331
what makes medicine a p.,
1777
Professional
question of p. etiquette, 519
real p. advises against
intrusive treatment, 1968
Professional development
politics and p., 2124
Professional help
telling us to seek p., 2069
Professional patient
role of full-time p., 90
Professionalism
ideals of p., 2131
Professions
medicine is many p., 2010
Professor
is productive scientist, 1771
Professors
salaries of clinical p., 1770
Profit
health care company in
business for p., 1732
is problem, 1620
Medicare is profit-driven
system, 2072
Prognosis
can be guided by statistics,
3141
giving favorable p., 2407
gloomy prognostications, 2698
make sure of the event first,
2697
not improved by screening,
3012
Prognostications
gloomy p., 2398
Progress
in treatment of fever, 3350
medical p. based on research,
1837

to know natural p. of disease,
510
watch p. of disease, 508
Progressive lenticular
degeneration
disease of nervous system,
1275
Prolapsus bulbi
differentiated from
exophthalmos, 1024
Prolong
does surgery enable us to
simply p. life, 3225
Promise
to the sick, 2370
Promises
be moderate in p., 2695
Proof
obtain a perfect p., 443
Property
disease as p., 2459
Prostate gland
cancer of p., 407
Prosthesis
polypharmacy is p., 899
Prostration
seized with great p. of
strength, 219
Protein
synthesis is a central
problem, 2701
Protoplasm
and plasma cells, 2616
Prove
true scientist doesn't set out
to p. something, 2944
Providence
the arrangements and
decreesof P., 163
Prudence
of surgeon, 3224
Pseudohypertrophic muscular
dystrophy
weakening of movements,
2706
Pseudo-science
consists of nomenclature,
1853
does not consist wholly of lies,
2956
Psoriasis
only the sun had power over
p., 2708
teaches merits of humility,
721
Psychiatrist
abuse of p., 2746
physician as p., 1952
Psychiatry
diffusion of psychotherapy
had nothing to do with p.,
2749
disparage labeling in p., 750
in p. patient has untold story,
1882
Psychic disorder
Korsakov psychosis, 1509

Psychic effect
p. consists of exhilaration, 562
Psychic influences
some maladies accessible to
p., 2395
Psychic state
will bring individual to
psychiatrist, 1405
Psychoanalysis
mystic sees the ineffable, 2730
Psychological effects
of cannabinoids, 1633
Psychological factors
of smoking, 3098
Psychologically
must understand patient p.
and physically, 2411
Psychologist
physician as p., 1952
Psychosis
no man can be born again,
2737
switch from p. to neurosis as
object of study, 2726
the psychotic has solutions,
2741
Psychotherapy
neurologist tends to turn to
p., 2007
Puberty
complaints do not appear
before p., 1369
gout never before p., 1141
Public good
health care as p., 1702
Public health
causes of public ill health,
1681
interference with important p.
questions, 3003
Publishing
authors are not what they
should be, 2778
can get his work published,
2770
faithfully recording their
experience, 2760
results unpublished are little
better, 2765
we are what we write, 2776
Puerperal fever
under p. are grouped very
different disease, 1429
Pulmonary artery
contraction of orifice of p.,
575
Pulmonary circulation
blood circulating in the lungs,
2783
blood is carried, 2781
Pulmonary edema
with normal heart, 1285
Pulsatile
one large p. vessel, 487
vessel which originates from
heart, 486
Pulsating

few r. are 90% correct, 3353
heart r. over all, 1229
of diet and regimen, 763
of malingering, 1609
young man knows r., 1661
Rushing
    sound of r. in mitral stenosis,
        2190

S

Sac
    lined by distinct membrane,
        171
    water in s. of heart, 2499
Sacred
    epilepsy as s., 970
Sacred space
    as circle of caring, 1705
Sacrifice
    peer review means s., 2473
Sailors
    suffer from scurvy at sea,
        3015-3017
Sal armoniac
    spirit of s. is excellent for
        scurvy, 3014
Salaries
    of clinical professors, 1770
Salvation
    surgery is s. of inner medicine,
        3235
Sanctity of marriage
    trampled upon and derived,
        1641
Sanitation
    overwhelming importance of
        s., 2752
Sarcoidosis
    groups of lymph nodes much
        swollen, 2930
    the nose has doubled in size,
        2929
Sarcoma
    of jaws of African children,
        360
Satisfaction
    more concerned about welfare
        of loved one than own s.,
        2732
Satyriasis
    is form of disease, 2687
    transition of s. to gonorrhea,
        1124
Savage
    has nothing to fear but his
        disease, 3336
Save life
    does surgery enable us to s.,
        3225
Scab
    is beautiful thing, 1167
Scalp
    phrenology picks pocket
        through s., 2518

Scanners
    main groups are readers, s.,
        and shirkers, 1903
Scars
    becoming nation of s., 3231
    experience leaves mental s.,
        1030
Schizophrenia
    designate a group of
        psychoses, 2936
    give the disease a new name,
        2937
    history of another self, 2935
    method of treating s., 2739
    the attack is almost
        imperceptible, 2934
School, medical, *see* MEDICAL
    EDUCATION
Schooling
    no one can understand
        surgery without s., 3195
Sciatica
    lumbago and s. frequently
        disappear, 34
Science, *see also* Medical
    science; MEDICAL SCIENCE
    a series of approximations,
        3004
    adopt for practical art
        standard applicable to
        applied s., 2809
    advancement of s., 2353
    almost anybody can have an
        idea, 2985
    anatomy and physiology as s.,
        1769
    anecdotes as emblem of
        human s., 1887
    application of mathematics is
        aim of s., 2960
    arch-martyr to s., 168
    art of engraving enhances s.,
        1894
    art of medicine and s. of
        medicine, 1942
    basis of the scientific method,
        2979
    better colleges founded on
        advancement of s., 1773
    biological s. in application to
        social problems, 1010
    certainty only when can apply
        mathematical s., 3128
    clinical epidemiology is name
        of new s., 504
    clinical medicine will never be
        exact s., 1847
    clinical practice is not a s.,
        1973
    danger to s. of statistics, 3159
    disconnection of medical s.
        from moral foundation,
        1701
    familiar with art and s. of
        past, 1293

find expression in art of
    medicine, 1932
first teach s., then
    detachment, 1798
French medical s., 1067
handicraft outruns s., 3237
healing not a s., 3354
how much s. do clinicians use,
    1788
how to wait is great s., 1306
in s. goes credit to person who
    publishes, 2762
is analytic, 1950
medical practice and s. move
    in opposite directions, 1973
medicine as applied s., 1946
medicine cannot be pure s.,
    1674
medicine is s., 2081, 2108
must keep in touch with s.,
    2031
nature of s., 2874
no opinion formulates whole
    truth in s., 2959
of disease is purely
    descriptive, 2025
of uncertainty, 2123
old art replaced by new s.,
    2107
phrenology as s., 2518
pretend modern medicine is
    s., 2125
principles of s. to diagnosis,
    1942
progress of art and s. of
    medicine, 274
relationship between s. and
    practice, 1962
resistance to anything that
    contradicts it, 2975
study of s. is great, 1974
tells us nature of disease, 1680
we see more and farther, 2938
what distinguishes ethics from
    s., 1833
Science faculty
    not interested in family
        practice, 1789
Science method
    in practice, 1941
Sciences
    have become too
        multilayered, 1745
    in natural s. necessary to
        create new classifications,
        498
    long process of education in
        s., 1805
    student must educated
        himself in exact s., 1748
Scientific
    discipline is gift, 2964
    error of s. truth, 2111
    growth of s. medicine, 2861
    has no foundation in s.
        observation, 1452

Super-power
  comes with knowledge and
    skill, 2571
Support
  emotional s. not easily
    quantified, 1704
  uses statistics as s., 3151
Suppuration
  in tuberculosis, 3376
Suprarenal capsules
  diseased condition of the s.,
    45
  functions of the s., 42
  yield to water, 981
Supreme Judge
  physician must render
    account to S., 1978
Surgeon, *see also* SURGEONS
  is great treasure in army, 2177
  patients survive s.'s mistakes,
    1870
Surgeons
  as s. and sexton, 3193
  judicious s., 3200
  no s. who is not also a
    physician, 3198
Surgery
  act with deliberation, 3217
  attempts to replicate
    perfection, 3247
  cured by the knife, 3211
  discovery of anesthesia, 3223
  knowledge of anatomy is
    essential to s., 1749
  military, 2182
  mitral valve, 2195
  nothing pleasing or attractive
    in it, 3218
  reconstructive s., 2837, 2838
  reporting on results of s., 1900
  speed or slowness are
    commended alike, 3212
  surgeons must be very careful
    in it, 3222
  tantamount to having a
    vicious bully, 3246
  those who look after the
    patient, 3210
  ulceration after s., 3522
  vascular s., 3422
  why not more women in s.,
    3480
Surgical diseases
  organic lesions on same plane
    as s., 738
Surgical operations
  I have performed s., 162
  mitigating the pain of s., 157
Surgical treatment
  epilepsy cured by s., 979
Surrogate
  food industry as s. physician,
    1202
Survival
  love necessary for s., 960
  of complex organisms, 2224
Survivor

death is more s.'s affair, 915
Susceptibility
  to tuberculosis, 3398
Susceptible
  to cancer, 383
Suture
  feasibility of cardiac s., 1248
Swallowing
  difficulty s. in tetanus, 3284,
    3287
Swamp
  precautions about, 1599
Swelling
  cancer is a s. or sore, 659
  cancer is an uneven s., 372
  cancerous s., 373
  considerable s. of wrist, 565
  deep s. causing compression
    of trachea, 772
  edematous s. of the skin, 187
  in groin, 354
  in legs, 938
  of mumps, 2203
  of myositis ossifcans, 2213
  of pus, 16
Swellings
  in biliary tract, 1559
  of throat are endemial in parts
    of England, 1389
Sympathetic pain
  disease can produce s., 2840
Sympathy
  in care of aged, 1114
  in women, 3475
  is sharing of feelings, 954
  time, s., and understanding,
    2408
Symptom
  do not doctor a s., 3347
  not every s., 3249
Symptoms
  cretinous s. following
    thyroidectomy, 3302
  fearful s. of bubonic plague,
    358
  headaches with deadly s. are
    fatal, 2692
  in psychiatry, s. are elevated to
    disease status, 2722
  inquire as to patient's s., 2380
  of approaching nervous
    breakdown, 3485
  of emphysema, 2787
  ofParkinsonism, 2341
  of peptic ulcer, 2487
  of pernicious anemia, 2506
  of rheumatic fever, 2904
  of valvular heart disease, 3421
  pain most common, 2324
  patient is not mere collection
    of s., 2414
  patients have s. not diseases,
    2461
Synapse
  such a special connection,
    3250
Syncope

angina pectoris is case of s.,
    612
  s. and chest pain, 609
Syndrome
  Munchausen, 2205
  person's name for designation
    of s., 986
  prevent the s. of symptoms,
    3251
  studies delineate a new
    clinical s., 125
Syphilis
  a venereal taint, 3261
  classification of the symptoms
    of s., 3260
  improvement in treatment of
    s., 2753
  irregular animal indulgence,
    3262
  is self-inflicted, 3058
  mercurials for treatment of s.,
    806
  this spirochetal form, 3264
  tuberculosis analogous to s.,
    3385
System
  in which there is no equity,
    1730
  medicine as elaborate s., 2129
  medicine as sprawling s., 2130
  patient and physician make
    up social s., 2409
  pharmacopeia as s., 2515
Systole
  ventricle made premature s.,
    1035, 1036
Systolic pressure
  elevated s. in dogs, 1351
  s. is the highest level sounds
    are heard, 314

T

T-cell
  defect, 27
T-wave
  early exaggeration of t., 626
Table
  statistical t., 3154
Tables
  statistical t., 3150
Take care
  begins to t. of health, 1182
Take charge
  the rascal t. as general
    factotum, 78
Take stock
  doctors do not t. often
    enough, 594
Talk
  begin to t. about health, 1187
Talking
  don't get paid for t. to
    patients, 1722
  too much t., 1873

characteristics of man, 37
no such thing as u., 3501
Universal
    education for both sexes, 3472
    tuberculosis infection u., 3397
University
    as proper home of medical
        school, 2033
    college or u. is sensitive to
        outside criticism, 2034
    medical school independent
        from u., 2040
Unknown
    scientist's thirst for u., 3006
Unnecessary operation
    doctors perform u., 1830
Unprejudiced approach
    each clinical problem calls for
        u., 2529
Unprepared
    mass of u. youth, 1762
Unsafe
    absolute diagnoses are u., 744
Unsociability
    smoking is u., 3094
Untreated group
    equalized between treated
        group and u., 542
Unwell
    presence or absence of disease
        has little to do with feeling
        u., 3248
Urea
    excretion proceeds at
        maximum speed, 1497
    volume of blood cleared of u.,
        1500
Urinary calculus
    new species of u., 646
Urinary excretion
    performed with ease, 3415
Urination
    frequent u. in prostatism,
        2699
Urine
    amount of sugar excreted in
        u., 730
    blood in, 2343
    can provide story of events in
        kidney, 3413
    collection of u. from frogs,
        1481
    evaporated to dryness, 726
    excretion of r., 1479
    formation of u., 1495
    kidney makes u., 1485
    melting down of flesh and
        limbs into u., 724
    percolation of u., 1478
    protein in u., 2383-2386
    sediment in u., 3414
    stone blocking flow of u., 3213
    total suppression of u., 1492
    volume above augmentation
        limit, 1497
    was sweet, 725

would become concentrated,
    1494
Usefulness
    are patients of use to
        themselves or others, 2460
    significance of university
        greater than u., 3411
Useless
    most treatments are u., 3357
Uselessness
    comparative u. of men, 76
Uterus
    arising from horn of u., 1037
    arrange u. and you fix
        hypochondria, 1371
    cancer attacks u., 376
    cancer most often in u. or
        breast, 372
    cancer of, 372-374
    pituitrin effects on, 2606
Utilitarian
    researchers don't want u.
        purpose to research, 2865
Utility
    of healing arts, 2083
Utopia
    hospitals in u., 1319

V

Vaccination
    as sure a preventive of
        smallpox, 3417
    smallpox v., 2716-2720
Vaccine
    for rabies, 2814
    poliomyelitis v., 2638
Vaginal route
    is blind method of operating,
        3203
Vaginal smear
    for cancer, 2332
Valetudinarians
    are too sedentary, 1019
Value
    real v. from relationships with
        family, 1042
Values
    questions about v. of his
        mentors, 41
Valve
    digital examination of mitral
        v., 1251
    mitral, 1937-1944
    mitral v. was much diseased,
        451
Valves
    cardiac thrill, 427
    if v. are source of fibrin, 947
    in heart failure, 1245
    indurated and ossified
        semilunar v., 214
    semilunar v. incapable of
        closing mouth of aorta, 635
Valvular

pulsus irregularis in v. heart
    disease, 255, 254
Van Slyke
    sought how to dispense
        mathematics, 1500
Vanity
    committed in custom of
        smoking, 3088
Variability
    is law of life, 785
    is reason for planned clinical
        trial, 549
Variable
    humans likely to be v., 3160
Variableness
    result is subject to v., 3140
Variables
    statistical correlation of v.,
        3158
Variation
    individual v. in homeostatic
        range, 802
Variations
    in fetal heart beat, 1046
Vascular resistance
    pulmonary v., 2784
Vasovesiculitis
    almost mistaken for
        appendicitis, 2839
Vein
    inflamed with cancer, 379
    pulmonary v., 2780, 2782
    remarkable pulsation in right
        jugular v., 418
    venipuncture of v., 3425
Veins
    blood flows by v., 490
    blood received into the man's
        v., 316
    cancer involved with v., 375
    hemorrhoidal, 1267
    injection of tepid water into
        v., 471
    v. which by thickening, 231
Veneration
    not most highly developed
        altruistic instinct, 1294
Venereal disease, 2692-2698
    see also Syphilis; SYPHILIS
    rejection of paper or proposal
        like v., 2475
Venous blood
    pressor and vasoconstrictor
        properties of v., 1354
Ventilation
    experiments on lung v., 2891
Ventricle
    blood turns back into v., 635
    falling back towards the v.,
        209
    in mitral stenosis, 2189
    it sent back into the left v. a
        part of the blood, 206
    made premature systole, 1035,
        1036
    nothing admitted into v.
        unless opened, 1001